Endorsements for HIV AND BREASTFEEDING:

"This book is a timely reminder that tragedy follows any ne
of all babies, maternal milk. Its lessons are needed in this late
unrecognised misogyny combine to separate mothers and babies. Meticulously researched, it is a must-read for anyone who cares about human health, especially those who know little about human lactation's critical role in creating immune memory across whole populations. I am delighted to see Pamela Morrison's lifework in print at last."

Maureen Minchin – pioneer lactation consultant,
author of *Milk Matters: Infant Feeding and Immune Disorder*

"A most sensitively written book. Pamela Morrison is to be congratulated on putting together such a well-researched and provocative masterpiece. This should be required reading for every student of public health policy. Pamela's experience of working on the ground, experiencing the lived experience of HIV infected mothers, has resulted in a wonderful resource for those supporting HIV infected mothers and their infants."

Anna Coutsoudis – Professor Emeritus, Nelson R Mandela School of Medicine,
University of Kwa-Zulu, Natal, South Africa

"Pamela Morrison provides a comprehensive examination of the aetiology of HIV, and – importantly – the history of its identification of mother-to-child-transmission (MTCT), the design of studies and policies from the beginning of the HIV pandemic to today. An important contribution of this book is the author's emphasis on the necessity of clear and consistent definitions, particularly of 'breastfeeding' and whether it is once-only, token, mixed, predominant, or exclusive. There is a difference, and shoddy or inconsistent definitions can seriously skew the results of any study. Sadly, as Morrison documents, policy-making has repeatedly followed uncritical acceptance of studies with flawed (or no) definitions and poor study design. The importance of cultural context in applying policies is amply illustrated, especially when the assumptions of the global north are transplanted inappropriately into other settings. Morrison provides numerous relevant tables, a glossary, and 66 pages of references. Lessons can be learned from this book for health workers, researchers, and policy-makers working in other disease contexts. These are the importance of definitions and study design, as well as the cultural contexts in which studies and policies are situated."

Virginia Thorley, OAM, PhD, IBCLC, FILCA –
International Board Certified Lactation, and Cultural Historian
of the History of Medicine, Ipswich, Queensland, Australia

"Part memoir, part research summary, Pamela Morrison's account of how HIV threatened breastfeeding and the lives of millions of children and how the public health response failed them is a must-read."

Dr Karleen Gribble – Adjunct Associate Professor,
School of Nursing and Midwifery, Western Sydney University, Australia

"I began following the HIV and infant feeding issue closely from 1985, attending international WHO expert consultations on the issue in 1987 and 2006, as well as several other meetings on the topic and publishing numerous relevant articles and letters in scientific journals, many of which in both cases are referred to in Pamela Morrison's new book *HIV and Breastfeeding: the untold story*. I had the pleasure of working closely with Pamela on this issue several times and we have collaborated closely many times on relevant publications. I have never come across anyone who was more meticulous and comprehensive in following and keeping track of the scientific literature on relevant issues. Over the years, I have often asked her for details and references on certain aspects and she has never taken long to respond with exactly what I needed.

Now she reveals in this impressive book that she was also keeping careful track of the relevant history, accurately documenting in the book the relevant events that shaped research, program and policy agendas, many of which most of us, even scientists and health professionals working in this field, are likely unaware. It is and surely will remain a unique documentation of what took place during a dramatic period when thousands of infant lives were at stake, with UN agencies and the global breastfeeding 'community' at odds for the first and only time. Much of the disagreement has now been bridged. For example, when former allies strongly objected and explained why, WHO rather swiftly changed its objective for its PMTCT program from 'minimizing postnatal HIV transmission' to 'optimizing HIV-free survival.' The need to ensure exclusive breastfeeding among HIV-infected mothers actually put it on the map in health policy spheres where most health workers were unaware that young babies did not need extra water or any other food or fluid. In Africa in particular (except in a couple countries), only a few percent of mothers practiced exclusive breastfeeding in the early 90s, but is now practiced at 40% of babies 0-6 months old (based on a 24-hour recall).

However, as Pamela emphasizes, further work remains to ensure that rational policies on HIV and infant feeding are not only promulgated by all relevant authorities, but also implemented at the level of patient care around the world, not just in poor countries. As she points out near the end of the book, we saw a graphic example of how quickly much of the professional health community is still ready to abandon breastfeeding in the unfortunate and scientifically unjustified advice that quickly emerged from many quarters when the COVID epidemic started."

Ted Greiner PhD – retired Professor of Nutrition, Hanyang University, South Korea

"If you're gazing at the cover, chances are you're not expecting the unravelling of a public health whodunit lasting over two decades that not only proved to be a totally false start but also contributed to the worst health outcomes, including death, for the children the policy was intended to succour and save. Having had the privilege of accompanying the author part of the way on her journey to defend breastfeeding in the face of HIV, I invite you to join her as she recounts her tireless efforts to expose and debunk bogus assumptions and to restore Mother Nature's reputation, as the author reaches the only valid conclusion that had, in fact, been hiding out in plain sight all along."

James Akre – author, speaker, reviewer and commentator
on breastfeeding's sociocultural dimension

HIV AND BREASTFEEDING

THE UNTOLD STORY

PAMELA MORRISON

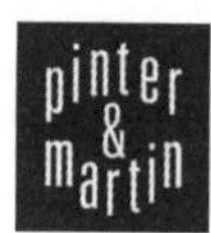

HIV and Breastfeeding: The untold story

First published by Pinter & Martin 2022

ISBN 978-1-78066-750-8
Also available as ebook

British Library Cataloguing-in-Publication Data
A catalogue record for this book is available from the British Library.

Index: Helen Bilton

Cover image courtesy of Maureen Minchin, previously used on the cover of ALCA News 1991, supplied by Sigi Frans of Sweden, source unknown.

Set in Adobe Garamond

Printed and bound in the EU by Hussar

Pinter & Martin Ltd
6 Effra Parade
London SW2 1PS

pinterandmartin.com

CONTENTS

Introduction	The untold story of breastfeeding and HIV	7
Chapter 1	What is HIV?	13
Chapter 2	The origins of HIV	20
Chapter 3	The rise and rise of the HIV pandemic	31
Chapter 4	Routes of infection of babies, mothers, fathers and others	42
Chapter 5	HIV testing and monitoring the stage of disease	56
Chapter 6	Breastfeeding: why it matters	69
Chapter 7	HIV in breastmilk	96
Chapter 8	Breast and nipple problems: do they increase the risk?	102
Chapter 9	The importance of exclusive breastfeeding: why definitions matter	118
Chapter 10	Components in breastmilk that protect against HIV	128
Chapter 11	Pasteurised breastmilk as a replacement feed for the babies of HIV-positive mothers	134
Chapter 12	Global policy on HIV and breastfeeding 1996–2009: formula for disaster	142
Chapter 13	Implementing the policy through the HIV and Infant Feeding Counselling Course	189
Chapter 14	Outcomes from the first PMTCT pilot sites	204
Chapter 15	Problems with counselling, but scaling up anyway	215
Chapter 16	What we don't know about the outcomes from the PMTCT sites	235
Chapter 17	Botswana, poster child of the PMTCT programme	248

Chapter 18	**Early cessation of breastfeeding**	**254**
Chapter 19	**Animal milks: errors, omissions and experiments**	**267**
Chapter 20	**Already HIV-infected infants and babies who escape infection**	**277**
Chapter 21	**HIV-free survival**	**283**
Chapter 22	**ART and breastfeeding**	**293**
Chapter 23	**EBF + ART, a winning combination**	**306**
Chapter 24	**International HIV and infant feeding policy comes full circle**	**317**
Chapter 25	**If undetectable equals untransmissable, what about breastfeeding?**	**333**
Chapter 26	**Breastfeeding by HIV-positive women in the global north**	**352**
Chapter 27	**Mothers' stories**	**372**
Chapter 28	**Helping an HIV-positive mother who wants to breastfeed**	**388**
Chapter 29	**Advocacy, politics, spillover and lessons learned**	**394**
	About the author	408
	Acknowledgements	408
	Glossary	409
	References	415
	Index	481

INTRODUCTION

The untold story of breastfeeding and HIV

This is the story of how the discovery that a deadly virus, passed through a mother's milk to her baby, came close to turning breastfeeding into an endangered practice, and how catastrophic that was for the babies of HIV-infected mothers. The dilemma that breastfeeding, in itself an act of nurturing which confers food, comfort and love, practised by most of the world's mothers and babies since the dawn of time, could be at once life-saving, yet lethal, has been called 'the ultimate paradox'.[1]

In my life I've lived in eight different countries, six of them in Africa, and I consider myself to be a White African. African babies are generally breastfed. I went to live in Kenya as a little girl and moved further south as a young adult, finally settling in Zimbabwe for 30 years. My own babies were born in Harare. In 1987 I was accredited as a voluntary breastfeeding counsellor with the mother support group La Leche League, so for over 30 years I've worked with the guiding vision that all mothers everywhere should be helped to breastfeed their babies for as long as they want. In 1990 I qualified as the first International Board Certified Lactation Consultant (IBCLC) in Zimbabwe, where circumstances had combined to ensure that breastfeeding was an idea whose time had come. Our Minister for Health was a signatory to the Innocenti Declaration on the Protection, Promotion and Support of Breastfeeding,[2] many of our hospitals were being accredited as Baby Friendly, and I was building a thriving private practice in a country which had one of the most progressive breastfeeding policies in the world.

In December 1995 I received a phone call that would turn out to have a major influence on the course of my career. The caller was a young mother whose accent told me that she was from the Coloured (an ethnic group in their own right[3]) community. She was distraught. She had been referred by a local La Leche League Leader because she had just tested positive for HIV (human immunodeficiency virus).[4] Her successfully breastfed baby daughter was eight months old, but her doctor had recommended immediate weaning from the breast, and the baby was refusing a bottle. She wanted to know if she really had to wean? Could her baby become infected with HIV through her breastmilk? She didn't know how she herself might have acquired the virus; she had been in a relationship with the baby's father for two years, but his HIV status, and indeed that of the baby, was unknown. The mother even wondered if there had been a mistake with her own test result because the doctor had ordered a second test to confirm the diagnosis. She wanted to continue breastfeeding, but needed to know the implications for her baby.

Lactation consultants do not give medical advice. Our role is to provide our clients with sufficient information and assistance to enable them to breastfeed easily, comfortably and effectively – and to make their own decisions about their breastfeeding goals. Sometimes we're able to clear up areas of 'myth-information' and prejudice, but we always encourage our clients to discuss any medical decision with their doctors. However, weaning a happily breastfed baby is a serious matter. Abrupt weaning can have extremely adverse consequences for the nursling as well as the mother. It was most likely that, if this mother was indeed infected with HIV, then the baby had already been exposed to the virus over many months. I promised to obtain the most current advice from the Ministry of Health, look up the literature, consult with local HIV support organisations and get back to her as soon as I could.

There was little coverage of HIV and its implications for breastfeeding in the lactation literature. Most texts were written by practitioners from the First World, where mothers infected with HIV were simply advised not to breastfeed at all. A sympathetic doctor at the Ministry of Health invited me to his office and discussed with me the pros and cons of breast vs bottle in this particular situation, but basically he said that not enough was known to provide a clear answer for my client. There was no official national policy. A very helpful counsellor at the Women and AIDS Support Network (WASN) in Harare gave me a generous amount of her time, and loaded me up with pamphlets and journal articles. Many of the WASN counsellors were mothers themselves, who had bottle-fed their own babies in order to protect them from HIV acquired through breastfeeding. The consensus was that if there was even a 1% risk of a baby becoming infected with HIV through breastfeeding then they would advise against it.

I read the articles and made copious notes but the real knowledge was sparse. I set out all the information I'd been able to glean in a three-page letter to my client. It was limited to confirming what the Ministry doctor had said – there was not enough known at this point in time to be able to provide a quantification of the risk of HIV transmission through breastfeeding for her particular baby in her unique circumstances. I gave information about gentle weaning and wished her well. I often wonder about this young mother and her baby.

Having been caught unawares by this first conversation, I soon realised that advice to wean wouldn't work for the majority of HIV-positive African mothers and, due to growing press coverage of HIV, it was going to be an increasingly common question. The discordance between the known life-saving benefits of breastfeeding, and its growing demonisation due to transmission of the virus through breastmilk, seemed all wrong. My African roots are strong. I bring to my work a vision that haunts me; the typical African mother trudging along a dusty track near her village, with a load balanced on her head, a baby tied to her back and another small child trailing behind her. Her vulnerability and gallantry, as she does the very best she can to live her life, to have her children survive and thrive, tugs at my heart. What would be best for her? Are we helping her to achieve these very ordinary, achingly human ambitions?

Piqued by the paucity of information, I continued to dig for more. Someone, somewhere must have looked at this? I slowly became aware that I was sleuthing in largely unknown territory. In trying to find the answer to the question, 'Should an HIV-positive mother breastfeed her baby?' it often felt as if I had stumbled into the pages of a detective story. So little was known. There were gaps in the narrative. Existing research went off at a tangent. Promising leads petered out and a strange prejudice clouded opinion when it came to breastfeeding. The search became as frustrating as it was fascinating. Each new fact only raised more uncertainty. Each new published paper posed even more questions, to which the answers became ever more ambiguous. Why did some babies become infected while others were spared? The trail began to seem like a maze with many blind alleys and several tantalizing but inexplicably dead ends. As my pile of paper and research articles grew, paradoxically there seemed to be scant real evidence to back up any suggestion that mothers on the world's largest, yet oft-forgotten continent[5] should abandon the age-old, life-saving practice of breastfeeding.

When I left Africa for Australia in 2003, Zimbabwe had the highest rate of HIV infection in the world, with an average prevalence among pregnant women of over 30%. In 2005 I went on to England. From 2005 and for several years afterwards, I was able to pursue my passion for protecting breastfeeding in the face of HIV as a paid consultant to the World Alliance for Breastfeeding Action (WABA), the Secretariat of which was located in Penang, Malaysia. Chasing the uncertainties to separate fact from fancy, to shine a light on the risk of HIV transmission to babies through breastfeeding, as well as the risk to breastfeeding posed by the fear of HIV transmission, has opened up opportunities to become friends and to collaborate with some of the most brilliant intellects in the field of lactation, to comment on hundreds of documents, and to work on projects collating background research that would inform policy on HIV and breastfeeding, both nationally and internationally. WHO acknowledged my input in one of their policy documents. One of my advocacy projects resulted in lunch with a Lord at Westminster Palace in London, and another led to a day assessing infant feeding conditions for failed asylum-seekers at Yarl's Wood detention centre in Bedford for the Children's Commissioner. Other projects have brought speaking engagements in the US, the Caribbean, Australia, Africa and Europe.

The politics of breastfeeding and HIV

Clearly, it has not always been politically correct to ask uncomfortable questions of the gatekeepers to the planet's health, even though subsequent research may have shown that the questions were valid. At various times, and sometimes in the most unexpected places, my words and writings have been effectively silenced; at international agency workshops on child hunger or at the field-testing of global HIV and infant feeding guidelines; by my own international professional association on several different occasions; by groups who commission me to write on a particular aspect of the topic, but then suffer from cold feet when it comes to publishing any criticism of the status quo. Other individuals or organisations don't want to be tainted by any controversy. A co-author who managed, finally, to get our joint paper accepted by a fourth reputable medical journal after three previous rejections, confessed that this was a first for him; one rejection was fairly common, twice was not unknown, but he'd never had *three* rejections before. The subject of HIV and breastfeeding stirs up all sorts of strong feelings.

There are many questions. Perhaps only a formal enquiry could uncover the full extent of what was surely a silent humanitarian disaster. While the AIDS industry I describe below has chugged relentlessly on, it's likely that more infants have died as a result of misguided efforts to prevent mother-to-child transmission of HIV, than ever fell prey to HIV-laced breastmilk. They died without a whisper of their fate ever becoming public knowledge.

As HIV spread out from the heart of the world's largest continent, already suffering from simultaneously high birth rates, high maternal and infant mortality and eye-watering poverty, life expectancy and national budgets plummeted. For the first time, it seemed as if formula feeding could not be dismissed as just a profit-making undertaking by an unethical industry. Finally it seemed that there was a valid medical contraindication to breastfeeding for thousands and possibly millions of babies on the continent most in need of its life-saving effects. The fear that so many mothers could pass a deadly virus to their babies through their milk, and incidentally facilitate onward transmission of AIDS down the generations, caused breastfeeding to be systematically undermined.

Conversely, research on every conceivable aspect of HIV and how it leads to AIDS has been so extensive that it has morphed into a separate growth industry, employing hundreds of thousands of privately and publicly funded investigators, researchers, social workers, scientists and experts of every kind, leading to the formation of hundreds of non-governmental organisations in almost every country, and consuming billions of dollars worldwide. During the first five years of UNAIDS' operations, from 1996 to 2001, the estimated global spending on AIDS grew from $292 million to $1.6 billion, a five-fold increase in as many years.[6] By 2020 the budget had swelled to $26 billion.[7]

Can HIV-positive mothers breastfeed?

There is still debate over the question of whether an HIV-positive mother can safely breastfeed her baby. The more we learn about the efficacy of modern antiretroviral treatment, the more frequently mothers in the high-income countries of North America, Europe and Australasia are asking this question. Notwithstanding the transforming results of research showing that horizontal transmission could be a thing of the past because 'undetectable' means 'untransmittable', many experts still doubt that the same reassurance can be extrapolated to vertical transmission through breastfeeding. Perhaps viral reservoirs in breastmilk are still capable of infecting the vulnerable infant, even when HIV testing shows that there is no detectable virus in the mother's blood.[8] Thus little has changed. Exaggerated fears of the risk of HIV transmission through breastfeeding, coupled with simultaneous complacency about the apparent safety of commercially manufactured breastmilk substitutes, serve to perpetuate the status quo.

There are many unanswered questions. Why did HIV/AIDS researchers seem to know so little about the physiology of lactation and the practice of breastfeeding that much of their research could have been so badly designed? Who decided that the evidence from the last 50 years demonstrating the hazards of formula-feeding in poverty-stricken environments could be ignored? Who selected topics worth researching? Why were so many promising leads not followed up? When policy was being decided, which criteria determined which research would be excluded? How could the importance of mother's milk to child survival be so casually dismissed? What were they thinking, these eminent and clever HIV experts, who were apparently persuaded to set up, facilitate and administer such poor infant feeding experiments? How could ethical review boards *not have known* that promoting formula-feeding for HIV-exposed babies on the world's least developed continent was going to have disastrous consequences? How could human rights be invoked to lend credibility to these experiments? Above all, how could pilot studies be meticulously planned and undertaken in the knowledge that there was no intention to ever monitor, or record, let alone publish, the health outcomes? Why did it seem that a political agenda was influencing such critical decisions? It would be naïve to expect that manufacturers of the competing product, infant formula, would not try to exploit the resulting fear and hysteria to their own advantage.

Quite early on, we were led to believe that support for new Prevention of Mother to Child Transmission (PMTCT) initiatives was widespread and popular because HIV was an 'emergency', which could not wait. A UNICEF official responded to my questions about the folly of plans to undermine breastfeeding by retorting, 'But the breastfeeding community is only speaking in whispers'. This was not entirely true. Many colleagues and friends in the lactation field had become increasingly uneasy about the likely repercussions of proposed recommendations discouraging breastfeeding, but such was the momentum to do something, anything, at whatever cost, to prevent HIV being passed to the next generation, that there seemed little that the lactation community could do or say to halt the juggernaut that was the PMTCT programme. This was an emergency that justified throwing caution to the wind.

Now that we know more, the impact of the ill-advised political decisions which resulted in a tragic betrayal of the world's most vulnerable babies can be pieced together. The role of those who should have known that undermining breastfeeding would be disastrous, but would heed neither the lessons from history, nor the warnings of breastfeeding advocates, can be scrutinised. The actions of those who wanted to help, and were persuaded into endorsing harmful practices through ignorance, can be tracked. A PubMed search can reveal the writings and findings of those researchers who courted the approbation of funding agencies, to endorse a desired outcome, or to provide the studies which justified an already-decided policy.

Mortality due to formula-feeding

Less easy to document are the fierce whispers of 'Those babies are dying like flies', heard in the corridors of African maternity units, mission hospitals and ministries of health, describing the fate of infants fed formula ostensibly to 'save' them from HIV acquired through breastfeeding. These warnings were ignored for years. It was only the unusually high number of deaths of bottle-fed babies during the 2005/6 flooding in Botswana and the subsequent brave reporting of this tragic loss of life by a few courageous scientists, which brought breastfeeding back from the edge of the abyss. In the following months, the full scale of the disaster, with its tragically high infant mortality, was widely reported. And then, suddenly, other reports were published showing that infant mortality due to formula-feeding exceeded mortality due to HIV-transmission through breastfeeding. What began as an isolated report of the dangers of formula-feeding in Botswana, turned into a steady stream of documented evidence from other southern and eastern African countries, accompanied by calls for policy change.

The story of the HIV pandemic as it impacts breastfeeding has taken place over the last four decades. The full extent of the global response, and the implications for child survival, has yet to be told. I believe it's important to piece together the discoveries and dead ends I happened upon as I sought to learn more. Early research led to the development of policy and programmes which seriously undermined breastfeeding in areas of the world where it was essential to child survival. In this book I attempt to set out the repercussions of a policy to promote replacement feeding. My sources are journal articles, unpublished literature, news media reports, and the words of counsellors, colleagues and mothers themselves. There are hundreds of cumbersome references because facts and figures concerning HIV and breastfeeding are so often met with scepticism that they always need to be meticulously backed up.

It is a tale of political intrigue, of fancies and fables, protagonists and victims, money and power, of deceit, fear and hope. It is a story of a humanitarian disaster, wrapped in layers of political rationalisation, delivered through a framework of human rights. It tells of how myth-information and hysteria led to the development of global strategies and public policies that cast real doubt on whether breastfeeding should continue to be promoted or supported at all.

This story is written to break the silence around what happened to the unknown number of HIV-exposed babies who died not only of the disease, but also due to ill thought-out prevention strategies. Their deaths were often unrecorded. It's also written in tribute to their gallant mothers, who were counselled not to breastfeed and complied against all cultural and intuitive norms in the desperate hope that their babies might live. Thus this account is written for the betrayed babies who were, and are, the most vulnerable victims of policy developed by those who should have known better. Here, in the following pages, is the untold story of breastfeeding and HIV.[9]

CHAPTER 1

What is HIV?

HIV stands for human immunodeficiency virus, identified in 1981 as the virus which causes AIDS.

The average virus is about one 1/100th the size of the average bacterium, with many viruses being among the most symmetric and beautiful of biological objects.[1] Viruses are the most common and abundant type of biological entity on earth, and there may be trillions of different viral species in the world, exceeding the number of cells 10 to 100-fold.[2] They populate virtually every ecosystem on the planet – ocean, water and soil, including the most extreme acidic, thermal, and saline environments.[3] Their diversity, and their number of distinct genes, substantially exceeds that of cellular life forms.

Viral diversity

Fortunately, only about 250 viruses are able to infect humans.[4] Otherwise they mainly infect bacteria, but also bats, beans, beetles, blackberries, cats, dogs, mosquitoes, pangolins, potatoes, ticks and the Tasmanian devil. They can give birds cancer and turn bananas black.[5] Of the trillions of viruses which exist, very few even have names. Described as the ultimate genetic parasite, viruses are unique because they are only alive and able to multiply inside the cells of other living things.[6] A virus, at heart, is a packet of genetic data that benefits from being shared with instructions to make more virus. Unlike a truly living organism, a virus cannot replicate on its own; it cannot move, grow, persist or perpetuate – it needs a host. Virus particles (known as virions) consist of two or three parts: genetic material made from either deoxyribonucleic acid (DNA) or ribonucleic acid (RNA), which are long molecules that carry genetic information; a protein coat that protects the genes; and in some cases an envelope of lipids that surrounds the protein coat when they are outside a cell.

In view of their huge diversity and numbers, it is a tribute to the cunning of the human immune system that so few viruses infect us. Not only are we almost always able to vanquish and overcome them, but we also have the capability to produce antibodies that recognise them in the future, thus preventing reinfection, and vaccines employ this mechanism to protect us. One notable exception is HIV.[7] Viruses are not technically alive, and in order to make new viruses, they must hijack a cell. Following invasion, a virus then uses the host cell's machinery to replicate its own genetic material. Once replication has been completed the virus escapes from the host cell by either budding or bursting out, causing lysis or cell death, only to enter other cells to multiply again. Like other members of this extremely diverse and evolutionarily successful family of viruses, HIV cannot live outside a cell, nor make new copies of itself except by using the cell's own genetic material.

What makes HIV so uniquely dangerous is that it binds itself specifically to and replicates within the very cells of the defence system that we use to fight disease. In a master stroke of stealth and camouflage, HIV is able to lay siege to the most important cells of the human immune system, CD4 T-cells and macrophages. The T-lymphocyte, or T-helper cell, is a white blood cell with proteins on its surface called CD4 receptors which warn the immune system that there are invaders in the system. So T-cells are often referred to as CD4 cells. Around 1/70th the diameter of the human CD4 cell it invades, with a diameter 60 times smaller than a red blood cell, HIV is a tiny round particle dotted with 72 spikes formed from the proteins gp120 and gp41 that can only be seen through an electron microscope. Deploying the spikes on its own surface, HIV uses receptors on the human CD4 cell as its docking station to fuse with the cell membrane and enter the host cell. Because of their central role in regulating the immune response, depletion of CD4 cells renders an HIV-infected individual incapable of adequately responding to micro-organisms which would ordinarily be harmless.[8] Once HIV binds to a cell, it hides HIV DNA inside the cell's DNA: as the virus replicates, this turns the cell into a sort of HIV factory.

The special risk of HIV

HIV is variously described as a lentivirus, an enveloped virus, a recombinant virus or a retrovirus. Sheathed in a fatty viral envelope which surrounds a matrix composed of protein p17 and with a bullet-shaped p24 inner core, are three enzymes required for the virus to replicate: reverse transcriptase, integrase and protease. Also nestled within the core is the virus's genetic material: two identical strands of RNA. This identifies HIV as a retrovirus, since most other viruses use DNA, an organism's hereditary material, for this purpose. Unlike other organisms which contain hundreds or thousands of genes, HIV has only nine, of which three (gag, pol and env) contain information needed to make structural proteins for new virus particles. The other six (tat, rev, nef, vif, vpr and vpu) code for proteins that control HIV's ability to infect a cell, produce new copies of virus, or cause disease.

Once inside the CD4 cell, the enzyme reverse transcriptase converts the single-stranded viral RNA into double-stranded DNA. Viral DNA is then transported to the cell's nucleus, where it is spliced into the human DNA by the HIV enzyme integrase. Once integrated, the HIV DNA is known as provirus. Infected CD4 cells become virus factories which, if activated, will produce viruses instead of triggering the production of more antibodies against HIV.[9] HIV destroys CD4 cells by means of direct killing of infected cells, by increasing rates of apoptosis (programmed cell death) and by destruction of infected CD4 cells by CD8 cytotoxic lymphocytes. In a contrary quirk, the greater our immune activation, the quicker our immune system will be destroyed. Thus HIV replicates throughout the course of infection, causing a persistent activation of the immune system that leads to a gradual attrition of immune-system resources, ultimately resulting in the group of symptoms, a syndrome, identifying an HIV-infected individual as having AIDS.

A secret disease

The ultimate irony of this tragically lethal infection, which brings disease and death in its distant wake, is that it is passed from person to person during the most compelling, intimate and joyous of all human connections; those that form bonds between those who are the most mutually beloved, essential to the very survival of the human race. HIV is passed through an exchange of body fluids between adults during love-making, and between mothers and babies during gestation, while giving birth, and during breastfeeding.

Although HIV can also be detected in cerebrospinal fluid (surrounding the brain and spinal cord) and synovial fluid (surrounding the joints between bones), it's generally believed to be either not present at all, or present in only minute amounts, in saliva, tears, blister fluid, urine, faeces, vomit or sweat. HIV's main routes of transmission are through blood, semen, vaginal fluid, amniotic fluid and breastmilk.[10] The virus is considered to be fairly fragile, and cannot be passed through kissing or by sharing cutlery. It can, however, sometimes survive in dried blood at room temperature for up to six days[8] and in saliva in pre-chewed food. It is not affected by extreme cold, but it is destroyed by heat, e.g. after 30 minutes at 60 degrees C, or by just a few minutes at 71 degrees C,[11] temperatures achieved during pasteurisation of breastmilk.

One of the most unnerving aspects of HIV is that transmission occurs in stealth. If symptoms of infection were severe and showed soon after infection, as they do with many other viruses, we could receive fair warning in time to take avoiding action. For instance, the symptoms of Ebola are so frightening that they provoke extreme quarantine measures; smallpox causes an ugly rash and leaves severe scarring in its few survivors; polio causes paralysis; even the common cold causes such visibly unpleasant symptoms that most people try and avoid becoming infected. SARS-CoV-2 has provoked worldwide robust avoidance measures. But HIV is a member of the family of lentiviruses, meaning that it is a slow virus with a time-lag of several years to active disease.

Although a new infection with HIV quickly leads to high levels of virus in an infected person's blood, if there are any symptoms at all they are usually mild, e.g. a dry cough and flu-like symptoms. A person living with HIV looks perfectly healthy and the virus is able to spread undetected and unchecked through concentric rings of intimate relationships. Paradoxically, as the immune system works to overcome the initial infection, viral levels may fall and the person living with HIV may be less infectious. An infected individual can more easily infect others when viral levels are high, either shortly after primary infection, or later when developing active AIDS, which may take a decade or more.

Detection

The life cycle of HIV can be as short as 1.5 days from viral entry into a cell, through replication, assembly, and release of additional viruses, to infection of other cells. The production of viruses does not last very long. After three weeks, a reservoir of white blood cells is formed and the infected white blood cells then become dormant.[12] During the period of acute primary infection, the virus multiplies rapidly, but until the number of viral particles or the antibodies reach sufficiently high levels to be detected on a blood test, there can be no way of knowing that infection has taken place. This undetectable window period can last anywhere from a few weeks to several months. Once 'sero-conversion' has occurred (which means that the body responds to HIV by making antibodies), HIV infection can be diagnosed by means of an antibody test, which will then show positive.

Another of the more insidious attributes of HIV is its formidable ability to mutate. The virus lacks proofreading enzymes to correct errors made when it converts its RNA into DNA via reverse transcription. Its short life-cycle and high error rate cause the virus to mutate very rapidly, resulting in a high genetic variability. Most of the mutations are either inferior to the parent virus (often lacking the ability to reproduce at all) or convey no advantage, but some of them have a natural selection superiority to their parent, enabling them to slip past human defences.

The genetic diversity of HIV is primarily caused by the fast replication cycle of the virus coupled with the high error-prone function of its reverse transcriptase. HIV can evolve around one million times faster than mammalian DNA. Additional genetic diversity is introduced as a result of recombination that takes place during HIV replication if the host cell is infected with multiple HIV subtypes, also known as co-infection or super-infection. Recombination allows for an even more rapid increase in viral diversity than does the accumulation of mutations through replication errors. This in turn allows for rapid adaptation to host immune responses, target cell availability, and antiretroviral therapy, which can lead to increased viral pathogenicity, infectivity, and decreased antiretroviral susceptibility. Clinical progression to AIDS might be more rapid in individuals with dual infection.

Because HIV uses several enzymes, including reverse transcriptase, proteases, ribonuclease and integrase to invade host cells and replicate, these are the targets of an increasing arsenal of medications known as antiretroviral drugs (ARVs) to treat, halt and, more recently to prevent the disease through pre-exposure prophylaxis (known as PrEP). The means to completely eradicate dormant reservoirs of the virus within infected but otherwise healthy treatment-adherent individuals, whose levels of virus are virtually undetectable, remains elusive. However, antiretroviral treatment typically inhibits viral replication in those cells and viral levels can be suppressed to the point that an individual's infectivity becomes nil.[13]

The more active the virus, the greater the possibility that one resistant to antiretroviral drugs will be made. Thus efforts to develop a vaccine against it, or to completely eradicate it, have been plagued with difficulty. The more diversity the virus has, the older it is, and this characteristic has enabled the origins of HIV to be traced (see Chapter 2).

The Berlin patient

A rare natural genetic abnormality, present in less than 1% of Caucasians in northern and western Europe, called the CCR5-Delta32 deletion mutation, means that the docking station which HIV uses to enter and infect CD4 cells can combat the disease. Individuals who inherit the mutation from a single parent are resistant to HIV, while those who inherit the gene from both parents are virtually immune. It was this gene profile that was responsible for the known cure for HIV, achieved in 2008. In 2007 Timothy Ray Brown, known as 'the Berlin patient',[14] had been suffering from HIV for 10 years when he received a bone marrow transplant to treat leukaemia. His donor had inherited the gene mutation from both parents, rendering the donated new white blood cells resistant to infection with HIV.[15] Three months after the transplant, Timothy Ray Brown's levels of HIV rapidly plummeted to undetectable levels, while his CD4 count increased, showing that his immune system was recovering. A second transplant was received from the same donor the following year, and today he remains free of leukaemia as well as HIV.[16,17] Debate continues about whether he is cured or whether he simply no longer needs treatment.

After many years of infection with HIV, a few individuals naturally develop broadly neutralising antibodies, by virtue of immune escape. How such antibodies arise, and the role of viral evolution in shaping these responses, is not yet known, but is the subject of ongoing research.[18] A 2012 ground-breaking paper describes how two HIV-infected women developed broadly cross-reacting neutralising antibodies to the tiny glycoprotein (gp120) expressed on the surface of the HIV envelope through immune escape from earlier strain-specific antibodies.[19] Anything which binds to gp120's target can block it from binding to a cell by being physically in the way. Thus the change in the outer covering of the virus enabled the women to make potent antibodies which are able to kill nine out of 10 HIV types from around the world. The viruses lacked a specific glycan, a sugar that coats the surface protein of HIV, forming a site of vulnerability in transmitted subtype C viruses. By tracing back the evolution of the virus that elicited these antibodies, the research team found that this particular weak point was absent from the virus that first infected these women. Under constant pressure from other less powerful antibodies that develop in all infected people, their HIV was forced to expose this vulnerability over time. This allowed the broadly neutralising antibodies to develop. Analysis of a large number of other viruses from throughout the world suggests that the vulnerability may be present at the time of infection in about two-thirds of subtype C viruses, which affect 46% of HIV-infected people globally and are the subtype most common in Africa.[20]

Long-term non-progressors and elite controllers

Years after the initiation of the 1981 AIDS pandemic, a small subset of HIV-positive individuals, called 'long-term non-progressors' (LTNPs), were discovered. They had a markedly slow disease progression to AIDS.[21,22] They comprise 2–5% of infected individuals who have never been on antiretroviral therapy (ART) and have been infected with the virus for 20–25 years. Throughout the course of their infection LTNPs maintain low levels of viraemia, and elevated CD4+ T-cell levels, and remain free of AIDS-defining illnesses, in contrast to rapid progressor HIV subjects who succumb to AIDS after a few years of infection if they don't receive ART. A small subset (<1%) called 'elite controllers' have undetectable viral loads, but generally lower CD4 counts than other LTNPs. Understandably, they have been the subject of intense investigation since they may hold the key to future treatment or prevention strategies.[23] Studies have shown that some LTNPs have unique genetic advantages: mutations that upregulate the production of the chemokines that competitively inhibit HIV binding to CCR5 or CXCR4. Immunological factors are crucial for providing LTNPs with a natural form of control, the most important being robust HIV-specific CD4 and CD8 T-cell responses that correlate with lower viral loads. LTNPs serve as an ideal model for HIV vaccine development due to their natural control of HIV infection.

Evidence is contradictory as to whether the virus infecting non-progressors and elite controllers is different from the virus infecting those who progress more rapidly to AIDS. Elite controllers make up less than 0.5% of the HIV-positive population. It is known that their method of control is based on viral, genetic and immunological components. Genomic sequencing shows that some are infected with attenuated strains of HIV and harbour mutant genes.[24] A lucky combination of several different characteristics – including defective HIV, a hypervigilant and specific immune response to HIV, and cells that are unusually resistant to infection – may all have a part to play. Elite controllers may not be unique – there may also be a larger population of people on long-term ART who would qualify as 'post-treatment controllers' – but the only way to find out would be to take them off ART. A study published recently in *Nature* has used novel gene-sequencing probes to investigate exactly how the one in 200 people with HIV who are so-called elite controllers manage the feat.[25] The study suggests that a dynamic process happens whereby a strong anti-HIV response by the CD8 cells of the immune system preferentially kills off cells that are more likely to produce active HIV. The low-level stimulus from the cells that are left – and which contain HIV genes that are much less likely to spring into action – is nonetheless enough to keep the anti-HIV CD8 response attuned to HIV.[26] In one individual, a 66-year-old Californian woman, among the 64 elite controllers studied, investigators were unable to find any replication-competent HIV genetic material in over a billion T-cells, and were also unable to grow any HIV from her T-cells. She has managed to clear all intact viral material from her system in what could truly be called a self-cure.

Intriguingly, a group of Kenyan sex workers who were apparently immune to HIV was identified in the 1990s.[27] Their resistance to infection was also associated with CD8 lymphocyte responses, but 11 prostitutes meeting criteria for HIV resistance seroconverted between 1996 and 1999. Ironically, the key correlation with late seroconversion to HIV was a reduction in sex work over the preceding year. In persistently uninfected women, a break from sex work leading to waning CD8+ responses seemed to occur as a result of reduced antigenic exposure. And continued exposure to HIV appeared to be necessary to maintain a robust immune response.

Meanwhile, for most untreated HIV-infected individuals, CD4 cells dwindle, cell-mediated immunity is lost, and the body becomes progressively more susceptible to opportunistic infections. A declining CD4 count and a soaring level of viral shedding into the body, taking approximately eight years on average, results in progression to the collection of symptoms known as AIDS.[28] This leads inexorably to an increasingly compromised ability to fight the other opportunistic viral, bacterial or fungal infections and cancers to which the severely immuno-compromised individual will eventually succumb. Furthermore, the higher the level of virus in the blood, the more infectious a person is. The HIV virus will die with the victim, but has already assured its own immortality by being passed in the previous decade to blood-brothers, lovers and children.

CHAPTER 2

The origins of HIV

'Progress in scientific research rarely follows a straight path. Generally, it entails many unexpected meanderings, with a mix of good and bad ideas, good and bad luck. The discovery of the human immunodeficiency virus (HIV) as the cause of AIDS did not avoid this pattern.'

Robert C. Gallo and Luc Montagnier, 'The Discovery of HIV as the Cause of AIDS', *New England Journal of Medicine*, 2003

The origins of the human immunodeficiency virus (HIV) have intrigued scientists ever since the disease was recognised as a separate entity in the early 1980s. Where did this lethal disease come from? How did it spread to affect almost every country in the world?

Some of the earliest known viral samples point to clues showing when it first appeared in humans and how it evolved. Due to the stigma and shame associated with HIV, political sensitivity has sometimes hindered attempts to trace its origins and in some cases, details have even been suppressed. Many pieces of the puzzle have been located by chance and as new testing techniques have been developed, sometimes what we thought we knew has been revised.

Animal immunodeficiency viruses

The story of how humans first became infected with HIV must begin with an examination of similar viruses which affect other vertebrates. All the organs and tissues of the human body are susceptible to infection by different viruses called zoonoses (diseases that spill over from animals to humans), with outcomes which range from no symptoms at all, to those which can be life-threatening.[1] They may cause an epidemic by overwhelming their new target group, which has not yet had time to develop immunity against them. Examples include rabies (from dogs or bats), the Hantavirus (from rodents), influenza (from birds or bats) and HIV (from primates). More than 1,200 species of bat, making up about a quarter of all mammalian species, are host to a significantly higher proportion of zoonoses than all other mammals.[2] Bats are linked to the most recent coronavirus pandemic, causing Covid-19, currently rampaging throughout the world.

Animal immunodeficiency viruses show many similarities to HIV in terms of incubation, infection and symptoms. These species-specific viruses can infect primates, sheep, goats, horses, cats, and cattle. Bovine immunodeficiency virus (BIV) was first isolated from a cow with a wasting condition in Louisiana in 1969.[3] By 1994 it had been found in the US, Canada, Europe and Australasia. BIV impairs the immune systems of cattle, just as HIV does in humans. Infection rates range from 4%–8% in the US. A *Wall Street Journal* article in 1991[4] confirmed that cooking or pasteurisation would kill the fragile virus and that it was not transmitted to humans. Sheep and rabbits have been experimentally infected with BIV and have seroconverted, with a high mortality rate in rabbits. However, in the laboratory, neither personnel who had accidental needle-stick injuries with infected cattle sera, nor a human cell line used to isolate HIV, have been infected by BIV. Other cell cultures have also failed to establish infection.

Cats infected with feline immunodeficiency virus (FIV) are also found worldwide. In the United States, infection rates vary from 1.5–3% in healthy cats and >15% in sick cats respectively.[5] Biting, rather than casual contact, appears to be the most efficient route of transmission. The course of disease is remarkably similar to HIV in humans, with the virus reproducing in white blood cells, spreading throughout the body and resulting in generalised but temporarily enlarged lymph nodes, accompanied by fever. This stage of infection may pass unnoticed so that infected cats may appear normal for years. However, secondary infection with the same normally harmless bacteria, viruses, protozoa, and fungi found in the everyday environment that will not usually cause disease in otherwise healthy animals, can cause severe disease in immunodeficient animals, to identify the cat as infected with FIV.

Simian (monkey) HIV

The discovery of simian immunodeficiency virus (SIV) in monkeys occurred almost by chance. Former director of UNAIDS, Peter Piot, whose early work with infectious diseases in central Africa led to the discovery of the Ebola virus, and later led him to research on HIV, describes in his book *No Time to Lose* how he and his group were stunned to discover that an apparently healthy chimpanzee had a virus almost identical to human HIV. While screening monkeys and apes for another retrovirus called human T-cell leukaemia virus (HTLV) that infects T-lymphocyte white blood cells, a colleague, Belgian microbiologist Martine Peeters, had found a strain of simian immunodeficiency virus (SIVcpz) in a pet chimpanzee named Amandine.[6] The chimp virus so closely resembled HIV that Martine's article describing the discovery was initially rejected for publication, the review panel assuming that there had been contamination of laboratory equipment. On her return to Belgium, however, Martine found a second simian virus (SIVcpz) in a chimpanzee named Noah, living in the Antwerp zoo. Clearly SIV is an older disease than HIV, and one which simians have learned to live with, since it is not nearly as fatal as its human cousin. Piot reports that Noah, now living in a chimpanzee hotel in the Netherlands, remains as healthy as Amandine.[6]

SIV jumps to humans

In 1999 Dr Peeters and colleagues succeeded in formally publishing what they had learned; the origins of HIV occurred nearly 80 years previously due to a strain of SIV in a chimpanzee (*Pan troglodytes troglodytes*) that was almost identical to HIV in humans.[7,8] Later, the location of this particular strain was narrowed down to wild chimpanzees found in the forests of southern Cameroon. The chimps were highly endangered and thus protected and could not be killed or captured for testing. However, by analysing hundreds of samples of chimp droppings, the researchers were able to obtain 34 specimens that reacted to a standard HIV DNA test. The results were virtually indistinguishable from human HIV. Chimp SIV was most likely transmitted to humans as a result of chimps being killed and eaten, or their blood getting into the cuts or wounds of local villagers in the course of hunting.

Because one of the enzymes the virus requires in order to replicate – HIV reverse transcriptase – is error prone, and the viral generation time is short,[9] having a half-life of only two days,[10] HIV evolves around one million times faster than mammalian DNA.[11] This characteristic has helped to show when and where the AIDS pandemic originated. Multiple zoonotic transmissions of SIV have resulted in different HIV lineages in humans. Natural hosts for SIV very rarely progress to AIDS, but several simian viruses have crossed the species barrier to great apes and humans, generating new pathogens. The high mutation and recombination rates during viral replication result in a great genetic variability of HIV within individuals, as well as within populations.

There are two strains of the virus, HIV-1 and HIV-2, which are genetically quite different; HIV-1 is closely related to chimpanzee SIV (SIVcpz). HIV-2 is closely related to a strain of SIV found in sooty mangabeys (SIVsmm), who do not seem to show AIDS independent of a strong cellular immune response in infected animals. Similarly, although HIV-2 is known to cause AIDS in humans, it is less virulent and less transmissible than HIV-1 M group viruses.[12] For this reason, this book focuses on HIV-1, which I refer to as HIV, unless otherwise indicated.

Lineages and where they occurred

Human–ape encounters in west central Africa have resulted in four independent cross-species transmission events.[13] HIV-1 is not just one virus, but comprises four distinct lineages, termed groups M, N, O and P.

- Group M, (for 'Major') which accounts for the world HIV pandemic, is descended from SIVcpz, with its reservoir in the species *Pan troglodytes troglodytes*, confined to Gabon, Congo Brazzaville, Cameroon, and a small range of northern Congo (now the Democratic Republic of Congo).[14]
- Group O (for 'Outlier'), discovered in 1990, accounts for less than 1% of all HIV-1 infections, and is largely restricted to Cameroon and neighbouring countries.[15,16]
- Group N was identified in 1998,[17] and only 13 cases have ever been documented, all in individuals from Cameroon.[18]
- Group P was discovered in 2009 in a Cameroonian woman living in France.[19] Only

one other person, also actually living in Cameroon, has been found to have this type of HIV.[18]

To add to the complexity, different subtypes can combine genetic material to form a hybrid virus, known as a 'circulating recombinant form' (CRF). Around 89 of these are known to exist.[20]

Interestingly, the regions of Cameroon and Congo where the HIV epidemics originated show the greatest diversity of subtypes of HIV. This means that these viruses had more time to mutate. Recent studies of SIV-infected monkeys show that geographically isolated sub-species have been infected with the same type of SIV for at least 32,000 years.[21]

The pandemic form, group M, likely originated in an area flanked by the Boumba, Ngoko and Sangha rivers in the south-eastern corner of Cameroon[22] before travelling down river to Kinshasa in the Congo and spreading for some 50 to 70 years before it was recognised. Rivers served as major routes of travel and commerce.[13] Leopoldville was the largest city in the region at that time and all current evidence points to Leopoldville/Kinshasa as the cradle of the AIDS pandemic.

When did HIV originate

Although primate lentiviruses were first identified in the late 1980s, the complexity of their evolution, geographic distribution, prevalence, natural history and pathogenesis in natural and non-natural hosts has only recently been appreciated. In the unfolding story of HIV, more recent research often clarifies and in some cases corrects previous misconceptions first touted as fact in earlier papers. Molecular clock analyses have dated the onset of the HIV-1 group M and O epidemics to the beginning of the 20th century (between 1915 and 1941).[23,24,25]

In 2003 Belgian researchers reconstructed the evolutionary history of HIV-2 to find that the approximate date of the most recent common ancestor of HIV-2 subtype A strain was 1940, and that of B strain was 1945. Their analysis provided evidence for a zoonotic transfer of HIV-2 during the first half of the 20th century and the beginning of the epidemic in Guinea-Bissau that coincided with the disruptive effects of the war of independence between 1963 and 1974.[26]

Taken together, international commissions and omissions likely set the scene for the spread of HIV in a way which could never have been foretold.

The earliest cases in the Congo

Edward Hooper, writing in the *British Medical Journal* in 1997, alleged that the earliest confirmed case of AIDS in the world was in a young Norwegian sailor who was infected with HIV-1 Group O, 'probably in Cameroon in 1961–2', but the earliest evidence of HIV-1 Group M is from 1959.[27]

A 2014 article in *Science* describes two HIV-1 sequences that substantially pre-date the discovery of AIDS, which were retrospectively recovered from blood and tissue samples collected in Kinshasa in 1959 and 1960.[28] In 1998 the very first verified case of HIV was reported from a blood sample taken in 1959 from a Bantu man living in Leopoldville, Belgian Congo (now known as Kinshasa, Democratic Republic of Congo).[29] The sample was retrospectively analysed and HIV was detected. A second case, from a woman living in Leopoldville in 1960, was recovered with great difficulty in 2008 from stored lymph node tissue samples.[30] Although there are numerous earlier cases where patterns of deaths from common opportunistic infections, now known to be AIDS-defining, suggest that HIV was the cause, these became the earliest blood samples that could verify infection.

Genetic analysis of infected blood and tissue samples collected in Kinshasa revealed that HIV-1 had already diversified into different subtypes when urban populations in west central Africa were expanding.[25] Using a database of HIV-1 sequences and an estimate of the rate at which these sequences change over time, researchers modelled when HIV-1 first surfaced. By taking tiny genetic fragments from lymph node tissue, work which took five years, they managed to almost completely reconstruct the HIV genome from a time before anyone even knew it existed.[31] Their results showed that the most likely date for HIV's emergence was about 1908, when Leopoldville was emerging as a centre for trade.[30]

In 1920, Leopoldville had just been made the capital of the Belgian Congo. The city became a very attractive destination for young working men seeking their fortunes. Nearly 400,000 people immigrated to Kinshasa between 1950 and 1967.[32] Growing prostitution may have played a part in the spread of HIV; during colonial times, a few 'free women' worked as prostitutes, but after independence in 1960 sex workers in Kinshasa may have had more than 1,000 clients each year.[33]

Nosocomial infection

HIV transmission was also facilitated by the use of syringes and needles that were merely rinsed between patients receiving daily injections for sexually transmitted diseases in the city's clinics. An outbreak of 'innoculation hepatitis' from 1951 to 1952 was spread by this route. Blood transfusions were widely used throughout sub-Saharan Africa during the crucial period of 1950–1970, when all epidemic strains of HIV first emerged. By 1955, 19 African colonies and countries reported transfusion programmes –with national rates of approximately 700–1,400 per 100,000 by 1964, and urban rates similar to those in developed countries. By 1970 an estimated one million transfusions per year were administered in sub-Saharan Africa, rising to two million per year by 1980.[34] Zimbabwe was reportedly the third country in the world to institute screening of blood donors in 1984 at the National Blood Transfusion Services of Zimbabwe,[35] yet it is unknown how many cases of HIV may have occurred through transfusions with infected blood before then, in a country which eventually attained an HIV prevalence of over 30%.

From the Congo to other African countries

The Congo shares borders with nine other countries. Movement of peoples in the early years was restricted by distance and lack of development, but the Congo's rapidly expanding colonial transportation system and rail links, used by millions of waged labourers, facilitated the spread of the virus to mining areas in south-eastern Congo and beyond. Most workers were men; sex work flourished, and the number of infections soon tripled. Group M viruses hitched rides, travelling from the commercial capital to the rest of the vast Congo basin and beyond.[36]

Edward Hooper adds another intriguing theory to the spread of HIV in his 1999 book *The River*. In a meticulously researched and detailed account he describes how an experimental polio vaccine being tested in the 1950s on chimpanzees in Lindi in the Congo may have inadvertently given rise to the lethal and infectious new disease.[37] In March 1957 the chimps had been sacrificed (killed), and their kidneys had been removed and sent in special flasks from Stanleyville to New York and then on to the Wistar Institute in Philadelphia. There, the CHAT vaccine, an attenuated Type 1 polio virus strain, was subjected to numerous laboratory procedures for selection of the least virulent particles. CHAT was produced in 'primary monkey cells' straight from the animal's kidney. Primary cells, in contrast to secondary and tertiary cells, are rich in lymphocytes and macrophages, the target cells for SIV and HIV. Shortly afterwards large pools of CHAT vaccine were manufactured for feeding in the Congo. Hooper maintains that there is very little published in the medical literature about the safety and effectiveness of polio vaccines that were later fed to over nine million people.

However, at a Royal Society meeting on the origins of HIV and AIDS organised by the Pasteur Institute and the Windeyer Institute, University College Hospital Medical School, in 2000,[14] one of the speakers confirmed that by good fortune, the process failed to lead to human contamination. There is thankfully no evidence that the oral polio vaccine is the cause of the AIDS epidemic, but it seems likely this may have been a near-miss. There are many examples of transfer of other retroviruses from animals to humans, including iatrogenic transfer of retroviruses. The Royal Society meeting was a welcome opportunity to review concerns about the potential role of medical science in causing or amplifying the HIV epidemic. The Covid-19 pandemic is another more recent example of how important this is and how easily things can go wrong.

Political events in the Congo in the 1950s may have also facilitated the spread of HIV, allowing it to become a world pandemic. As a Belgian colony, Congo had a waged labour force twice as large as that in any other African colony. By the time of the Congo Crisis in 1960, when many Belgians left the country, there was no proper national economy or Congolese middle class. As a child in Kenya, I was witness to Belgian refugees arriving traumatised and penniless in my little town after fleeing the violence in Congo. Little did any of us realise the profound implications these events would have in the next few decades. Between 1960 and 1964 the United Nations' first peacekeeping mission, comprising some 20,000 troops and commanded by a Haitian, was sent to help restore stability.[38]

As early as 1958, the United Nations had begun recruitment efforts to replace European administrators of African bureaucracies. The Congo recruited French-speaking professionals and technicians from overseas to help establish the country's infrastructure and to supplement the small Congolese leadership class. Hundreds of Haitians – teachers, professors, engineers, and doctors – went to Africa. By 1962,

Haitian émigrés constituted the second largest contingent of UN experts working in the Congo. The Chief of UNESCO's Africa Division was Haitian, as was the Director of the WHO medical team that included several Haitian doctors. Immigration from Haiti to Congo in the 1960s had in part been helped by events at home, coinciding with Papa Doc Duvalier's promotion of emigration to the newly independent countries of French-speaking Africa. Eventually, an estimated 7,500 Haitians spent time in African countries. Some spent career lifetimes with their families in Congo, while others returned to Haiti, but their experiences often went undocumented. Nevertheless, between 1985 and 1988, there are reports from Haiti of medical investigations and clinical observations of deaths, suspected to be due to AIDS, of retired Haitian managers who had lived and worked in Zaire (as Congo was renamed in 1971) and then returned to Haiti. A dynamic propagation of this virus may have been made possible by this movement of Haitians between Haiti and Africa.[39] Thus HIV crossed the Atlantic in Haitians returning home. From those early events, a pandemic was born.

The very first Haitian AIDS patient was identified in 1978, the same year the disease was first seen in the United States, but the prevalence of HIV in Haiti turned out to be much higher. The speculation is that either the virus was introduced into Haiti from the United States at a very early stage in the epidemic, possibly through gay sex tourism (Haiti was a popular holiday destination for gay men), or it came to Haiti via migrant workers from Congo/Zaire, and spread to the US homosexual population via sex tourism. Since 85% of Haitian patients were male it was commonly assumed at the time that homosexual contacts formed the 'HIV bridge'. All 82 Haitian sequences then available were found to be of subtype B, (subsequently identified as the homosexual 'signature').

Subtype B is carried to North America

A fascinating paper by Carla Kuiken and colleagues in 2000 provides a slightly different theory for the introduction of HIV into the Western world.[40] Based on available data, the most plausible scenario was that subtype B virus was carried out of Africa and introduced into the Western homosexual community by one person. It's possible that this person was 'Patient Zero', a Canadian gay airline steward who was infected in the late 1970s and allegedly subsequently infected a number of his sexual partners. A sequence of this patient's virus showed subtype B with viral characteristics consistent with homosexual transmission (as distinct from transmission due to intravenous drug use or heterosexual contact). However, it was later concluded that Patient Zero was probably not solely responsible for the initial spread of the virus in the United States; anecdotal evidence showed that he was part of a cluster of homosexual men who travelled frequently, were extremely sexually active, and died of AIDS at a very early stage in the epidemic (around 1980–82).

At the Fourteenth Conference on Retroviruses and Opportunistic Infections (CROI) held in Los Angeles in March 2007, the Haitian connection was made again. Data was presented by a group of international scientists based on complex genetic analysis of 122 early samples of the most common strain of HIV found in the US and in Haiti. HIV had probably been brought to Haiti from Africa by a single person in around 1966, when many

Haitians would have been returning from working in the Congo.[41] A single mutation from the Haitian source samples in or around 1969 (1966–72) was ancestral for almost all non-Haitian subtype B infections around the world. One exception was the subtype B epidemic in Trinidad and Tobago, which was linked to a separate, single-patient introduction from Haiti. The molecular modelling established the infection in Haiti as the oldest HIV/AIDS epidemic outside sub-Saharan Africa. The migration of Haitian professionals to work in the newly independent Congo during the 1960s pre-dated US tourism to Haiti in the mid-1970s. The CROI presentation was clear. HIV did *not* start in Haiti, but the clade-B subtype did slowly evolve there before moving to the US and beyond.[42] Other conclusions from this research included that HIV was clearly circulating in the United States for over a decade before its recognition in 1983. It also seemed clear that the global spread of HIV involved major outbreaks hinging on rare, single transmission events, rather than widespread multiple sources of the first infections.

Global spread of different subtypes

Group M HIV, the first to be discovered, accounts for more than 90% of HIV/AIDS cases worldwide, infecting millions of people in virtually every country of the globe. The extreme variability of HIV-1 makes it possible to conduct transmission studies on the basis of genetic analysis and to trace global and local patterns in the spread of the virus.[40] Dissemination involved a number of population bottlenecks – founder events – which led to the predominance of different group M lineages, now called subtypes, in different geographic areas (see Table 1).[13]

Subtype	Area
A	East Africa
B	North & South America, Europe, Japan, Australia, Middle East, North Africa
C	South & East Africa, India, Nepal, China
D	East & Central Africa,
E	South East Asia
F	Central Africa, South America and Eastern Europe
G	East and West Africa and Central Europe
H	Central Africa
J	North, Central West Africa & Caribbean
K	Congo & Cameroon
L	Congo

Table 1: Different geographical locations of HIV subtypes

Subtype B, which accounts for the great majority of HIV infections in Europe and the Americas and is found among gay men, is the most studied subtype. Arising from a single African strain spreading to Haiti in the 1960s and then onward to the US and other western countries,[43] subtype B viruses are infrequently found in Africa.

Subtype C currently accounts for around 50% of HIV-1 infections worldwide. It originated in the Congo in the mining regions, from where it spread south and east, probably through migrant labour. It predominates in southern Africa from where it spread to India and other Asian countries. Genetic and historical data indicate independently that the Congolese transportation network provided the key connection between the Kinshasa region and other human population centres in sub-Saharan Africa, including neighbouring Zambia and Angola.

Subtype D originated in central Africa, but moved to eastern Africa. It is associated with greater pathogenicity,[44] cognitive impairment and AIDS dementia.

Subtype E, now called CRF01, probably first occurred in central Africa. This viral lineage arose from a recombination event and is one of the most intensively studied of the regional epidemics, being first noted in the late 1980s as causing a heterosexual epidemic in Thailand. Today it dominates in heterosexual populations in south-east Asia.[45]

Subtype F1 viruses were first recognised after seeding an epidemic of paediatric infections in Romania.[46]

Viral complexity

In some European countries (e.g. Scotland and Germany) homosexual men tend to be infected with a subtly different variant of the same strain of HIV compared to intravenous drug users. In other areas (e.g. Norway and Sweden), a distinction is also found between the two risk groups; but it is a different distinction. There is a tendency for homosexual men in many different geographic regions around the world to carry HIV subtype B, the variant that is most prevalent in the Americas, Europe and Australia. In contrast, people infected via other routes (mostly heterosexual contact) in those same countries carry a mixture of other subtypes. Biologic differences between the viruses infecting different risk groups have not been found, so the most likely explanation for the findings is different epidemiologic patterns. Both the genetic and biological diversity of HIV-1 group M subtypes and CRF is increasing,[13] and these patterns help to reconstruct the worldwide spread of the HIV epidemic.

Importantly, while subtype C is responsible for nearly half of all infections worldwide, and is the most common subtype affecting heterosexual couples in Africa, most clinical research has been conducted in populations where subtype B predominates (i.e. in America, western Europe and Australasia), even though these areas are home to only 12% of HIV-infected people.[47] This presented special challenges when early decisions were being made about whether HIV-infected mothers should breastfeed. While HIV-positive mothers lived in areas where subtype C predominated, early tests for infants were not powered to identify HIV subtypes other than B, making determination of infant HIV status especially problematic.

History of the US epidemic

In the United States, the AIDS epidemic was first recognised in June 1981 with the report of an outbreak of pneumocystis pneumonia among homosexual men.[48] Increasing numbers of young gay men in New York and California were succumbing to an unusual syndrome of opportunistic infections and rare malignancies such as Kaposi's sarcoma, a rare cancer, and a lung infection called pneumocystis pneumonia.[49] It was concluded that the cause must be an infectious 'disease'. Patient Zero, Gaëtan Dugas, the Canadian flight attendant described earlier, was part of an early CDC study that showed HIV could be transmitted through sexual contact. He provided the names of a greater number of his previous sexual partners than others involved in the study, and was therefore central to the transmission network analysis. His story has provided an intriguing narrative in Randy Shilts's book *And the Band Played On* of how the virus was able to spread unknown and unchecked in men who frequented the gay bath houses in New York and San Francisco.[50]

By mid-1982 the disease was also being experienced by haemophiliacs and intravenous drug users. In September that year the CDC finally named the syndrome as acquired immune deficiency syndrome (AIDS).[51] But it was only in 1983 that the HIV virus was isolated and identified by researchers at the Pasteur Institute in France. Originally called lymphadenopathy-associated virus (or LAV), the virus was confirmed as the cause of AIDS. Finally the virus was named human immunodeficiency virus type 1 (HIV-1), and was eventually identified as the causative agent of what has become one of the most devastating infectious diseases to have emerged in recent history.[52,53]

Using HIV subtype B information obtained from seven HIV-infected US individuals in 1981 and one from the infected Canadian Patient Zero in 1982, which were subjected to nucleotide analyses, and phylogenetic testing (a methodology within the field of molecular virology that compares partial DNA or RNA sequences from different sources to infer evolutionary relationships between them), researchers in 2003 gave the date of origin of the US epidemic as approximately 1968. The dating results suggest a US introduction date (or date of divergence from the most recent common ancestor) that precedes the date of the earliest known AIDS cases in the late 1970s.[54]

As a postscript it is well to remember that nothing about HIV is ever straightforward. In a paper published in *Nature* in 2016,[55] a team of scientists presented the first comprehensive study of pre-1981 HIV in north America. Using blood samples taken from 1978 and 1979, and using molecular clocks and phylogenetic analysis, they determined that the virus arrived in New York city from Haiti in around 1970, then spread to San Francisco and elsewhere in the country during the mid-1970s. One of the blood samples came from the man widely identified as Patient Zero, but in fact the virus recovered from Patient Zero's blood falls in the middle of the US HIV evolutionary tree, not at the base, clearing him as the culprit for initial HIV transmission in the US. Going back to look at archived samples from gay men in New York city and San Francisco, the team made an attempt to recover the HIV genome.

By painstaking comparison the researchers were able to construct an evolutionary tree of subtype B. HIV genomes from patients in San Francisco were nested in the tree as descendants of the viruses found in patients from New York city. In addition, the

New York city strain was more genetically diverse than the San Francisco one, indicating that the former variant was likely older. The researchers found that subtype B genomes from Haiti were the most diverse of all, indicating that they were likely ancestors of the US strains. Molecular clocks thus date the arrival of HIV in Haiti from Africa, where the virus originated, to the 1960s. The precise point of transmission from Haiti to New York city remains an open question.

Global spread

From the United States, the virus was presumed to have spread from one Western country to the next, most likely via homosexual contact. There were some isolated early cases of group O virus in Europe: the Norwegian sailor and his family, infected with the African group O virus, and two possible cases in homosexual men in Germany and Austria. However, the epidemic did not gather momentum in Europe until several years after it appeared in the United States. In 1982, there was a 43% prevalence of HIV among homosexuals in San Francisco, but only 7.5% in Amsterdam. The first AIDS patients in the US and western Europe, and in most other countries where subtype B predominates, such as Australia, Taiwan, and Korea, were homosexual men. Because subtype B was so rarely found in Africa, the odds of a second independent introduction from Africa with the same rare subtype were considered to be very low. It seems that the epidemic among intravenous drug users (IDUs) in a given country usually lags several years behind that among homosexuals. Aside from epidemiologic evidence, this hypothesis is supported by genetic data.

It is hard to conceive that, from such chance beginnings, a virus that jumped species almost 100 years ago has infected 75 million people worldwide and that about 33 million people have died.[56] While approximately 5,000 individuals still become newly infected every day,[57] HIV continues to be a deadly threat to us all.

CHAPTER 3

The rise and rise of the HIV pandemic

'No one should be blamed for the spread of a virus that nobody even knew about.'
Michael Worobey, *Los Angeles Times*, 26 October 2016

On 3 July 1981, the *New York Times* alerted the world to an unusual new disease, affecting 41 homosexual men in New York and San Francisco.[1] What made this noteworthy was that they were suffering from a rare cancer called Kaposi's sarcoma, normally only seen once in 1.5 million people, and never before outside of equatorial Africa. Most cases occurred in New York. A lesser number had been found in San Francisco. Many cases had gone undetected because of the rarity of the condition and the difficulty even dermatologists may have had in diagnosing it.

A month before the *New York Times* article, the US Centers for Disease Control and Prevention (CDC) had issued a warning about a relatively rare form of pneumonia among a small group of young gay men in Los Angeles.[2] Accompanying the report the editors wrote:

> *'Pneumocystis pneumonia in the United States is almost exclusively limited to severely immunosuppressed patients. The occurrence of pneumocystosis in these five previously healthy individuals without a clinically apparent underlying immunodeficiency is unusual. The fact that these patients were all homosexuals suggests an association between some aspect of a homosexual lifestyle or disease acquired through sexual contact and pneumocystis pneumonia in this population.'*

In their intriguing book, *Tinderbox*, about the spread of HIV, Craig Timberg and Daniel Halperin write that AIDS was initially thought to be fundamentally an affliction of gay American men, and this persistent idea would shape impressions of the epidemic in the United States and elsewhere for decades to come.[3] In a $100-million industry stretching across America and Canada, the gay liberation movement of the 1970s had spawned a business of bathhouses and sex clubs. The bathhouses were a horrible breeding ground for disease. The average bathhouse patron in 1979 typically had 2.7 sexual contacts a night, and risked a 33% chance of walking out of the tubs with syphilis or gonorrhea.[4] By 1980, on any one night, there could be up to 20,000 men having sex in New York's bathhouses or parks, as well as in backroom bars, bookstores, porno theatres and a wide range of other places. A public health problem was in the making. Having held its first Gay Parade in June 1978, San Francisco was not far behind.

The airline steward from Quebec, Gaëtan Dugas, known as Patient Zero, stepped into this milieu with his boyish blond good looks, his fabric-covered address book, and his self-professed opinion that he was 'the prettiest one'. Indulging a voracious sexual appetite while travelling between Toronto, Paris, London, Mexico, the Caribbean and San Francisco,[5] the spread of the disease outwards from North America is often attributed to his promiscuity.

The risk of acquiring HIV is 27 times higher among men who have sex with men.[6] Scientists initially called the new disease 'the Gay Plague' or 'Gay-Related Immune Deficiency' (GRID). Patients with symptoms of AIDS were stigmatised and ostracised. They had to deal with accusations of receiving just retribution, or a judgement from God for going against nature. There can be little doubt that the belief that AIDS was confined to gay men created a curious kind of complacency among those outside the gay community, which persists even to this day. Early reports of AIDS were confined to four main risk groups within the US: homosexuals, haemophiliacs, heroin addicts and Haitians. Even as the scale of the disaster became clearer, there were always hopes for the prospect of a cure, or a vaccine, or some medical solution capable of saving the world from what was becoming increasingly characterised as an epidemic. This complacency was about to be challenged.

AIDS spreads to Europe

The first clues about the true cause of AIDS stemmed from careful immunological investigations. One consistent manifestation was a rapid decrease in levels of circulating CD4 T-cells[7], specialised cells in the immune system which help to coordinate a response to outside threats of infection. Once those levels fell below roughly 200 cells per cubic millimetre, patients became vulnerable to myriad opportunistic infections and various malignancies. Exactly a year after Lawrence Altman's first report in the *New York Times*, came news in the *British Medical Journal* of 3 July 1982 that AIDS had crossed the Atlantic to Europe.[8] Four previously healthy Danish homosexual men were showing symptoms that were slightly different from each other, but with a common pathogenic pathway consistent with AIDS – fever of unknown origin, opportunistic infections, ulcers and Kaposi's sarcoma. Three of the men had never visited the USA, but all four had had sexual contact with homosexual men who had.

Infection in women

Then, in January 1983, the CDC released a report of two women who had contracted AIDS. Other than being in a close relationship with an infected male partner, neither woman had any other risk factors, and both had specifically denied drug abuse. But this now meant that AIDS could be transmitted between men and women.[9] The CDC speculated that the mechanism of transmission was an 'infectious agent' that could be passed sexually between both heterosexual and male homosexual couples. It also reported aspects of an additional 43 cases in previously healthy females which today we now recognise as being consistent with the natural history of the disease and not in any way unusual; 13 of the women were neither Haitians nor drug abusers. Four were either married or in steady sexual relationships with male intravenous drug users who themselves did not seem to be sick, but whose blood specimens showed evidence of disease. Perhaps these men could be 'carriers' of the infectious agent; it had not made them ill, but had caused AIDS in their infected female partners.

Infection through blood transfusion

Barely two months later, in March 1983, came the first report of infection through blood transfusion.[10] A previously healthy patient with classic haemophilia, who was receiving Factor VIII concentrates, developed an acquired immunodeficiency syndrome. He had lost 47kg over the previous 12 months, showed reduced immune function, and suffered opportunistic fungal and viral infections. Alarmingly, he was not homosexual and had no history of drug abuse.

We now know that in the 1970s and 1980s blood and blood products infected with HIV and hepatitis viruses sourced from the US were given to British people with haemophilia and other bleeding disorders.[11] The UK had struggled to keep up with demand for Factor VIII, so much of the human blood plasma used to make it was sourced from the US, where high-risk prison inmates and drug users sold their blood. Contamination risk was raised further because Factor VIII was made by pooling and concentrating plasma from up to 40,000 donors. Between 1981 and 1984, approximately 15,000 American haemophiliacs became infected with HIV as a result of transfusion. The subsequent infection of up to 30,000 Britons with contaminated blood has been called the biggest treatment disaster in the history of the National Health Service. Thousands died. Court cases brought by victims or their families seeking compensation are ongoing. By the mid-1980s, once it was clear that HIV was blood-borne, the products started to be heat-treated, to kill the virus, but questions remain about how much was known before this time. Contaminated blood products remained in circulation and continued to be used. Screening of all blood products did not begin until 1991. Without a test for AIDS, blood banks had difficulty safeguarding the blood supply. Millions of dollars have been paid out in out-of-court settlements by companies that supplied infected products in the US. Other countries that imported blood products included France, Ireland, Portugal and Italy. In Japan, Canada, Iran and Iraq, politicians and drug companies have been convicted of negligence.

Many were transfused with contaminated blood. One such person was Elizabeth Glaser, who became an AIDS activist and criticised underfunding of research and inadequate action in tackling the AIDS crisis.[12] Elizabeth had contracted HIV in 1981, early in the epidemic, after receiving a contaminated blood transfusion following the birth of her daughter Ariel. Ariel acquired the virus through breastfeeding and died in

1988. The Glasers' son Jake, born in 1984, contracted the virus *in utero*, but lived into adulthood. Elizabeth herself died in 1994, and her death triggered an outcry for more research and ultimately led to the formation of the Elizabeth Glaser Pediatric AIDS Foundation.

Randy Shilts notes that nearly five years passed from the time the first isolated gay men began falling ill from strange and exotic ailments in 1980 until the disease was finally taken seriously by medical, public health, federal and private scientific research establishments.[5] Intravenous drug users were also at high risk due to exchange of blood during needle sharing. The first needle exchange programme was set up in Amsterdam in 1984; such programmes would rapidly spread in Europe but not within the US. Before the mass media and the gay community's leaders mobilised, the story of those years in America is a drama of national failure played out against a backdrop of needless death. It was not until October 1984 that the authorities finally closed the bath houses and private sex clubs of San Francisco due to high-risk sexual activity.[13] The following year, city officials in New York and Los Angeles followed suit, but an untold number of infections had taken place before they were able to acknowledge that these venues were facilitating the spread of AIDS on a massive scale.

Rock Hudson's death on 2 October 1985, and his bequest of $250,000 to set up the American Foundation for AIDS Research, finally proved to be the game-changer. A matinée idol since 1954, Hudson had come out 10 weeks before his death to let people know that he was homosexual and infected. The extensive publicity surrrounding his death drew attention to the disease in a way that nothing else had. Whereas before, AIDS was something that happened to someone else, Rock Hudson's revelation meant that AIDS became familiar to almost every household in the Western world, although the full implications would not become apparent for another few years.[5]

Naming of the causative agent of AIDS

Dr Françoise Barré-Sinoussi, a young French virologist at the Pasteur Institute, who had received her PhD eight years earlier and had interned at the US National Institutes of Health, was especially interested in retroviruses. In May 1983 she reported the discovery of a new retrovirus that could be the cause of AIDS.[14] She found that the lymphadenopathy-associated virus (LAV) was a retrovirus with reverse-transcriptase activity, belonging to a family of recently discovered human T-cell leukaemia viruses (HTLV). These viruses were horizontally transmitted in humans and could be involved in several pathological syndromes, including AIDS. Years later, after she had become a Nobel Laureate jointly with Dr Luc Montagnier, Dr Barré-Sinoussi described how hard it had been, at the time, for a woman, especially a relatively young woman, to be convincing about this discovery. In fact, several years later a dispute arose about whether the virus was first identified by the Pasteur Institute or the US National Cancer Institute. Dr Barré-Sinoussi knew that it was an important virus that had not been identified before, but neither she nor her colleagues had had any idea of the sheer magnitude of the epidemic, nor of the complexity of the interaction between the virus and the body.[15]

Almost a year later, in April 1984, Robert Gallo and colleagues at the National

Cancer Institute in the US announced that they had isolated HTLV-III retroviruses from both men and women, as well as children, with pre-AIDS. They also found that serum samples from a high proportion of AIDS patients contained antibodies to HTLV-III, which differed from HTLV-1 and HTLV-II. They concluded that HTLV-III was the primary cause of AIDS.[16] An editorial in *Science* reported, 'It is very likely that this virus is associated with the disease'.[17] Identification of the agent that caused AIDS had enormous clinical implications. In a joint conference Luc Montagnier's group at the Pasteur Institute and Robert Gallo and colleagues from the National Cancer Institute announced that LAV and HTLV-III were identical and the likely cause of AIDS. A blood test was created to screen for the virus in the hope that a vaccine would be developed within two years.

With the perspective of almost 20 years, Gallo and Montagnier wrote in 2003 that the year 1984 was a time of both intense excitement and harsh discussions between members of their two groups.[18] Identifying the cause of AIDS presented a unique challenge, because unlike other viral diseases responsible for past epidemics, AIDS was characterised by clinical signs that developed years afterwards, and by then patients usually had numerous other infections. Thus, an exceptional linkage of agent to disease had to be established. This linkage was made through the repeated isolation of HIV from patients with AIDS and, more importantly, through the development of a readily reproducible blood test.

Finally, in May 1986, five years after the new disease was identified among gay men in the US, the International Committee on the Taxonomy of Viruses urged adoption of a new name for the virus. They decided that the virus that causes AIDS would henceforth officially be called the human immunodeficiency virus (HIV).[19]

Eastern Europe and Asia

Until 1991, eastern Europe was still mostly free from HIV. The epidemic began in 1995 in Ukraine, and spread to Belarus, the Republic of Moldova and the Russian Federation in 1996, Latvia in 1998, Estonia in 2000, Lithuania in 2002 and central Asia in 2003.[20] By 2001, eastern European and central Asian countries had the fastest-growing epidemic, concentrated in key affected populations – those who inject drugs, and gay men. Armed conflict and displacement of people in eastern Europe in the 1990s had provided the perfect storm to fuel the rapid spread of the disease. Conditions reflected a climate of desperation among youth in the former USSR, with many resorting to commercial sex work to survive, some to injecting drug use and some to both. Fully 70–90% of all HIV infections in eastern Europe were due to sharing contaminated drug-injecting equipment.

Countries in the East (including Russia) saw rates of new infections double in 10 years. By 2016 cases reached one million.[21] The increasing overlap of injecting drug use and commercial sex work explained rising rates of heterosexual transmission; the epidemic was spreading from drug users to women. A few years ago, on the website which is home to the series of documents I helped to write on HIV and breastfeeding, known as the WABA HIV Kit, I noticed a very dramatic rise in the number of hits from

Russia. The increased interest was mystifying, but in light of the subsequent exploding epidemic among women in Eastern Europe, it fitted with an increased interest in whether HIV is transmitted during breastfeeding.[22]

The Middle East and north Africa

This area has one of the world's lowest HIV prevalence rates at 0.1%. However, new HIV infections have risen by 26% since 2000 and AIDS-related deaths have increased by 66% since 2005, largely due to the fact that ART coverage is only 11%, the lowest rate of any region in the world.[23]

AIDS in Africa

On the continent which was to be so badly affected by HIV/AIDS, the first reports coming from America caused hardly a ripple. New York, California and Europe seemed a long way from Nairobi, Cape Town or Entebbe. Furthermore, a syndrome of diseases which affected gay men seemed to pose little threat to most Africans. Homosexuality was almost never seen, and in many countries that would become hardest hit, it was in fact illegal.[24] Early complacency was misplaced, however; when it arrived in Africa, HIV would turn out to cause a different but much more severe epidemic.

West Africa

Initially there were high levels of infection of both HIV-1 and HIV-2 in the geographical area where the virus had originally jumped from monkeys to humans, although in nowhere near the proportions found in other areas of sub-Saharan Africa. The HIV-1 epidemic initially began with reported cases in Ivory Coast, probably due to rapid urbanisation, immigration and prostitution. By 1986 HIV prevalence among sex workers in Abidjan was already 38%. All of the west African states identified infection by 1990. Guinea-Bissau had the world's highest level of HIV-2 by 1986, with 26% of paid blood donors, 8% of pregnant women and 36% of sex workers testing positive, but HIV-2 was not infectious enough to generate an epidemic beyond this region.

East Africa

East Africa, where I spent my childhood from 1958 to 1970, was among the first areas in Africa to be affected by HIV-1. Uganda was hit particularly hard. Phylogenetic analysis, allowing the reconstruction of viral history over time, shows that subtype A HIV originated in the rural south-west in 1960 and subtype D in 1973, with subsequent spread to Kampala.[25] By 1982 doctors at the Uganda Cancer Institute began to recognise a new disease in rural areas called 'slim disease' due to its symptoms of weight loss and diarrhoea.[26] They thought it might be associated with HTLV-III infection because there were clinical features similar to those of an enteropathic acquired immunodeficiency syndrome previously seen in neighbouring Zaire (Congo). But in Uganda it affected females nearly as frequently as males, occurring predominantly in the heterosexually promiscuous population, and there was no clear evidence to implicate other possible means of transmission, e.g. insect bites or reused injection needles. Doctors suspected that the disease came from Uganda's east African neighbour, Tanzania. That these reports took three years to be published in the *Lancet* is regrettable. David Serwadda, the first author, recalls 'We just could not connect a disease in white, homosexual males in San Francisco to the thing that we were staring at.'[27] By 1990 HIV prevalence among pregnant women in Uganda's capital had peaked at over 30%.

By now I was living in Zimbabwe, where we heard that whole Ugandan villages were inhabited only by grandparents and children, with all the young adults having been wiped out by this new disease. Truck drivers – alongside other migrants such as soldiers, traders and miners – were identified as groups who facilitated the initial rapid spread of HIV as they engaged with sex workers and spread the infection on the transport and trade routes. It was found that 35% of tested Ugandan truck drivers were HIV-positive, as were 30% of military personnel from General Amin's Ugandan army. By 1986, 85% of sex workers in Nairobi were infected. In 1988 the second highest prevalence rate of HIV in all of Africa was found on the Tanzam road linking Tanzania and Zambia.

Southern Africa

The east African epidemic, first noted in Uganda, continued relentlessly south through Kenya and Tanzania to Mozambique, Zambia, Malawi, Zimbabwe, Botswana and Namibia, to finally arrive in the northern province of South Africa. After crossing the Limpopo it rolled on south through Swaziland and Lesotho until it reached the southern tip of Africa where it was stopped by the Atlantic and Indian oceans. I remember hearing from a paediatrician in Cape Town, who anxiously described the first AIDS cases he was seeing in his small patients, realising that South Africa had not escaped, and in fact that things were going to get worse. Eventually the numbers became eye-watering: while southern Africa had less than 2% of the world's population, it was home to about 30% of all people living with HIV/AIDS. Colleagues in Zimbabwe had been seeing an escalating number of cases for several years. By the end of the decade the countries of Malawi, Zambia, Zimbabwe and Botswana were overtaking east Africa as the focus of the global HIV epidemic.

The beginning half of the 1990s was a bleak time. Even as new HIV infection rates were rocketing, there were few new ideas about how to deal with generalised epidemics in poor countries. For a long time people laboured under numerous misconceptions, for instance that being overweight or obese (a sign of great beauty in some African societies) was evidence of not being infected, or that having sex with a virgin would cure AIDS. Public anxiety was high. Fear quickly bred stigma. HIV was often associated with prostitution, promiscuity and high-risk lifestyles. Doctors never wrote AIDS as the cause of death on a death certificate. Obituaries asserted that the deceased had 'died after a short illness'.

The situation continued to deteriorate as governments in the worst affected countries seemed unwilling to acknowledge that there was a problem and were powerless to take any action. By 2000 AIDS accounted for 25% of all deaths. Even as the country's neighbours ramped up prevention and treatment efforts, the South African president, Thabo Mbeki, influenced by a group of AIDS dissidents from overseas, publicly challenged the scientific consensus that HIV causes AIDS, blaming poverty for the spread of the virus.[28] His health minister, Manto Tshabalala-Msimang, promoted herbal remedies, including beetroot, garlic and lemon, as alternatives to antiretroviral medication. In 1997 the South African president had officially supported a treatment called Virodene that was later identified as an industrial solvent with no benefit. Thus for several years the South African government denied the cause of AIDS and succeeded in delaying provision of standard treatment to HIV-infected people. Under relentless pressure from the activist group Treatment Action Campaign, and a Constitutional Court judgement ordering the government to make drug treatment universally available to pregnant women infected with HIV, South Africa finally launched a program in 2003 to prevent mother-to-child transmission of HIV, and initiated a national antiretroviral program the following year. But, according to Dr Pride Chigwedere, a Zimbabwean doctor affiliated with Harvard University who investigated the consequences of the disastrous government policy in South Africa, this was too late to save the more than 330,000 people who died prematurely from HIV/AIDS between 2000 and 2005.[29] In addition, at least 35,000 babies were born with HIV infections that could have been prevented.

Writing retrospectively in the *New England Journal of Medicine* in 2011, Peter Piot, who helped discover HIV, wrote that without access to antiretroviral drugs in low and middle-income countries, there were 2.4 million deaths and more than 3 million new infections reported in 2001. Of these new infections, two-thirds occurred in sub-Saharan Africa. HIV had become hyperendemic, with an overall prevalence among adults of up to 31% in Swaziland, 25% in Botswana, and 17% in South Africa. In Swaziland, the prevalence among women between the ages of 30 and 34 was an astonishing 54%.[30]

The special risk of women

By the late 1990s it was clear that Africa had very different patterns of infection compared to America and western Europe where most patients were gay men. The overwhelming route of transmission was between men and women in heterosexual relationships. Women began to account for more cases than men, and peak infection rates occurred in young women, those aged 20–24. Eighty percent of all infected women in the world lived in Africa. HIV infection became the most common medical complication of pregnancy in Zimbabwe and other sub-Saharan countries.[31] Maternal HIV sero-prevalence was monitored by means of anonymous sentinel surveillance testing and the numbers of mothers infected continued to rise, from 18% in 1990[32] to over 30% in urban referral hospitals in 1996.[33] Indeed, in one town on the Zimbabwe-South African border, HIV prevalence in pregnant women shot up from 32% in 1995 to 59% in 1996.[34]

More often than not, HIV entered a family through the woman's male sexual partner and it was understood by many that one of the biggest risk factors for HIV infection was to be a married woman. Women are more vulnerable to HIV-infection than men because biologically, a larger mucosal surface is exposed during sexual intercourse and semen carries a greater concentration of the virus than vaginal fluid.[35] Other factors include immaturity of the genital tract, sexually transmitted diseases[36] and certain sexual practices such as 'dry sex' (the use of intravaginal herbs, or other preparations, for alleged enhancement of sex), which can cause swelling or peeling of the vagina.[33,37,38] I attended a joint WHO/Health Action International workshop on the Rational Use of Drugs in 1989 at which one of the speakers graphically described how women would use chemical fertilisers inside the vagina with the aim of facilitating dry sex. Damaged tissue facilitated transmission of the virus.

African women, unlike women in other regions, were 1.2 times more likely to be infected with HIV than men. The ratio was even higher – 2.6 times as likely – among young women.[39] Cultural, economic and social influences meant that African girls tended to marry or have sex with older men who had had more sexual partners in the past. They may have had little or no choice about whether and with whom they had sex, whether or not condoms were used, or whether their partners were currently indulging in risky unprotected sexual activity with multiple other partners.[33,35] It was normal for both men and women to conduct several sexual relationships at the same time.[3] Younger women were more likely to have transactional sex with more financially well-off older 'sugar daddies', often in exchange for food, clothes, cell phones and other favours. In South Africa the practice of 'survival sex' helped to spread the virus: young women in the townships, often migrants from impoverished rural areas, used their bodies as an ordinary economic resource outside the context of prostitution.[28] A pattern started to develop: older men infecting young women, while young men remained HIV-negative until they got married. Then the married men would become infected by their young wives, and later infect new girlfriends. And so the cycle continued. Unfaithful men did not expect to use condoms, nor discuss sex, with their wives, and in fact in traditional African families talking about sex was taboo.

In those early years, there was an unwillingness to take an HIV test. If there was no treatment, only stigma, what was the point in knowing that you might have a lethal disease? If you didn't know, you could hope that you weren't infected. Seeming good health was taken as a marker of negative HIV status. A young dental nurse I chatted to while waiting for an appointment confessed to me her relief at the recent birth of a healthy baby boy, which she took to be evidence that she must be free of HIV.

When I left Zimbabwe in 2003, 32% of pregnant women in Harare were testing HIV-positive on anonymous sentinel surveillance testing; we had the highest HIV prevalence in the world. Carol Bellamy, Director of UNICEF from 1995 to 2005, aptly described the reality when she said 'AIDS has a woman's face'. It was terrifying to know that more than half the women in some of the little villages were going to die, leaving their children as orphans. We heard of grandmothers who were struggling to feed, clothe and send as many as 12 orphaned grandchildren to school.

Speaking at the International AIDS Conference in Toronto, which I attended in 2006, Stephen Lewis, Special UN Envoy, gave an impassioned speech about the impact of HIV on women and their children, and on so many orphaned children being cared for by their grandmothers:[40]

'The monumental numbers of orphans, so many of them now adults because the pandemic has gone on for so long, pose a bracing, almost insuperable challenge for the countries which they inhabit. I appeal to everyone to recognize that we're walking on the knife's edge of an unsolvable human catastrophe. Inevitably we're preoccupied with the here and now, but the cumulative impact of these orphan kids, their levels of trauma, their overwhelming personal needs, their intense collective vulnerability strikes at the heart of the human dynamic, creating a sociological rearrangement of human relationships. ...It is impossible to talk about orphans without talking about grandmothers. Who would ever have imagined it would come to this? In Africa, the grandmothers are the unsung heroes of the continent: these extraordinary, resilient, courageous women, fighting through the inconsolable grief of the loss of their own adult children, becoming parents again in their fifties and sixties and seventies and eighties. I attended a grandmothers' gathering last weekend on the eve of the conference: the grandmothers were magnificent, but they're all struggling with the same anguished nightmare: what happens to my grandchildren when I die?'

An unimaginable pandemic

The fight against AIDS has been aptly characterised as a war. Nobody could have imagined that within 30 years, this new disease would kill over 33 million people. Author Susan Hunter wrote in 2003 that if current trends continued, by 2010 HIV/AIDS would take as many lives as the First and Second World Wars, the Vietnam and Korean wars, the American Civil War, the Bolshevik Revolution, the first Chinese Communist War, the Spanish Civil War, the Taiping Rebellion, the Great War in La Plata and the Partition of India put together.[41]

Earlier in 2006, Stephen Lewis had spoken at the United Nations in New York[42] to say:

'Swaziland continues to have the highest prevalence rate in the world at 42.6%. In its recent antenatal survey of pregnant women between the ages of 25 and 29, the prevalence rate was 56.3%. That's the highest prevalence I have ever seen registered in any age group anywhere. The mind fractures at the thought of it... Lesotho is only now beginning to confront the numbers, and hardly knows where to begin. Swaziland is faced with the apparent inevitability that between ten and fifteen per cent of its entire population will consist of orphans by the year 2010. While I was in the country, I encountered a primary school of 350 students, 250 of whom were orphans... 70 per cent of the total. How in the world is the educational system expected to cope?... The legacy is an omnibus catalogue of women's vulnerability... the litany never ends. It is impossible to traverse the continent of Africa, it is impossible to visit countries like Lesotho and Swaziland, without an enveloping sense of horror and despair at the carnage amongst women. And in very large part, this carnage took root and has been allowed to rage because the voice of women is the voice that is still not heard. We're losing millions of young women in Africa...How will we ever explain what we have wrought? What a universe this is... It is my contention that years from now, historians will ask how it was possible that the world allowed AIDS to throttle and eviscerate a continent, and overwhelmingly the women of that continent, and watch the tragedy unfold, in real time, while we toyed with the game of reform.'

HIV infection is not distributed evenly, nor is it a generalised epidemic. At the end of 2019, 38 million people were living with HIV, an estimated 0.7% of adults aged 15–49 years worldwide. Social exclusion, discriminatory cultural practices, political upheaval, war and natural disasters all take their toll and demonstrate that marginalised members of society are always most at risk. Lest we should imagine that this is a disease which only affects citizens of developing countries, it is sobering to realise that in parts of New York city the burden of HIV disease is as high as some countries in sub-Saharan Africa, with African-American women and gay men being disproportionately affected, while the impact on white middle-class heterosexuals who don't inject drugs is minimal. Similar patterns exist in Europe. In eastern Europe it is the young urban men in their twenties who inject drugs, whose opportunities are already extremely limited due to the upheaval their societies have experienced since 1991, who carry an enormous burden of the area's HIV epidemic and an intolerable risk for infection.

In Africa nearly 1 in 25 of all adults (3.7%) have HIV, accounting for more than two-thirds of those infected worldwide.[43] The rapidly spreading virus affects men and women in heterosexual relationships. Not all of them live in poverty, though being poor places them at special risk. The most vulnerable are young women. This has terrifying implications. Unlike other groups, when women are infected the virus can be passed on down the generations. No wonder then, that the international community took mother-to-child transmission of HIV so seriously.

CHAPTER 4

Routes of infection of babies, mothers, fathers and others

The alarming news came at the end of 1982 that four babies, one black-Spanish, two Haitian and one white, seemed to have been infected with the 'AIDS agent'. The CDC reported that infants in New York, New Jersey and California had suffered unexplained immunodeficiency and opportunistic infections such as those previously believed to infect only gay men.[1] The children had presented with conditions such as oral thrush, enlarged liver, skin infections and chronic pneumonia. Their mothers were described as Haitian, prostitutes or intravenous drug abusers – groups at increased risk for AIDS – although not all had shown symptoms. Transmission of the infection from mother to child, either *in utero* or shortly after birth, might have caused the early onset of immunodeficiency in these infants.

First report of HIV through breastfeeding, April 1985

Just over two years later, the news that the lactation community had been dreading arrived through an impeccable source. In April 1985 the *Lancet* carried a report of maternal infection with subsequent vertical HIV transmission to a breastfed baby.[2] A 34-year-old Australian mother giving birth to her third child through caesarean section suffered a haemorrhage. Following a 1,200ml blood loss, she received a transfusion of two units of whole blood. She started breastfeeding on the day of her baby's birth and continued for six weeks. From three months onwards, the baby suffered from eczema and inadequate weight gain and the mother had enlarged lymph glands. While both mother and baby subsequently tested positive for HIV, the baby's father and two siblings were not infected. On investigation it was found that the second unit of blood received by the mother had been donated by a homosexual man who, although healthy at the time, developed AIDS-related illnesses 13 months later. The mother could only have been infected by the contaminated blood transfusion. Since she was transfused after the birth, the baby could only have acquired the virus through breastfeeding.[3]

Five months later, Belgian researchers isolated the HTLV-III virus from five breastmilk samples taken from three mothers. All had connections to either Rwanda or the Congo, and had breastfed babies ranging in age from 1– 5½ months.[4] In 1988 the virus was reported to have been detected in breastmilk by electron microscope, which further supported the hypothesis that breastmilk could carry the virus.[5,6] The discovery that HIV could be transmitted through breastmilk was to have enormous repercussions, particularly in areas of the world where large numbers of women were becoming infected, and where breastfeeding, being a cornerstone of child survival, was almost universal.

There is considerable overlap in the risk of infection *in utero*, during birth or postnatally during breastfeeding. This makes it difficult to pinpoint exactly when transmission happens. Did the infant acquire the infection during early or late pregnancy, during birth, during early breastfeeding, or during 'extended' breastfeeding after six months? Or did the baby become infected by contaminated equipment such as unsterilised needles used during hospital procedures or immunisations? Does it make a difference when the mother herself first became infected? Ascertaining the timing of transmission is difficult due to inherent problems in HIV testing techniques, and these will be explored below.

But there are other problems. Members of a group of researchers in Nairobi, Kenya, describe why distinguishing the route of transmission of HIV to the baby is so difficult.[7] The majority of transmission events are believed to occur across infant mucosal surfaces, such as the gastrointestinal tract and nasopharyngeal surfaces. These mucosal barriers are in contact with HIV-infected maternal fluids throughout gestation, delivery and the breastfeeding period, providing ample time and opportunity for transmission to occur. For systemic infection to take place, maternal HIV must infect susceptible cells within or underneath the epithelial barrier and then traffic to underlying layers to disseminate the virus to lymphatic and blood vessels. But in the majority of cases, the polarised epithelial barrier that overlies mucosal surfaces contributes to the infant's protection so that most babies do not become infected.

Infection during pregnancy (*in utero* transmission)

Research on HIV transmission from mothers to infants is bedevilled by conflicting findings. *In utero* transmission is generally accepted as the least common route of mother-to-child transmission (MTCT), but not all research confirms this. A baby testing HIV-positive at birth is deemed to have been infected *in utero* via the placenta. While HIV has been detected in foetuses as early as eight weeks, the majority of transmission occurs during the third trimester and only 5%–10% of infants born to HIV-infected mothers become infected via this route.[7,8,9] Cells that provide nutrients to the embryo form a polarised epithelial barrier between maternal and foetal blood supplies. A number of early in vitro studies suggested that cell-free HIV can infect these cells. Later research shows that while cell-associated virus can cross the placenta and cause productive infection in target cells, cell-free virus cannot. Animal models show cell-free HIV transmission through amniotic fluid; direct injection of simian immunodeficiency virus (SIV) into the amniotic fluid of pregnant macaque monkeys resulted in infant infection in two different studies. However, research in humans is limited and conflicting; if HIV is present in amniotic fluid, it is likely rare or present at low levels. Given the difficulty of sampling viral reservoirs and infected tissues during pregnancy, as well as the challenge of accurately estimating the time of infection in the foetus, the roles of cell-associated and cell-free virus during pregnancy are still largely undefined. Whether cell-associated or cell-free virus occurs through breastfeeding is also unclear, and this question will be explored further in Chapter 25.

During birth, genital secretions also pose a risk of transmission to the unborn baby.[10,11] A 1997 paper from Nairobi, Kenya, showed that 32% of infected women shed virus from the cervix during the last trimester[12] and that simultaneous shedding from multiple sites may be due to a high total virus burden. Zimbabwean research from 1998, looking at the route of transmission in babies who had died within two years of birth, found that 70% had acquired HIV *in utero*, 19% were infected at delivery and only 11% were considered to have been infected postnatally, i.e. showed their first positive result at the 10-week test.[13]

Then research published in 2010 showed that when women received antiretroviral therapy (ART) during pregnancy, their babies were much less likely to become infected.[14] Women who became pregnant after they were already receiving highly active antiretroviral therapy (HAART) had an eight-fold reduced risk (0.7% vs 5.7%) of their baby being born infected; the longer they received the drugs the lower the risk: 9.3% with less than four weeks of HAART, 5.5% with 4–16 weeks of HAART, and 3.5% with 16 to 32 weeks. Especially importantly, there were no transmissions among women who were on HAART for more than 32 weeks before they gave birth.

Birth (intra-partum transmission)

We've known since 1983 that HIV can be transmitted during pregnancy *and* birth.[15] The older studies in untreated non-breastfeeding mothers whose babies were infected attributed risk as 30% *in utero* and 70% during labour and delivery.[16] In fact the risk is as great during the 24 hours surrounding birth as it is during 24 months of breastfeeding.

Transmission during pregnancy, or labour and delivery, can occur if a breach in the maternal-infant blood barrier, a placental microtransfusion, occurs.[7] The exact cause is unknown, but may be due to contractions during the early stages of labour when membranes rupture, resulting in the exchange of small amounts of maternal and foetal blood.[17,18] One researcher concludes that the majority of infant infection occurs close to the time of delivery due to the presence of viral shedding in the birth canal.[19] Cervical shedding, correlated with viral load, occurs in more than 30% of infected women and vaginal shedding in 10–17%.[20] During labour and delivery, the infant is exposed to and swallows cervical and vaginal fluids infected with HIV. HIV has been isolated from gastric/oropharyngeal aspirates. Neonatal skin and mucous membranes are not effective barriers against infective organisms. Direct invasion of the skin, eyes, oral and gastric mucosa during labour allows the virus to gain access to the bloodstream.[21]

Vaginal delivery, artificial rupture of membranes, especially if longer than four hours before birth, episiotomy,[22] duration of labour >12 hours, and especially emergency caesarean section following a difficult labour, all increase the risk. Sexually transmitted diseases assist both horizontal and vertical transmission.[12,23]

A new maternal infection during the pregnancy greatly increases the risk of MTCT, so that if mothers test HIV-negative during early pregnancy, the recommendation is for repeat testing nearer the time of delivery.[24]

The twin phenomenon

Twins provide a special insight into the random nature of infant infection with HIV. Research on MTCT nearly always excludes twin babies. Intriguingly, in multiple pregnancies, the first-born baby is 2–7 times more likely to be infected[25-28] even when both are breastfed or both babies have received antiretroviral therapy. This lends support to the hypothesis that it is passage through the birth canal which poses the greatest risk of infection, rather than breastfeeding. A Ugandan study comparing different methods of antiretroviral therapy to reduce transmission during birth in babies breastfed for a median of nine months included 13 sets of twins (four sets receiving zidovudine, eight nevirapine, one placebo). Siblings had concordant infection results, except for three sets of twins, in all of whom the first-born (one from each group) was infected and the second-born was not.[29]

An analysis of 115 HIV-exposed twin pairs prospectively studied to assess concordance, birth order, route of delivery and other factors for HIV infection showed that HIV transmission occurred in 35% of vaginally delivered first-born compared to only 15% of second-born twins, and in 16% of first-born vs only 8% of second-born twins born by caesarean section.[7] Three-quarters of the transmission risk was related to vaginal exposure, possibly due to having spent a longer time in the birth canal. Infected second-born twins had slightly more rapid progression to AIDS. It was concluded that HIV infection of second-born twins occurs predominantly *in utero*, whereas infection of first-born twins (and, by implication, singletons) occurs predominantly during labour and birth. The authors proposed that intrapartum transmission was responsible for the majority of paediatric HIV infections and that reducing exposure to HIV during birth could reduce MTCT.

Thus the twin phenomenon raised the possibility that there might be a role for caesarean delivery in the prevention of MTCT of HIV.[30] In 1998, women allocated to elective caesarean delivery had an 80% reduced rate of MTCT.[19]

These findings underpinned new US guidance to recommend that HIV-positive mothers be offered elective caesareans.[31] But there were concerns about the feasibility of providing caesarean sections for HIV-positive women in resource-limited settings with variable degrees of medical infrastructure.[32] Emergency caesareans performed after the onset of uterine contractions also carried a greater risk. Later, for women in resource-rich countries who had a low viral load as a result of treatment with HAART, recommendations for vaginal delivery were once again instituted.

Postnatal transmission, through breastfeeding

Several studies published between 1991 and 1994 estimated the risk of HIV transmission through breastfeeding by comparing infection rates among formula-fed and ever breastfed infants. Using this approach, early reports showed that the risk attributable to breastfeeding ranged anywhere from 0–46%.[33] An early paper suggested that a high transmission rate in the first month of life might be explained by the large number of HIV-infected cells present in colostrum and early milk.[34] From 1995 onwards, new HIV detection technologies enabled closer scrutiny of the role of breastfeeding in mother-to-child transmission.

Between 1994 and 1997, Miotti and colleagues looked at the transmission rates according to the duration of breastfeeding for babies of untreated mothers in Blantyre, Malawi.[35] Infants who were found to be HIV-positive on viral testing at six weeks were excluded on the assumption of infection during pregnancy or birth. The remaining babies were exclusively breastfed for four months and then partially breastfed thereafter. The cumulative risk of infection for infants continuing to breastfeed was:

3.5% at the end of five months,
7.0% at the end of 11 months,
8.9% at the end of 17 months, and
10.3% at the end of 23 months.

The decline in the rate of new HIV infections over time during the first two years of life was considered to be statistically significant. The conclusion was that an uninfected infant, breastfed by an HIV-positive mother for 23 months, had at least a 10.3% risk of becoming infected.

Increased risk to the baby with primary infection of the mother

The earliest case reports documenting that breastfeeding could be a mode of HIV transmission involved mothers who were given blood transfusions shortly after birth. Their children were therefore exposed to HIV during their mothers' seroconversion phase, during which HIV viraemia and risk of infectivity is particularly high.[2]

Very little research on vertical transmission of HIV documented when the mothers' primary infection was acquired, but an early study conducted in Kigali, Rwanda, where researchers attempted to pinpoint the timing of infection by intensive follow-up, showed fairly conclusively that transmission by newly infected mothers shortly after birth was high. Rates ranged from 25%– 53% and seroconversion of the baby in each case occurred within three months of the mother's seroconversion. Transmission was attributed to the mother's high viral burden during primary infection.[36] During the first 30 days of acute infection, the ZVITAMBO project also found that breastmilk viral load peaked in the same range as plasma viral load. New infections placed both mother and baby at severe risk.[37]

When talking about early estimates of MTCT through breastfeeding, three studies are most often cited, even today, as evidence for the risks of breastfeeding with HIV:

- A 1992 meta-analysis by Dr David Dunn and colleagues: of 42 women with new infections and 1,772 women with established infection; the additional risk of transmission from breastmilk was approximately 14% in cases of established infection, and 29% in newly infected women. However, breastfeeding duration was very short;

the majority of the women had breastfed for only 2–4 weeks, too short a time to differentiate transmission occurring *in utero* or during birth from transmission occurring due to breastfeeding (see the window period of testing techniques, outlined in the next chapter). Only 6% of mothers breastfed longer than six months.[38–40] According to another group involved in research on HIV and breastfeeding, the Dunn meta-analysis was methodologically flawed.[41] Definitions of 'breastfeeding' were problematic. Out of the 1,772 breastfed babies, only 28 had been exclusively breastfed. Breastfeeding lasted nearly 10 months in one study, but in others only seven weeks, four weeks or two weeks, and no measure of breastfeeding duration at all was given for another. In fact, most babies were breastfed for less than the 90 days required at that time to distinguish postnatal from *in utero* transmission.[42]

- The Nduati trial: between 1992 and 1998, Dr Ruth Nduati in Nairobi, Kenya, randomised babies of untreated HIV-positive mothers to either breastfeeding or formula-feeding.[43] She found that the risk of HIV transmission through breastfeeding, over and above that occurring *in utero* or during labour/delivery, was 16.2%, and that the majority of infections occurred early during breastfeeding. She concluded that the use of breastmilk substitutes prevented 44% of infant infections and was associated with significantly improved HIV-free survival. These results were startlingly unexpected and have thus been subjected to close scrutiny.
- The De Cock Review: this oft-cited paper, published in 2000 by the highly respected Dr Kevin De Cock,[44] who had worked for both the Centers for Disease Control in Nairobi, and for the World Health Organization, highlighted the stark contrast in the response of industrialised countries to the risk of MTCT of HIV compared to that of the developing countries. By 2000, an estimated 590,000 infants acquired HIV from their mothers each year, mostly in developing countries unable to implement interventions to reduce breastfeeding, now standard elsewhere, eroding hard-won gains in infant and child survival.[45] Reviewing five previous clinical trials, including both the Dunn meta-analysis and the Nduati randomised controlled trial, De Cock observed that the risk of MTCT of HIV through breastfeeding was substantial; near-universal breastfeeding was probably the most important reason for high HIV transmission rates in developing countries. In untreated mothers and babies the route, timing and risk of MTCT was estimated as follows:

Timing	**Risk**
During pregnancy	5–10%
During labour and delivery	10–15%
Overall without breastfeeding	15–25%
Overall with breastfeeding to six months	20–35%
Overall with breastfeeding to 18–24 months	30–45%

From these papers we learned that in the story of breastfeeding and HIV, definitions can be crucial. We know that the protective effects of breastfeeding against other infections are often seen as a dose response; the more breastmilk the infant receives, the higher the protection. Both the Dunn and Nduati papers illustrate the confusion that can occur when breastfeeding is loosely defined. Researchers who critiqued the Nairobi study[45] noted that 30% of the women in the formula-feeding arm also reported breastfeeding, and that possibly up to 60% of women randomised to breastfeeding were also giving formula. Cumulative mortality at six weeks and three months was higher in the formula-fed group compared with the breastfed group (3.9% vs 1.0% at six weeks and 6.4% vs 4.1% at three months). In the first six months increased rates of sickness and death were most obvious in the uninfected formula-fed infants. Mortality was 5% for formula-fed vs 0.8% for breastfed infants. No analysis was done to compare infection rates of mixed-fed with exclusively breastfed infants. More discussion of the importance of breastfeeding definitions is found in Chapter 9.

Louise Kuhn and Grace Aldrovandi, who conducted exhaustive research on HIV and breastfeeding in Zambia, looked back in 2012 at the Nduati research.[46] It seemed unclear to them why so few adverse outcomes of formula-feeding had been reported when no other study had been able to replicate such good outcomes. All studies in later years recording shifts away from breastfeeding, many of them considerably larger and some of them randomised and with at least equivalent methodological rigour, had reported at best no benefit and in fact worse HIV-free survival with formula-feeding. Kuhn and Aldrovandi speculated that maybe strict selection of study participants from unusually good socio-economic circumstances and extensive monitoring and support during the trial limited its generalisability. They also noted that due to public pressure, WHO policy had shifted towards support of formula-feeding and had disregarded the dangers of withholding breastfeeding due at least in part to the results of the Nairobi study (as will be further discussed in Chapter 12).

In spite of criticisms from highly respected researchers, the Nduati paper has been cited over 230 times. The Dunn, Nduati and De Cock papers are frequently offered in current guidance documents as incontrovertible evidence that breastfeeding transmits HIV, notwithstanding that the women in these studies did not receive antiretroviral therapy and that risk estimates when mothers *do* receive antiretroviral therapy are almost zero, as will be explored in Chapter 23.

In a 2004 document written for the World Health Organization,[47] summarising how often and by what route babies are infected with HIV, Ellen Piwoz wrote that transmission occurs during pregnancy, at the time of delivery, and after birth through breastfeeding, but that it is by no means universal. In the absence of interventions to prevent transmission, only 5 to 20% of babies are infected through breastfeeding.[44] Several conditions are known to increase the breastfeeding-associated risk. These include the mother's immune status[48,49] and blood viral load,[50,51] the duration of breastfeeding,[52] the presence of bleeding nipples,[49,53] breast inflammation, mastitis, abscesses,[49,51,53,54] and oral thrush in infants.[53] Mixed feeding may also increase the risk of HIV transmission.[55,56] Women who become infected with HIV while they are breastfeeding are also more likely to infect their infants because of the higher viral load that occurs at this time.[38]

In 2002, presenting an extremely thorough update to delegates attending the WABA-UNICEF HIV Colloquium in Arusha, Tanzania, Ellen Piwoz had attributed the risk of MTCT through the different routes as follows:[57]

Pregnancy	7%
Delivery	15%
Breastfeeding	15%
Uninfected	63%

In 2005, Ellen Piwoz and Jay Ross further generalised their figures.[58] In the absence of interventions to prevent transmission, such as antiretroviral therapy, their generalised risk estimates were as follows:

During pregnancy	5 to 10%
During delivery	10 to 20%
During breastfeeding	10 to 20%

When researchers and experts are writing about the risk of vertical transmission, they often round off or average out the figures. Since there was a correlation in both the Dunn and the Nduati figures at 15–16% risk during breastfeeding, and De Cock's important review lent further credibility to this estimate, this figure was more or less agreed by researchers and policymakers. Based on these estimates, it can be seen that even if *no interventions are made* to reduce MTCT, a full 85% of HIV-exposed babies would *not* be infected through breastfeeding.

We've come a long way since the end of the 20th century when the only strategy to avoid postnatal transmission of HIV was avoiding breastfeeding. Yet the old estimates, using poor breastfeeding definitions, are still being cited by some organisations as if this is up-to-date information. It's not. It's crucial that present-day mothers have accurate information about the risk factors for MTCT through breastfeeding and how to avoid them.

Importantly, as will be explored in future chapters, mothers also need to know that when exclusive breastfeeding is supported in the early months, in the same way that it should be for all babies outside the context of HIV, the risk of HIV transmission could be reduced by two-thirds and mortality from all other causes could be reduced by more than half even for mothers who cannot access antiretroviral treatment.[59] For those who can obtain highly active antiretroviral treatment (HAART) it has been a game-changer (see Chapter 23). When HIV-positive mothers receive and are adherent to their medications, when they have been taking ART for long enough to achieve an undetectable viral load, in accordance with current guidance in place since 2010, and when they combine ART with exclusive breastfeeding (EBF), the risk of HIV transmission by any route, including through breastfeeding, is vanishingly small. The answer is ART+EBF. To withhold this information from mothers, or to mislead them about it, is unethical.

Child to mother transmission

Low on everyone's radar is the possibility of a baby infecting a mother with HIV through breastfeeding. Although rare, it can happen and this question really should be considered in any situation involving wet-nursing, cross-nursing or lactation for an adopted baby.

In 1990 a Russian medical journal reported that a nosocomial (hospital acquired) infection of HIV had occurred in Elista, the capital of the Kalmykia Republic, 1,250km south-east of Moscow.[60] The infection was traced to a man who had brought it home from a trip abroad and then infected his wife and subsequently their baby. The newborn had been admitted to Elista Hospital, from where she was transferred to the regional centre. In the course of investigating the epidemic, 83,000 Elista inhabitants underwent planned examination, and 65 cases of HIV infection (in 56 children and nine adults) were detected. All were traced to individuals who had been admitted to either of the two hospitals in Elista, where they had received intravenous or intramuscular injections using multi-dose syringes. The infection spread from the infant department of the regional paediatric hospital to four more departments and to the infectious diseases hospital. Transmission was maintained for several months by the use of nonsterile syringes. But the seven women who became infected contracted the infection from their infected children in the process of breastfeeding.

A further mishap occurred in Libya. In one of the darker moments of the country's recent history, in 1998, 402 children at the Benghazi Children's Hospital were found to be infected with HIV.[61] Italian medical investigators found that although the infected children had not received any blood or blood products, they had been treated with intravenous fluids, antibiotics, steroids or bronchodilators. Five Bulgarian nurses and a Palestinian doctor were accused of deliberately infecting the children and were sentenced to death. They were subsequently released in 2007 in exchange for a debt-forgiveness package. Researchers presenting at the International AIDS Conference which I attended in Toronto in 2006 had already described how the Libyan children had been infected with a monophyletic strain of HIV (CRF2-AG).[62] The mothers of 20 infected babies were infected through breastfeeding. To exclude the possibility of sexually transmitted infection of the mothers by the fathers, all fathers had been tested and their results had come back negative. The association between the mothers' serostatus and breastfeeding during hospitalisation led to the conclusion that HIV can be acquired by breastfeeding an infected child.

In 2012, Kirsten Little and colleagues published the most comprehensive review to date of child-to-mother transmission of HIV.[63] They identified five studies beginning with the 1988 cases in paediatric Soviet hospitals following nosocomial HIV outbreaks. A total of 152 children and 12 mothers (8%) were found to be HIV-infected. An epidemiologic investigation established that none of the women's sexual partners were infected, but all had breastfed their infants after the earliest dates of possible infection. Transmission rates were high, ranging from 40% to 60%. An additional study also reported that another 11 of 18 (61%) of women who breastfed their children after their child's admittance to another hospital tested positive for HIV. Similar cases of hospital-acquired infections of babies and subsequent transmission to breastfeeding mothers in Kazakhstan and Kyrgyzstan were documented between 2006 and 2007. Poor infection control practices, especially in areas of high HIV prevalence, had led to infection in the babies, and had put breastfeeding women at risk.

Little and colleagues also outline the risk of child-to-wet-nurse transmission when orphaned babies are breastfed. Acceptability for the practice of wet-nursing ranged from less than 37% in Côte d'Ivoire to 74% in Burkina Faso and was highest where women felt that an orphaned baby would ideally be wet-nursed by a female relative.

Mothers may also cross-nurse infants other than their own. Cross-feeding typically occurs on a more informal basis, although research on the topic is limited[64] and there is variable acceptability by country. A survey done in Gabon found that 40% of respondents breastfed up to four additional infants other than their own, and that 40% of the infants in the study had been breastfed by as many as three women in addition to their biological mothers.[65] In contrast, a South African study found that only 3.5% of women reported breastfeeding a non-biological child.[66,67] Cross-nursing may involve multiple infants and women over long periods of time. Even when knowledge of HIV transmission through breastmilk from mother to child is high, women may not take on board their own risk of HIV acquisition from an infected infant. In cross-nursing situations, the direction of causation may be difficult to determine, although HIV could potentially be passed from one infected individual to multiple infants and mothers.

Current infant feeding guidelines and HIV prevention messages do not address child-to-mother transmission. The World Health Organization guidelines in 2003 had suggested the use of a wet-nurse for HIV-infected mothers who chose not to breastfeed their infants.[68] In fact emergency preparedness guidance continues to suggest wet-nursing as a feeding option for babies in refugee camps if formula is unavailable.[69] When women are considering adoption or wet-nursing, we need to be aware that unfortunately HIV can be transmitted from an HIV-infected infant via breastfeeding.

In African countries, where grandmothers typically bear the responsibility for childcare if a mother is ill or absent, non-puerperal-induced lactation is sometimes practised. Induced lactation may be undertaken through nipple stimulation, such as infant suckling. This means that grandmothers and other older female relatives may place themselves at risk for HIV infection if they breastfeed HIV-infected orphans. This is especially worrying where a grandmother is caring for many orphaned grandchildren.

The lack of recognition of breastfeeding as a risk factor for HIV transmission to women contemplating breastfeeding an adopted baby, or wet-nursing in either social or emergency situations, mirrors the attitudes and beliefs I've encountered while working with breastfeeding women and/or supporting my colleagues in the lactation community.

When generous women with kind hearts see breastfeeding as a way to care for a vulnerable and needy baby, the risk of HIV transmission is frequently overlooked. The risk needs to be gently raised with women who might be considering inducing lactation for an adopted baby, or breastfeeding the baby of a refugee, sister, cousin or friend in the mother's absence, to help out. Questions need to be asked about whether the birth mother has been tested for HIV and, if she was HIV-infected, has the infant been tested, and has the infant received prophylactic antiretroviral therapy?[70] Some ask if creating a barrier between the wet-nurse and the baby would prevent infection. But a nipple shield is unlikely to be a sufficient barrier to ensure that saliva from the baby's mouth is not absorbed up into the breast at the end of nursing, a physiological mechanism that 'innoculates' the breast tissue to produce antibodies to various infections suffered by the baby, and to pass them back in the milk.[71]

In any scenario where a woman contemplates nursing a baby not her own, everyone needs to acknowledge that the risk extends not only to the lactating woman, but also to her other breastfed baby or babies and her sexual partner, and indeed her other non-nursing older children who also depend on her continued good health for their care. The possible risk of child-to-mother transmission may be as high as 40–60% if a baby is newly infected. It's an unpalatable fact that such women will be potentially virally connected not just to the baby, but to the baby's mother and her sexual partner, and all their sexual partners.

The possibility of group or shared wet-nursing may be raised in emergency situations, but the risk of cross-infection will increase incrementally depending on how many people are involved. For the new baby's safety, each wet-nurse would need to have her HIV-status checked beforehand and at periodic intervals and be able to guarantee that neither she nor her sexual partner were placing themselves at risk for a new HIV infection. The risk to the wet-nurse is undiagnosed and untreated HIV infection. If there is one breach in this linked group, then, in theory, every wet-nurse, every baby, and every sexual partner might be at risk.

Nevertheless, breastmilk would be of huge value to an orphaned or adopted baby, and especially if that baby is infected with HIV. Would an adoptive mother, or a donor in a refugee camp, consider expressing milk for a baby in need? In cases of uncertainty, a baby could be fed donor breastmilk by another method, perhaps by bottle or by cup, pending testing to show that the baby has definitely escaped infection. If the tests come back negative, then the baby could be transitioned to the breast and then breastfeed directly. If the tests return positive, then breastmilk-feeding by bottle for as long as possible (i.e. exclusively for six months and partially for several years) would be of immense value to a baby with a compromised immune system.

Father-to-child transmission

It seems that the virus still has the means to surprise us. In a recently reported case of father-to-child transmission the four-year-old son of an HIV-negative mother in Portugal was found to have been infected as a newborn by contact with his newly infected father's chickenpox blisters. Transmission was likely accidental and occurred during the seroconversion period when the father was unaware of the infection.[72,73] Based on comparative analysis of genetic, phylogenetic, and serologic data from father and son, researchers concluded that the virus was accidentally transmitted to the baby during the first days of his life. During the time of seroconversion, the father was being treated for infection with syphillis and *varicella zoster* virus (chickenpox) when he developed large vesicles all over his body that profusely leaked fluids. The high virus production early in HIV infection would have made the fluids leaking from the father's skin blisters highly infectious. These infectious fluids could have come into contact with the newborn child, causing this atypical HIV transmission event. The editorial accompanying the report warned that although this type of infection is rare, it is important that the general public realise that HIV is present in most bodily fluids and can be transmitted in atypical and unexpected ways. In this case, the circumstances of fluids leaking from skin blisters with the high amount of HIV present in the first months of HIV infection led to the unfortunate infection of a newborn child.

Transmission through saliva during pre-mastication of food

In February 2008, the US Centers for Disease Control and Prevention (CDC) reported that between 1993 and 2004 it had identified three cases of paediatric HIV transmission through the mechanism of pre-chewing a child's food.[74] In 1993 a 15-month-old boy whose mother was not infected was fed pre-masticated food by his HIV-positive great-aunt. The boy's mother did not know that the aunt had been infected with HIV until after she died of AIDS. The boy is still alive and receiving ART. In 1995 a three-year-old boy had been fed pre-chewed food by his infected mother and had died a year later. In 2004, a nine-month-old girl was diagnosed with HIV after her HIV-positive mother reported giving her pre-chewed food. This child is also still alive. There had been a thorough investigation to rule out alternative modes of transmission conducted by primary care staff and Health Department investigators. Blood samples from the cases and suspected sources were sent to the CDC for HIV DNA extraction, amplification, sequencing, and genetic and phylogenetic analysis. The latter showed strong relatedness of the virus from the infant and mother in two of the cases and ruled out a household contact, the aunt's partner, as a source of infection of the aunt, although she had died before her blood could be collected. Perinatal and breastfeeding-associated infection having been ruled out, the evidence was compelling that pre-mastication of foods had been the route of transmission of the virus. The conclusion was that this route of infection has important global implications, and deserves further investigation.[75,76]

Publication of these findings generated some consternation among international nutritionists, doctors and epidemiologists working in the field of child malnurition. Some said that pre-mastication generates a second potentially major channel for postnatal HIV transmission. Others urged against a knee-jerk reaction to prohibit the practice, asserting that pre-mastication and tasting and testing of young children's foods by caregivers happens in the West too, although it isn't talked about because of the more common use of commercially manufactured weaning foods.[77] Improving the identification of women who are HIV-positive so that they can be provided with antiretroviral medications was the most important need, for their own treatment as well as to reduce the viral load in their saliva. Others asked how much paediatric HIV – currently attributed to breastfeeding – might have been due to pre-mastication? Perhaps breastfeeding would prove to be safer than was previously thought?

Experts from Cornell University responded by letter in the *Journal of Pediatrics*,[78] asserting that pre-mastication had been a prerequisite for human evolution and survival in the past, and is currently a crucial global behavioural adaptation enabling nutritional adequacy for young children when milk alone is no longer adequate, yet children do not yet have sufficient dentition to consume the family diet. They said that saliva transmits HIV very poorly unless there is a portal of entry, such as a sore in the mouth of the infant.

In March 2011, the CDC reported that from December 2009 to February 2010 it had conducted a cross-sectional survey at nine paediatric clinics in the US to assess the prevalence of pre-mastication among caregivers of both HIV-positive and HIV-perinatally-exposed infants.[79] Thirty-one per cent of children had been fed pre-masticated foods. The CDC recommended that public health officials and healthcare providers educate the public about the risk for disease transmission via pre-mastication and advise HIV-infected caregivers against the practice.

These concerns were partly endorsed by researchers in Cape Town, South Africa, who published their findings on pre-mastication of food in the August 2011 issue of *Pediatrics*. They interviewed 154 caregivers (92% biological mothers) about pre-mastication.[80] Nearly half of the babies were teething, and the other half had mouth sores. Just over half of the caregivers also reported oral conditions, e.g. bleeding gums, mouth sores and thrush, and 40% reported seeing blood in the food they chewed. Reasons given for chewing the babies' food were to pre-taste, encourage eating, estimate the food temperature and homogenise the food. A press report on this study in the *Swazi Observer*[81] said that more than two-thirds of mothers and other caregivers in the southern Africa region pre-chew food for their infants. They were not aware of any risk involved. The study authors noted that 'Due to its long history and cultural acceptance, pre-mastication (the pre-chewing of food that is then consumed by another person) seems to be considered so harmless and natural by caregivers that they tend not to mention it during health interviews, or suspect there could be something wrong with this feeding method.' It was believed that pre-chewed food might be a good source of nutrition for infants whose families do not have access to processed baby food or in places of poverty where malnutrition is common.

In a case reported in 2013 from Chile, where paediatric HIV is rare, a single finding of infection in a child was thoroughly investigated.[82] Late transmission was traced to pre-masticated food.

Whether there was a danger of HIV transmission through the saliva was tested in court the following year.[83] A court in Albany, New York, determined that an HIV-positive man who had admitted to biting a police officer attempting to arrest him could not be found guilty of aggravated assault. In a previous hearing the court had ruled that while teeth could not be considered a deadly weapon, saliva could. In throwing out the previous conviction, the court ruled that body parts, saliva or anything that 'comes with' a person cannot be considered deadly weapons under state law. However, the court declined to determine whether HIV could be spread through biting. A number of studies have found that saliva does not contain sufficient concentrations of HIV to transmit the virus to other people. According to the CDC, 'contact with saliva alone has never been shown to result in transmission of HIV'. Gay rights activists characterised the ruling as an important step forward for HIV-positive people, decriminalising the disease itself.

HIV-infected cells have been identified in salivary glands and HIV RNA has been detected in saliva. A 2010 study found that most patients with plasma virus >50 copies/ml had detectable saliva HIV RNA, and the data was highly concordant between saliva and plasma. In fact researchers concluded that in patients with high levels of plasma HIV RNA, saliva might be useful in identifying viraemia and evaluating drug resistance.[84,85]

In fascinating research to investigate whether HIV can be transmitted via saliva and can infect an infant's oral mucosa, Grace Wahl and colleagues from the University of North Carolina, Chapel Hill, in the US, conducted exhaustive tests on BLT (bone marrow, liver, thymic) mice. [86] These 'humanised' mice are created by implanting mice with a piece of human foetal liver sandwiched between two small pieces of human foetal thymus to effectively develop a human immune system with dramatically high human T-cell and other cell counts in virtually all of their tissues.

Wahl and colleagues established that reconstitution of the oral cavity and upper gastrointestinal (GI) tract of their BLT mice with human leukocytes, including the human cell types important for mucosal HIV transmission (i.e. dendritic cells, macrophages and CD4+ T-cells), renders them susceptible to oral transmission of cell-free and cell-associated HIV. Once infection was confirmed in the plasma of the mice, they also determined the presence of viral RNA in the saliva of four out of five infected BLT mice examined. Consistent with the previous research in humans,[84,85] the viral load in the saliva of each BLT mouse was lower than the viral load in plasma. The presence of viral RNA in the saliva of BLT mice was consistent with the productive infection of human cells within the oral mucosa and/or salivary glands. Taken together, these findings demonstrated that BLT humanised mice were susceptible to oral HIV transmission that results in systemic infection, as demonstrated by the presence of HIV RNA in plasma and saliva. Thus saliva appears to be a viable route of transmission after all.

CHAPTER 5

HIV testing and monitoring the stage of disease

In 1983, doctors at the Albert Einstein College of Medicine in the Bronx, New York, first described a new syndrome of acquired immunodeficiency in seven children whose mothers they had labelled as sexually promiscuous and/or drug-addicted.[1]

The question of whether a baby has become HIV infected, and if so, by which route – whether during pregnancy, birth or early breastfeeding – has been complicated by the inadequacy of the testing and monitoring techniques used over the years. Early on it was observed that 'unanswered questions exist because of limitations in HIV test technology, which make it impossible to determine the precise timing or mode of transmission to newborns at the time of delivery and during the first two months of life, and because of other issues related to the design, analysis, and interpretation of studies on this issue.'[2] Nearly 25 years later, many of these constraints persist.

To add an extra layer of complexity to an already confusing situation, maternal antibodies persist in an HIV-exposed baby's blood for 18–24 months. An antibody test before this time will always show positive, although the baby may not actually be infected. Nevertheless, in order to definitively conclude that a baby has escaped infection, clinicians will hold out for a negative antibody test at 18–24 months before giving the all-clear.

Establishing HIV-infection in adults

Compounding the many difficulties in untangling the uncertainties surrounding mother-to-child transmission of HIV is the fact that two individuals are involved, a mother and a baby, and different tests with different characteristics and limitations are used on each member of the dyad.

After infection with the HIV virus, which multiplies rapidly, a mother's immune system will respond by producing antibodies. This is known as seroconversion.[3] Antibodies continue to increase in the months after infection. Six to 12 weeks after primary infection a woman will experience a rapid rise in virus in all body fluids lasting for several weeks, i.e. in blood, plasma, genital secretions and, if she is lactating, in breastmilk. After initial infection an immunologic response ensues resulting in a reduction of systemic virus to a steady set point lasting 7–10 years before the onset of symptomatic AIDS. Higher levels of systemic plasma viral load, occurring immediately after infection and during the late stages of AIDS, increase the risk of transmitting HIV to her baby either before, during or after birth through breastfeeding.

Various tests and ways of monitoring the course of an individual's disease have been developed:

ELISA

The enzyme-linked immunosorbent assay (ELISA) was the first screening test commonly employed for HIV. It has a high sensitivity (meaning it can correctly identify a high percentage of people who have the condition). In an ELISA test, if antibodies to HIV are present in diluted serum they bind to the HIV antigens. ELISA results are reported as a number, and the most controversial aspect of this test is determining the cut-off point between a positive and negative result. There is a window period between exposure and before seroconversion (when infection takes place), during which antibodies (markers of infection) are still absent or too scarce to be detectable on a test. The window period for antibody tests is three weeks to three months. Up to 95% of people will have antibodies after six weeks, and 99% of people will have antibodies after three months.

Indirect fluorescent antibody (IFA)

This test detects HIV antibodies using a special fluorescent dye and a microscope. This test may be used to confirm the results of an ELISA test.[4]

P24 antigen

One distinctive HIV antigen is a viral protein called p24, a structural protein that makes up most of the HIV viral core. High levels of p24 are present in the blood serum of newly infected individuals during the short period between infection and seroconversion, making p24 antigen assays useful in diagnosing primary HIV infection.[5] Antibodies to p24 antigen are produced during seroconversion, rendering p24 antigen undetectable after seroconversion in most cases. Therefore, these assays are not reliable for diagnosing HIV infection after its very earliest stages. However, HIV infection can be more reliably diagnosed earlier with combined antibody/antigen tests than with purely antibody-detecting tests, and fourth-generation antibody/antigen tests are now the standard screening assay in the UK and some other countries.

Fourth-generation, antigen-antibody combination tests

These are good screening tests because they can detect both the p24 antigen and anti-HIV antibodies.[6] By 20 days after infection most people have detectable levels of p24 antigen, which is generally earlier than antibodies can be detected. However, levels of p24 antigen in the blood begin to decrease 3–4 weeks after infection and *are no longer detectable* after 5–6 weeks. This is why HIV tests were designed to also detect anti-HIV antibodies, as antibodies are usually present for the entire course of HIV infection. These tests can detect HIV infection in 50% of people by 18 days after infection (range 13–24 days); 95% of people by 34 days after infection; and 99% of people by one and a half months after infection. They are recommended in the UK and the US. Some countries recommend retesting 90 days after a possible exposure to HIV.

NAAT (nucleic acid amplification test)

This test looks for the genetic HIV material in the blood. It is also known as the 'early HIV test' or 'RNA test'. Ninety percent of NAATs are positive 10 to 12 days after a person acquires HIV, and over 99% are positive after six weeks. The RNA NAAT can be specially ordered by doctors or nurses if someone has had a recent high-risk exposure to HIV and/or they are having symptoms that are highly indicative of HIV. WHO strongly recommends the use of this testing technique when possible for babies.

Polymerase chain reaction (PCR)

This test finds either the RNA of the HIV virus or the HIV DNA in infected white blood cells. PCR testing is not done as frequently as antibody testing, because it requires technical skill and expensive equipment. Genetic material may be found even if other tests are negative for the virus. The PCR test is very useful to find a very recent infection, to determine if an HIV infection is present when antibody test results are uncertain, and to screen blood or organs for HIV before donation.[4] PCR has the shortest window period and can be used to detect very early infections before antibodies have developed, just days or weeks after exposure to HIV. But because it's less accurate, PCR testing is not recommended for testing of adults except in specific circumstances. Viral load is usually very high within the first four weeks after infection. However, some people have undetectable viral load even without treatment, so a negative result does not guarantee that an individual is not infected.

Rapid tests

These are usually reliable for long-standing infections, but are sometimes unable to detect recent HIV infections acquired in the past few weeks.[7]

Third-generation tests

A few third-generation rapid point-of-care tests are available. They are described this way because the test can be done and the result can be obtained in a doctor's office without specialised lab equipment. The estimated window period for these is 26 days (range 22–31 days) and 99% of infected individuals would be detectable within 50 days of exposure. These tests do not detect p24 viral antigen.

Second-generation tests

Many rapid, point-of-care tests are described as second-generation, in that they can detect IgG antibodies, but not IgM antibodies of p24 viral antigen. As these two substances are detectable sooner after HIV infection than IgG antibodies, second-generation tests have longer window periods. Half of all infections can be detected within 26–37 days, with a median of 31 days, and 99% of HIV-positive individuals would be detectable within 57 days of exposure.

Self-test kits

These are modified versions of rapid point-of-care test kits originally designed for healthcare professionals. Most are based on second-generation testing and are likely to have relatively long window periods.

Most positive tests in the West are repeated to confirm the result due to the window period – the time between acquiring HIV and the time that the test will show positive. Understanding the window periods for HIV testing is important because it helps in obtaining the most accurate results.

Newer methods of testing are more efficient and accurate than those employed in the past, but when looking at vertical transmission of HIV, particularly postpartum transmission through breastfeeding, the window periods in testing techniques have proved to be problematic, and there is still a way to go.

It's hard to say exactly how long the window period lasts, as there are variations between individuals and it's a difficult topic to research. To be accurate, recently infected people would need to know exactly when they were exposed to HIV and then give multiple blood samples over the following days and weeks. A study conducted to determine the window period of various tests, reported at the 2018 Conference for Retroviruses and Opportunistic Infections, looked at the infection date based on changes in viral load, reported symptoms of acute HIV infection, and HIV risk history, and described, based on plasma samples, the distribution of time from infection to first detection with each test and specimen type combination.[8] Dates of infection ranged from 21 to 60 days before enrolment. Median time to first detection ranged from 33–43 days, and most tests were reactive in all participants by 90 days. Window periods are likely to be several days longer when testing samples of finger-prick blood or of oral fluid, as might be used for rapid, point-of-care tests and self-testing devices. Precise figures for how much longer the window periods are have yet to be published.

Sensitivity and specificity are measures of the accuracy of an HIV test.[6] Sensitivity refers to the probability that a test will correctly indicate that an HIV-positive person is infected with HIV. Lower sensitivity increases the chance of false negatives (testing negative when actually HIV positive). Specificity refers to the probability that a test will correctly indicate that an HIV-negative person is not infected with HIV. Lower specificity increases the chance of false positives (testing positive when actually HIV negative).

CD4 T-cell count

This measure does not check for the presence of HIV, but rather determines the number of CD4 T-cells in the blood, so it is used to monitor immune system function. As the disease progresses and viral load increases, the number of CD4 cells declines. A normal CD4 count can range from 500 cells per cubic millimetre (500 cells/mm^3) to 1,000 cells/mm^3. A low CD4 T-cell count is also associated with many other viral, bacterial and parasitic infections, such as sepsis, tuberculosis, malnutrition, pregnancy and other conditions which weaken the immune system. This test is also used occasionally to estimate immune system function for people whose CD4 T-cells are impaired due to blood diseases, several genetic disorders, and as a side-effect of many chemotherapy drugs. In general, the lower the number of T-cells, the lower the immune system's function will be. Women tend to have somewhat lower counts than men.

In HIV-infected individuals, AIDS is officially diagnosed when the count drops below 200 cells/mm^3. When certain opportunistic infections occur together as a 'syndrome' this will alert physicians to the possibility that HIV infection may have progressed to AIDS. The use of a CD4 count for this purpose was introduced in 1992; the value of 200 was chosen because it corresponded with a greatly increased likelihood of opportunistic infection. The CD4 count is usually inversely related to a person's viral load, i.e. the lower the CD4 count, the higher the viral load, and vice versa. Lower CD4 counts are indicators that prophylaxis against certain types of opportunistic infections should be instituted. Until fairly recently, the CD4 count was used as a marker for when an infected individual would benefit from antiretroviral therapy, which was sometimes only provided for a limited time period, especially to prevent MTCT. However, for the last several years universal treatment of all individuals who test HIV-positive has been recommended on diagnosis and continued for life, and the use of CD4 counts to determine the stage of disease is not considered to be as useful today as a viral load test. Much of the research on MTCT, however, describes CD4 counts as a way of assessing a mother's disease progression, as a marker for infectivity or for eligibility for antiretroviral drug therapy.

Viral load

HIV viral load refers to the number of viral particles found in each millilitre of blood.[9] The more there are, the faster the progression toward AIDS. WHO recommends that viral load tests should consistently detect and measure virus levels down to 50 copies/ml, have a high specificity and provide reproducible results.

Current technologies are very sensitive for measuring the amount of HIV genetic material present in the blood, but different research studies have historically recorded very differing viral loads, and set different safety criteria for intra-partum or post-partum transmission based on those numbers. Sometimes those criteria are still applied and sometimes they're not. For instance, international guidance promoted caesarean section after a 1999 review found that infant contact with virus in cervical secretions during vaginal birth was a risk factor for MTCT.[10] Nine years later it was shown that when a mother was treated with sufficient ART to reduce her viral load to <50 copies/mm^3, the risk of MTCT with vaginal delivery could be reduced to less than 0.1%.[11] This major success is attributed to the achievement of such a low viral load that it was effectively 'undetectable'. Opinion on the role of viral load in transmission of HIV is divided, however. It was found in Botswana that reducing maternal viral load to 400 copies/mm^3 was effective in reducing breastfeeding-associated MTCT to 0.3%.[12] Yet in the UK, while a level of 50 copies/mm^3 is considered to be low enough to permit a vaginal birth, it is still not considered safe enough to encourage breastfeeding, notwithstanding the Botswana findings. In other words a low/undetectable viral load does not receive the same acknowledgement when it comes to breastfeeding as it does when it comes to intrapartum transmission. This is just one of the double standards in place where breastfeeding is concerned. This will be further explored in Chapter 25.

In acknowledgement that HIV-positive mothers may wish to breastfeed in spite of formal recommendations for formula-feeding, the US and UK HIV and infant feeding guidance contains the suggestion that the mother's viral load should be monitored monthly until after the baby is weaned.[13,14]

In considering whether HIV tests are always accurate in identifying HIV-infection, two further complications need to be borne in mind: individuals who are taking pre-exposure prophylaxis (PrEP) or post-exposure prophylaxis (PEP) may have a delayed antibody response which extends the window period. There are suggestions that the window period for accurate test results may be a little longer for newborns whose mothers are receiving ART compared to those who are not.

Phylogenetic testing

One of the defining features of HIV is its ability to rapidly evolve and persist within individuals despite continued pressure from the host immune response. This struggle between virus and human has resulted in one of the most genetically diverse pandemics in recorded history. Phylogenetic analysis is a methodology within the field of molecular virology that compares partial DNA or RNA sequences extracted from different sources to track evolutionary relationships between them.[15] By identifying shared genetic sequences, an evolutionary 'gene tree' is constructed based on the relatedness of the samples via a common ancestor. Phylogenetic testing has the potential to show the direction of HIV infection between two individuals.[16] Phylogenetics are improving understanding of HIV diversity within individuals and populations, to improve ways of preventing and treating the disease.[17]

Testing babies

Identifying babies infected with HIV has been one of the most challenging tasks for those working in countries in which most paediatric infections occur. The relative role of breastfeeding in the epidemiology of HIV remained uncertain for several years,[18] in part due to the difficulty in establishing when babies became infected.

It quickly became apparent that not all HIV-infected mothers passed the virus on to their babies. Why did some babies become infected, and others did not? Why did some babies grow and thrive after birth when others quickly sickened and died? What determined maternal infectivity? Furthermore, exactly when did transmission of the virus to the baby take place? Did it happen during pregnancy, and if so, at what stage? Did babies become infected during labour and birth? The *Lancet* report from Australia had already shown that babies uninfected at birth could become newly infected through breastfeeding – how many were infected in this way, and how could we determine which ones were in fact HIV-free at birth in order to determine that the route of transmission was definitely mother's milk?

The industrialised countries quickly responded to the *Lancet* report by banning breastfeeding, so the answer to how much postpartum transmission of the virus occurred through breastfeeding would have to come from the developing countries, where breastfeeding was universal. However, distrust of research done outside the global north created a credibility gap that was difficult to bridge.

Using HIV testing to identify the timing of infection could also identify the route of infection, but this was easier said than done. Because of uncertainty about the different testing techniques it became apparent that the possibility of overlap between infection occurring *in utero*, during birth or during breastfeeding could not be excluded.

Due to the presence of circulating maternal antibodies, techniques to detect the virus itself by PCR are considered more definitive. However, PCR tests were often too complex and expensive for widespread use in the early years of research into MTCT of HIV.[19]

Perinatally-infected infants have plasma HIV viral RNA that increase rapidly in the first two months of life and then gradually fall. Even with this type of test, initially there is often insufficient virus in the baby's bloodstream, or the virus is sequestered in the baby's lymphoid tissue, so that a PCR test will only be capable of identifying infection 4–6 weeks after it happened. For HIV-exposed babies, testing should occur in the newborn period (i.e. before the infant is 48 hours old), at 1–2 months, and again at 3–6 months. Testing at 14 days may allow for earlier detection of HIV in infants who had negative test results within the first 48 hours of life. By approximately one month, PCR testing has a 96% sensitivity and 99% specificity to identify HIV.[20]

Opinion is divided on the length of the window period for PCR testing. Curiously, the accepted window period for breastfed babies in developing countries, to rule out infection having occurred at birth, may be as short as four weeks, but the American 2010 Panel on Antiretroviral Therapy and Medical Management of HIV-Infected Children confirms that HIV infection can only be ruled out if DNA HIV PCR results are consistently negative in an infant older than four months in the absence of breastfeeding,[21] i.e. four times longer. Of interest is that this long interval is required in the US, where the last possible exposure to the virus would have been at birth, whereas in studies to determine whether babies have been infected by breastfeeding, the window periods are very much shorter (usually 4–6 weeks).

Testing for antibodies to HIV

In adults, for reasons of cost, and because specialised laboratory facilities were needed, the most commonly used test was initially the ELISA,[21] which identified antibodies to the virus and not the virus itself. Antibody tests cannot be used for babies, because maternal HIV antibodies cross the placenta and persist in the baby for about 18 months,[22] meaning that even an uninfected baby will test positive in the early months. An ELISA test is not used until a child is 18–24 months old, or until at least three months after weaning, whichever is the later, and only a positive ELISA test after 18 months means that an infant is definitely infected.

Thus the window periods of various testing techniques complicate diagnosis according to:

- when a mother or baby is exposed to sufficient virus to become infected
- whether there are sufficient copies of the virus or sufficient measurable antibodies in the blood
- what type of testing technique is used
- the technology available
- the subtype of HIV being tested for

Efforts to devise effective intervention strategies to reduce MTCT of HIV to infants have used the timing of a first positive assay to determine the route of infection and thus suggest appropriate interventions.

Initial evidence for transmission around the time of birth was obtained from an intriguing early Swedish study showing that infectious HIV was detectable during pregnancy in infected women, was not isolated from any of their newborn babies at birth, but was present in 26% of them at six months. Postpartum transmission would not have been considered as a route of transmission because Sweden had effectively prohibited breastfeeding by HIV-positive mothers since 1985. The researchers concluded that in most cases, transmission occurs close to or at the time of delivery.[23]

In breastfeeding populations, the inaccuracy of tests to determine when an individual infant may have become infected obscures the route of transmission. Breastfeeding advocates point out that there is no method of testing which can conclusively determine that a newborn baby is not *already* infected. After 1997, the World Health Organization used the opposing negative argument to rationalise discouraging breastfeeding by saying that, given the limitations of testing methods, it was necessary to act on the assumption that the infant of an HIV-infected mother was *not* infected at birth (which would be true for 70–85% of infants, even without any preventive measures). Where the mother had received antiretroviral drug prophylaxis during pregnancy or labour, this assumption could be made with even more confidence: >90% per cent of babies would have been born uninfected.[24]

In an attempt to address the uncertainty, experts were reduced to making assumptions. A paper published in 1992 by Yvonne Bryson and colleagues attempted to create a working definition for *in utero* infection vs intrapartum transmission. On the basis of data then available, the consensus was that an infant would be considered to have been infected during pregnancy if they tested positive on a PCR test within 48 hours of birth or, in the case of a non-breastfed infant, to have been infected during birth if the test showed positive any time from day 7 to day 90.[25]

Tests and HIV subtypes

A further difficulty concerns the sensitivity of early testing techniques used to determine the route of transmission. Most tests are designed to identify infection with HIV subtype B, the form of HIV most commonly found in Western countries and the subtype most often found in infected gay men. It is possible that these tests are less sensitive to other subtypes. For example, it is subtype C which is most often found in populations where heterosexual and vertical transmission are the main forms of infection. A full three-quarters of HIV-positive women living in the UK are immigrants from areas of high HIV-prevalence, specifically east, central and southern Africa, where subtype C is the main form of HIV.[26]

The National Institutes of Health confirmed in an October 2006 update that HIV PCR tests manufactured in the United States to identify subtype B, the predominant viral subtype most commonly found in the US, and the subtype for which all initial assays were targeted,[27] were less sensitive in the detection of other subtypes. For example subtype E is the strain of HIV found in much of south-east Asia, and subtype C predominates in regions of Africa and India where most heterosexual transmission of the virus – and infection of babies – occurs. False negative results had initially been reported in 2001–02 in infants infected with non-subtype B newly arriving in New York State from outside the country. This raised the question about whether at least some babies infected with other subtypes, especially subtype C, who tested negative on a test designed to identify a subtype B virus, but who subsequently tested positive during the period when infection was attributed to breastfeeding, may actually have acquired the virus prenatally or during birth, and not during breastfeeding at all. Caution was urged in the interpretation of negative HIV PCR test results in the babies of mothers infected with non-subtype B HIV.

Perhaps more attention needs to be paid to the types of tests used in research pointing to breastfeeding as the cause of transmission of HIV. In 2007, Tracy Creek wrote that a variety of commercial and in-house processing methods for DNA PCR testing exist worldwide, but not all tests are equally accurate with all HIV subtypes.[19] One commercially available PCR test, Amplicor HIV-1 DNA PCR (version 1.5, Roche Molecular Systems, Branchburg, NJ), is highly accurate in detecting the multiple HIV-1 subtypes circulating in Africa, is standardised and supported for use in Africa, and has been used by researchers and pilot infant diagnosis programmes in several countries. The cost for each PCR test in developing countries varied between $8 and $18. An earlier version of this assay, the Roche Amplicor version 1.0, was slightly less sensitive in detecting non-B subtypes. The choice of assay should have been dictated by the prevailing subtypes in the country.

Ruling out HIV infection in an exposed baby

Information given by the National Institutes for Health in the US in 2011[28] stated that HIV may be presumptively excluded with two or more negative tests, one for babies aged 14 days or older and the other at age one month or older. Definitive exclusion of HIV in non-breastfed infants could be based on two negative virologic tests at ages one month and four months or older. Many experts confirmed HIV-negative status with an HIV antibody test at age 12–18 months. Alternative algorithms exist for presumptive and definitive HIV exclusion. Again, this testing algorithm applies mainly to exposure to HIV subtype B, the predominant viral subtype found in the United States. Non-subtype B infection may not be detected by many commercially available nucleic acid tests, particularly HIV DNA PCR. Many of the newer HIV RNA assays have improved detection of non-subtype B HIV, but there are still variants that are either poorly detected or undetectable. If non-subtype B HIV infection is suspected based on maternal origins, then newer HIV RNA assays that have improved ability to detect non-subtype B HIV should be used as part of the initial diagnostic algorithm. Exposed infants should also be closely monitored and undergo definitive HIV serologic testing at age 18 months.

Current British HIV pregnancy guidelines recommend that a series of diagnostic tests should be undertaken to determine the HIV infection status of HIV-exposed babies. These should include three HIV proviral DNA PCRs conducted at birth, and again when the child is six and 12 weeks old. Infants are also recommended to have an HIV antibody test at 18 months. Antibody testing is delayed due to the persistence of maternal antibodies.[29]

However, the unsettling possibility that ELISA testing may need to be extended to two years was raised in a Malawi study published in 2007. Maternal antibodies persisted longer than was previously thought in a small but significant number of children born after 1999 and the trend was increasing over time. Significantly, about 2% of 18-month-old Malawian children were falsely classified as HIV-positive by serological testing.[30] The age of seroreversion, at which maternal antibodies disappeared and there was reversion to an HIV-negative status in HIV-free children born to HIV-infected Malawian women, increased between 1989 and 2003. The proportion of children at 18 months of age with persistent maternal antibodies increased from 0.2% between 1989 and 1991, to 0.5% between 1993 and 1996, and to 1.9% between 2000 and 2003. This trend was similar for children aged 15 and 21 months. The investigators believed that the current policy of HIV serological testing in children of HIV-infected mothers needed to be urgently revised.

Nastouli and colleagues also found in 2007[31] that newer, fourth-generation HIV antibody tests with enhanced sensitivity and specificity had shown value in the earlier detection of HIV in adults, but the use of fourth-generation assays was more problematic in infants. Eight of 18 infants tested negative using the most recent assay, but 10 tested positive. Nine tested again using the fourth-generation assay a few months later tested HIV-negative. The remaining child was not available for repeat testing, but didn't show any clinical signs of HIV infection. The researchers suggested that a fourth HIV PCR test should be considered after six months, and if an HIV antibody test at 18 months is used, it 'should be undertaken with a standard assay rather than an assay of enhanced sensitivity for antibody detection'.

Timing and infectivity

The timing of maternal primary infection will determine maternal infectivity to the baby, whether that happens during pregnancy, during delivery, or during the course of breastfeeding.[32] The hypothesis was made in 1993 that it might be possible to identify those HIV-positive women who were more likely to infect their children through breastfeeding, e.g. those with clinical AIDS, low CD4 counts at delivery, or positive cells in early milk.[33] The Nairobi group found that viral loads in breastmilk samples of mothers who had tested HIV-positive at 32 weeks of gestation decreased to zero nine months after delivery.[34] And Dunn et al in 1992[35] suggested that breastfed children of mothers newly infected prior to conception or early in pregnancy could be at lower risk of infection several months later from breastmilk because their mothers, unless symptomatic, were probably less infectious.

Several researchers were able to demonstrate a strong correlation between maternal immunosuppression and prevalence and quantity of breast milk HIV DNA. For example, during the later stages of a mother's disease, when viraemia increased again, the risk of transmission via breastfeeding was also more likely.[36] Women who had been infected for a longer time, with consequently lower CD4 cell counts, had an increased likelihood of shedding virus in breastmilk, which is consistent with higher levels of viraemia seen with advanced HIV disease.[37] HIV DNA correlated with CD4 depletion, which suggested a later stage of maternal infection. Malawian researchers, studying the effects of Vitamin A deficiency on vertical transmission, found that breastfeeding practices were not significantly associated with increased mother-to-child transmission of HIV, but that maternal CD4 cell counts and the CD4/CD8 ratio were.[38,39] Ekpini and colleagues described the risk for babies breastfed beyond six months as 'substantial', although information about how long before delivery the mother herself became infected was not given. CD4 T-lymphocytes were significantly lower in transmitting than in non-transmitting mothers of breastfed babies who seroconverted after 11 months of age, indicating that their mothers were at a later stage of the disease.[40]

Long window periods in definitively establishing HIV infection in an HIV-exposed baby raise the possibility that transmission attributed to breastfeeding in early research may have actually occurred during pregnancy or during the birth process. This meant that the risks of breastfeeding could be exaggerated. Over-inflation of breastfeeding-associated transmission has had the unprecedented potential to endanger breastfeeding on a global scale. Accurate identification of the route of transmission was crucially important when developing strategies for risk avoidance and adoption of various interventions to safely navigate those risks.

In research attempting to quantify the risk of vertical transmission in untreated mothers there were gaps in knowledge about the risk of acquiring the virus through breastfeeding. Advice to untreated women that suggested that there was an increased risk of HIV transmission with increased duration of breastfeeding may or may not have been correct. On the one hand, maternal viral load falls as antibodies increase. However, over time, viral levels increase again with the onset of active AIDS. Thus it was possible that the reason that breastfeeding didn't consistently lead to infection could have been due to the window period of comparatively low viral load, beginning sometime after the high level of viraemia which accompanies maternal primary infection has fallen, and before viraemia climbs again in the final stages of the disease.

Another study from the ZVITAMBO project[41] looked at MTCT according to the timing of maternal infection. Breastfeeding-associated transmission was responsible for about 9% of infections among babies of untreated mothers who tested HIV-positive at baseline and whose infant tested HIV-negative with PCR at six weeks. Infant transmission varied little over the breastfeeding period. However, breastfeeding-associated transmission for babies whose mothers seroconverted postnatally averaged nearly 35% during the first nine months after maternal infection, then declined to 9.5% during the next three months and was zero thereafter. Among women in whom the precise timing of infection was known (defined as <90 days between the last negative and the first positive test), over 60% of transmissions occurred in the first three months after maternal infection. In these cases breastfeeding-associated transmission was nearly five times higher than in mothers who tested HIV-positive at baseline and whose infant tested HIV-negative with PCR at six weeks. Both plasma HIV concentration and breastmilk viral load declined rapidly in the following three months. Among women whose plasma sample collected soon after delivery tested negative for HIV with ELISA but positive with PCR, 75% of their infants were infected or had died by 12 months. An estimated 18–20% of all breastfeeding-associated transmission observed in the ZVITAMBO trial occurred among mothers who seroconverted postnatally. Thus it can be seen that the risk is high during primary maternal HIV infection (when the mother's plasma viral load is high) and is mirrored by a high but transient peak in breastmilk HIV load. Yet, worryingly, around two-thirds of breastfeeding-associated transmission by women who seroconvert postnatally may occur while the mother is still in the 'window period' of an antibody-based test, when she would test HIV-negative using one of these tests.

Ultimately, we have to ask what importance was placed on establishing the timing of infection – and thus the route – for HIV-exposed babies. At the 11th International Conference on AIDS in Vancouver back in 1996, Dr David Ho, of the Aaron Diamond AIDS Research Center, New York, and Dr George Shaw, of the University of Alabama at Birmingham School of Medicine, presented viral dynamics data showing that the average person with HIV infection produced an alarming 10 billion virions/day, bringing into sharp focus the fact that this was a viral infection that required antiviral treatment. At the same event, Dr John Mellors of the University of Pittsburgh also presented data showing that HIV viral load predicted progression as well as CD4+ cell decline rates, and the HIV viral load test with a threshold of detection at 15–25 copies/ml was introduced.[42] Why was this sensitive technology never used to help determine early infection status in mothers or their babies?

Michael Latham and Pauline Kisanga, writing a four-country report in 2001 about how support for breastfeeding was being negatively impacted by the response to HIV/AIDS,[43] put their finger on why establishing the route of transmission of MTCT was so important:

> *'We believe it would be useful in discussions, but also in policy considerations, to separate the modes of transmission of HIV from mother to baby. They call for very different actions. We cannot think of a truly appropriate analogy. But consider the use of amniocentesis,*

or similar methods to diagnose congenital abnormalities like Down Syndrome in the foetus. These diagnostic methods, and decisions about what to do prior to birth, are completely different from post-delivery treatment of the infant who has the syndrome. A different set of specialists deals with each half of the problem. So should we not devise language, and options, that separate (these two different) means of MTCT of HIV: (1) In utero and during childbirth and (2) through breastfeeding. Perhaps MTCT (IUC) and MTCT (BF) could be used. Virologists and obstetricians might be the major specialists dealing with MTCT (IUC). Lactation specialists, nutritionists and paediatricians with knowledge of breastfeeding are specialists best placed to deal with MTCT (BF).'

Later research looking at postnatal transmission of the virus to the babies of mothers who have received ART has noted that the timing of initiation of maternal therapy is important in reducing viral load in breastmilk. And it is the quantity of virus in breastmilk which appears to be the key factor governing whether an individual baby will become infected or not. This will be explored further in Chapter 7.

Finally, the importance of identifying an infected infant cannot be understated. Because mortality in the first year of life is very high among untreated HIV-infected infants, early HIV testing, prompt return of results and rapid initiation of treatment are essential. According to WHO, infants who have a positive test at birth are likely infected *in utero*, will progress to disease rapidly and, in the absence of treatment, experience high mortality in the first few months of life. Infants infected at or around delivery may not have detectable virus for several days to weeks. The ability of testing techniques to detect virus in the blood may be affected by ARV drugs taken by the mother or infant for postnatal prophylaxis, resulting in false negative results. This includes any drug that is present in the breastmilk as a result of maternal ART during breastfeeding. However, the sooner an infected baby can receive treatment with antiretroviral therapy, the more likely they are to survive.[44–46] And, as further discussed in Chapter 20, babies born already infected should continue to be breastfed in order to receive maximum immunological protection from other opportunistic infections.

CHAPTER 6

Breastfeeding: why it matters

'If a multinational company developed a product that was a nutritionally balanced and delicious food, a wonder drug that both prevented and treated disease, cost almost nothing to produce and could be delivered in quantities controlled by the consumers' needs, the very announcement of their find would send their shares rocketing to the top of the stock market. The scientists who developed the product would win prizes and the wealth and influence of everyone involved would increase dramatically. Women have been producing such a miraculous substance, breastmilk, since the beginning of human existence.'

Gabrielle Palmer, *The Politics of Breastfeeding: When Breasts are Bad for Business*, 3rd Ed., Pinter & Martin, 2009

Breastfeeding is the biological continuum of pregnancy. After birth, breastmilk synthesis happens automatically, even if a mother chooses not to breastfeed. For as long as milk is drained from the breasts, 99.99% of mothers will produce ample quantities of milk.[1]

During the early weeks and months after birth, a mother's breastmilk fulfils two of the primary functions previously undertaken prenatally by the placenta: to provide both perfect, species-specific nutrition and immunological protection to the vulnerable, immature infant. Tonse Raju, writing in *Breastfeeding Medicine*,[2] says:

'An infant suckling at his or her mother's breast is not simply receiving a meal, but is intensely engaged in a dynamic, bidirectional, biological dialogue. It is a process in which physical, biochemical, hormonal, and psychosocial exchange takes place, designed for the transfer of much needed nutrients, as well as for building a lasting psychosocial bond between the mother and her infant. Among mammals, breastfeeding has evolved over millions of years as a multi-tiered interaction to meet the biological and psychosocial needs of the progeny, enhancing its well-being and survival chances, as well as complementing the nurturing role of the mother. Thus, this unique, dynamic process benefits both the mother and her infant. Breastfeeding needs to be considered quintessentially as a continuation of the more intense, intrauterine dialogue, mediated through the placenta and the umbilical cord between the mother and her fetus.'

The first report in 1985[3] that HIV could be transmitted to the vulnerable human baby through breastmilk sounded the death-knell for continued universal promotion of breastfeeding. The implications of the *Lancet* report were especially devastating for countries being ravaged by HIV – particularly those in eastern, central and southern Africa. Here, heterosexual, not homosexual, transmission was the main route of infection. Being both the cultural norm and a cornerstone of child survival, breastfeeding was universally practised. Since the 1970s and 1980s, growing knowledge about the importance of breastfeeding[4] had underpinned WHO and UNICEF efforts to promote, protect and support breastfeeding as a strategy to combat young child malnutrition and mortality. But after 1985, faith in the wisdom, or even the ethics, of promoting breastfeeding when it could transmit a lethal virus, was seriously questioned. Paediatricians would say, 'Breastfeeding? Ah yes, but what about HIV?' For the first time, there was a medical indication for formula-feeding for millions of babies throughout the world. The HIV pandemic threatened to 'knock breastfeeding off its pedestal as a pillar of child survival'.[5]

What's so special about breastfeeding?

Why is breastfeeding so important? Isn't formula-feeding just as good? Mothers could be forgiven for believing that artificial baby milks are equivalent to breastmilk, when Western media and even healthcare providers often trivialise breastfeeding as little more than a lifestyle choice[6,7] and when marketing of breastmilk substitutes is so cleverly undertaken by huge multinational corporations who befriend newly pregnant women offering special offers, 24-hour advice lines and the latest in infant nutrition – which they say is almost as good as the real thing.[8]

Milk is a baby's sole food for several months, at a time when they are growing and developing faster than at any other period of life. Breastmilk is a complete food and drink, containing all the nutrients in the right quantities to enable a baby to grow and thrive. World Health Organization guidelines recommend that the newborn is put to the breast within an hour of birth, that they are exclusively breastfed for the first six months of life and that breastfeeding should continue with the addition of other foods and liquids for up to two years or beyond.[9]

Maureen Minchin, who describes the consequences down the generations when breastfeeding is abandoned, has also called the feeding of artificial baby milk in the developed world, 'one of the largest uncontrolled in vivo experiments in human history'.[10] Her latest book, *Milk Matters: infant feeding & immune disorder*,[11] is the last word on the need for human babies to receive their own mothers' milk. She argues that 'milk is the necessary bridge from the womb to the world'. The first 1,000 days of feeding are the single most important factor determining a child's health outcomes. Any excesses or inadequacies in a breastmilk substitute, exacerbated over and over, can have life-long consequences. There are substantially higher rates of mortality among infants never breastfed compared to those who are,[12] or even among babies for whom breastfeeding is delayed more than an hour after birth compared to those who are breastfed immediately.[13] Breastfeeding is truly a pillar of child survival, reducing morbidity and mortality in children worldwide, in every country and every environment.[14]

Keith Hansen, a Vice President for Human Development at the World Bank, writing in the *Lancet* in 2016,[15] observed:

> *'If breastfeeding did not already exist, someone who invented it today would deserve a dual Nobel Prize in medicine and economics. Breastfeeding is a child's first inoculation against death, disease, and poverty, but also their most enduring investment in physical, cognitive, and social capacity. Breastfeeding is one of the highest impact interventions providing benefits for children, women, and society. It reduces infant morbidity and mortality, increases IQ score, improves school achievement, and boosts adult earnings – all essential for reducing poverty. It also contributes to equity by giving all children a nutritional head start for success in life. For many people living in poverty, malnutrition remains a prime contributor to stunted development, and ...breastfeeding can make a lasting difference... The challenge now is to scale up breastfeeding.'*

We knew the risks of not breastfeeding

When the first doubts were raised about whether breastfeeding would continue to be safe, there was already in existence a huge amount of research on breastmilk and breastfeeding and in particular, the morbidity and mortality risks of *not* breastfeeding.

According to doctors Ruth and Robert Lawrence, who have written successive editions of *Breastfeeding: A guide for the medical profession*,[16] the biochemistry of human milk encompasses a mammoth supply of scientific data and information, most of which has been generated since 1970. In a pivotal publication looking at the importance of breastfeeding worldwide, published to assist discussions about development and adoption of an International Code to limit the marketing activities of manufacturers of breastmilk substitutes,[17] Dick and Patrice Jelliffe wrote in 1978 that an abundance of new information had accumulated in the previous 10 years.[4] In a way never attempted before, based on modern scientific research into all aspects of the subject including, for example, biochemistry, immunology, nutrition, endocrinology and psychophysiology, the Jelliffes brought together comparative information from all over the world, including the logic of considering breastfeeding as a biological and ecological system. Their book reviewed and evaluated the scientific information for health professionals on a wide range of different aspects of human milk and breastfeeding. Looking at the unique properties and functions of human milk, they asked what the consequences would be if breastfeeding in the world was to decline.

Well-documented concerns about the use of breastmilk substitutes in low-income settings had been available for 50 years. Dr Cicely Williams, pioneer and first head of Maternal and Child Health in the new World Health Organization in Geneva from 1948–1951[18] had worked with thousands of severely malnourished young children in Ghana and Gold Coast, and her findings had been published by the Royal College of Paediatrics and Child Health in 1933. Transferred to Malaya in 1936, Cicely Williams then campaigned against artificial infant feeding. Incensed by milk companies sending girls in white coats around the tenements of Singapore, selling tinned milk as though they were nurses promoting infant health, in 1939 she delivered a stinging speech entitled 'Milk and Murder' to the Singapore Rotary Club, whose chairman was also the president of Nestlé,[19] asserting 'Misguided propaganda on infant feeding should be punished as the most miserable form of sedition, these deaths should be regarded as murder.' Thus by 1985, the value of breastfeeding was well acknowledged by experts in infant and young child nutrition.

Mothering through breastfeeding

Breastfeeding a baby is one of the most rewarding and joyful experiences a woman can have. Women want to breastfeed for all sorts of personal reasons as well as for the health benefits.[20] Little babies are infinitely vulnerable. Having the means and the sole responsibility for keeping her very own tiny human alive until he grows old enough to take care of himself, is as terrifying as it is empowering. From the moment of birth, the breast continues the work of the placenta, providing for the baby's complete immunological and nutritional needs. The biological expectation of the newborn is to have constant access to the warmth and security of the mother's body and continuous nutrition from her breast – literally 'a womb with a view'.

The breast is the all-purpose mothering tool, enabling a mother to nourish and nurture her baby anywhere, any time. I haven't met a single mother who regrets having breastfed her babies, whether breastfeeding lasted a couple of days, a couple of months, a couple of years, or longer. Older baby-children can and do describe, often very eloquently, how much they love breastfeeding. It's right that mothers are sobered by this responsibility because breastmilk is awesome. It's almost impossible to put a true value on this once-in-a-lifetime gift that only a mother can bestow on her child.

Helping mothers breastfeed

The accumulation of knowledge about the crucial importance of breastfeeding has underpinned development of a whole new profession, lactation consulting. Coincidentally, the first International Board Certified Lactation Consultant (IBCLC) was certified in 1985; the same year that the *Lancet* reported on the first case of transmission of HIV through breastmilk. Thirty-six years later, over 33,000 IBCLCs practice in 122 countries.[21] An IBCLC is an allied healthcare professional whose area of expertise focuses solely on providing evidence-based information and skilled assistance in routine and special circumstance lactation and breastfeeding.[22] In order to keep up-to-date in such a fast-changing field, IBCLCs are required to recertify every five years. Not only do we know why women should be recommended to breastfeed their babies, we also have the skills and expertise to help them succeed.[23,24] We know that there are only about five drugs which preclude breastfeeding.[25] We know how to help mothers to bring in an adequate breastmilk supply after birth, and how to help them recognise that the baby is transferring milk at the breast. We know how to work around and through the little and large difficulties women face in initiating and maintaining breastfeeding and we know that, in spite of assertions to the contrary by women who had difficult breastfeeding experiences, for various stated reasons, there is almost no problem that cannot actually be overcome. We can distinguish between real and perceived breastmilk insufficiency, and we can identify when a mother or baby is really struggling, and how to resolve their difficulties. While we know that breastmilk substitutes might occasionally be needed, and how much and when to use them in emergency situations, we also know that these emergency situations can be almost completely avoided if mothers are given enough help and information to effectively manage their own lactation. Because we know so much, we have difficulty with the ethics of supporting infant feeding choice as if the differences in health outcomes between breastfeeding and bottle-feeding did not matter.[26]

The unique specificity of breastmilk

Researchers from the University of Western Australia, whose past work has exploded so many myths surrounding breast anatomy and the synthesis of human milk, write:

> *'The potential to secrete milk is a characteristic common to the females of all 4000+ species of mammal. However, the great variation that exists between species in maturity of the young at birth has resulted in the nutrient composition of milk being uniquely adapted to complement the young of each species. Furthermore, the maturity of the infants' systems (such as digestion, hepatic, neural, renal, vascular, visual, skeletal and immune) varies between species. Thus, the composition of milk varies with stage of lactation specific to each species, so that the infant receives nutrition appropriate to its stage of development.'*[27]

Evidence is accumulating about the importance of the gut microbiota in health and allergy.[28] There is an important 'window of opportunity' in early life, during which interventions altering the gut microbiota induce long-term effects, both directly and indirectly, via maternal milk factors that affect bacterial growth and metabolism. A link between gut microbial dysbiosis in the first 1,000 days of life and an increased risk of asthma was demonstrated. Healthy microbiota is highly diverse, i.e. above 600,000 bacterial genes, mostly involved in the control of inflammation and innate immunity.

Never before in science history has so much been known about the complex significance of breastfeeding for mothers and their children.[29] Lactation is an ancient adaptation perhaps 300 million years old. Each species of mammal has its own variety of milk and even each mother has her own variety, allowing mammalian mothers to signal biochemically to their offspring over an extended period, guiding the development of their young. In humans, exclusive breastfeeding for the first six months of an infant's life, with continued breastfeeding for up to two years or longer, is recognised as the 'gold standard' for infant feeding because human milk is uniquely suited to the human infant, and its nutritional content and bioactivity promote healthy development. The composition of human breastmilk is complex, containing factors that interact with the infant immune system and intestinal milieu including allergens, cytokines, immunoglobulins, poly-unsaturated fatty acids, and chemokines.

A whole special issue of *Nutrients*, published in April 2019 and reviewed by Donna Geddes and Sharon Perella, contains 30 manuscripts that cover a wide range of areas in lactation research.[30] Most address factors influencing milk composition, or relationships between composition and infant development. While breastmilk is traditionally thought of primarily as a source of infant nutrition, the evidence shows a diverse range of functions, including protection from infection and disease, and programming of future health and development of both mother and infant through microbial and hormonal signalling.

Other mammals' milk

Milk composition is largely a function of evolutionary history, maternal nutrient intake and duration of milk production. Natural selection and breast evolution over some 160 million years[31] has culminated in milks uniquely suited to nourish and protect infants of each species. Antimicrobial, anti-inflammatory and immunoregulatory agents and living leukocytes are different from those in other mammalian milks. Typically, a mother invests much more of her energy into making milk for her babies than she does in feeding them during pregnancy. Looking at the differences in the milk of different species, and what that milk needs to contain in order that the young will survive and thrive, provides a fascinating insight into what selective pressures have been exerted over time. Across species there is substantial variation in the proteins, fats and sugars in different mammal milks.

For example, a hooded seal mother produces milk with the highest fat content in the world at 60%.[32] She gives birth to her pup on floating ice in the freezing and highly unstable environment of the North Atlantic, nursing him for only four days before weaning. During that short time he doubles his birthweight, while consuming about 7.5 litres of super-creamy milk, so that he can gain a thick layer of blubber as insulation against the cold. Conversely, the milk of species that lactate for longer durations tends to have lower fat and proteins. Black rhinos, born into hot arid environments, produce watery milk with the lowest fat content of any mammal, only 0.2%, but they nurse their young for almost two years. Camels and zebras also produce more dilute milk. Notwithstanding that humans have drunk the milk of domesticated cows for the last 8,000–10,000 years, it is zebra milk which most resembles human milk.

From birth through puberty, pregnancy and lactation, no other human organ displays such dramatic changes in size, shape and function as does the breast.[33] In a marvel of design efficiency, the human embryo secures his own continuing food source after birth. During pregnancy, the placenta, which is foetal tissue, not only nourishes the baby, supplying sufficient food and oxygen for him to develop and thrive, but also secretes the hormones oestrogen and progesterone, which act on the mother's breasts to cause proliferation of the ducts and alveoli, little grape-like bunches of milk-producing cells, which will be the baby's sole food-source for the first six months of life. As the pregnancy progresses the mother's pituitary gland also begins to secrete the milk-making hormone prolactin. The breasts are ready to make milk from approximately the 16th week of
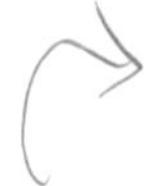
pregnancy – way before the infant is viable – and it is only the presence of high levels of progesterone produced by the placenta which puts a brake on milk production. With delivery of the placenta after birth, there is a sharp drop in progesterone, and it is the fall in progesterone levels, together with high levels of prolactin, which causes lactogenesis-II, the copious secretion of milk, beginning within 36–72 hours of birth. This event is often referred to in the lay literature as 'the milk coming in'. Colostrum, the initial

scanty, high-protein, high-sodium, low-sugar secretion produced by the breasts during late pregnancy and in the first three days after birth, is high in protective antibodies, and has been called the first immunisation.

Human milk has the highest lactose content (6.8%– 7.2%) of any mammal milk[34] and this small fact is often underestimated. Lactose is broken down into glucose and galactose by the enzyme lactase in the baby's gut. Galactose is responsible for rapid brain development, crucial to the survival of our species. Unlike other animals whose unique survival mechanisms include sharp claws, strong teeth, or fur to camouflage them from predators, the main survival mechanism of *Homo sapiens* (coincidentally Latin for 'wise man') is our very clever brain. Lactose is brain food. Baby humans are among the most helpless of all mammals at birth and they grow and mature very slowly. There is no doubt that parents are sometimes overwhelmed by the long-term needs of babies and toddlers, but the idea that the timing of birth optimises cognitive and neuronal development was first proposed by Swiss zoologist Adolf Portman in the 1960s.[35] More time to mature ensures a longer period of learning before the young are expected to function independently. Infants grow new synapses, or neural connections, in their developing brains, at a rate of 40,000 new synapses a second. The brain more than doubles in volume during the first year,[36] taking approximately five years to reach 85–90% of its final size. To achieve this neurodevelopment the baby's brain requires constant energy and nutrition. Children who consume mother's milk in the early weeks of life have an 8.3 point advantage in IQ at 7½–8 years compared to those who don't. The difference is due to breastmilk alone, rather than variability in their mothers' education, social class and interactions with their small infants.[37]

What about babies who are not breastfed? Governments who provide financial assistance to low-income mothers to formula-feed have probably overlooked the fact that on a population basis breastmilk substitutes harm babies' intellectual development to such an extent that it is possible to detect the impact on the gross domestic product of a predominantly bottle-fed population.[38]

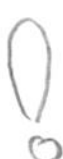

Human milk oligosaccharides

Breastmilk contains more than 200 complex sugars called oligosaccharides. Human milk oligosaccharides (HMOs) are found in abundance in human milk, but not in cows' milk, from which infant formula is made. The formula industry is eyeing the possibility of including them in its products,[39,40] but each mother produces a unique set of HMOs that cannot be duplicated.[41] Many factors, such as duration of lactation, environment and genes influence the amount of HMOs in a mother's milk at any one time. Intriguingly, these bioactive components are metabolically inert, indigestible by the developing infant[42] and significant amounts are excreted intact. HMOs promote healthy gut colonisation, including stimulation of beneficial bifidobacteria (prebiotics). They also act as decoy receptors to block pathogenic microbes adhering to the infant gut,[43] prevent infections entering the bloodstream, promote brain structure and function and reduce the risk of brain inflammation.[44] In premature infants they protect against necrotising enterocolitis, candidiasis and several other immune-related diseases. While bacterial resistance to antibiotics causes 23,000 deaths annually, oligosaccharides in human milk not only possess antibacterial properties of their own, but also enhance the effectiveness of the antibacterial proteins, killing bacteria directly and physically breaking down the biofilms that bacteria form to protect themselves. The sugars have a one-two punch which biologists call 'synthetic lethality'; sensitising and then killing the target bacteria. There is a major push to develop new antimicrobial drugs with this capability, yet mothers produce it automatically.

Fats

A mother who breastfeeds for the first six months mobilises some 35,000kcals to provide her baby with almost 4kg of fats through her milk.[45] A healthy, thriving breastfed baby will gain approximately 4.5kg in the first six months of exclusive breastfeeding, i.e. 30g per day from birth to three months and 20g per day from 3–6 months. Breastfed and formula-fed infants lay down different types of adipose tissue.

Lipids average 3–5% of human milk, the second greatest constituent,[16] though it is also the most variable, since the fat content of milk changes throughout a breastfeed, according to the time of day or night, and even the sex of the baby.[46] The frequency of the baby's demand for milk influences the degree of fullness or emptiness of the breasts, which in turn affects the fat content – the emptier the breast the more creamy the milk.[47] The fat is contained within milk fat globules composed of a core and a membrane consisting of phospholipids, cholesterol, proteins, and glycoproteins. Both membrane and core components provide protection against microorganisms. As well as energy, the lipid portion supplies fat-soluble vitamins, essential fatty acids and bioactive compounds which fulfil a host of crucial functions in growth and development. Lipids also serve as carriers of messages to the infant, allowing maximum intestinal absorption of fatty acids. The supply of long-chain polyunsaturated fatty acids improves cognitive development and reduces the risk of asthma. Milk fat globule lipids provide considerable amounts of free and esterified cholesterol, resulting in a total cholesterol content of 90–150mg/l. Cholesterol has received some bad press in the popular health literature, but in infancy it's an indispensable building block for all cell membranes, being incorporated in considerable amounts into myelin in the nervous system during the period of rapid brain growth, and in the synthesis of bile acids, lipoproteins, vitamin D, hormones, and oxysterols that modulate lipid and glucose homeostasis. This early exposure to the high cholesterol content of breastmilk may programme fat metabolism, improving the body's ability to metabolise fat and providing long-term benefits for cardiovascular health in later life.[48]

Water content

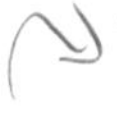

The versatility of breastmilk contributes to the convenience of breastfeeding. Breastmilk is approximtely 87% water, and babies don't need extra fluids, even in hot, dry climates.[49] In fact, extra water may be harmful since the delicate balance of fluids to electrolytes may be disturbed; water displaces milk that contains nutrients needed for growth and may also contain pathogenic bacteria. Most research shows that the higher the degree of exclusivity of breastfeeding, the greater the protective effect against disease.[50] When the breasts are fuller the milk is more watery. A thirsty baby will just want a quick snack. A hungry baby will want to suck for longer or may want to cluster-feed, especially in the evenings. With increasing emptying of the breast (either towards the end of a single feeding, or if there has been a short interval between feedings) the milk becomes creamier. A mother who is worried about whether a baby has had enough milk during breastfeeding can express a drop or two to check its colour and consistency. If she can express blue, watery jets, she can be reassured she still has plenty of milk left in the breasts for the baby. However, if she finds that she can express only creamy drops, then the baby has done a good job of draining the breast, though he may well want to continue sucking for comfort because breastfeeding just feels blissful.

Proteins

Differences in the content of human milk vs the milk of other mammals are shown in their respective feeding intervals, which in turn are influenced by the protein content of the milk. Rabbit milk has 15% protein, the highest percentage in the animal kingdom. Mother rabbits who cache their young, leaving them unattended for long periods of time, feed their babies only twice in 24 hours. While human milk contains more than 1,600 different proteins, the total protein content is less than 1%, demonstrating why we are a continuous-contact species who, like other primates, feed our babies often. The proteins in human milk are made up of amino acids and nucleotides, all serving different functions such as development of the gastrointestinal tract, the immune system and the brain.[51] Nucleotides and cytokines in breastmilk help with T-cell maturation and immune system modulation, and evidence of this function is the unexpected finding that breastfed babies mount a more robust immune response following vaccination than do babies who have not been breastfed.[52] Breastfeeding can also double the size of the infant's central immunological organ, the thymus.[53]

The importance of human proteins for human babies is crucial. Most infant formulas are manufactured from cow's milk. Early exposure to foreign proteins can set up a sensitivity which can last for life. With formula-feeding being so common, the most ubiquitous allergen in the Western world is bovine protein. Recommendations for six months exclusive breastfeeding are underpinned by the immaturity of the baby's intestinal mucosa. The gut is porous so that immunological components from mother's milk can be easily absorbed to boost the baby's own immune system. Gut closure doesn't normally occur for about 4–6 months. It's sensible to avoid exposing the vulnerable baby to foreign proteins during this time. The Western diet comprises a very large quantity of dairy products and recent thinking is that we may be eating too much of them. Public Health England recently halved its recommendation on the percentage that should be included in the British diet, from a whopping 15% down to 8%.

Against this background, it's not hard to see why autoimmune diseases are increasing. Asthma prevalence has been increasing over decades and is one of the most common chronic conditions of childhood, associated with significant effects on quality of life. Asthma is the leading cause of morbidity in children globally, as measured by emergency department visits, hospitalisations and days of missed school.[54] Exclusive breastfeeding protects against respiratory symptoms and asthma and protects against atopic disease throughout childhood and into adolescence.[55–57]

Maureen Minchin, who has written the definitive book on infant feeding and immune disorder,[10] describes how allergy leads to inflammation that forms the basis of many autoimmune disorders. High intakes of immunologically active animal milks during pregnancy expose a foetus to antigens. After birth, continued exposure directly through formula-feeding, or indirectly through mother's milk, when mothers are themselves already sensitised to certain proteins, allowing them to be secreted into their milk, can lead to allergy in the baby which can manifest as eczema, hives, flaky skin, asthma, hay fever, colic, prolonged crying, gastrointestinal problems, vomiting, reflux or impaired growth. Sometimes single symptoms are quite subtle and sometimes they are multiple and undeniably obvious. Maureen asserts that artificial feeding of infants is the single greatest avoidable negative input into normal human development and health, with immediate and long-term harms. Western epidemics of allergy and autoimmune disease are the inevitable and predictable result of generations of infant dysnutrition, mainly artificial feeding. Recovery requires exclusive human milk feeding of infants for the first few months of life, preferably six months or more, with continued breastfeeding for many months longer.

In practical terms, not breastfeeding increases the risk of allergy. Spend time on any cyber support group for mothers of babies whose young children suffer allergies and the case histories and images of little ones manifesting severe eczema are heart-wrenching. Truly terrifying are accounts of babies and toddlers who experience severe reactions to ingestion of even tiny quantities of a food that they are known to be allergic to, most frequently cow's milk. Stories of babies needing hospital treatment for anaphylactic shock are frequent and chilling. Surely every mother would want to avoid this life-threatening danger for her child. But much of the research is ambiguous, and input from industry is accepted by journals and professional associations and even charities providing support to those with allergies.

In a beautifully written article about the immunological function of breasts,[58] K.K. Prameela and A.E.K. Mahommed of the University of Sains Islam Malaysia in Kuala Lumpur write:

> *'The lactating mammary gland is an integral part of the common mucosal immune system which stands as a sentinel in combating pathogens that enter the body via the mucosal route. The common mucosal immune system also competently controls tolerance mechanisms to innocent proteins and is involved in surveillance of carcinogenesis. The diverse roles of general mucosal immunity are nearly well established but the specialised functions of breast tissue and breast milk in boosting the immune responses need more emphasis and highlighting... In humans, the production and functions of sIgA are not optimum until four years of age, however breast milk is able to compensate for this when it confers sIgA passively to the suckling infant, providing a robust local immunity. sIgA in the breast milk, mainly colostrum, is a developmental bridge until the infant's intestines secrete its own.*

> *...The lactating mammary glands are integral parts of the common mucosal immune system as evidenced by the milk composition of lymphocytes derived from precursor immuno-competent cells present in breast-associated lymphoid tissue and gut-associated lymphoid tissue. Breast milk is a complex mixture of interacting compounds that differ in composition not only between women but also within the lactation period. It is a species specific product which contains proteins, non-protein nitrogen compounds, carbohydrates, lipids, minerals and vitamins. Many of the milk components are non-nutritive elements, designed particularly to support immune development, tolerance, and to regulate inflammation.'*

According to eminent immunologist Armand Goldman, the immune system in human milk, refined by evolution, forms the major basis for encouraging breastfeeding.[59] It consists of three overlapping groups of bioactive compounds: antimicrobials, anti-inflammatories and agents which modulate or regulate the immune response. It has four classes of immunoglobulins (IgA, IgM, IgG, IgD). Similar antibodies are found in other secretions, e.g. tears, saliva, the respiratory tract, the genito-urinary tract and the gut, but the star of the show is secretory immunoglobulin A (sIgA). During early infancy about 0.5 to 1.0g of secretory IgA (sIgA) is transferred daily to the infant by breastfeeding. By binding microorganisms sIgA is able to keep bacteria from attaching to mucous membranes and thereby invading tissues to cause infection. Infants fed human milk have increased concentrations in their urine. Secretory IgA antibodies are produced in the breast to protect the baby against gastrointestinal and respiratory pathogens, which migrate from cells in the small intestine (the enteromammary pathway) or the bronchial tree (the broncho-mammary pathway.)

The human baby is delayed in the production of immune factors and the mother's immune system is able to compensate for this vulnerability until the baby matures.[60] Protection against infections such as acute and prolonged diarrhoea, respiratory tract infections, otitis media, urinary tract infection, neonatal septicaemia and necrotising enterocolitis has been well documented.[61] Interestingly, there is also evidence for an enhanced protection for years after lactation against diarrhoea, respiratory tract infections and otitis media, *Haemophilus influenzae* type b infections and wheezing illness, and the longer a mother breastfeeds, the longer the protection lasts. Studies that show better vaccine responses among breastfed compared to non-breastfed infants show that factors in breastmilk stimulate the infant's own immune system to function more efficiently, and this protection may last for life. Such an enhanced function explains why breastfeeding is protective against autoimmune conditions like coeliac disease and allergy.

Breastmilk contains three million germ-killing cells per teaspoonful.[62] In some instances, the baby's mouth inoculates the breast, stimulating on-demand antibodies to a specific infection to which the baby has been exposed. When a baby suckles, a vacuum is created. Within that vacuum, the infant's saliva is sucked back into the mother's nipple, where receptors in her mammary gland read its signals. This 'baby spit backwash' is one of the ways that breastmilk adjusts its immunological composition.[63] When breastmilk mixes with baby saliva a chemical reaction happens that produces hydrogen peroxide and the combination produces a strong enough reaction to 'inhibit growth of the opportunistic pathogens *Staphylococcus aureus* and *Salmonella*',[64] also promoting the growth of beneficial bacteria. Lactocytes respond to saliva exposure by producing particular macrophages. If the baby has been exposed to an infection, at the next feeding they will receive leukocytes and antibodies to fight that specific infection.[65] Research from the Queensland University of Technology in Australia shows that the growth of some microbes is inhibited for up to 24 hours following breastmilk and saliva mixing. The interactions of these breastmilk components boost innate immunity by acting in synergy to regulate the oral microbiome of newborn babies.[66] Thus when the mother is exposed to pathogenic organisms, she will start to produce specific antibodies to those bacteria and pass them back to the baby in her milk.

Antibodies are present in human milk throughout lactation, so that there is no age at which they 'run out'; rather, a mother's body works to protect her baby-child from infections which they will meet in their day-to-day environment for as long as they receive any breastmilk at all.[67] Some immune factors actually increase in concentration as the baby gets older and nurses less. In other words, as the quantity of milk decreases during normal gradual weaning, the concentration of immunities increases (as in colostrum) – it depends on the amount of milk that a baby is removing from the breast rather than their age.[68] Even 5ml per day is valuable.[69] Expressed breastmilk can be used as eye drops to treat conjunctivitis, and for ear infections. Breastmilk contains neutrophils and stem cells, and a recent study with cerebral ultrasound suggested that intranasal application of breastmilk could have a beneficial effect on neurodevelopment in preterm infants who have experienced intraventricular haemorrhage (brain bleeds).[70]

When breastfed babies do fall prey to infections, the duration of illness is often shorter and the severity is decreased.[71] Breastfed babies are able to recover more quickly because the mother's body produces ideal nutrition and fluids as well as antibodies specific to the baby's infection. If a sick baby can have anything at all by mouth, it should be breastmilk. If a sick older baby with diarrhoea is receiving about 600ml per day of breastmilk then he may not also require oral rehydration therapy; in fact, feeding with water instead of with nutrient-rich breastmilk may lead to greater weight loss than is necessary.[72] It's hard to describe the relief of a mother with a sick baby or toddler who is still breastfeeding, in the knowledge that as they seek the comfort and solace of the breast more often because they are not well, she can also provide them with the best nutrition, continued fluids, and antibodies to their specific infection. Considering that diarrhoeal diseases and pneumonia are the greatest causes of infant mortality worldwide, and that breastfeeding is protective and therapeutic against both, it can be seen how very valuable breastfeeding is.

Enzymes, hormones, and multitasking protective components

According to a group of parents who set out to make a promotional video listing its components, as well as food for the baby, human milk contains hundreds to thousands of distinct bioactive molecules that protect against infection and inflammation and contribute to immune maturation, organ development and healthy microbial colonisation.[73]

Many host defence agents in human milk have more than one function. Secretory IgA, lactoferrin and lysozyme are examples. Lactoferrin, an iron-binding protein common to many external secretions, present in high concentrations in breastmilk, protects against certain viruses, and enhances the antimicrobial effects of other agents in breastmilk. Lactoferrin is not digested by the infant. A substantial proportion remains intact throughout the baby's gastrointestinal tract and some whole lactoferrin molecules and proteolytic fragments are absorbed and excreted into the baby's urine where they protect against urinary tract infections. Breastmilk also contains components such as glycoconjugates, glycosylated proteins and cytokines, phospholipids, glycolipids, and glycoproteins which multi-task.[60] Breastmilk also contains hormones, neuropeptides and growth factors that affect growth and self-regulation of food intake, e.g. leptin, which suppresses appetite, and ghrelin which stimulates it, the latter being found in higher concentrations in foremilk, the more watery milk at the beginning of a breastfeed. This concentration difference may also cause the breastfed baby to better self-regulate his intake compared to formula-fed infants, leading to lower rates of obesity.

There is a dizzying array of substances in breastmilk. Enzymes are species-specific and mother's milk also contains lysozyme, lipase, amylase, growth factors and hormones, epidermal growth factor, human milk growth factors, insulin-like growth factor, thyroxine and thyrotropin-releasing hormone, cholecystokinin, beta-endorphins, prostaglandins and taurine.[33] Human milk also contains key compounds such as erythropoietin, antioxidants, other bioactive factors and multiple cellular elements, with new components and interactions being discovered regularly.[16] Transforming growth factor β is a cytokine in human milk involved in maintaining intestinal homeostasis, inflammation regulation and oral tolerance development.[29]

In 1995 Sweden's Dr Catharina Swanborg discovered a substance in human milk called human α-lactalbumin made lethal to tumour cells (HAMLET), which killed bladder or colon cancer cells, two of the most common cancers in the world.[74] HAMLET is formed by two molecules naturally present in breastmilk. When extracted, subsequent trials have shown α-lactalbumin, the most common protein in human milk, to be effective against a variety of tumour cells without harming healthy cells.

Flavours

Breastmilk is a unique food that a mother produces for her individual baby. The flavours a mother offers to her baby through her milk are as diverse as her diet and the taste changes according to what she eats. This accustoms her breastfed baby to the kinds of foods that they will one day consume at her table. Maternal diet alters the aromatic profiles of mother's milk and early flavour experiences affect food preferences during weaning and childhood. We know that babies enjoy a variety of flavours. In addition, a breastfed baby experiences textural variations, such as viscosity and mouth coating, so 'breastfeeding provides an even richer variation in oral sensory stimulation'.[75,76] Unsurprisingly, one study found that babies like the taste of vanilla. More interestingly, if a mother eats garlic she will produce garlic-flavoured milk – not only will her baby enjoy the taste, but given the choice between garlic and plain, the baby will drink more of the garlic variety.[77]

Infant oral development

Breastfeeding is believed to have positive effects on the development of an infant's oral cavity, including improved shaping of the hard palate resulting in proper alignment of teeth and fewer problems with malocclusions.[78,79] An old New Zealand study found a distinct relationship between breastfeeding and clarity of speech, and a dramatic effect of breastfeeding on the development of speech and reading ability, especially in boys, suggesting that breastfeeding accelerates the rate of maturation in the male infant.[80]

Autism

A systematic review published in the December 2019 issue of the *Asian Journal of Psychiatry* reported on the role of breastfeeding status in autism spectrum disorder (ASD).[81] Nutritional status in newborns, and the duration of breastfeeding, plays a key role in the pathogenesis of ASD. Seven case-control studies were found in which the association between ever breastfeeding and risk was investigated. There was a 58% decrease with some breastfeeding and a 76% decrease with exclusive breastfeeding. Breastfeeding for six months was associated with a 54% reduction. Breastfeeding for 12–24 months was even more significant.

Stem cells in breastmilk

For several decades it has been known that stem cells were a part of mother's milk, capable of becoming any cell of the human body. Foteini Kakulas of the University of Western Australia describes how stem cells are able to cross the gut and migrate into the blood.[82] From the blood, they travel to various organs including the brain, where they turn into functioning cells. This is more than just a random event. The stem cells survive the neonatal gut, migrate into the blood and from there travel and integrate into various organs such as the thymus, liver, pancreas, spleen, kidneys and brain. In the brain they can be coaxed by specific brain micro-environmental cues to become specialised into the two main brain cell types: neurons and glia. What makes this finding all the more exciting is the presence of the blood-brain barrier, which only allows very selective cells to pass to and from the brain, due to the obvious need to protect this important organ. However, in the neonate this barrier is leaky, allowing more trafficking than we see in adults. This phenomenon of transfer and integration of foreign cells into an organism is called micro-chimerism. Chimerism has been previously demonstrated to occur reciprocally between the mother and the embryo during pregnancy, with embryonic cells found alive and integrated within the mother's brain and other organs many years after the birth of her child. In turn, maternal micro-chimerism, the transfer of maternal cells to the offspring, can happen not only *in utero,* but also during lactation. This had been previously shown for either immune-like cells of milk or indeterminate cells. Now, for the first time two independent groups have shown this for stem cells of breastmilk. The fact that chimeric cells persist in the offspring suggests that maternal micro-chimerism is not a random event, but rather a well-designed and specifically orchestrated integral characteristic of breastfeeding, aimed at boosting and multilaterally supporting the optimal development of the infant, to protect against infectious diseases.

This raises important questions about what happens to infants who are not breastfed or who are not fed fresh own mother's milk. What happens if vulnerable infants are deprived of breastmilk stem cells and immune cells, components that can potentially offer them a multitude of benefits, both developmentally and for their survival?

Cognitive development

There has always been controversy about whether it is breastmilk itself or the act of feeding at the breast which confers beneficial effects on breastfed babies, with some suggesting that those mothers most likely to breastfeed will have more intelligent babies anyway. Intriguingly, a recent study tested the hypothesis, and found that nutrients in breastmilk may improve general child cognition, but breastfeeding had a positive influence on memory.[83] In other words, babies bottle-fed breastmilk had better cognition than babies bottle-fed with formula. But babies who were nursed directly at the breast had better memory outcomes than either group. Furthermore, the benefits seem to last into adulthood; a Brazilian study looking at cognitive development, educational attainment and income tracked almost 3,500 participants for 30 years.[84] Adults who had been breastfed for 12 months or more as babies had 4-point higher IQ scores, one more year of education and higher monthly incomes than those who had been breastfed for less than one month. Higher IQ led to more education, which in turn was responsible for 72% of the effect on higher income at age 30.

Nutritional adequacy

George Kent, Professor Emeritus of Political Science at the University of Hawai'i, an expert on the human right to food, writes extensively about the differences between mother's milk and breastmilk substitutes. Citing a WABA document, '21 Dangers of Infant Formula',[85] he asks, 'Does infant formula do what it is supposed to do?'[86] George is able to show that there are serious risks to not breastfeeding, and they have been well documented. Even formula manufacturers recognise that at the population level, feeding with formula generally leads to worse health outcomes than breastfeeding for both mother and child, as demonstrated by many highly regarded studies.[87–99]

The list of formula ingredients specified in the global guidelines and in national law is described as *nutritionally adequate*. This is not good enough. The gold standard against which infant formula should be compared is not another formulation of a breastmilk substitute, but against optimal breastfeeding. The comparison should be based not on examination of formula's ingredients, but on examination of its performance. Does feeding with any particular type of infant formula protect the health of infants and their mothers as well as breastfeeding? If not, it is not *functionally adequate*. Some might argue that while infant formula is not quite as good as breastfeeding in protecting infants' health, it's not much worse. George contends that families might have their own reasons for feeding their infants with formula, but there is a need for serious discussion of the gap between breastfeeding and formula-feeding and of the degree to which considerations other than the infant's health might play a role.

Emotional benefits of breastfeeding for mother and baby

A 2009 Australian study involving over 7,000 mother-baby pairs that explored maternally perpetrated maltreatment of children discovered that breastfeeding was protective, particularly against neglect.[100] Substantiated child protection agency reports of 512 children showed that >60% experienced at least one episode of maternally perpetrated abuse or neglect and the risk of maternal maltreatment increased as breastfeeding duration decreased. Babies who had not been breastfed were almost five times more likely to have suffered maternal maltreatment than babies breastfed for at least four months.

The benefits of breastfeeding are threefold. As well as nutritional and immunological protection, there are also emotional advantages to both mother and baby which are less often mentioned. When a mother is breastfeeding her child many times a day there is a physical closeness which lets her know how her baby is feeling. Are they happy, playful, content? Are they hungry, tired, irritable, bored, frightened? Putting the baby to the breast will satisfy a hungry baby, comfort a distressed toddler, or send a grouchy pre-schooler off to sleep in minutes. Breastfeeding will calm a tantrum, and soothe a child in pain. Breastfeeding is quite literally the all-purpose mothering tool. A breastfeeding mother has the means to keep her child fed and well hydrated in an emergency. It is a huge comfort to a mother to have the means to keep her child happy and healthy wherever they are, particularly if they are sick or they are both living in challenging circumstances. Such competence builds a mother's self-confidence. Young children who are developing new skills, or who are coming down with a new infection, often seek more frequent solace at the breast and a mother can follow her baby's lead knowing that breastfeeding is always an appropriate response. It's been said that a mother doesn't need to count how often she breastfeeds her child any more than she needs to count how often she kisses them. What she finds herself doing almost by instinct is underwritten by real hormonal and physiological responses. In spite of magazine articles and social media blogs urging mothers not to spoil their babies, and to allow themselves enough 'me-time', Julie Smith, the Australian researcher who looks at the economic value of breastfeeding, found that although time spent with a baby when a mother is breastfeeding exceeds time spent by formula-feeding mothers, this is clearly advantageous to both members of the dyad.[101]

The effects of oxytocin

For women, two of the major hormonal influences during breastfeeding are oxytocin and prolactin. Oxytocin is a hormone produced by the posterior pituitary gland. Oxytocin release assists in delivery of the placenta after the birth of the baby, and works to minimise postpartum bleeding,[102] which is one reason why breastfeeding is recommended from birth.[103] Oxytocin acts on muscles called myoepithelial cells surrounding the milk-producing cells within her breasts, to cause contractions known as the milk ejection reflex (MER), making milk available to the baby. Oxytocin also causes the uterus to contract, so that in the early postpartum period it returns to its pre-pregnancy size and shape more quickly and this in turn minimises blood loss, protecting a new mother's iron levels. The let-down reflex becomes well established within two or three days of birth and once it has become conditioned to respond to the baby, it is almost impossible to disturb, notwithstanding the popular myth that an emotional shock will cause a woman to 'lose' her milk.

Each MER causes fat droplets to be squeezed into the milk, making the milk more creamy the longer the baby feeds. Oxytocin causes the mother to feel thirsty as her milk lets down so that she replaces her fluids ready to synthesise more breastmilk for later. It enhances her enjoyment of the baby and her feelings of protection and closeness to them, and finally it makes her feel sleepy so that after breastfeeding she is able to rest more easily. Contrary to popular belief, breastfeeding mothers not only get more sleep than mothers who formula feed, but they also feel happier and are protected from depression. Oxytocin plays no small part in these outcomes.[104]

Often called 'the love hormone', or 'the mothering hormone', oxytocin is responsible for many feel-good emotions. Released by both men and women in response to touch, during eating and other pleasurable activities, oxytocin is important to social relationships, bonding, trust and love, and is the hormone responsible for orgasm and closeness between lovers. While oxytocin lowers stress and blood pressure, increasing relaxation, it enhances maternal protective behaviour.[105] It appears in the brain as a neurotransmitter, or signalling substance, working through a large network of nerves that connect with many different areas of that organ. Oxytocin is thus able to influence many vital operations in the body. The same brain and nervous system that produce the fight or flight mechanism sometimes generate entirely opposite responses when oxytocin is involved.[106]

Oxytocin released in babies and young children during pleasurable experiences increases the number of oxytocin receptors in the brain, particularly in the first three years of life, and enables them to better cope with stress when they are older. Maternal care changes the activity of a gene that regulates the baby's physiological response to stress, specifically release of the hormone cortisol. Breastfeeding causes decreased DNA methylation and decreased cortisol reactivity in infants. In other words, there is an epigenetic change in babies who are breastfed, resulting in reduced stress compared to those who are not.[107]

The effects of prolactin

The other hormone crucial to lactation, released by the anterior pituitary, is prolactin. Secreted in response to nipple stimulation during breastfeeding, prolactin causes more milk to be made ready for the next breastfeed. Prolactin is also the hormone that we all make to help us cope with stress, and in fact many anti-depressants work by increasing prolactin levels. Not surprisingly, several of these drugs (metaclopramide, chlorpromazine, domperidone, sulpiride) also act as galactogogues (drugs which increase breastmilk production). Prolactin produced in response to infant suckling helps mothers to feel calm. For mothers who elect not to breastfeed, and in the absence of breast drainage (either by the baby, by pump or by manual expression of breastmilk), prolactin levels will plummet. In physiological terms, the mother's body acts as if the baby has died. The grief that many women experience when their nursling is finally weaned from the breast is often unacknowledged, but it is nevertheless very real, and may have an hormonal basis.[108] Mothers who plan to breastfeed, and fulfil their ambitions, have a reduced risk of postpartum depression, compared to mothers who plan to breastfeed but do not succeed.[109] Kathleen Kendall-Tackett, who has been studying the effects of breastfeeding on maternal mental health for over 20 years, maintains that, *'Breastfeeding does not deplete mothers, nor does it cause depression. Breastfeeding problems certainly can do both of these things – all the more reason why women need good support and accurate information. But it doesn't make sense for something so critical to the survival of our species to be harmful for mothers. And it is not.'* [110]

Extended breastfeeding

Breastfeeding is often described as being 'extended' if it lasts beyond the first 6–12 months, in spite of the recommendation by the World Health Organization that continued partial breastfeeding should be practised for up to two years or beyond. In an Information Note released by the UNICEF Baby Friendly Initiative in December 2018, the World Health Organization highlights the importance of safeguarding breastfeeding for children up to three years of age.[111,112] Breastfeeding beyond 12 months has a profoundly positive impact on infant and maternal health:

- Children who are not breastfed from 12–23 months of age are about twice as likely to die as those who are breastfed in the second year of life
- Breastfeeding for more than 12 months reduces breast cancer by 26%
- Breastfeeding longer than 12 months reduces in ovarian cancer by 37%
- In a large study among low-income children in the United States, those breastfed for at least 12 months were 28% less likely to be overweight at four years of age than those never breastfed
- In a meta-analysis of 17 studies conducted in seven countries, each additional month of breastfeeding reduced the risk of childhood obesity by 4%
- Each additional year of lifetime duration of breastfeeding is associated with a 9% protection against type 2 diabetes.

We need to recognise that breastfeeding might permanently shape an individual's life course. Prolonged breastfeeding appears to have an impact on factors associated with modulation of the immune system as well as metabolic programming. Matylda Czosnykowska-Lukacka, writing about macronutrient components in prolonged lactation for healthy mothers from the first to the 48th month after birth, confirms that the concentrations of proteins, carbohydrates and lipids change during lactation stages.[113] The variability of the macronutrient content of human milk is very wide. Its composition is specifically tailored by each mother to precisely reflect the requirements of her infant. Fat and protein content increase after 18 months, and carbohydrates decrease significantly compared with the milk of women with babies up to 12 months of age. Macronutrient concentrations remain at a stable level from the 24th to the 48th month, but are correlated with the amount of feeding. While carbohydrates play a greater role in infant nutrition in the early stage, the source of calories in breastmilk for older children is mainly fat, no doubt an adaptation to the increased energy demand of the intensively growing child. Furthermore, the baby is able to tailor some of the components of mother's milk according to specific need. Girl babies get more fat, boy babies get more salts. The difference in the milk components may reflect the differences in metabolic substrate needed for optimal growth and development in female and male infants, with boys, and especially first-born boys, getting milk which is much higher in fat and protein.[114]

Mothers in tribes that still follow infant feeding patterns practised by our ancient ancestors, such as the !Kung hunter-gatherers of the Kalahari, usually feed their babies roughly four times an hour for 2–3 minutes each time.[115] Thus the infant is comforted and nourished by almost constant food and body contact. Short feeding intervals with continuing elevated prolactin levels inhibit maternal ovulation, ensuring that the next baby will not be born before the nursling is weaned. For the !Kung this is normally at about four years of age. So while a newborn assures his own future milk supply, so too the breastfeeding toddler, if permitted to breastfeed until they outgrow the need, assures their own ideal birth spacing, which assures them, as well as the younger sibling, an improved chance of survival.

Breastmilk for preterm babies

Breastmilk is the source of many unique and dynamic bioactive components that play a key role in the development of the immune system and could be especially important for very vulnerable premature infants. These include essential microbes, human milk oligosaccharides (HMOs), immunoglobulins, lactoferrin and dietary polyunsaturated fatty acids. These components all interact with intestinal commensal bacteria and/or immune cells to play a critical role in establishment of the intestinal microbiome and ultimately influence intestinal inflammation and gut health during early life.[116] Exposure to breastmilk has been associated with a decreased incidence and severity of necrotising enterocolitis (NEC), a devastating disease which can affect up to 10% of pre-term non-breastfed infants.[117] NEC is characterised by overwhelming intestinal inflammation, and breastmilk is protective against NEC in a dose-dependent manner. The intestine, which plays a critical role in the overall inflammatory response, is the largest immune organ in the body and, due to its large surface area, has the greatest exposure to the outside environment. The newborn intestine is equipped with all the basic functional structures, but is immature. In order to fully mature, it undergoes rapid mucosal differentiation and development with exposure to enteral nutrition, namely human breastmilk containing maternal passive antibodies, especially secretory immunoglobulin A (sIgA) in the first weeks of life. It has its own unique microbiome, providing 25% of a breastfed infant's intestinal microbiota by one month of age as a result of exposing the infant to over 700 species of bacteria daily. The interaction among the intestinal microbiota, human milk oligosaccharides, immunological factors and metabolic components fosters optimal intestinal biology and a healthy functioning gastrointestinal tract, free of overt inflammation and infection. For breastmilk-fed infants, additional inflammatory regulation is not only protective in the preterm period, but also likely has implications in decreasing the risk of acquiring long-term chronic inflammatory illnesses. Emerging evidence suggests that providing human milk is crucial to optimising both short-term and long-term health outcomes for newborns.

As an IBCLC who often worked with mothers and their pre-term infants in Harare, I had never heard of a case of NEC. In the neonatal intensive care units, babies were fed exclusively with their own mother's milk. Infant formula was sometimes used in tiny quantities in the first two days of life if the babies needed more milk than their mothers could yet express, but it was quickly phased out as mothers' milk increased in quantity. The use of so-called human milk fortifier (a commercially manufactured cows' milk product marketed to boost the calorie content of human milk for pre-term infants and containing additional micronutrients) was unknown. The quantity of breastmilk feeds was tailored to the age and condition of each baby, but once a baby was stable, and simply waiting to grow bigger before being allowed home, the paediatricians would authorise them to receive up to 300ml/kg/day of breastmilk. Babies on this regimen would gain up to 75g/day. They were discharged home at 34 weeks corrected gestational age, or when they weighed 1,800g and were gaining at least 30g/day on exclusive breastfeeding. They received needed iron, vitamin D and calcium as additional separate medications, but no formula or fortifier.

Formula mishaps

Occasionally mishaps and mistakes which harm formula-fed infants are reported. There are cases of contamination, mistakes in mixing, and findings that formula contains larvae, worms or foreign bodies. One of the largest disasters, reported in the *Lancet* in 2009, happened in China.[118] Mothers unwittingly fed their babies infant formula that was contaminated by a potentially toxic chemical, melamine. The toxic effects included obstructive uropathy and acute renal failure, resulting in more than 50,000 babies being admitted to hospital. The epidemic spread to neighbouring countries in south-east Asia, and melamine was detected in formula milks in the USA and South Africa, but the full extent of the calamity may never be known. Professor Anna Coutsoudis, author of a *Lancet* article, asked why formula milk was being so widely used, and breastfeeding avoided? Although breastmilk is well known to be economically and physiologically crucial to child survival, voracious global marketing by the formula milk industry over the past 60 years has methodically dislodged breastfeeding as a viable and desirable strategy for infant feeding.

The 'Voldemort effect'

In 2008, Julie Patricia Smith and two colleagues examined journal titles and abstracts to see if they accurately convey findings on differential health outcomes between breastfed and formula-fed infants.[119] They found that in 30% of cases, titles imply misleadingly that breastfeeding raises health risk. Examples include:

> *'Breastmilk and Neonatal Necrotising Enterocolitis'*
> *'Breast Feeding and the Sudden Infant Death Syndrome in Scandinavia'*
> *'Breastfeeding and Childhood Obesity'*
> *'Breastfeeding and the Risk of Postneonatal Death in the United States'*

This skewed terminology reduces health professionals' knowledge and support for breastfeeding and normalises bottle-feeding, and these attitudes are in turn communicated to mothers. In an analysis of the titles and abstracts of 78 studies reporting poorer health among formula-fed infants, Julie Smith examined whether formula feeding is actually 'named' as the risk factor in published research, or whether – like 'Voldemort' in *Harry Potter* – it is 'He Who Shall Not Be Named'.

Patents

The value of breastmilk's individual components has been receiving increasing attention from the formula industry over the last several decades. Valerie McClain, a well-known blogger in the lactation world, has uncovered some 2,000 patents and applications in the US Patent & Trademark Office taken out on the components of human milk.[120] Her investigations make morbidly fascinating reading. In 2001, she wrote that the human milk fat globule was being used to help produce monoclonal antibodies, a multibillion dollar industry, and that human milk components would have a huge potential in the healthcare industry, involving billions of dollars in profit for those who hold the patents.[121] Writing in May 2020,[122] Valerie sets out informaton on Patent #7893041, 'Oligosaccharide compositions and use thereof in the treatment of infection':[123]

> *'Consumption of human milk is one of the most cost-effective strategies known to medicine for protecting infants against morbidity and mortality due to infectious disease. Human milk may be considered a natural and efficacious 'nutriceutical', i.e., a model food that conveys immunologic benefits. Protection against infectious diseases occurs through a variety of complementary mechanisms found in human milk, including oligosaccharides and their related glycoconjugates. Significantly enhanced immunologic protection by breastfeeding has been demonstrated for diarrheal diseases, respiratory tract illnesses, bacteremia, meningitis, and necrotizing enterocolitis. Protection by breastfeeding is especially efficacious against diarrheal disease.'*

While most of the patents are geared toward the genetic engineering of human milk components, there are a few that propose use of the real thing. Are the scientists or companies registering the patents trying to create a monopoly on human milk? A number are owned by Abbott, which uses human milk oligosaccharides (HMOs) to improve its product.[124] This begs the question, will patenting, with its need for profits and monopoly, result in more or less encouragement, protection and promotion of breastfeeding? Way back in 2001 Valerie wrote, 'It is ironic but not surprising that it is the infant formula and drug industry, who have so much faith in human milk that they are willing to patent its properties. This patenting can only be detrimental to the understanding, promotion, support, and encouragement of breastfeeding.'

Melissa Bartick, who comments on the risks of not breastfeeding for women, writes in a recent blog:[125]

> *'The biggest recent application has been the synthesis of HMOs, which have been patented and added to formula, now for sale on supermarket shelves where they cost at least 30%*

> *more than formulas without HMOs. It is unclear if these products are actually better for babies, even though they might technically resemble human milk slightly more than formula without HMOs. But given that genuine mother's milk has unique HMOs for a unique infant, it's unclear which HMOs a manufacturer should even be adding to a formula. So, is this product actually better, or is this just a marketing ploy and an excuse to mark up the price?... No company can provide a mother's own living cells, her unique antibodies, or the change between the watery foremilk and creamy hindmilk during the course of a feed. And nothing on a shelf can substitute for the act of breastfeeding itself. No improvements in infant formula are likely to approach the differences in childhood health outcomes seen with breastfeeding. Finally, even if it were possible to create the perfect infant formula that mimicked mother's milk, that would still have no impact on maternal health due to breastfeeding, in terms of lowering the risk of maternal diabetes, cardiovascular disease, breast and ovarian cancer. And nothing on a shelf would substitute the experience of breastfeeding for mother and child.'*

Also of interest to those registering patents on the components of human milk is the human milk fat globule membrane (HMFGM), a structure of lipids and proteins that surround the milk fat globule made in the milk producing cells.[126] Milk fat globule membrane proteins are known to be a source of multiple bioactive compounds including phospholipids, glycolipids, glycoproteins and carbohydrates that are important to the health of the brain and gut. Almost half of these proteins have trafficking or cell signalling functions to influence circulating lipid levels later in life. These components have been repeatedly targeted by the formula industry and prominent researchers due to the reported beneficial effects on cognition, behaviour, gut and bacterial composition, fever incidence, diarrhoea and otitis media, cardiovascular health, regulation of cholesterol uptake and reduction in blood pressure. Ironically, a lot of money is being spent on trying to make infant formula more like breastmilk. But although mothers themselves produce the real thing, breastfeeding rates are falling.

The value of human milk is often unacknowledged. Julie Smith, the Australian researcher cited above, who is an expert on the economic value of breastmilk, has been working on having breastmilk included in the gross domestic product (GDP).[127] She writes that the production of breastmilk is a major investment in healthcare, nutrition and nurture, as well as lifetime risk reduction in health and education. It doesn't require plastic and doesn't make waste. Julie's research on the Australian Time Use Survey of New Mothers found that having an infant added 44 hours a week to a woman's unpaid workload and exclusive breastfeeding took 17–20 hours of mothers' time. Her value estimate of this annual food production is AU$2.1 billion per year. The GDP loves breasts when they are part of the vast international market for pornography, but apparently doesn't count them in relation to food production. Milk from sheep, goats, cows and buffalo appears in national accounts, but not women's milk. There are markets for breastmilk bags, bottles, storage cups, containers for freezing expressed milk, and lots of advice on expressing milk, storing milk, or reusing frozen milk. Some websites offer it for sale, and some as a free donation. But human milk currently has no value in the GDP. Food for thought!

When breastfeeding is not the norm

At the turn of the millennium, 92.5% of babies were born in the global south, where breastfeeding was the cultural norm. Which means that only 7.5% of babies were born into countries where bottle-feeding was seen as usual.[128]

The United Kingdom has the dubious distinction of having the very lowest breastfeeding rates in the world. Four out of five British mothers start off breastfeeding, but only one in 100 babies is exclusively breastfed for the recommended duration of six months, and only one in 200 is receiving any breastmilk at one year.[129] Furthermore, within the UK it is low-income mothers who breastfeed least.[130]

In the bottle-feeding cultures of the global north, many reasons are given for not breastfeeding. But only one in 1,000 mothers does not lactate following the birth of her baby.[1] For bottle-feeding to become popular, it needs only two pre-conditions: formula must be both socially acceptable and easily accessible. Due to tepid government support for breastfeeding, both have existed for many years in the resource-rich settings which set infant feeding trends. Low-income mothers, whose babies are likely to battle poverty and deprivation all their lives and most need the health and cognitive advantages conferred by breastmilk, receive free formula through the government Healthy Start voucher scheme in the UK[131] or the WIC Program in the USA.[132] Nurseries and crèches in the UK that look after babies of working mothers can feed them free formula through the Nursery Milk Scheme.[133] At the same time past government austerity measures have led to funding cuts to breastfeeding support groups, and suspension of monitoring of national breastfeeding rates, while healthcare personnel receive inadequate training to assist mothers to breastfeed and professional associations, including the Royal College of Paediatrics and Child Health, and the Royal College of Midwives, have a long history of accepting funding from formula milk companies.[134,135]

The high-income countries of the global north, with their low breastfeeding rates, are the trend-setters of tomorrow. Viewed as the most progressive and up-to-date nations, protecting babies' health and acting as the gatekeepers of women's aspirations and human rights, these are the countries most likely to have influence over global health policy.[136] And while the British healthcare system is held in such high regard and British hospitals help to train overseas medical personnel, these kinds of attitudes and the normalisation of formula-feeding have been exported to the global south where they can do untold damage.

Formula marketing is widespread and uses powerful emotional techniques to sell a product that is vastly inferior to breastmilk.[137] The formula industry is dominated by a small number of extremely powerful multinational corporations with the resources to buy the best global marketing expertise. Like all corporations they are governed by the fiduciary imperative, which puts the pursuit of profits ahead of all other concerns. This mix of fiscal power, sophisticated marketing and single-mindedness is causing great harm to public health. The campaigns use emotional appeals to reach out to mothers and build relationships with them. Evocative brands give their overtures a human face. The advent of social media has made it easier to pose as the friend and supporter of parents; it is also providing companies with a rich stream of personal data with which they hone and target their campaigns. Worldwide, breastfeeding rates continue to drop.

James Akre, long-time breastfeeding advocate, who worked for 30 years at the World Health Organization, listed the increased risks to infant and maternal health of not breastfeeding:[138]

For *children*, increased risk of:

Asthma
Behavioural or mental health problems
Cardiovascular disease in later life
Cognitive and visual development
Child mortality
Celiac disease
Cholesterol concentrations elevated
Crohn's disease
Delayed development
Diabetes
Diarrhoeal disease
Hypertension
Leukaemia
Lung function reduced
Metabolism impaired
Necrotising enterocolitis
Obesity greater risk
Otitis media (ear infection)
Pathogens in the gastrointestinal tract
Respiratory ailments
Sepsis in very low birth weight infants increased risk
SIDS rates increased
Urinary tract disease increased risk

For *mothers*, increased risk of:

Breast cancer
Birth spacing shortened
Child neglect/maltreatment
Diabetes
Gallbladder disease
Haemorrhage
Hypertension increased
Myocardial infarction (middle to late adulthood)
Osteoporosis and hip fractures
Uterine cancer
Weight retention
Rheumatoid arthritis
Multiple sclerosis, postpartum relapses

Source: James Akre, 2009

The cost of not breastfeeding

It takes 20kg of powdered infant formula to bottle-feed one baby for the first six months of life.[139] In England, excluding the price of bottles and sterilising equipment, the cost of feeding a typical 2–3 month old infant artificial baby milk varies from £1 to £4 per day.[140] But the cost to the NHS every year of treating just five illnesses linked to *not* breastfeeding, i.e. ear, chest, gut infections (including those in premature babies) and breast cancer in adult women is at least £48 million.[141] If only 45% of mothers breastfed their babies at four months, the UK could save nearly £22 million.[38]

When formula-feeding is seen to be perfectly normal, concerns about maternal guilt frequently prevent information about the negative consequences of not breastfeeding from being articulated. Since the 1970s, increasingly rigorous and positive research findings have led to the rediscovery of breastfeeding as a valid and evidence-based health intervention for infants. A clear pattern of positive improved short and long-term health outcomes for mothers is also being identified.[142] In general, there's a dose response in health risks due to not breastfeeding; the younger the baby, the greater the negative health outcomes with no breastfeeding at all, and gradually improving outcomes proportional to the duration and exclusivity of breastfeeding.[143]

There have been several modelling exercises conducted to estimate the cost of not breastfeeding in terms of maternal and infant health and the increased rates of morbidity and mortality to the US economy:

- In 2002 the cost of breast cancer, hypertension and heart attack for two million women aged 15–70 due to suboptimal breastfeeding was estimated to be $17.4 billion for deaths and $734 million in extra illness.[144]
- In 2005, if 90% of American mothers could have been encouraged to breastfeed their babies, over 900 deaths would have been avoided or reduced due to necrotising enterocolitis, otitis media, gastroenteritis, lower respiratory tract infections, eczema, asthma, sudden infant death syndrome, leukaemia, type 1 diabetes and obesity, saving $13 billion.[86]
- In 2012, suboptimal breastfeeding and health outcomes were estimated for nine paediatric and five maternal diseases. Once again, if 90% of infants had been breastfed according to medical recommendations, 3,340 deaths would have been avoided, 78% of them in mothers due to nearly 1,000 heart attacks, and over 800 cases of breast cancer and diabetes. There were over 700 excess deaths in babies, with nearly 500 due to sudden infant death syndrome and nearly 200 due to necrotising enterocolitis. Medical costs were $3.0 billion for mothers. The cost of premature death was over $14 billion. For every 597 women who optimally breastfeed, one maternal or child death is prevented.[87]
- Breastfeeding has a protective effect against Alzheimer's disease in later life. Women who breastfed had a 64% reduced risk compared with women who did not breastfeed at all. Breastfeeding for a year had a 78% reduced risk compared to breastfeeding for only four months. It was hypothesised that ovarian hormone deprivation and/or insulin sensitivity benefits were responsible for the reduced risk.[145]

Formula-fed babies experience higher morbidity and mortality wherever they are born, costing the global economy over US $300 billion every year.[146] The importance of breastfeeding is well set out in two sets of articles published in the *Lancet* in 2016[94] and 2018.[146] Increasing breastfeeding to near-universal levels for infants and young children could save over 800,000 children's lives a year worldwide, equivalent to 13% of all deaths in children under two. Low breastfeeding rates are attributable primarily to poor policymaking, lack of investment, low levels of community support and education, and aggressive marketing of formula. Contrary to the popular narrative of there being 'too much pressure to breastfeed', the real picture of breastfeeding is one of reproductive disruption and insurmountable barriers preventing women from being able to attain biological norms in caring for their infants.

These kinds of results translate to wide, far-reaching implications for society in terms of health and economic costs. In global terms, the costs of not breastfeeding are substantial. Breastfeeding is estimated to prevent almost 100,000 deaths from breast and ovarian cancer and type 2 diabetes in women each year. The economic losses of premature child and women's mortality are estimated to cost US $53.7 billion. However the largest economic loss is cognitive loss, estimated to equal US $285.4 billion annually. Aggregating these costs, the total global economic losses are estimated to be 0.70% of global gross national income.[147]

Breastfeeding is vital where there are few social safety nets

It's not hard to see that if there are such important implications due to breastfeeding for the babies of mothers in the industrialised western world, how much more vital it is that babies in resource-poor settings continue to breastfeed in the age-old way that has maximised child survival since humankind first walked out of the Rift Valley. Only easy access to good medical care, hospitals and antibiotics to treat the greater number of infections experienced by formula-fed babies make it possible for a mother living in the industrialised world to have her infant survive if she does not breastfeed.[26] In parts of the world where these social safety nets are not available, mothers who do not breastfeed put their infants' survival in jeopardy. Policies exported from the West, encouraging mothers to abandon breastfeeding, have a lot to answer for.

Fortunately, the taboos, social stigma and negative traditional beliefs surrounding failure to breastfeed in low-income countries help to ensure infant and young child survival. To have many children and to be seen to successfully breastfeed them demonstrates that a woman is a good wife and mother and elevates her position in society. Far from being characterised as a burden which ties her down, or violates her rights to bodily integrity (as it is often portrayed in the West), breastfeeding is seen as both a duty and a privilege.

Thus in 1985, when breastfeeding was shown to be a vector of HIV-transmission to the next generation, it was immediately recognised that the implications would be very grave indeed.

When UNICEF and WHO sought to impose a policy of informed infant feeding choice on HIV-positive mothers living in resource-poor settings, those who were being targeted for replacement feeding of their babies did not have access to the research so they were never able to provide informed consent. But the international agencies knew the risks of not breastfeeding. What were they thinking? The influences behind development of the 1997 international policy on HIV and infant feeding to move mothers away from breastfeeding, using a rights-based approach, will be explored in Chapter 12.

'Lactation is an ancient physiological process, dating back almost 200 million years. Human lactation and human milk have evolved to meet the needs and address the vulnerabilities of the human young. Milk intended for a four-legged, cud-chewing, nonverbal species may cause human infants to grow, but their growth and development will take a different trajectory than that of their breastfed counterparts. Infant formula

and human milk components are not interchangeable. Artificial diets are not the same as human milk. The immuno-nutrition provided by human milk has no equal.'

Marsha Walker, 2014[148]

CHAPTER 7

HIV in breastmilk

The virus that led to development of AIDS was first found in specimens of cell-free breastmilk in 1985.[1,2] In 1988 it was detected by electron microscope, which further supported the hypothesis that breastmilk could carry the virus.[3]

Much of the very early research on HIV in breastmilk was conducted at the University of Nairobi in Kenya by expatriate researchers and former Kenyan students who had studied and qualified at overseas universities. The first study began in 1986,[4] the year after the first *Lancet* report appeared showing that HIV could be passed through breastfeeding. Financial assistance for the early work was received from several national research groups in Canada, the National Institutes of Health in the US and the European Community in Brussels. The Nairobi group was headed by Dr Ruth Nduati. Other members included Peter Piot, Marleen Temmerman, Grace John, Paul Lewis, Julie Overbaugh, Barbara Richardson, Joan Kreiss, Pratibha Datta, Joanne Embree, Dorothy Mbori-Ngacha and others. The group also had close links to the University of Washington in Seattle, where Ruth Nduati had studied and met Peter Piot, who subsequently also spent time at the University of Nairobi. The Nairobi group was hugely influential in the AIDS community. Peter Piot was appointed the first Director of UNAIDS in 1994 and Ruth Nduati went on to write the first background document which underpinned the 1996–97 WHO change in policy on HIV and breastfeeding (explored in Chapter 12).

In 2003, Barbara Richardson and colleagues in the Nairobi group reached the startling conclusion that the probability of infection per litre of breastmilk ingested by the baby of an HIV-infected mother is equivalent to the amount of virus passed in one act of unprotected sex.[5] Richardson found that the probability of infection was .00064 per litre of breastmilk, or .00028 per day of breastfeeding (vs .0003–.0015 per sex act). While this seemed alarming, to put it in perspective, it would actually correspond to approximately one infection per 1,500 litres of breastmilk ingested. The average baby consumes roughly 750–900ml of breastmilk per day, so this would be the amount of milk consumed by one baby in about five years.

In 1992, WHO had recommended that HIV-positive mothers in developing countries should continue to breastfeed their babies because the risk of death due to breastfeeding was likely to be less than the risk of death when breastfeeding was withheld.[6] However, when bottle-feeding of formula in the West seemed like such an easy solution, HIV clinicians were not persuaded and more research showing the risks of breastfeeding continued to be published.

Breastfeeding as a risk factor for MTCT

- A 1993 paper found HIV-infected cells in breastmilk at 15 days postpartum; a defective maternal IgM response was the strongest predictor of infection of the infant.[7] After ingestion of virus in breastmilk, infant gut mucosal surfaces were the most likely site of transmission.
- In research published in 1994 to see whether cell-free virus could traverse intact neonatal mucosal surfaces, researchers administered simian immunodeficiency virus (SIV) to four rhesus monkey neonates within an hour of caesarean section delivery, thus ruling out the possibility of infection occurring during labour and delivery. They found that the monkeys could be infected orally and that tonsillar cells were capable of viral replication.[8] All neonates developed viraemia and subsequently tested HIV positive.
- In 1995, an analysis to define the prevalence, concentration and determinants of virus-infected cells (HIV DNA) in breastmilk from which the lipid layer had been removed (which inhibited antiviral activity) found that during the first few days of life an infant would ingest a daily dose of 25,000 HIV-infected cells, and at six months 24,000 HIV-infected cells per day. Researchers asserted that 'there is compelling evidence that breastfeeding contributes substantially to vertical transmission'.[9]
- The concentration of virus in breastmilk was considerably lower than in blood. If no antiretroviral drugs were used, the plasma of most HIV-infected individuals contains 10,000–1,000,000 copies of HIV/ml.[10] Although breastmilk samples contained only 240–8,100 copies/ml,[11] the baby would consume a large volume every day.
- Even though technically it was impossible to distinguish transmission occurring during labour and birth from transmission occurring a day or two later, one paper said that 'colostrum would provide an effective route for transmission of HIV'.[12] Another suggested that viral shedding in mature milk does not support of the concept of withholding colostrum from infants;[10] there would be no point – although almost 40% of cell-free breastmilk specimens contained HIV RNA, prevalence did not decrease as the milk supply matured.
- Procedures which could cause damage or lesions in the infant's mouth, e.g. oral suction, or frenulotomy of the baby's tongue, should be identified as factors which could increase transmission risk, by allowing contact between virus in breastmilk and the infant's bloodstream.[13,14]
- While studying the relationship between viral shedding of HIV in the cervix, vagina and in breastmilk, Grace John suggested that simultaneous shedding from multiple sites may be due to a high total virus burden.[15]

Cell-associated vs cell-free virus

There was a lot of research looking at the likely infectivity of cell-associated HIV compared to cell-free HIV, a lot of it conflicting:

> *Cell-associated virus* refers to HIV which lives inside the cell, measured as HIV DNA
>
> *Cell-free virus* refers to parts of the virus (virions) not associated with a cell, measured as HIV RNA

- There was a strong correlation between maternal immunosuppression (CD4 cell count <400/ml^3) and prevalence and quantity of breastmilk HIV DNA. Above-average viral load in plasma meant a 2–4-fold increased risk of viral shedding in blood, genital secretions and breastmilk, leading to a higher risk of infecting the baby by all routes, including breastfeeding.[16,17]
- In a Ugandan study detection of HIV-infected cells in breastmilk was *not* associated with transmission. Although 80% of transmitting mothers had detectable virus in their breastmilk, so too did 72% of non-transmitting mothers; the presence of HIV DNA in the cells of breastmilk did not result in increased late breastmilk transmission.[18]
- Cell-free and cell-associated virus varied in their prediction of HIV transmission at early and late lactation stages.[19] High levels of cell-free virus in maternal plasma and breastmilk led to a high risk of HIV transmission during breastfeeding, *and* with cell-associated virus in breastmilk, suggesting that both cell-free and cell-associated virus were involved.[20]
- A South African group, which included the highly respected researchers Anna Coutsoudis and Nigel Rollins, quantified the relationship between HIV RNA shedding in breastmilk, cumulative RNA exposure, and postnatal transmission, relating timing of infection in the infant to estimated total volume of milk exposure.[21] Cumulative exposure to RNA particles in breastmilk significantly increased the risk of HIV acquisition postnatally, independently from maternal antenatal CD4 cell count, plasma HIV load, and duration of breastfeeding.
- Previous research had shown that while ART leads to undetectable levels of cell-free virus in breastmilk, cell-associated virus was still detected.[22,23] Cell-associated virus per ml was more important than cell-free virus for early postpartum transmission at six weeks. Each 10-fold increase was significantly associated with transmission. However, at six months, cell-free rather than cell-associated virus posed the higher risk.[24]
- Certain factors in breastmilk blocked the transmission of HIV from mother to child during breastfeeding when the virus was outside of cells, but had little effect on the transmission of the virus once it had entered them.[25] However, the inhibitory effect on cell-free virus was lost during extended culture, while the effect on cell-associated virus was not. Antiretroviral therapy (ART) made no difference to virus in cell-associated milk and direct co-culture of HIV-infected CD4 T-lymphocytes with susceptible target cells revealed that breastmilk was ineffective at blocking cell-associated HIV infection.

Early findings on the effects of ART on virus in breastmilk

- Single-dose nevirapine reduced intrapartum transmission of HIV but also selected for non-nucleoside reverse-transcriptase inhibitor (NNRTI) resistance in breastmilk and plasma.[26] Median eight-week breastmilk RNA levels were half the level identified in plasma. Breastmilk samples from women with laboratory-diagnosed mastitis were >5 times more likely to have HIV RNA levels above the median.
- HIV persisted in breastmilk cells despite ART to prevent MTCT.[27] Cell-associated HIV RNA levels in breastmilk were suppressed by antiretroviral regimens used to prevent MTCT. However, even with HAART, there was no significant reduction in the reservoir of infected cells, which could contribute to breastmilk HIV-transmission.
- Women randomised to receive highly active ART (HAART) vs zidovudine/nevirapine[28] had similar prevalence of undetectable breastmilk HIV RNA 3–14 days after birth. But from 15–28 days afterwards, women in the HAART arm had significantly lower levels of breastmilk HIV RNA than women randomised to ZDV/NVP. HAART resulted in lower breastmilk HIV RNA than ZDV/NVP; however, ZDV/NVP yielded comparable breastmilk HIV RNA levels in the first two weeks post-partum. Breastmilk HIV RNA remained suppressed in the ZDV/NVP arm despite increased plasma HIV levels, which might reflect local drug effects or compartmentalisation.

Finding HIV in breastmilk

In the quest for answers about HIV in breastmilk, and HIV transmission through breastfeeding, there's a confusing amount of research containing often conflicting results. It's always wise to read the fine print. How was a particular piece of research done: do the researchers appear to be familiar with ordinary, common-or-garden, day-to-day lactation management techniques; do the results seem plausible? Have the breastmilk samples been stored or prepared in a particular way so as to conserve their anti-infective properties? Several researchers have battled with identifying the virus in breastmilk because of its intrinsic properties, which destroy HIV. These questions will be further explored in Chapter 10.

When research reports that breastfeeding posed a risk of HIV-transmission for a particular population of babies, it can be important to note how 'breastfeeding' was defined. Was mixed feeding common in this population of babies? Did mixed feeding affect breast fullness and thus viral levels in the milk? The importance of breastfeeding definitions will be more thoroughly discussed in Chapter 9.

A literature review published in January 2021 on human milk collection for Covid-19 research, which could equally be applied to research on HIV in breastmilk, describes what selected factors impact the concentration and/or stability of milk components that are particularly pertinent to research, e.g. those affecting potential transmission of pathogens from mother to infant through human milk and/or breastfeeding. They include viral DNA and RNA, bacterial DNA, microbial viability, immunoglobulins, cytokines and other soluble components, and immune cells. Importantly, these questions inform what should be considered, controlled for, or at least reported when human milk is being collected, handled and stored for this type of research. The authors note that the state of the science for many of these factors is insufficient, and additional research is urgently needed to fill these knowledge gaps.[29]

The timing of maternal infection also plays an extremely important part in whether the baby will become infected or will escape infection. If mothers are newly infected while still breastfeeding, the risk of transmission through breastmilk is nearly twice as high as for women infected before pregnancy. This increased risk is due to the high viral load in a mother's system shortly after initial infection,[30] which will also affect viral levels in her milk. Over time, if she is not receiving treatment, her viral load will increase as her immune system is destroyed by HIV and she develops clinical symptoms of AIDS. Thus the timing of maternal primary infection may be the most important factor in the transmission of HIV from mother to infant, whether this is during pregnancy, during delivery, or during the course of breastfeeding. Very little of the early research on vertical transmission of HIV, on which we still base current risk estimates given to mothers by organisations keen to dissuade them from breastfeeding, even mentions when the mothers' primary infection was acquired.

An increased risk of transmission via breastfeeding is also more likely if mothers remain untreated during the later stages of disease, when viraemia increases again. Several of the Nairobi researchers demonstrated a strong correlation between maternal immunosuppression and prevalence and quantity of breastmilk HIV DNA.[14] Joan Kreiss concluded that 'prolonged breastfeeding' (>15 months) doubles the risk of infection, and also noted that the presence of HIV DNA correlated with CD4 depletion (a marker for immune dysfunction), which could indicate a later stage of maternal infection.[31] Ekpini described the risk of transmission for babies breastfed beyond six months as 'substantial',[13] although information about how long before delivery the mother herself became infected was not given in either his or Kreiss's studies. The Nairobi group also found, intriguingly, that the viral loads in breastmilk samples of mothers who had tested HIV-positive at 32 weeks of gestation decreased to zero nine months after delivery.[8]

Guidelines which suggested that there was an increased risk of HIV transmission to the baby with increased duration of breastfeeding may or may not have been correct. On the one hand newly infected mothers appear to become *less* infectious with time as the viral load decreases and antibodies increase. On the other hand, untreated mothers with long-standing infections may have become *more* infectious as viral loads increased in the later stages of the disease or with the onset of active AIDS. Overall, however, despite apparently consuming 60,000 HIV-infected cells and more than half a million cell-free HIV virions per day,[10] over 85% of infants breastfed by HIV-positive mothers, even those who received no treatment, did *not* become infected through breastfeeding[32] and most HIV-positive mothers fell inside the 7–8 year window period when viral levels in both blood and breastmilk were no doubt comparatively low. When this old research is still being cited in support of discouraging HIV-positive mothers from breastfeeding today it needs to be challenged.

The success of ART

The major miracle of antiretroviral therapy lies in its ability to reduce the amount of virus in all body fluids, including breastmilk, to undetectable levels, thus greatly minimising the quantity of virus delivered to the breastfed baby. Once again, timing is everything. The effectiveness of ART depends on the duration of treatment. Later research has identified that the duration of maternal drug regimens is crucial in protecting babies from MTCT of HIV through breastfeeding. Many months of treatment with combined drugs produces better results than single-dose or short-course therapy. The effects of antiretroviral therapy for HIV-positive mothers and their infants will be explored in chapters 22 and 23.

CHAPTER 8

Breast and nipple problems: do they increase the risk?

The interplay between a baby's need for milk and a mother's ability to produce it – the demand of the baby and the response of the mother's breasts – is one of the most fascinating facets of the study of lactation and breastfeeding, simultaneously subtle and robust. When and how a mother breastfeeds her baby affects the nutritional and immunological components in her milk. And this in turn impacts whether breastmilk can transmit HIV. In other words, breastfeeding can either pose a risk or provide lifesaving protection.

Exclusive breastfeeding for the first half-year of life, and continued breastfeeding with the addition of household weaning foods for up to two years or beyond, is the global recommendation for all babies.[1] There's a widespread, but mistaken belief that breastfeeding is only recommended for babies in developing countries, whose mothers don't have the kinds of conditions in the global north that make formula-feeding safe – or at least not as unsafe – as it is in the global south, but this is not true. Breastfeeding is recommended for *all* babies everywhere including in the context of HIV, as further discussed in Chapter 24.

Exclusive breastfeeding means feeding the baby no other foods or liquids, not even water, for the first six months. This greatly reduces the risk of all infections for the baby, compared to complete or partial formula-feeding, or feeding solid foods before six months of age.

Breastfeeding is one of the most fulfilling experiences a woman can have. It should commence within an hour of birth and continue for as long as the baby-child wants. Breastfeeding is not always easy, especially in societies where bottle-feeding has become the norm and breastfeeding is seldom actually seen. Mothers can experience difficulties such as sore or abraded nipples, or breast infections, or under- or over-production of breastmilk. These problems are not inevitable, but they're fairly common during the early days after the birth, and in fact they can happen at any time. Mothers should be able to count on skilled and prompt help to resolve these problems, so that breastfeeding can be enjoyable and successful for as long as both partners in the relationship desire.

In the context of HIV there's an additional motivation to resolve difficulties quickly because breast and nipple problems have been estimated to double the risk of postpartum transmission of HIV.[2]

How the breasts make milk

The physiology of breastmilk synthesis is key to whether breastmilk transmits the virus. During the last weeks of pregnancy and the first 36–72 hours after birth, the breasts produce colostrum, the first milk, which is low in volume, but rich in antibodies. Delivery of the baby and placenta causes a sharp drop in maternal progesterone levels, signalling the onset of copious milk production (lactogenesis-II). From making approximately 30ml of colostrum on the baby's first day of life, breastmilk production increases rapidly to about 600ml/24 hours by day four.

Before lactogenesis-II there are large gaps between the cells in the breast (the mammary epithelial cells) which, as a safety mechanism, allow for the exchange of components between blood and milk. Lactogenesis-II brings a profound, orderly and rapid series of changes in the activity of differentiated mammary epithelial cells from a resting state to a fully active secretory state.[3] Epithelial permeability is increased during the immediate postpartum period as lactogenesis is established, and again during weaning as milk production diminishes. The early changes start with closure of the tight junctions (gasket-like structures which join the cells tightly to one another) between the epithelial cells, followed by a transient increase in the secretion of the protective proteins sIgA and lactoferrin. After about 36 hours a rapid increase in the synthesis of all the components of mature milk begins that is complete by about day five postpartum.

During full lactation, the passage of substances between alveolar cells is stopped by the tight junctions. An understanding of this physiology is important, since later events in lactation can cause the tight junctions to reopen, and in the context of HIV ideally this is to be avoided, or at least minimised. Tight junctions act to regulate the movement of material through the paracellular pathway, forming barriers between adjacent epithelial and endothelial cells in the breast that restrict passage of serum components into the milk. Being impermeable during established lactation, the tight junctions allow milk to be stored between nursing periods without leakage of blood components into milk.[4]

Mammary epithelial tight junctions are dynamic and can be regulated by a number of stimuli. They are leaky during pregnancy. During established lactation, the tight junctions are usually closed, but increased permeability can occur during extended periods of milk stasis (immobility, if the milk is not being drained out of the breast),[5] with high doses of oxytocin, or during periods of inflammation such as breast infections or mastitis. The tight junction state appears to be closely linked to milk secretion. An increase in tight junction permeability is accompanied by decreased breastmilk production, and conversely a decrease in tight junction permeability is accompanied by an increase in milk production.

Starting immediately after birth, the first change to occur is a fall in the sodium and chloride concentrations in the milk and an increase in the lactose concentration. These modifications are largely complete by 72 hours postpartum. With blockage of the paracellular pathway, lactose – made by the epithelial cells – can no longer pass into the plasma. Sodium and chloride can no longer pass from the interstitial space into the lumina of the mammary alveoli. As the breasts become fuller, the taste of the milk changes from salty to sweet.

What does this have to do with HIV transmission? Permeability of the milk cells, occurring as a result of postpartum breast engorgement and opening of the tight junctions, or in conjunction with inflammation, is a likely reason for elevated HIV viral levels. This phenomenon is more likely during the first few days postpartum as breastmilk synthesis increases, particularly if the baby is not breastfeeding effectively (i.e. during milk stasis). Permeability stabilises as milk synthesis down-regulates according to the baby's demand (as the baby drains the milk more effectively during breastfeeding).[6,7] Conversely, permeability may also occur if the breasts become too full during mixed feeding, mastitis and particularly following abrupt weaning.[8] Thus breast permeability is a likely cause of elevated HIV viral levels in breastmilk, leading to an increased risk of transmission of HIV to the breastfed baby.

Elevated breastmilk sodium may be a marker for inadequate breastmilk drainage, which in turn precipitates breast engorgement and/or blocked ducts, predisposing to mastitis, in itself a risk factor for breast abscess. More specifically, breast permeability:

- is related to an oversupply of milk.
- increases at days five and 14 postpartum, in conjuction with postpartum breast engorgement, often experienced by mothers when the milk 'comes in' after the birth.[6,7]
- stabilises between days 30–90 as breastmilk synthesis down-regulates according to the baby's demand.
- occurs if the breasts become too full following abrupt weaning.[8]

Delayed lactogenesis

Milk that continues to taste salty after day four or five postpartum suggests that lactogenesis-II has not occurred, and will need medical investigation. A common reason for delayed milk production is retained placenta. The breasts do not 'fill' in the expected way, the exclusively breastfed baby shows increasing hunger, and the mother may need a surgical procedure known as a dilation and curettage to clear the retained placental fragments. Lactogenesis will occur in the usual way once any retained tissue has been removed.

Breast overfullness or engorgement following lactogenesis-II

After the breasts start producing larger quantities of milk, and if the milk is not drained efficiently, the tight junctions may remain open, causing a mother to secrete lactose in her urine, and this can be measured. Cathy Fetherston looked at the excretion of lactose in urine as a measure of increased permeability of the lactating breast during inflammation.[9] Another study from Western Australia[6] followed mothers at a private hospital who were assessed to be at risk for breast problems, e.g. a history of mastitis in previous lactations, or nipple trauma, attachment difficulties and either an uncomfortable oversupply or engorgement at lactogenesis-II. Milk from both breasts and 24-hour urine samples were collected. There were a total of 22 episodes of mastitis, suffered by 14 mothers, occurring after day five postpartum. Twenty-four-hour lactose excretion in urine was found to be significantly higher during mastitis, peaking at the beginning of symptoms and decreasing over time until there was no significant difference at follow-up compared to the mothers with no symptoms.

Fetherston found that mean excretion of lactose in 24-hour urine samples provided a reliable marker of breast permeability.[9] Associated changes in milk composition decreased from days 5–14 postpartum, and then remained fairly constant over the next eight weeks. The significantly higher amounts of lactose excreted at days five and 14 accorded with previous research,[6] which suggested that an increase in permeability of the paracellular pathway related to an oversupply of milk,[7,8] often experienced by mothers at lactogenesis-II, which then downregulates according to demand. A relatively low, stable excretion rate for urinary lactose from days 30–90 indicated that milk supply had stabilised in response to demand. The use of 24-hour excretion of lactose in urine provided a reliable laboratory marker for changes occurring in breast permeability. In mastitis, the larger the area of inflammation of the breast, the greater the increase in lactose excretion in urine; this provided a useful clinical predictor for an increase in breast permeability and resulting changes in milk composition.

In the presence of milk stasis, mammary tight junctions become leaky, and following 24 hours of milk stasis women were found to have elevated concentrations of milk sodium.[9] Thus during mastitis, or during weaning, the milk may once again taste salty. Opening of the paracellular pathways during established lactation leads to oedema of the interstitial tissues from the leakage of proteins from both blood and milk. Increased paracellular permeability and a consequent decrease in lactose concentration is associated with decreased milk production. Importantly, Fetherston comments that 'although several studies have used an increase in breastmilk sodium as an indicator for mastitis, raised sodium, in isolation from physical signs and symptoms, cannot be accepted as a reliable indicator for infection or subclinical infection because there are known confounding factors where sodium concentration in milk is normally raised, such as initiation of lactation, involution and pregnancy'.

Early lactation management

For the next several days after the onset of lactogenesis-II the mother's breastmilk supply often exceeds infant demand, resulting in breast overfullness. This time is most likely from day four to day nine after birth. Conventional wisdom (and advice on internet mother-to-mother support groups) suggests that mothers should not relieve the pressure of the extra milk by expressing it or by pumping, for fear of continuing to over-produce milk, thus exacerbating the problem. This single piece of myth-information is often responsible for a whole cascade of difficulties which can severely impact the mother's and baby's health, leading to what has been called 'the domino effect of lactation failure'.[10] Crucially, in the context of HIV, this avoidable calamity can increase the risk of postpartum transmission. Every mother wants to do the best she can to ensure that her baby is happy, healthy and survives, if only she knows how. The help and assistance that an HIV-positive mother receives during breastfeeding, and particularly to relieve postpartum breast fullness, is key.

There can be many factors, either maternal or infant, resulting in over-production of milk (which, if severe, is known as breast engorgement). Often the baby's appetite in the first few days of life hasn't caught up with his mother's breastmilk production. Or the baby may be sick or small or too weak or sleepy to latch to the breast. Or perhaps an inexperienced mother needs help in learning how to breastfeed. Postpartum breast engorgement can be a risk factor for sore nipples, milk stasis and mastitis. Unrelieved pressure on the milk producing cells within the breast can cause pain and damage, to the extent that whole lobes of breast tissue may become non-functional for the whole of that lactation. This is especially detrimental in view of the recommendation for exclusive breastfeeding, with no supplementation, for a full six months in order to reduce the risk of postpartum transmission of HIV associated with mixed feeding.

Whatever the cause, the immediate remedy is always the same – and urgent. Mothers need to be helped, as soon as possible, to drain the breasts of the extra milk. They should breastfeed the baby often, look for swallowing and do everything to encourage the baby to breastfeed more effectively and for longer. They can hand-express or pump any milk that the small or sick baby is unable to take. If a baby cannot latch, or is too sleepy to suck, he may need to receive the milk in another way, e.g. by spoon, or tube or bottle until the difficulty is addressed or resolved. But even if the baby is drinking well, a new mother may over-produce milk for a few days and she should drain the breasts of the extra milk whenever she feels slightly too full. It's been said that Nature doesn't know that she didn't have twins. Failure to drain the breasts has serious consequences, especially in the context of HIV.

The interplay of mother-or-baby influence, each on the other, provides a glimpse into the intersection between maternal HIV infectivity and infant susceptibility to infection. Exclusive breastfeeding is clearly protective for the baby, and mixed feeding is clearly risky, as will be discussed in the next chapter.

Maternal risk factors for breastfeeding transmission include breast pathologies such as overfullness, sore nipples, engorgement, mastitis and abscess, down-regulation of breastmilk production, 'not enough milk' followed by premature supplementation and mixed feeding of the baby.[2] Many of these consequences are preventable. In this beautifully interdependent relationship any factor which affects one member of the couple can impact the health and comfort of the other.

Risk factors for HIV transmission during breastfeeding

Mother

- Nipple damage/abrasions
- Inadequate drainage of milk from breasts, e.g. stasis
- Mastitis
- Breast abscess

Baby

- Oral thrush (may be first symptom of an already infected baby)
- Mixed feeding (other foods and before six months of age)
- Drug therapy which alters/damages intestinal flora/mucosa, e.g. oral antibiotic treatment

Sore nipples

Sore nipples are a frequent cause of breastfeeding difficulties and if nipples are abraded, infant contact with maternal blood may increase the risk of HIV transmission. Outside the context of HIV, nipple lesions have been found on clinical exam in 10–13% of mothers.[11] Damage can take the form of abrasions, or cracks either on the face or along the shaft of the nipple, allowing ingestion of maternal blood by the infant.

The majority of women experience an increase in nipple sensitivity during the first week postpartum and nipple pain is the most common lactation problem for which mothers consult health professionals. Nipple trauma occurs as a consequence of several factors:[12]

- poor positioning of the infant at the breast, or shallow latching techniques
- overfull breasts, leading to a short latch, creating unrelieved negative pressure on the face of the nipple leading to abrasions and cracks
- a fungal or bacterial infection
- nipple anomalies
- oral anomalies in the infant

Two studies observed higher proportions of infected infants among mothers reporting cracked or bleeding nipples, but a history of colostrum intake or cracked nipples without bleeding were not associated with higher transmission.[11,13] The risk of transmission was not significant in another study that assessed breast problems after six months postpartum.[14]

Bacterial infections

Bacterial infections can contribute to breakdown of the nipple epithelium[15] and can be very painful and slow to heal. A mother whose nipples are becoming sore or damaged should seek help quickly from a lactation consultant or experienced breastfeeding counsellor to identify the cause and facilitate healing. If standard recommendations such as improving positioning and attachment techniques do not quickly resolve the problem, the mother should be referred to her doctor for a culture of the milk and/or a nipple swab and advice on appropriate antibiotic therapy.

One of the most common, but frequently unidentified causes of sore nipples is a bacterial infection. A 1996 study showed that mothers with infants younger than one month who complained of moderate to severe nipple pain and who had cracks, fissures, ulcers, or exudates had a 64% chance of having positive skin cultures and a 54% chance of having *Staphylococcus aureus* colonisation.[16] In Harare I worked with a series of mothers who developed *Staphylococcus pyogenes*, never identified as a cause of nipple pain before, and the laboratory initially wanted repeat tests because they thought the samples had been contaminated. When treated with an appropriate antibiotic, sometimes requiring two or three courses, each of these cases eventually resolved. While the nipple heals, the affected breast should be kept well drained to reduce the increased risk of mastitis and provide milk for the baby.

Frenulotomy for Ankyloglossia is contraindicated

In recent years, infant tongue-tie, lip tie or even buccal tie have become popular diagnoses as a cause of maternal nipple trauma. However, due to the risk of HIV transmission if virus in the milk comes into contact with the baby's bloodstream, every effort should be made to avoid oral surgery or frenulotomy, and to focus on improving positioning and latching techniques in order to reduce or work around sore nipples.

Thrush

Dr Rose Kambarami, a well-known paediatrician in Harare, looked at the prevalence of nipple disease among breastfeeding mothers whose babies were showing symptoms of HIV and had been admitted during a six-month period in 1992–93 to Harare Central Hospital general paediatric wards.[17] Oral disease was present in 58.8% of all symptomatic breastfeeding HIV-infected infants. Ninety percent of the babies were suffering from pneumonia and many had malnutrition, so it's likely that the majority had progressed to active AIDS, with the common symptom of oral thrush. Thirty per cent of mothers experienced sore nipples. Nipple eczema was seen in 22.1%, cracked nipples in 10.6% and sore nipples in 10.6% of the mothers. The major risk factor for the mother to develop sore nipples was infant oral disease.

Whether maternal nipple lesions are a cause of infant HIV infection by ingestion of maternal blood, or whether an already-infected infant suffering from oral thrush may be more likely to cause cracked or bleeding nipples for the mother is difficult to determine, but either member of the breastfeeding couple can transfer thrush to the other. Nipple thrush can cause severe pain for the mother. It's a common cause of cracked nipples, particularly in the fold of skin where the nipple meets the areola. Oral thrush in the baby can transfer to the mother's nipple, making the skin friable. The following points should be considered when determining risk:

- Pregnant women are increasingly susceptible to vaginal candida as pregnancy advances, due to hormonal influences. The infant's mouth can become infected during vaginal birth to infect the mother's breast and nipple during breastfeeding.[18,19]
- Women with diminished immune function may be prone to persistent fungal infections. Candida may be a significant problem for them.
- Oral infant thrush or maternal vaginal or nipple thrush may follow antibiotic therapy of mother or baby.
- A suppressed immune system increases susceptibility to thrush infections, especially in premature or sick babies. Oral thrush may be one of the first symptoms shown by an HIV-infected baby.

Thrush can be treated by effective antifungals applied to the baby's mouth, and oral or topical antifungal medications for the mother's nipples. Medical advice will be needed as well as prescription medications. Both members of the nursing couple should be treated for two weeks past the end of all symptoms, and the whole family needs to observe strict hygiene to prevent the spread of thrush back and forth between them.

Escalation

Sore nipples are frequently a cause of delayed breastfeeds, lengthened feeding intervals and supplementation (mixed feeding) as a mother attempts to avoid the pain of breastfeeding. Disruption of the integrity of the nipple can also allow entry of bacteria into the breast followed by bacterial proliferation, leading to breast inflammation, induration (hard lumpy areas), blocked ducts, with or without without pain and fever, symptoms of mastitis, and ultimately, if still neglected, to breast abscess.[20]

Blocked ducts/subclinical mastitis

The healthy lactating breast has a cobblestone texture. A blocked duct is a hard area of the breast which feels uncomfortably full, and may become painful but without inflammation. A blockage occurs when one overfull lobe presses on another, making drainage difficult. It should be dealt with promptly, by breastfeeding more often, massaging the affected breast down towards the nipple and expressing again until the indurated area becomes drained and feels soft and no longer feels tender. Massaging and expressing in a basin of warm water, or in a warm bath, may also help the milk to 'flow' and speed resolution. Placing cool cabbage leaves over the affected area, in between expressing the breast, may help to suppress lactation in that area. A blocked duct (subclinical mastitis) should not be ignored, since it can progress to mastitis if not dealt with promptly.[21]

Mastitis and subclinical mastitis

Mastitis can affect 20%– 30% of women, usually in the first seven weeks after delivery.[22] Mastitis is an inflammatory process in the breast characterised by an opening of paracellular pathways in the mammary alveoli and an abnormal increase in inflammatory cells and sodium in milk. The breast is lumpy, inflamed and painful. The mother's temperature is elevated and she feels as if she has flu.

In 1979 a correlation was made between elevated breastmilk sodium and clinically apparent mastitis.[23] For the purposes of research, subclinical mastitis was defined as elevated breastmilk sodium >12 mmol/l because this concentration is greater than three standard deviations above the mean for normal human milk at one month.[24] Thus clinical and subclinical mastitis were hypothesised as important risk factors for HIV transmission.

In 1990, Abakada, Hartmann and Grubb in Western Australia reported that sodium was sometimes elevated in both symptomatic and asymptomatic breasts, and that it may reflect the presence of either subclinical infection or involution.[25] In animals, elevated milk sodium concentrations are considered to be sensitive indicators of mastitis, accompanying permeability of the tight junctions, and are used to detect subclinical mastitis. In humans, elevated sodium helps to protect the breast from infection, and during mastitis, or at any time that the breast is not draining well, the milk can taste salty, e.g. during lactogenesis-II when the milk first comes in after birth, or during involution of the breast that occurs during weaning. Coincidentally, these are all recognised times when there can be an increased risk of transmission of HIV from breastmilk.

During mastitis, breast permeability:

- is significantly high
- peaks at commencement of symptoms
- correlates to the area of breast inflammation
- decreases over time as symptoms of mastitis resolve.

In the context of HIV, breastfeeding during mastitis is considered to be risky. In addition, the theoretical risk of suffering mastitis, or subclinical mastitis, is always put forward as a reason why HIV-positive women should not breastfeed. Ellen Piwoz, speaking at the WABA-UNICEF HIV Colloquium in Arusha in 2002, estimated that by raising viral levels in breastmilk, or by exposing the baby to maternal blood during breastfeeding, breast and nipple problems doubled the risk of HIV infection.[2] Notwithstanding that concentrations of protective immunological factors such as lactoferrin and lysozyme increase,[26,27] the presence of plasma-derived components and inflammatory cells in breastmilk, such as HIV-infected lymphocytes, could raise breastmilk HIV load and add to the risk of transmission.[28]

Semba and colleagues in Malawi published a series of papers in 1999,[28–31] reporting on mother-baby pairs studied at six weeks postpartum, to examine 'subclinical mastitis' as a risk factor for vertical transmission. They were especially interested in the relationship between elevated human milk sodium levels, milk immunological and inflammatory mediators and viral load in milk and plasma, on the rationale that during mastitis, inflammatory cells enter the milk, and inflammation is accompanied by an opening of tight junctions between breast cells and the maternal bloodstream, allowing intercellular fluid and plasma to enter the milk through paracellular pathways between alveolar cells.

The Semba research is very often cited, even today, to paint breastfeeding with HIV as risky. Semba found that at six weeks postpartum, about 16% of all lactating women, including those without HIV, had elevated sodium concentrations in breastmilk which were consistent with subclinical mastitis. These findings matched other research suggesting that clinically apparent mastitis occurs in about 20 to 33% of lactating women at some time during lactation, mostly within the first two months after delivery. Although levels of cell-free HIV were similar to those in the Lewis research from Kenya,[32] and HIV load in breastmilk was much lower than that found in plasma,[28] nearly half of babies of HIV-positive mothers with elevated milk sodium were found to be infected at six weeks, compared to only a quarter of babies whose mothers had normal breastmilk sodium levels. Median breastmilk HIV load was 700 copies/ml among women with infected infants versus undetectable (<200 copies/ml) among those with uninfected infants respectively. Among those with elevated breastmilk sodium levels, the median milk HIV load was 920 copies/ml.[28] Treatment with oral antibiotics resulted in a decrease in breastmilk leukocyte counts and a significant decrease in inflammation of the breast, but breastmilk HIV load remained elevated despite a significant decrease from baseline.[33] The conclusion was that mastitis and breastmilk HIV load could increase the risk of vertical transmission through breastfeeding, since an extremely high number of virions may overwhelm its immunologic mechanisms.

Semba had reported in 1999 that, given the lack of access to clean water, hygiene problems and privacy issues, universal breastfeeding was encouraged for all Malawian women, regardless of HIV status. He thought that other causes of increased breastmilk sodium such as early weaning and poor feeding by a malnourished and dehydrated infant were unlikely because women were exclusively breastfeeding at six weeks postpartum, and none of the infants were noted to be malnourished or dehydrated at the time of examination. However, exclusive breastfeeding rates in Malawi had been only 3.2% in 1992, rising to a reported 62.7% in 2000.[34] It's likely therefore that a significant percentage of the babies included in his research had in fact been mixed fed. It's also important to note that the HIV status of infants was only estimated when they were six weeks of age, which makes it difficult to distinguish intrapartum from postpartum transmission.[35] How many were infected during labour and birth? In addition, microbiological cultures of breastmilk were not done, and clinical symptoms were not recorded.

The timing of publication (in 1999) and the volume of the Semba papers (four in one year) on elevated sodium in breastmilk as a marker for 'subclinical mastitis', with the implication that this phenomenon was a more-or-less unavoidable risk factor for breastfeeding mothers, is interesting. Was it coincidental that publication occurred on the eve of implementation of global recommendations for HIV-positive mothers to stop breastfeeding, as will be more fully discussed in Chapter 12? The Semba findings warned of a phenomenon which had no symptoms and was thus unavoidable, except by not breastfeeding. Effectively the papers endorsed the change of WHO HIV and infant feeding policy (to avoid postpartum MTCT of HIV by avoiding breastfeeding), announced in 1997 and about to be implemented.

Acknowledging that MTCT had been associated with symptomatic and asymptomatic mastitis and with the quantity of HIV RNA and DNA in maternal milk, Zimbabwean researchers conducted a highly technical study from 2005–2007, to examine the relationship between indicators of inflammation and HIV viral loads in breastmilk.[36] Eighty-five percent of the mothers had received single-dose nevirapine to prevent MTCT during birth, but no other antiretroviral therapy. Laboratory indicators of mastitis (breastmilk sodium concentration, sodium/potassium ratio and leukocyte count) were evaluated to see if they could predict viral loads in milk. Mastitis was present in 15%, 15% and 18% of 412 milk specimens as defined by sodium concentration, sodium/potassium ratio and total leukocyte counts respectively. Each indicator was associated with an increased milk HIV RNA load but not with HIV DNA load. Neutrophils correlated better with milk HIV RNA load than total leukocytes. However, neither neutrophil count, sodium concentration, nor sodium/potassium ratio displayed a threshold that was both sensitive and specific for the detection of HIV RNA in milk. Nor were HIV DNA loads increased in breastmilk during mastitis. The group concluded that the simple and inexpensive tests most commonly associated with breast inflammation, such as electrolyte concentrations or cell counts, had 'poor predictive value' and would not be useful as surrogate markers of milk HIV RNA or DNA loads for individual women.

The importance of exclusive breastfeeding to protect against MTCT

Investigating whether subclinical mastitis among breastfeeding women in South Africa was related to high milk viral load or increased infant gut permeability, Durban researcher Juana Willumsen concluded that subclinical mastitis among HIV-positive women may increase the risk of vertical transmission through breastfeeding by increasing milk viral load.[37] Causes, such as local infection, sterile inflammation, systemic infection, micronutrient deficiencies, or poor lactation practices differed at one week from later times. Further analysis of breastmilk by Willumsen and colleagues in 2001[38] showed that the virus was undetectable in approximately one-third of samples, that it was shed intermittently and that the number of virus may differ considerably between breasts of an individual woman at any given time.

Simple lactation counselling interventions improved lactation practice in Bangladeshi women in 2002. Nutritional supplementation increased the sodium/potassium ratio in breastmilk and concentrations of the immune factors secretory immunoglobulin A (sIgA), lactoferrin, lysozyme and interleukin-8 in 25% of 212 women at 1–3 weeks postpartum and 12% of women at three months.[27] The counselling messages included the importance of exclusive breastfeeding and feeding on demand while achieving good positioning and attachment[39] – the kinds of strategies outlined at the beginning of this chapter.

In 2003, Willumsen further investigated breastmilk RNA viral load among HIV-positive South African women.[40] Low blood CD4 cell count (<200 cells/mm^3) during pregnancy and raised milk sodium/potassium ratio were significantly associated with raised milk RNA viral load at all times, but there were no consistent associations between infant feeding mode. The six infants known to be infected postnatally (vs 88 uninfected infants) had been exposed to breastmilk of higher viral load at each time point. Willumsen concluded that breastmilk HIV RNA viral load in the first 14 weeks of life varied; high levels were associated with both subclinical mastitis and severe maternal immunosuppression.

Nusenblatt and colleagues reported on further research in Blantyre, Malawi,[41] in 2005. HIV-infected women were followed from two weeks to 12 months postpartum. The prevalence of subclinical mastitis, as assessed by breastmilk leukocyte counts, was highest at two weeks and 14 weeks and 27.2% of women had at least one episode. The proportion of women with positive cultures decreased during follow-up at later times.

Not surprisingly, a lower prevalence of subclinical mastitis in early lactation was reported among women who exclusively breastfed than among those who mixed-fed with breastmilk and other foods or liquids. As part of the ZEBS study in Zambia, Katherine Semrau and colleagues published a paper in 2011 looking at the relationship between breastfeeding patterns, markers of maternal HIV and breast pathology in women making nearly 6,000 clinic visits.[42] From birth to six months, one in five women had a breast problem, one in 10 suffered mastitis, and 3% had an abscess. There was an increased risk of breast problems in women not exclusively breastfeeding. Women with a low CD4 count (i.e. their HIV infection had progressed closer to AIDS) had an increased risk of abscess. Semrau and colleagues concluded that exclusive breastfeeding is not only optimal for babies' health, but also benefits mothers by reducing breast problems.

It would seem wise, in order to avoid over-exaggeration of risks of HIV transmission during breastfeeding, to endorse the global recommendations for exclusive breastfeeding for all babies, by all mothers, regardless of HIV infection. Prevention and treatment for breast engorgement (from any cause), blocked ducts, subclinical mastitis, true mastitis and abscess also needs to be recommended for all.

Increased maternal infectivity due to mixed feeding

The possibility of breast problems and their relationship to mixed feeding as a risk factor for HIV transmission has received inadequate attention in the literature on HIV and infant feeding, where the advice has often been simply to suspend breastfeeding and discard the milk from an affected breast to avoid risk of transmission of HIV.[43,44]

In ways that are often unrecognised, it is the baby who exerts the major influence on the mother's synthesis of breastmilk, to 'drive' both the quantity of milk produced, and its individual nutritional and immunological components. This delicate symbiotic relationship is disturbed when other foods and liquids are fed to a baby too early. The displacement of breastmilk

- profoundly affects the milk-producing cells within the mother's breasts, as well as the quantity and composition of her breastmilk
- exerts major effects on the infant gut, as well as disturbing the interaction of the components of breastmilk ingested by the baby, to alter or destroy many of their nutritional and disease-protecting effects

Lactation consultants and others working with breastfeeding mothers and babies have long been aware of the domino effect of inappropriate displacement of breastmilk by other foods and liquids in the diet of young babies, which leads to missed feedings and long breastfeeding intervals, in turn resulting in maternal breast engorgement[10] and then mastitis and sometimes even abscess. Yet the possibility of mixed feeding, occurring either as a consequence or a cause of these conditions and identified as a risk factor for HIV-transmission in breastfed infants, received little attention.[45]

Mohrbacher & Stock, co-authors of *The Breastfeeding Answer Book*,[46] report that, as well as being a *cause* of mastitis, mixed feeding may also be a *consequence*, since reduced breastmilk output often accompanies unrelieved areolar and/or peripheral engorgement in the presence of a blocked duct or mastitis, and may be a motivating factor for mothers to initiate inappropriate supplementation of the breastfed baby.

In 2000, Melanie Smith and Louise Kuhn gave a very full explanation of how breastfeeding practices influence mammary epithelial permeability in the context of HIV.[5] In 2007 Louise Kuhn and colleagues[47] further reported on the additional processes including elevations in breastmilk HIV viral load as a result of decreased frequency of infant suckling. Small changes, such as a missed feed or an infant not suckling as much as usual, can lead to milk stasis. If this is not reversed within a short period of time, epithelial permeability may increase, allowing more efficient paracellular transfer of both cell-free and cell-associated HIV as discussed before.

Risk factors for mastitis relating to breastfeeding management and epidemiological factors are thoroughly reviewed by Fetherston,[48] who notes that blocked ducts, mastitis and breast abscess as a continuum had been described by another Australian expert, Wendy Brodribb,[49] and that non-infective (inflammatory) mastitis occurs with ineffective milk drainage from the breast. This may be related to engorgement or blocked ducts which can result in a local inflammatory response occurring at the site of the blockage.

Kevin Lunney and colleagues, in another arm of the ZVITAMBO study, which had originally been set up to look at the protective effects of antioxidants (vitamin A) against transmission of HIV to infants, (but which later found that they made no difference), found that plasma viral load was what influenced viral load in milk.[50] When the quantity of HIV in plasma was high, elevated sodium was associated with an increased risk of transmission of HIV to the baby. Because sodium is a marker of mammary permeability, as well as of mastitis, either non-pathological or pathological processes could be implicated in recruiting immune factors into breastmilk. Importantly, mastitis was associated with postnatal transmission *only* when maternal plasma HIV load was high. Lunney confirmed that unnecessary supplements given to babies (resulting in mixed feeding) disrupted the physiological balance between milk production and removal. Irregular and/or infrequent suckling resulted in milk stasis, leading to breast engorgement, possible mastitis and high quantities of HIV in breastmilk, thus increasing the risk of postnatal HIV transmission.

Lactation management for mothers

Lactation management is a technical term used in the breastfeeding world to mean the body of skills and expertise needed by a healthcare provider in order to assist breastfeeding mothers and babies. It is used here more specifically to mean ways and means that mothers themselves can 'manage' their own breastmilk production after the birth of their babies in order to control how much milk they are able to produce so as to avoid elevated viral levels in their milk.

Consequences of breast overfullness

Once a mother understands how the breasts make milk easily and efficiently, and how she herself can monitor that her baby is 'getting enough', then she will not need to rely on out-of-date guidance that may come her way from others.

At various times, a mother may wish to:

- successfully initiate lactation
- maintain current breastmilk production in order to breastfeed one or more babies
- provide enough expressed breastmilk for her baby to receive her milk by another method of delivery (called breastmilk-feeding)
- increase the amount of milk she makes, if she thinks or actually knows that she doesn't have enough milk
- decrease the amount of milk produced, if she is making too much, e.g. past the newborn stage, or during gradual weaning to solid foods
- completely suppress lactation if she decides not to breastfeed at all

Effective lactation management strategies should include teaching women about:

- Positioning and attachment techniques to reduce nipple trauma and facilitate breastmilk removal by the baby
- Manual expression and/or pumping of breastmilk to prevent and/or promptly and thoroughly resolve breast engorgement
- Breastmilk synthesis and down-regulation of milk supply in the presence of engorgement, as well as the risk of mastitis if this is neglected
- The protective effects against all infections for their babies of exclusive breastfeeding for six months, and how this works
- The necessity of minimising the risk of breastfeeding-associated HIV-transmission through exclusive breastfeeding for a full six months

Mothers can be warned about what will happen, and given information about how to manage potential postpartum engorgement, as follows:

1. Breastfeed the baby as soon as possible after birth.
2. Breastfeed the baby very frequently in the first few days, for as long as they want. Whenever the breasts start to feel even slightly too full, wake the baby to breastfeed.
3. Make sure the baby is able to attach easily and that breastfeeding is comfortable. Ask for help with positioning and attaching the baby to the breast if
    a. The baby is difficult to latch
    b. If the baby is not swallowing milk (long, slow sucks followed by a pause to swallow) in sucking bursts of 10 or so swallows, followed by a small rest, and then more swallowing
    c. If there is pain, or damage to the nipple
4. Milk transfer/drainage (from the breasts to the baby) can be assisted by 'breast compression': cup the breast with one hand during breastfeeding, gently compress the breast between fingers and thumb whenever the baby takes a pause in swallowing longer than just a few seconds, i.e. gently squeeze or massage the breast, being careful not to disturb the baby's latch (i.e. do not pull the nipple out of the baby's mouth), and then watch for the baby's swallowing again. Keep the breast still while the baby drinks, but use breast compression again at the next sucking pause.
5. Express or feed the baby whenever the breasts feel even just a little too full, especially from day 4–9, even if this is very often. It is very important to keep the breasts soft and comfortable and well-drained. The expressed milk can be stored in the fridge, or frozen.
6. If the baby is not breastfeeding, the expressed milk can be fed by cup or spoon.
7. After day 10, it is usual for:
    a. The baby's appetite to have caught up with the mother's milk production
    b. The breasts to have stopped feeling overfull.
8. By day 14, most mothers find that their breasts are much softer, but still producing enough milk for the baby. Thereafter, if the baby is taking enough, they should be fed 'on demand' (as often as they want, for as long as they want).

Management of a blocked duct or mastitis

Milk stasis underlies the development of mastitis and other breast problems and is nearly always preventable by avoiding overfullness of the breasts. Mastitis may be infective or non-infective. An area of the breast becomes hard, inflamed and painful in a blocked duct, and the mother may start to run a fever in mastitis. At the first signs of these symptoms, the mother should make every attempt to drain the whole breast very thoroughly every two hours during the day and every three hours during the night, expressing and massaging, and expressing again after breastfeeding. She can also place raw cabbage leaves on the affected area, tucked inside the bra, and change them after every expressing session. If there is no very noticeable improvement within 24 hours she should seek medical advice about the need for an antibiotic, and continue to keep the breast very well drained until all pain/induration/inflammation and fever have resolved. The expressed milk can be heat-treated before being fed to the baby.

Stopping breastfeeding

For the HIV-positive mother, rapid weaning is specifically not recommended, since it has been shown to greatly increase viral levels in the milk, posing an increased risk of transmission to the HIV-exposed baby if breastfeeding takes place sporadically. Kuhn and colleagues in Zambia followed HIV-infected women and their infants for 24 months, and tested whether minor and major changes in feeding frequency influenced breastmilk viral concentrations.[51] Women were randomised to wean abruptly at four months or continue breastfeeding for as long as they liked. Two weeks after breastfeeding cessation at 4.5 months, HIV concentrations in breastmilk were substantially higher than if breastfeeding continued. HIV levels were also higher with early mixed feeding and led to higher rates of HIV transmission. Changes in the frequency of breastfeeding during weaning and with non-exclusive breastfeeding influenced milk viral concentrations. The researchers suggested that this may explain the reduced risk of HIV transmission associated with exclusive breastfeeding and why early weaning does not achieve the magnitude of HIV prevention predicted by models. The Zambian results supported continuation of maternal ART over the full duration of any breastfeeding.

As we have seen, when considered with existing knowledge of mother and/or infant causes and consequences of breast and nipple pathology, a review of lactation physiology can provide greater insight into factors influencing both maternal HIV infectivity and infant risk factors during breastfeeding. Most importantly, knowing what these causes might be can alert mothers to how to avoid them.

Availability of clinical breastfeeding support for women to prevent or quickly resolve breastfeeding problems is critical for reducing HIV transmission through breastfeeding. It's not inevitable that women will experience sore nipples or breast infections, as is often implied in literature written for new HIV-positive mothers.[44] When they receive assistance and up-to-date preventive care and advice from knowledgeable lactation consultants, breastfeeding supporters or health workers, sore nipples, breast engorgement, mastitis and abscess are largely preventable. These calamities happen on a continuum, not suddenly. Avoiding action and strategies to resolve problems can be taken at the earliest symptoms instead of waiting until a nipple or breast problem becomes a full-blown emergency requiring weaning from the breast.

Research can provide insight into factors influencing both maternal HIV infectivity and infant susceptibility to infection during breastfeeding, but researchers in the AIDS community have seldom included or collaborated with lactation practitioners who would have been able to save valuable time by sharing their knowledge and expertise of normal day-to-day lactation physiology. Most importantly, knowing what these causes are and how breastfeeding works, might have suggested how mothers could avoid them without abandoning breastfeeding altogether.

CHAPTER 9

The importance of exclusive breastfeeding: why definitions matter

> *'Breast milk is the best food but has the worst marketing. Why is it that breastfeeding, so obviously beneficial for children and for the child survival agenda, continues to be low priority, under-supported or neglected, controversial, misrepresented, under-taught and countered by many forces? Unlike infant formula... breastfeeding has no significant commercial advocate.'*
>
> Miriam Labbok, University of North Carolina

Exclusive breastfeeding – meaning that the young baby receives only mother's milk with no other foods or liquids at all, not even water – has been shown to greatly reduce the risk of *all* infections, compared to either mixed breastfeeding or exclusive formula-feeding. Outside the context of HIV, exclusive breastfeeding is one of the most effective strategies for preventing infant morbidity and mortality.[1] In the unlikely event that an exclusively breastfed baby does pick up an infection, both the severity and the duration will be reduced. For this reason, to achieve optimal infant growth, development and health, WHO recommends exclusive breastfeeding for the first six months of life. Thereafter, babies should be given nutritious complementary foods and continue breastfeeding up to the age of two years or beyond.[2,3]

In spite of this very clear global guidance, rates of exclusive breastfeeding around the world, including in countries of high HIV prevalence, are quite low.[4] Promotion and teaching about exclusive breastfeeding doesn't receive nearly as much attention as it deserves.

For babies exposed to HIV, exclusive breastfeeding during the first six months of life can mean the difference between escaping the infection completely, or acquiring a lethal disease for which there is currently no known cure. Exclusive breastfeeding also facilitates normal physiological regulation of milk production, which depends on regular infant suckling, allowing for a healthy balance between the infant's needs and the mother's milk production.[5–7]

In 2001, the World Health Organization outlined in a research tool potential mechanisms that could explain a reduced risk of MTCT of HIV when children are exclusively breastfed.[8] They included:

- Reduction in dietary antigens and enteric pathogens to maintain integrity of the baby's intestinal mucosal barrier and limit inflammatory responses within the baby's gut
- Promotion of beneficial intestinal microflora to facilitate resistance to infection and modulate the infant's immune response
- Modulation of anti-microbial, anti-inflammatory and immuno-modulating properties of breast milk
- Maintenance of mammary epithelial integrity to viral load in breastmilk

Mixed feeding and compromised infant gut integrity

Outside the context of HIV, the mechanisms by which babies are protected by exclusive breastfeeding have been well described. Inappropriate supplementation with other foods or liquids interferes with the integrity of the infant gut mucosa even within the first week of life.[9] The younger the baby, the more immature the gut lining, and the greater the risk.[10] Premature babies fed only raw breastmilk have lower rates of infection than those fed either pasteurised breastmilk or those supplemented with formula. Infants fed formula have more than three times the rate of infections (33%) of infants exclusively fed raw human milk (10%).[11]

Rebecca Black wrote about the antiviral properties of human milk and the significance of exclusive breastfeeding in an early paper on HIV and breastfeeding published in 1996.[12] Preble and Piwoz[13] described in 1998 how mixed feeding can involve unhygienic food preparation, and ingestion of contaminated water, fluids and food, leading to gut mucosal injury and disruption of immune barriers. Bacteria and other contaminants introduced into the gut with mixed feeding can result in inflammatory responses and subsequent damage. Maintaining the health and integrity of the gastrointestinal mucosa will thus be protective against HIV.

In their ground-breaking 1999 paper, Coutsoudis and colleagues discovered that exclusive breastfeeding by untreated mothers posed a similar risk of HIV transmission as exclusive formula-feeding.[14] They outlined how once the integrity of mucosal surfaces has been compromised by infection, allergens or trauma, the passage of HIV across mucous membranes into body tissues is facilitated. The importance of Anna Coutsoudis's paper will be further discussed later in this chapter.

The crucial importance of exclusive breastfeeding was further taken up in a paper published in 2000 by Melanie Smith and Louise Kuhn[15] and later by others. HIV-infection of infants by 14 weeks had been significantly associated with increased gut permeability,[16] which occurred with premature introduction of other foods, liquids or the use of antibiotics,[17–19] to cause disturbances of normal gastrointestinal flora, exposure to dietary antigens,[20] inflammation resulting from infection with pathogens, small sites of trauma and inflammation in the infant's intestinal mucosa[21] and contact of HIV with the infant's blood supply and leukocyte population. Damage to the infant gut as a result of premature exposure to solid foods was found to pose a 4–10 fold greater hazard than exposure to other liquids.[22,23]

The diagram below shows how the combined effect of mixed breastfeeding on the infant gut (infant susceptibility) and on the mother's milk production (maternal infectivity) both exacerbate the risk of mother-to-child transmission of HIV through breastfeeding.

Mechanism for HIV transmission through mixed breastfeeding

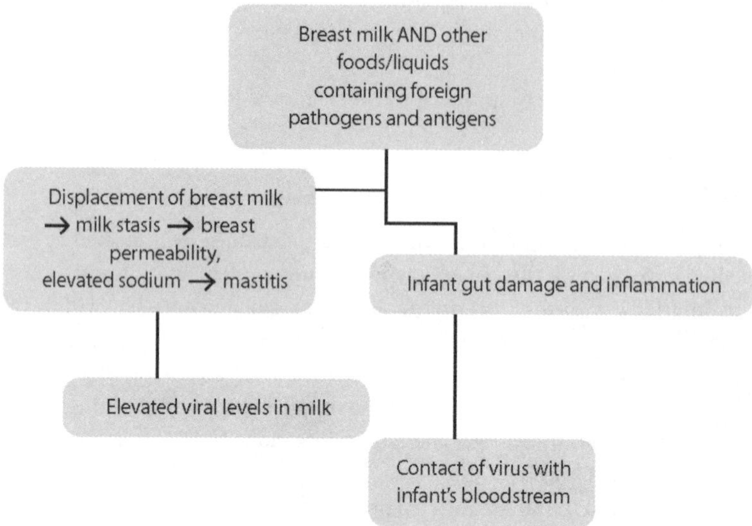

Adapted from: Pamela Morrison's presentation, Mother's milk and HIV: risks, rights and responsibilities, given at the Australian Breastfeeding Association Seminar for Health Professionals, Breastfeeding: Science and Experience, 2004, Sydney, Brisbane, Melbourne, Adelaide and Perth, Australia.

The most common reasons for mixed feeding

While women in most low-income countries breastfeed, rates of exclusive breastfeeding are low, particularly in Africa (though they are increasing there now more than elsewhere). The belief among health workers, family members and mothers themselves, universally, in the inadequacy of breastmilk alone to sustain a baby for the first six months of life, is the most common reason for supplementation of the breastfed baby.[24] Many reports from Prevention of Mother to Child Transmission project (PMTCT) sites have shown that mothers did not believe that they could make enough breastmilk and expected to give their babies extra drinks. Traditional practices demand that new babies are given little sips of water, either in the belief that they are thirsty or to preserve the shape of the fontanelle. Older babies are given porridge or 'real food' in case they are hungry. Cultural norms, passed down the generations, sometimes require babies to be given other special foods and liquids, often from birth. Customary traditional beliefs that babies need other foods and liquids besides breastmilk place HIV-exposed babies at risk for transmission of HIV, and lead to reduced breastmilk production by displacement of breastmilk.

For many years after the discovery that HIV could be transmitted in breastmilk, health workers, counsellors and women themselves believed that these practices could not be changed, and that mixed feeding was inevitable, but fortunately further research was able to show that this is not the case. Several studies now attest to the efficacy of mother support in achieving exclusive breastfeeding.[25,26] My own experience working with HIV-positive breastfeeding mothers confirms that once they have information about the rationale for the recommendation for exclusive breastfeeding, and how to achieve it, and especially how to know their babies are getting enough breastmilk by being able to access regular weight checks for their babies, and seeing their babies achieving good weight gain, they are able to easily exclusively breastfeed for a full six months and combat conflicting information from family members and friends.

A priority for counsellors and mothers is a clear understanding of how the breasts make milk, and factors which interfere with that process. For example, there is a responsibility to explain that breastmilk is in fact 87% water, so the babies do not need extra drinks.[27,28] It's also vital to teach them that extra foods and fluids are not only unnecessary, but dangerous for a young baby, increasing the risk of pneumonia, diarrhoea and other infections, as well as HIV. Mothers need to know how to watch their babies for signs of developmental readiness for solid foods, and also how to recognise that their babies are still too immature for them. The tongue protrusion reflex,[29,30] whereby immature babies offered solid foods too soon spit the food out on to their chins, is a very reliable sign that mothers find intriguing. It's not difficult to teach mothers *how* to exclusively breastfeed and especially how to make enough milk, so that they have the confidence to exclusively breastfeed for the full first six months of life. This how-to information was set out in Chapter 8.

Breastfeeding definitions

The degree of exclusivity of breastfeeding, and what it means, has been an aspect of the HIV and breastfeeding story which has received little recognition. When health outcomes for 'ever-breastfed' compared to 'never-breastfed' babies don't seem to be very different, we need to question how the study was done and why researchers were able to arrive at such a conclusion. Clinicians who receive little training or are just too busy to read more than the abstract and conclusion of a journal article can easily be lulled into complacency about the safety of formula; it may not be clear that formula-feeding is more than just a lifestyle choice. Nor that optimal health for mothers and babies really does depend on optimal protection, promotion and support of breastfeeding. While there will always be individual babies who seem to thrive even if they are not breastfed, at a population level the differences in health and cognitive outcomes between never-breastfed, ever-breastfed and exclusively breastfed babies are real and measurable. Closer scrutiny of research which appears to gloss over these distinctions nearly always reveals problems with the definitions. Nowhere does this have more life-changing implications than in the context of HIV.

For many years the late, great Miriam Labbok, a staunch advocate for children, who had at one time worked for UNICEF, campaigned for breastfeeding definitions to be more accurately described in the lactation literature.[31] Merely describing a baby as 'breastfed' could mean that they were put to the breast only once or twice in their life, or it could mean that they had only ever received their own mother's milk, unadulterated with other foods and fluids. In recognition of the growing problem in interpreting research on breastfeeding Miriam wrote the report from a global meeting held in April

1988 to examine how breastfeeding was defined. Sponsorship came from the Interagency Group for Action on Breastfeeding (IGAB), comprised of different UN groups, with input from the breastfeeding community and others concerned with infant feeding. The definitions were completed and submitted for publication in October 1989[32] after further review and input from more than 50 other breastfeeding research and programme experts from developed and developing countries, including the Jelliffes, Margaret Kyenkya-Isabirye, Ted Greiner and many other well-known individuals and organisations from the breastfeeding movement. The schema divided breastfeeding into two main categories, and additional descriptive parameters enabling more accurate definition.

Categories

1. *Full:* full breastfeeding is divided into exclusive and almost exclusive
2. *Partial:* partial includes three levels of feeding – medium, high, and low.
3. *Token breastfeeding:* non-nutritive

Additional parameters

1. time postpartum or child's age;
2. frequency;
3. intervals;
4. duration;
5. artificial nipples or other devices;
6. type, timing, and amount of other feedings;
7. expression of breast milk and later use and
8. other influences.

Definitions

Exclusive breastfeeding: no other liquid or solid from any other source enters the infant's mouth.

Almost exclusive: allows occasional other tastes of liquids, traditional foods, vitamins, medicines, etc.

Full breastfeeding: includes exclusive and almost exclusive.

Full breastmilk-feeding (or fully breastmilk-fed): receives expressed breastmilk, in addition to breastfeeding

Partial: mixed feeding, designated at high, medium or low. Methods for classification suggested include percentage of calories from breastfeeding, percent age of feeds that are breastfeeds, etc. Any feeding of expressed breastmilk would fall under this category

Token: minimal, occasional breastfeeds (for comfort or with less than 10% of the nutrition thereby provided.)

From this, one can fully describe breastfeeding behaviour at a single point in time and make useful distinctions between different types of breastfeeding in research studies.

One can also immediately analyse whether research apparently showing the risk of transmission of HIV through 'breastfeeding' has any merit. How long were babies breastfed? Was it long enough to distinguish a route of transmission? Did infants receive other foods and liquids, and if so what, and when?

The importance of exclusive breastfeeding had in fact been recognised for many years. For instance, my first baby was born in Zimbabwe in 1977 and shortly afterwards I went to live in Malawi where healthcare was quite sparse. Having been exposed to La Leche League literature,[33] I knew full well that he should be exclusively breastfed for six months, even though advice in the popular literature for mothers at the time suggested starting weaning foods much earlier.

Taking a new look at the old research on postpartum transmission of HIV

It took until 2001 for WHO to issue a formal recommendation (outside the context of HIV) that all babies should be exclusively breastfed for the first half-year of life.[34] By that time, 'breastfeeding' had been recognised as an important route of vertical HIV transmission for 16 years. But early studies paid little attention to the connection between the common practice of supplementing the immature newborn with other foods and liquids and the consequences for an increased risk of MTCT of HIV. In initial research, 'breastfeeding' was often not well defined, often of very short duration, and included infants who were receiving other foods and liquids.[35,36] Preble and Piwoz noted in their 1998 review[13] that the risk attributable to breastfeeding varied from 0–46%, and it's entirely possible that such a wide estimation of risk may have been due to very hazy definitions of what it meant to be breastfed.

Two of the most influential studies of all time, still quoted by reputable AIDS support organisations to illustrate that breastfeeding is a risk factor for HIV transmission, are the 1992 Dunn meta-analysis[37] and the Nduati randomised controlled trial[38] discussed in Chapter 4. Looking at how breastfeeding was defined in these papers throws some light on how unreliable these estimates were. The poor definitions raise questions about how much infection was actually due to breastfeeding. Certainly the researchers did not distinguish between mixed and exclusive breastfeeding.[39]

The Coutsoudis paper: exclusive breastfeeding

In 1998, well before WHO made the recommendation for exclusive breastfeeding in 2001, Anna Coutsoudis and colleagues in Durban, South Africa, had hypothesised that exclusive breastfeeding would be protective against transmission of HIV to the breastfed baby.[40] The rationale was that breastmilk contains components, such as epidermal growth factor, which may enhance the maturation of the gut epithelial barrier, thus maintaining its integrity and hindering passage of the virus. They noted that existing analyses of HIV-transmission via breastmilk were flawed because they failed to account for the effects of different types of breastfeeding practices: exclusive or mixed (with or without water, or other fluids that might contaminate and injure the immature gastrointestinal tract). Two earlier studies, one from South Africa[41] and one from Brazil[42] had attempted to examine the effect of different breastfeeding patterns on mother-to-child transmission, but both had limitations.

Anna Coutsoudis and colleagues' study prospectively examining the impact of different patterns of breastfeeding on MTCT of HIV[14] found that by three months, 18.8% of 156 never-breastfed HIV-exposed babies became infected compared with 21.3% of 393 breastfed children. But importantly, the *exclusively* breastfed babies had almost half the rate of transmission of those who received *mixed* feeding before three months (14.6% vs 24.1 %). Exclusive breastfeeding carried a similar risk to no breastfeeding at all. The results didn't accord with conventional wisdom because they suggested that the vertical transmission of HIV through breastmilk was dependent on the *pattern* of breastfeeding and not simply on *any* breastfeeding.

When the Coutsoudis paper was published in the August 1999 issue of the *Lancet* the results electrified the breastfeeding world, finally raising hopes that breastfeeding would once again receive international support. I had received a pre-publication copy a full four months earlier, while I was attending the March 1999 field-testing of the WHO-UNICEF HIV and Infant Feeding counselling Course, which focuses on counselling HIV-positive mothers to feed their babies breastmilk substitutes in order to avoid the risk of postpartum HIV transmission. We had high hopes that the findings of the Coutsoudis study would motivate policymakers to wind back some of their promotion of replacement feeding. But WHO were not persuaded on the basis of one study originally designed to test whether vitamin A would reduce the risk of MTCT and where transmission rates associated with exclusive compared to mixed breastfeeding hadn't been the main purpose of the research. Officials at WHO and UNICEF said that the findings needed to be replicated. It took another six years before that happened.

Meanwhile, Anna Coutsoudis published a follow-up paper in 2001[43] showing that the protective effect of exclusive breastfeeding against HIV lasted even beyond its duration: by 15 months, the cumulative probability of transmission remained lower among those babies who had been exclusively breastfed for three months or more compared to those who had been mixed fed.

ZVITAMBO confirms the effect of exclusive breastfeeding

In 2005, the landmark ZVITAMBO project published results from a very large and extremely thorough study in Zimbabwe.[22] The ZVITAMBO study had opened in 1997, with a huge budget and access to HIV-positive mothers giving birth at four of the Harare City polyclinics. My friend, Clare Zunguza, the Senior Nutritionist at the City of Harare, was a Wellstart graduate, with impeccable breastfeeding credentials who had the responsibility of overseeing the protection, promotion and support of breastfeeding in the polyclinics, all 13 of which had obtained the UNICEF Baby Friendly Hospital Initiative credential since 1992. We were very worried that breastfeeding promotion would be undermined by the 'infant feeding counselling' to be put in place by ZVITAMBO staff. My friend was able to vet the ZVITAMBO materials developed for staff and mothers before they were released and she asked me to collaborate with her on this. She would send the materials to me, I would provide input on the text or in short typed reports, and return them to her. I don't know how much of my commentary she used, but when the ZVITAMBO results came out, we were overjoyed. This was how it was supposed to work! Peter Iliff and colleagues showed very clearly in their 2005 paper that exclusive breastfeeding substantially reduced the risk of postpartum HIV infection, even in the absence of antiretroviral therapy. When mothers had received extensive and repeated opportunities to learn about the importance of really exclusive breastfeeding in accordance with the national policy for *all* mothers outside the context of HIV, they were more successful in breastfeeding exclusively. HIV infection attributable to exclusive breastfeeding was only 1.3% compared with 4.4% for infants who received mixed feeding.[22] Even feeding the infant with water and other non-milk liquids increased the risk. Mixed breastfeeding led to a four-fold increase in postnatal transmission, compared with exclusive breastfeeding. Or to phrase it another way, early exclusive breastfeeding (feeding only breastmilk) compared to early mixed feeding (feeding both breastmilk and non-breastmilk liquid or solid foods) led to a 75% reduction in postpartum transmission in babies tested at six months. And lastly, babies of mothers who had *not* received the special 'HIV and infant feeding counselling' had lower rates of HIV-infection and mortality (better HIV-free survival) than those who had.

The Coovadia study

Gerry Coovadia and Nigel Rollins published a third paper in 2007 looking at exclusive vs mixed breastfeeding.[23] From September 2001 to March 2003, they had assessed HIV transmission risk associated with exclusive breastfeeding and other types of infant feeding. The key finding was that early introduction of animal milks or solid foods increased the risk compared with exclusive breastfeeding from birth. Eighty-three percent of HIV-positive mothers had exclusively breastfed their infants for the first six months. The rate of postnatal transmission in exclusively breastfed infants who were negative at six weeks of age (i.e. those who were infected through breastfeeding) was 4.04% at 20–26 weeks of age. Babies who received both breastmilk and formula were twice as likely to become infected by 26 weeks compared to those who received only breastmilk. Babies who received breastfeeding with solid foods were 11 times more likely to acquire HIV than those who were exclusively breastfed. In addition, cumulative three-month mortality was more than twice as high, at 15.1% for infants given replacement feeds compared to only 6.1% in the exclusively breastfed group.

The lactation community was disappointed by the transmission rate attributed to really exclusive breastfeeding in the Coovadia and Rollins paper. It was roughly the same as for the mixed-fed babies in the ZVITAMBO project. Would this rather poor result be used to show that even when breastfeeding is apparently practised 'exclusively' there was still an unacceptable risk of transmission? In order to avoid the stated 4.04%, even with exclusive breastfeeding, would it still be 'safer' to use formula-feeding? As always, when there's a strange research finding, it's wise to look closely at the small print. An explanation for the disappointing Coovadia results can be found in the Methods section, in the definition of 'exclusive breastfeeding':

> *'Exclusive breastfeeding was defined as the infant receiving only breastmilk from birth (including expressed breastmilk) from his or her mother and no other liquids or solids, with the exception of drops or syrups consisting of vitamins, mineral supplements, or*

drugs.[16,17] ***Our protocol, however, allowed water or formula milk to be given for up to a total of 3 days, either on separate or continuous days, without exclusion from the group*** *(this allowance was included since we were unsure how well participants would be able to adhere to the strictest definition of exclusive breastfeeding). Periods of exclusive breastfeeding ended on the fourth day of a child receiving either water or formula milk. Infants who received porridge or other solid foods, even if only once, were excluded from the feeding group... Replacement feeding was defined as provision of any non-human milk and the exclusion of all breastmilk, with or without other liquids or solids. Mixed breastfeeding was defined as giving breastmilk with non-human milk, other liquids, or solids.'*[17,18*]

Citation of WHO documentation by Coovadia and Rollins implies WHO endorsement of inclusion within the definition of 'exclusive breastfeeding' the addition of other fluids or solid foods for up to three days. But the Coovadia study took place between September 2001 and March 2003, several months *before* a WHO meeting which endorsed lapses in the definition. The subject of allowable lapses was on the agenda at a WHO HIV and Infant Feeding Data Analysis Workshop from 12–14 November 2003,[44] seven months after the Coovadia and Rollins study ended. From the text emanating from the workshop, it almost seems as if the Coovadia and Rollins study definitions were being approved retrospectively, but before publication, which was not actually until 2007. The recommendation for the new definition of exclusive breastfeeding, and the acceptability of lapses, contained on pages 5 and 21 of the WHO 2003 document, reads:

'Defining and classifying feeding practices
Consistent definitions of feeding patterns should be used to ensure comparison of findings across studies. It is also desirable to specify allowable lapses and provide complete information about how feeding patterns are defined for analysis. An important issue to consider is whether to use a single classification for an infant or to use time varying classifications for different periods. This choice would depend on the research question being addressed. In addressing the issue of HIV transmission through breastfeeding, it might be appropriate to use a hierarchical definition of feeding status with some allowable lapses. For example, an infant classified as partially breastfed at 6 weeks of age, who has been given formula on more than 3 occasions, would not be classified as predominantly breastfed at 10 weeks even if the mother stops giving formula.

Recommendation for research studies:

Existing WHO definitions of exclusive, predominant and or partial breastfeeding given above should be used in HIV and infant feeding studies. Studies should clearly specify allowable lapses, if any.

---

* *WHO quote references:*

16. WHO. *Indicators for assessing breastfeeding practices. Report of an informal meeting. Division of Child and Adolescent Health.* WHO/CDD/SER/91.14.ed. Geneva: World Health Organization, 1991.
17. WHO. *Breastfeeding and replacement feeding practices in the context of mother-to-child transmission of HIV: an assessment tool for research.* WHO/RHR/01.12 (WHO/CAH/01.21) ed. Geneva: World Health Organization, 2001.
18. WHO, UNICEF, UNAIDS. *HIV and infant feeding: guidelines for decision makers.* WHO/FRH/NUT/CHD/98.1 ed. Geneva: World Health Organization, 1998

The definition of exclusive breastfeeding (EBF) will be the WHO definition but will apply some limits... The protocol acknowledges that some mothers will temporarily lapse from EBF and yet comply with an exclusive pattern for the majority of the study. ***If the mother interrupts EBF for a short period she may remain in the feeding arm to which she self-selected. A maximum of 3 lapses but EBF for the remaining duration of the study will be accepted. A lapse represents a day when either water or formula milk is given.*** *Porridge or other solid foods, even on one occasion, will represent non-compliance with the intervention and exclusion from the EBF group.'*

Was there a dose response with 'allowable lapses'?

Work with babies who are exposed to allergens indicates that it can take 2–4 weeks of subsequent exclusive breastfeeding for the gut to recover from even one insult. The introduction of just one bottle of artificial feeding product can decrease the acidity of the stomach.[45] HIV is an acid labile virus. Therefore a decrease in the acidity of the stomach or intestine might enhance survival of any maternal HIV-infected cells found in breastmilk and facilitate entry into the infant's bloodstream.

In the Coovadia study up to three such insults were allowed. It is perhaps not surprising that the rate of infection in the exclusive breastfeeding arm of the Coovadia study (4.04%) was three times higher than the rate of infection for the exclusively breastfed babies in the 2005 ZVITAMBO study (1.3%).[22] But looking more closely at the ZVITAMBO babies we see that even in this study, there was one allowable lapse:

'Exclusive breastfeeding (EBF) – the infant consumed only breast milk and no other liquids, milks or solid foods except vitamins or prescribed medicines, according to mothers' reports at all three timepoints, or at two of three timepoints. ***One lapse in the exclusivity of EBF at one of the three timepoints was allowed only if the non-breast milk item consumed was a non-milk liquid. Allowing one lapse in the definition of EBF is consistent with other studies.****'* A. Coutsoudis, N. Rollins, personal communications

It's disappointing that these permitted lapses have been overlooked by editors of the medical journals in which research on breastfeeding is published. This sort of oversight – that lapses are permitted within a careful definition and will not affect research results – is similar to the trivialisation of the importance of breastfeeding that occurs with the Voldemort effect described by Julie Smith. It can, and does, mislead clinicians and mothers about the risk of transmission of HIV, or the protection from many other diseases for the breastfed baby.[46]

To breastfeeding advocates, who noted that it took another two years before the global guidance from the UN agencies would be changed to once again stand behind breastfeeding for HIV-positive mothers, it seemed that the cards were often stacked against us. Even when the research was favourable, it was ignored, or delayed, or sabotaged in some way, to discredit trust in mother's milk.

Whether breastfeeding is exclusive or not makes a difference in the context of HIV. The way breastfeeding is defined helps us to read and interpret the research in a more accurate way.

CHAPTER 10

Components in breastmilk that protect against HIV

'Based on the evident protective capacity of breast-feeding, it has been suggested that not breast-feeding may be the most common immunodeficiency in infancy.'

Lars Hanson, expert in the immunobiology of human milk, 1998

Human milk has long been known to possess antimicrobial properties and to protect newborns from enteric pathogens. A long list of scientific-sounding components in breastmilk help protect an HIV-exposed baby from becoming infected; secretory immunoglobulins, maternal leukocytes, lactoferrin, lactoperoxidase, lysozyme, protease/protease inhibitors, other protein fractions, receptor-mimetic oligosaccharides and lipids, alone or in concert, have been identified with direct or indirect antimicrobial activity depending on the microbe under study.[1] Breastmilk also contains non-specific immune factors that have antiviral and anti-HIV effects *in vitro* (when examined in a laboratory). Breastmilk also contains epidermal growth factor and transforming growth factor β, which may enhance the maturation of the gut epithelial barrier, thus maintaining its integrity and hindering passage of virus.[2,3]

Some milk factors may be specifically protective against postnatal transmission of HIV. In 1992 Newburg and colleagues demonstrated that human milk glycosaminoglycans inhibited binding of HIV glycoprotein gp120 to host-cell CD4+ receptors, helping to block the first step that is critical for infection of a target cell. This inhibitory activity was found in colostrum and mature milk samples from both HIV-positive and HIV-negative populations of women.[4,5] In 1994, anti-HIV IgG and IgA antibodies were also identified in colostrum from HIV-positive women, but not from HIV-negative women.[6] Van de Perre suggested in 1993 that HIV IgM in breastmilk could be protective against postnatal transmission of the virus in three ways: (a) by compensating for a defective secretory IgA response and by directly coating viral particles, (b) because they are strong potentiators of complement-mediated cytotoxicity, of which at least nine components have been identified in human milk, and (c) by taking part in the lysis (breakdown) of infected cells by a mechanism of antibody-dependent lymphocyte cytotoxicity.[7]

Researchers looking at pasteurisation of breastmilk in 1993[8] to see whether it managed to inactivate HIV wrote, 'Human milk has long been known to possess antimicrobial properties and to protect newborns from enteric pathogens. ...Antiviral agents may destroy the infectious integrity of virions (inactivation) or block steps in the viral life cycle of attachment, penetration, replication and release.'

Antiviral properties of breastmilk

As early as the 1960s and 1970s a number of researchers looked at the antiviral properties of breastmilk, which showed the dual nutritional and antiviral role of lipids[9–12] including those that inactivated enveloped viruses.[13,14] In the late 1980s and early 1990s other researchers continued these investigations, looking at this phenomenon by different classes of free fatty acids in milk.[8,15,16] The fatty acids were found to cause leakage and, at higher concentrations, a complete disintegration of the envelope and the viral particles. They also caused disintegration of the plasma membranes of tissue culture cells resulting in cell lysis and death. Various enveloped viruses exposed to antiviral milk lipids or milk stomach contents were inactivated, including HIV.

The antiviral activity, which reduced titres of virus by as much as 10,000-fold, only affected enveloped viruses and was localised in the milk lipid fraction. Milk and stomach contents that were antiviral also lysed cultured cells by disruption of their plasma membrane. Cell lysis was caused by purified linoleic acid, which is a normal constituent of human milk triglycerides.[15] The HIV inactivating property was heat stable and remained after heating at temperatures consistently used by milk banks.[8] As will be discussed in the next chapter on breastmilk pasteurisation, McDougal noted the antiviral activity of milk lipids against HIV in spiked milk samples that sat on the counter as controls while other samples were being heat-treated.[17] Orloff noted that input HIV titre could not be recovered from control human milk preparations that were innoculated with HIV, but not heated.[8] This was due to inactivation of HIV infectivity by the human milk, rather than to cellular toxicity or interference with detection of viral replication. Isaacs and Thormar stated that the appearance of this antiviral activity occured only in stored milk in which the lipase had had a chance to break lipids down into free fatty acids.[18] The activity of the free fatty acids was cumulative (the more that are present, the more effective the antiviral activity) and viral killing was rapid when the free fatty acids came into contact with the envelope of the virus. In cases such as HIV infection, in which the virus may be found in the acellular fraction of the milk as well as the cellular fraction, these antiviral lipids reduced the risk of viral transmission by destroying the free virus. Milk concentrations as low as 10% had some antiviral activity. Titre reduction occurred rapidly, within 5–10 minutes, and was more efficient at high rather than low temperatures.[8] Although the study was done to assess the effectiveness of Holder pasteurisation, inactivation could not be attributable to heat alone.

This helps to explain why later research by the Nairobi group[19,20] and others to determine the quantity of HIV in breastmilk, or the quantity of virus that would be consumed by the breastfed infant, appears to have consistently used breastmilk that had the lipid layer removed and discarded. Culture detection of replicating HIV virus in breastmilk remained a challenge because of breastmilk's inhibitory factors. In order to isolate the virus the aqueous supernatant fraction must be prepared by centrifugation of freshly expressed milk for 20 minutes, then the lipid layer must be removed and discarded.[20] However, identification of the virus in what was effectively skim breastmilk in a petri dish may not tell us all that we need to know about how the virus behaves in whole milk ingested by an infant.

Researchers attempted to address that question in 2003. Hoffmann and colleagues conducted a study to determine which of the four components of breastmilk (whole milk, skim milk, the lipid layer, or breastmilk cells) had the highest sensitivity and concentration of HIV RNA.[21] The probability of detection of HIV (sensitivity) and the concentration of HIV RNA were associated with the choice of milk component, CD4 cell count, concentration of blood serum HIV RNA, and the presence of breast inflammation. Whole milk demonstrated higher sensitivity and mean concentration than any other single component. Sensitivity was enhanced by analysing all of them.

When research peters out

Many human milk components are such effective antimicrobial and antiviral agents that, according to Valerie McClain, who devotes her blog to examining industry interest in breastmilk,[22] over 2,000 patents have been taken out on them for commercial use by the pharmaceutical and food industries. Most favoured are human milk lipids, which serve not only as nutrients, but also as antiviral agents that constitute a defence system for mucosal surfaces against infections like HIV.

After reading about how difficult it was to isolate the HIV virus from human milk, a friend and I became interested in trying to find out more. My friend, Dr Hilary Cadman, was a lecturer in biochemistry at the University of Zimbabwe. Of particular interest to us was the research on the fatty acids in human milk and their ability to destroy the viral envelope, and how this was more likely at room temperature.[15,16] We also explored ways that working African women without refrigeration in their homes could safely store their milk at room temperature (about 15–20°C). We wanted to know how long expressed breastmilk would safely keep without too high a level of bacterial contamination. We tried to interest a lady researcher at the University of Zimbabwe in doing a little project with us on expressed breastmilk, but she was very dismissive of the idea, saying that hand-expression of breastmilk was too hard – she herself had never managed to do it successfully. Nevertheless my friend and I persisted in trying to find out more and were intrigued and not a little frustrated that this promising direction of research came to a dead end. Inexplicably, the line of enquiry pursued by researchers like Newburg, Isaacs and Thormar, which had looked so promising, appeared to peter out.

Later it was found that several of the researchers who had been working on identifying the protective components in breastmilk were registered as inventors of the patents on human milk oligosaccharides of human milk fat globules and had formed companies to commence manufacturing them.[23,24] Valerie McClain shared with me her finding that one of the researchers was also involved with the Human Milk Banking Association of

North America.[25] Another was listed as inventor of a patent #7253143 called 'Peptides based on the sequence of human lactoferrin', which was owned by Pharmasurgics AB of Sweden. He won the Nutricia Foundation Award in 2004 (approximately $400,000). One object of the invention was for use in infant formula, and use of human lactoferrin against AIDS was also mentioned. At least one prominent university, which itself funded research into transmission of HIV through breastfeeding, owned two patents, and the US government was also registered as having some rights to them.

David Newburg, who did so much research on the antiviral capacity of lipids in human milk against enveloped viruses, wrote in 2007[26] that:

> *'The most widely recognised element of the adaptive immune system is sIgA. The innate immune system is the sum of physical barriers, chemical barriers (including secretions), and reactive elements of local cells and cells recruited to a threatened site. The gut epithelium creates a tight barrier that separates luminal antigens and gut microbiota from invading the host while activating underlying lymphoid elements. Activation of reactive cellular elements can also stimulate responses by the adaptive immune system. The epithelium is a first responder of the mucosal immune system. The strong acid, proteases, and peptides secreted into stomachs of adults are major components of this barrier. In the infant, in whom these secretions are not as well developed, lingual and gastric lipases digest human milk triglyceride into free fatty acid and monoglyceride, which, at concentrations found in stomachs of breast-fed infants, are known to be highly toxic to many human pathogens, especially enveloped viruses.'*

Why do so few babies become infected with HIV through breastfeeding?

Lars Bode and colleagues in Zambia investigated whether human milk oligosaccharide concentrations were associated with a reduced risk of postnatal HIV transmission. Infants were followed from birth to 24 months of age.[27] Milk samples were collected at one month from HIV-positive women who transmitted the virus to their infants, from HIV-positive mothers who did not transmit, and from HIV-negative women. Higher concentrations of human milk oligosaccharides were associated with protection against breastfeeding-associated transmission independent of other known risk factors.

Alpha-defensins, observed to have anti-HIV activity, were detected in 79% of milk samples as measured by Louise Kuhn and colleagues to test whether they were associated with HIV-transmission.[28] The concentration increased as breastmilk HIV RNA quantity increased, and was a strong and significant predictor of infection. After adjustment for milk HIV RNA quantity, alpha-defensin concentration was significantly associated with a decreased risk of intrapartum and postnatal HIV.

Breastmilk cellular responses are potentially influential in decreasing MTCT of viruses. The intestinal mucosa of children exposed to HIV by breastfeeding produces HIV-specific antibodies harbouring major functional properties against HIV. A study published in 2012 found that the levels of total IgA and IgG were increased in milk of HIV-infected mothers and stools of HIV-exposed children, indicating the activation of B cell-derived mucosal immunity.[29] Palaia and colleagues assessed the HIV-inhibitory activity of HIV subtype A and D in breastmilk of Ugandan women and found that milk inhibited p24 production by ≥50%, and more effectively neutralised subtype A than D. Breastmilk from HIV-infected women showed homotypic and cross-subtype neutralisation of HIV by IgG-dependent and independent mechanisms.[30]

Maria Miller and Peter Iliff of the ZVITAMBO project noted in 2002 that one-third to one-half of 1.5 million HIV-positive children in the world acquired their infection via breastfeeding. They asked, what protects the 85% of breastfed babies of HIV-infected mothers who do not become infected? They postulated that erythropoietin (EPO), a hormone in human milk secreted by the kidney that stimulates red blood cell production, had a role in the prevention of HIV transmission during breastfeeding. Perhaps erythropoietin might maintain mammary epithelium integrity, thereby reducing viral loads in milk, or maintain intestinal epithelial integrity in the breastfed neonate, thus preventing ingested milk-borne virus being infective.[31] Eight years later researchers in Tanzania tested this hypothesis among HIV-positive ART-naive women.[32] The risk of MTCT was inversely related to breastmilk erythropoietin concentration, suggesting that breastmilk erythropoietin does indeed have cytoprotective properties which promote the integrity of the mammary epithelium – necessary to prevent leakage of HIV particles from blood into milk. Mammary gland leakiness associated with subclinical breast inflammation is a risk factor for MTCT and erythropoietin promotes gut integrity in infants, as already proven for premature infants whose risk of necrotising enterocolitis is reduced when they receive recombinant human erythropoietin.

In 2017, reviewing the role and significance of the innate immune factors in infant susceptibility to HIV infection, Henrick and colleagues wrote that the majority of infants breastfeeding from their HIV-infected mothers do not acquire HIV infection despite exposure to cell-free virus and cell-associated virus in HIV-infected breastmilk. Paradoxically, exclusive breastfeeding has led to a significant decrease in mother-to-child transmission (MTCT) compared with non-exclusive breastfeeding. Although it remains unclear how HIV-exposed infants remain uninfected despite repeated and prolonged exposure to HIV, the low rate of transmission is suggestive of a multitude of protective, short-lived bioactive innate immune factors in breastmilk such as lactoferrin and elafin, among many others. Their lab was the first to show that soluble toll-like receptor 2 (sTLR2) directly inhibits HIV infection, integration, and inflammation which directly binds to selective HIV proteins, including p17, gp41, and p24, leading to significantly reduced HIV infection in a dose-dependent manner.[33]

The Malaysian author K.K. Prameela, who has written a series of fascinating articles on the protective components of human milk, notes that the predominant lymphocytes in breastmilk are CCR5-expressing memory CD4 T-cells. CCR5 is the main HIV co-receptor, involved in virus entry and cell-to-cell spread.[34] Natural antibodies to CCR5 inhibit infection of macrophages and dendritic cells with HIV and may limit the transmission of HIV through breastfeeding. Viruses other than HIV can potentially also induce the formation of anti-CCR5 antibodies. It may be postulated that the breastfeeding mother who is not HIV-positive could be exposed to other such viruses with capacity to induce anti-CCR5 antibodies in host cells; such environmental exposure could thus lead to the passage of these viruses into breastmilk, potentially provoking the production of blocking antibodies against HIV, a mechanism that could be taken advantage of.

Prameela cautions that this re-emphasises the need for exclusive breastfeeding in all mothers not infected by HIV. Could this have implications for mothers who are newly infected during breastfeeding, where the risk of transmission is as high as 30%, but where the remaining 70% of infants still do not become infected?

Since HIV has so many dysregulatory effects on the human immune system, theoretically the immunologic quality of breastmilk from HIV-infected women might be compromised. However, reassuring research from Botswana showed that HIV-infected and uninfected women had similar quantities of the immunologic components, suggesting that despite HIV infection, breastmilk immunologic quality is not compromised.[35]

Louise Kuhn and Grace Aldrovandi wrote in 2012 that breastmilk contains a vast spectrum of immunologically active components including antigen-specific antibodies and cellular immune components, as well as almost every soluble factor known to have immunologic activity to protect against disease.[36] Passive transfer of maternal antibodies across the placenta is now well known to be an important means by which the infant, whose immune system is not fully mature at the time of birth, is protected immunologically. A substantial part of this activity happens by dampening the immune response, creating 'tolerance' in the infant and preventing activation after exposure to pathogens. They also noted:

> *'For low resource settings, women face a double whammy: the absolute background rates of mortality are several fold higher, so even small elevations translate into large numbers of infant deaths, and the relative risks are higher too because environmental deprivation and barriers to health care exacerbate the biological inferiority of formula. Benefits of breastfeeding are multifactorial. Although a strong public health program may be able to minimize risks of environmental contamination and poor nutrition, programs can do nothing to mitigate the risks conferred by the absence of the immunologically active components of breast milk. The fact that breastfeeding confers benefits to infant health even in wealthy countries suggests that there is a biological threshold below which it is not possible to go even with the strongest programs.'*

CHAPTER 11

Pasteurised breastmilk as a replacement feed for the babies of HIV-positive mothers

'Some argue that expressing and heat-treating breastmilk is too difficult, or not feasible. These are often the same people who are in favour of formula feeding by HIV-positive mothers. We agree that successful use of heat-treated expressed breastmilk is not easy, but we might argue that it is not more difficult than formula feeding, and it has other advantages. These include a secure supply of a superior product, and one that is available at all times, is locally manufactured and does not require careful mixing. A great advantage for poor families is that it does not require purchase, which may further impoverish the whole family. Formula requires an adequate good supply of water. Both methods require fuel, utensils and some skills.

Mothers who are HIV-positive and who choose not to breastfeed because of the risk of HIV transmission to their infants would be well served if the possibility of using their own heat-treated expressed breastmilk could be made possible. There seems no good reason why, in the near future, it could not be a realistic option; clearly, feeding expressed breastmilk is very much superior to infant formula, the product is locally manufactured, the procedure will have benefits to the mother's health and will reduce her likelihood of an early pregnancy.'

Latham and Kisanga, 2000[1]

Breastmilk is pasteurised by milk banks using a method called Holder pasteurisation, to inactivate viruses and bacteria and render donor milk safe for feeding needy babies whose mothers don't produce sufficient breastmilk. Holder pasteurisation involves heating milk to 62.5°C for 30 minutes. Banked milk can be lifesaving for small, sick or premature babies, providing optimal nutrition, immune protection and reducing the risk of necrotising enterocolitis, a killer of tiny babies. Banked heat-treated donor milk has also been used in the treatment of immunoglobulin-A deficiencies and immune-depressed states related to bone marrow transplants or leukaemia therapy.[2]

A fascinating little paragraph about the innate ability of human milk to inactivate HIV caught my eye in a 1993 article about the Human Milk Banking Association of North America.[3] Researchers were examining the effect of Holder pasteurisation on human milk that had been inoculated with cell-free HIV and HIV-infected cells to see if it would be practical and safe for milk banking. Input HIV titre could not be recovered from control human milk preparations that were inoculated with HIV, but not heated. This was apparently due to inactivation of HIV infectivity by the milk itself, rather than to cellular toxicity or interference with detection of viral replication.

Three years earlier another researcher had also noted the antiviral activity of milk lipids against HIV. The virus could not be recovered in spiked milk samples that sat on the counter as controls while other samples were being heat-treated.[4]

In an African country where refrigeration wasn't readily available, the intriguing possibility that just storing expressed breastmilk at room temperature could inactivate HIV was tantalising. How could this hypothesis be tested? As mentioned in the previous chapter, a friend and I discussed it endlessly.

In 1999, quite out of the blue, I received an email from a researcher called Dr Caroline Chantry at the University of California, Davis, in Sacramento. She had some funding and she asked if there was any topic of research that might be useful for women in Zimbabwe. It felt like Christmas! I put to her the possibility of looking at HIV virus levels in breastmilk that was allowed to stand at room temperature. I sent her reams of excerpts, ideas and references. And so began a line of needed research that has grown to further our understanding of how pasteurised breastmilk can be provided safely for needy babies in many countries.

Dr Chantry put together a small study in Puerto Rico and our research was published the following year.[6] Four HIV-positive mothers provided 17 samples of their breastmilk, which were analysed qualitatively for HIV proviral DNA and quantitatively for HIV RNA by polymerase chain reaction (PCR). Although the study mothers went into the study knowing they would not be breastfeeding their own babies, they pumped for the African mothers who might benefit from their efforts. Firstly, although an inhibitor was present in the milk, proviral HIV DNA was not destroyed by lipolysis as a result of standing for six hours at room temperature. Fifteen of 17 fresh breastmilk samples (88%) had measurable proviral DNA in the cellular fraction and 83% were positive after lipolysis. However, when the milk samples were placed in a water bath, and the water was brought to boiling point as quickly as possible and then removed from the heat source – a method called 'flash-heating' – proviral DNA was destroyed. Thirdly, a high prevalence of cell-associated HIV proviral DNA was detected in breastmilk despite combination antiretroviral therapy and low or undetectable plasma viral loads.

Although it was disappointing to find out that standing breastmilk at room temperature didn't inactivate the virus in all samples, these were the first findings to document that HIV could be inactivated by the use of boiling water. This method of heat-treatment could be replicated in resource-poor areas over cooking fires or stoves. Further research would be needed to rule out any negative nutritional impact on the breastmilk, and to see whether immunoglobulins, lipase and other anti-infective properties were altered, but it was the start of a line of enquiry which has had important benefits worldwide.

Shortly afterwards, one of Dr Chantry's students, Kiersten Israel-Ballard, came to Zimbabwe to conduct follow-up research on the feasibility of expressing and heat-treating breastmilk in an African setting as part of her Master of Public Health thesis requirement. Her plan was to conduct focus group discussions for breastfeeding mothers, fathers, grandmothers and midwives in Harare city and in Glenview, a high-density, low-income suburb. Kiersten and I spent many happy hours sipping tea or wine on my verandah as she outlined her plans and shared her findings. I also introduced her to my friend Gill Browne, a breastfeeding counsellor for La Leche League who lived on a tea estate in Chipinge, a beautiful rural area in the Eastern Highlands. Gill took Kiersten off to her home where she could interview conservative rural folk, who lived very simply, about the value they placed on breastfeeding. Kiersten's work in Zimbabwe resulted in a brilliant paper detailing the cultural attitudes and traditional beliefs of African people towards breastfeeding, and how they felt about the use of expressed breastmilk.[7]

Since then, Kiersten's research in Zimbabwe and elsewhere has contributed much knowledge to the possibility of using pasteurised breastmilk as a replacement feed for the babies of HIV-positive mothers worldwide. Her work now helps vulnerable babies, including AIDS orphans, to receive donor pasteurised human milk in Kenya, South Africa, Tanzania, Zimbabwe, Rwanda and India.[8]

Scepticism and prejudice

There is considerable negativity among health professionals about the use of home-pasteurised expressed breastmilk as a feeding method for HIV-exposed babies. I spent many months lobbying Helen Armstrong when she worked for UNICEF, trying to persuade her that more attention should be paid to this feeding option, rather than artificial formula. As a lactation consultant, I had a lot of experience with mothers who wanted to feed their expressed breastmilk to their babies rather than formula. They were mothers who either had difficulty in actually breastfeeding directly, or did not want to for various reasons, yet they really did want to give their babies the 'best' milk. I sent Helen no fewer than 30 carefully recorded and documented case histories from my own files to show how my clients had managed to achieve this. But Helen was not persuaded, merely saying that case histories (clinical experience) didn't equate to published research.

Even after the research had been published, the use of home-treated expressed breastmilk remained unacceptable in the opinion of Australian paediatricians who reported on a case history in 2010 of an HIV-positive mother who wanted to breastfeed her baby.[9] Not only was the mother prevented from breastfeeding on pain of having her baby removed from her custody, but the paediatricians were adamant that she could not feed her own pasteurised expressed breastmilk either, even if it was heat-treated in accordance with flash-heating or Pretoria pasteurisation methods, described later in this chapter. Their opinions were clear:

'The WHO lists pasteurisation of expressed breast milk as an option for prevention of MTCT in resource-poor countries. Several techniques for safe pasteurisation in the home have been developed and laboratory studies suggest they are effective in inactivating HIV in infected breast milk. However, there are no clinical trials evaluating the feasibility, safety and efficacy of these methods in preventing MTCT. These methods are time-consuming and inconvenient when compared with breastfeeding. There is also a risk that mothers may not be able to sustain this method of feeding over time and introduce mixed feeding. Until further information is available, outside of resource-poor countries, pasteurisation of breast milk cannot be recommended as an alternative to formula feeding.'

Those of us who worked with mothers in African countries were familiar with the negative bias surrounding the use of expressed breastmilk outside the hospital setting. Even educated African health workers believed that expressed breastmilk was open to witchcraft, and thus taboo, so that HIV-infected mothers would be reluctant to use this feeding method. Many also believed that mothers would be unable to maintain a good supply of expressed breastmilk for very long. While formula-feeding was often portrayed as easy and acceptable, expressing breastmilk was seen as difficult. Was this prejudice simply due to ignorance?

A visit to any premature or neonatal unit at any major hospital in Africa will show that mothers of sick or premature newborns are encouraged to hand-express their milk until breastfeeding is well-established. With practice, it becomes an extremely quick and useful skill. Mothers may be able to hand-express 120ml in 10 minutes. Some mothers of extremely low birthweight babies express breastmilk for many weeks. Working mothers of bigger babies express breastmilk to leave with childminders for feeding the baby during working hours.

IBCLCs know that many mothers who are unable or don't wish to breastfeed directly at the breast, are able to feed their babies exclusively on expressed breastmilk – a practice called 'breastmilk feeding'. I've worked with clients who breastmilk-fed for many months, and sometimes for years. Sometimes a mother will breastmilk-feed several consecutive babies in this way.[10] Ideally, the HIV-exposed breastmilk-fed baby would receive only breastmilk for the first six months of life, followed by partial breastmilk-feeding, with the addition of complimentary weaning foods for up to two years or beyond, in line with current global infant feeding recommendations for breastfed babies.[11]

In 2000 the Zimbabwe Ministry of Health officially endorsed the use of expressed breastmilk as a primary feeding option to be considered by HIV-positive mothers.[12] As Kiersten Israel-Ballard found, given its affordability and its potential to protect infants from HIV infection, heat-treated human milk could have been a feasible infant-feeding option which could have been more widely used.[7] Her focus-group discussions with mothers and healthcare staff revealed that once parents knew that pasteurised breastmilk was safe, and when they received accurate information about how they could provide it, they became enthusiastic about it.[7]

In 2006 Israel-Ballard and colleagues investigated the ability of flash-heating to eliminate bacteria such as *E.coli*, *S.aureus* and Group A and B *Streptococci*. No pathogenic growth was observed in the flash-heated samples. Storage was safe at room temperature for up to eight hours.[13] A further 2007 study done in Durban, South Africa, again confirmed that flash-heating can inactivate HIV in naturally infected breastmilk.[14]

Emotional and hormonal implications

The mother who provides her own milk for her baby has absolute control over her own milk supply and can assure her baby's food security for the whole time that she lactates. This is important in resource-poor settings and in natural disasters where access to breastmilk substitutes can suddenly fail. In addition, the hormonal impact on a mother who continues to lactate is likely to result in less stress, increased enjoyment of her baby and longer lactational amenorrhea (pause in menstrual periods while breastfeeding), which, in the absence of other methods of contraception, contributes to a longer interval before the birth of the next child. That this method of feeding HIV-exposed infants is not more widely known may be due to the fact that it hasn't been well promoted in the media and by local healthcare systems.[15]

Nutritional effects of flash-heating

A 2008 study to determine the effect of flash-heating on vitamin content found that vitamin A was not significantly affected and that vitamins B,^{12} C and folate increased significantly. Vitamins B_2 and B_6 were decreased to 59% and 96% respectively of levels found in unheated milk,[16] showing that most vitamin concentrations are retained.

Immunological and anti-infective components

Chantry and colleagues attempted to ascertain the effect on breastmilk immunoglobulins in order to ensure the milk would continue to offer passive immune protection. They reported in 2010 that flash-heating induced decreases in some immunoglobulins, e.g. polio, and increased others, e.g. influenza and *Salmonella*. They found that a similar proportion of IgA survived as occurred with traditional Holder pasteurisation used in breastmilk banks.[17]

Further research published in June 2010 found that flash-heating inactivates a high titre of cell-free and cell-associated HIV. Assays on spiked human milk demonstrated that new infectious virus did not replicate, and that residual viral particles and residual inoculum were non-infectious, thus predicting that latently infected lymphocytes would not transmit HIV after heating.[18]

In 2011, Chantry and colleagues reported on flash-heating's effect on antimicrobial properties of lactoferrin, lysozyme, and whole milk.[19] There was no difference in rate of growth of *E.coli* or *S.aureus* in flash-heated versus unheated whole milk. Antibacterial activity of lactoferrin was diminished by 11.1% and of lysozyme by up to 56%. Digestion of lysozyme was unaffected but 25% less lactoferrin survived digestion. Bacteriostatic activity of whole milk was unaffected. Flash-heated breastmilk likely had a similar profile of resistance to bacterial contamination as unheated milk.

The ZVITAMBO project in rural Zimbabwe[20] ascertained the feasibility of expressing and heat-treating all breastmilk fed to HIV-exposed, uninfected infants following six months' exclusive breastfeeding. Mothers successfully sustained flash-heating of their breastmilk for 4.5 months (range, 1–11 months), feeding 426 ± 227ml/day to their babies together with weaning foods. Stigma was not a major deterrent, likely due to a social marketing campaign to sustain breastfeeding for all women. This research confirmed that given family and health systems support, even resource-poor rural women can initiate and sustain pasteurised breastmilk-feeding for their babies.

In a further prospective longitudinal trial published in 2012,[21] data was collected on 101 Tanzanian HIV-infected breastfeeding mothers who were encouraged to exclusively breastfeed for six months and then feed flash-heated expressed breastmilk to babies who tested HIV-negative. Mothers received in-home counselling and support from 2–9 months postpartum. They provided a daily milk volume of 322ml per day (range 25–1,120ml). No flash-heated milk contained bacterial pathogens. The researchers found that flash-heating was a simple technology that many mothers could successfully use after exclusive breastfeeding ended, so as to provide the benefits of breastmilk while avoiding MTCT of HIV associated with non-exclusive breastfeeding. Furthermore, the high-temperature, short-time method used in home-pasteurisation preserved more of the immune properties in the milk.

Pretoria pasteurization

In 2000 and 2001, Dr Bridget Jeffery in South Africa described and researched the Pretoria method of home-pasteurisation using very simple implements available in the homes of ordinary women living in resource-poor settings.[22–24] Pretoria pasteurisation was begun at Kalafong Hospital, South Africa, at the end of 2001 for feeding HIV-exposed pre-term infants. Mothers found the method acceptable and easy to perform.[25] Pretoria pasteurisation avoided placing at least 25% of the infants on to formula feeds and there were fewer cases of necrotising enterocolitis, from 11 in the preceding year to three in the 11 months following the introduction of Pretoria pasteurisation. By August 2002, 38 infants had been followed to three months of age. After leaving hospital, 20 mothers claimed to have continued with pasteurising. Others had stopped using the method due to fear of stigma about HIV disclosure.

In an earlier South African study, however, only 6% of mothers ever used heat-treated expressed breastmilk in the first six months.[26] The low uptake was due to mothers worrying that there was no official endorsement of or media coverage of the method. They believed that a reduced amount of milk would be expressed and therefore the baby would not be satisfied. Some were concerned about the possibility of stigmatisation or associations being made in the community with witchcraft; finally, and perhaps most practically, mothers found it too time-consuming, especially when formula was readily available as an alternative.

Method: Flash-heating

A glass jar containing up to 150ml of expressed breastmilk milk is placed in a pan with water two finger-widths above the level of the milk. The water is heated over high heat. Once the water reaches a rolling boil, the milk is removed from the water, and cup-fed to the infant when cooled. Milk typically reaches a peak temperature of 72.9°C.[21]

Method: Pretoria Pasteurisation

Pretoria pasteurisation makes use of passive heat transfer from boiling water to milk that is contained in a glass jar standing in the water. The milk is poured into a clean glass peanut butter jar, which is then placed into a one-litre aluminium cooking pot. Boiling water is then poured into the cooking pot, and the jar and milk are left to stand until the water is a comfortable temperature, approximately 25 minutes. The desired temperature range is between 56–62°C as this will maintain a large proportion of the secretory IgA within the milk.[27] The method was tested and found to be reliable under a wide range of conditions.

A 2005 study comparing the safety of flash-heating and Pretoria pasteurisation found that flash-heating was more efficient and conserved more of the milk's components.[28] A 2008 paper showed results of viral, bacterial and nutrition assays; both flash-heated and Pretoria pasteurised milk achieved temperatures sufficient to inactivate HIV, yet retain most nutrients, but the flash-heat high-temperature short-term method was more inhibitory to bacterial growth than Pretoria pasteurisation, in destroying *E.coli* or *S.aureus* contamination.[29]

A 2009 systematic review of expressed breastmilk as an in-home procedure to limit MTCT of HIV[30] found that heat-treated breastmilk should be emphasised as a safe alternative for feeding HIV-exposed infants (where the mother is HIV-positive, of uncertain HIV status, or during weaning if the mother cannot afford formula or cows' milk), with appropriate information to the individual mother, her family and the community.

Heat-treated expressed breastmilk is:

- Physiologically normal
- Nutritionally superior to other replacement feeds
- Nutritionally perfect (some components slightly changed)
- Retains some immunological protection
- Non-allergenic
- Helps maintain a normal maternal postpartum hormonal profile
  - » Promotes maternal-infant bonding
  - » Likely to maintain some lactational amenorrhea/reduce fertility
- Safe

- Free
- Feasible
- Mother has absolute control over supply/sustainability/baby's food security
- After pasteurisation, breastmilk may be safely stored for eight hours at room temperature
- Mixed breastfeeding and heat-treated breastmilk-feeding are likely to carry no increased risk of transmission of HIV to the baby than exclusive breastfeeding
- Mixed pasteurised breastmilk-feeding with early cessation of breastfeeding; this feeding method is likely to be safe for an HIV-infected mother who wishes to supplement her own milk supply with formula, or when she intends to prematurely wean her baby from the breast on to other foods/liquids/formula.

It's possible for HIV-positive mothers to heat-treat or flash-heat their *own* milk at home in order to inactivate HIV:

- for those mothers who wish to absolutely avoid all possibility of exposing a baby to virus in breastmilk, yet wish to provide them with the most physiologically suitable milk for human infants (having all the benefits with none of the risks),
- for mothers who need to avoid the effects of mixed feeding if the baby has to also receive extra formula supplementation for any reason,
- as a temporary measure if there is a concern about elevated HIV levels in breastmilk due to mastitis or sore nipples or during weaning.

CHAPTER 12

Global policy on HIV and breastfeeding 1996–2009: formula for disaster

Shortly after the first report in April 1985 claiming that the virus that causes AIDS could be transmitted during breastfeeding,[1] and on the rationale that infant formula was safe, affordable, and culturally acceptable, the US Centers for Disease Control and Prevention (CDC) recommended that women testing HIV-positive in the United States avoid breastfeeding.[2]

Breastfeeding had already enjoyed several decades of unprecedented promotion and support. During the 1970s a flood of research into the unique properties of human milk, coupled with concerns about the negative consequences of formula-feeding on the health and survival of babies in developing countries, had underpinned the value of supporting breastfeeding.[3] Formula-feeding, particularly for babies in the developing world, was one of the factors contributing to infant mortality and malnutrition. A May 1974 World Health Assembly resolution[4] urged intensification of the promotion of breastfeeding, calling for mothers, the general public and health personnel to be educated accordingly.

In 1981, following a concerted campaign against unethical marketing, a set of recommendations was adopted by the World Health Organization to limit the promotion within the healthcare system of breastmilk substitutes and associated paraphernalia (bottles, teats and dummies). Known as the International Code of Marketing of Breastmilk Substitutes, the recommendations were overwhelmingly approved by 118 countries, with the US casting the only opposing vote.[5] Nevertheless, even today, healthcare institutions are traditionally seen by industry as effective places to exert influence on maternal infant feeding choice, and the love affair between industry reps and healthcare personnel is long-standing and well known.[6]

It seemed logical that in the early years of the HIV pandemic, in spite of the possibility that the virus could be transmitted through breastmilk, the UN agencies should continue to support universal breastfeeding. To the relief of the lactation community, the first formal WHO/UNICEF recommendation on HIV and infant feeding in 1987 followed a pragmatic, public health approach. On the rationale that the risk of death from transmission of HIV through breastfeeding was likely to be less than the risk of death if breastfeeding was withheld, the agencies favoured continued breastfeeding. The policy statement clearly

Provisions of the Code

The WHO/UNICEF International Code of Marketing Breastmilk Substitutes 1981: a summary

The aim of the Code is to contribute to the provision of safe and adequate nutrition for infants, by the protection and promotion of breastfeeding and by the proper use of breastmilk substitutes, when these are necessary, on the basis of adequate information and through appropriate marketing and distribution.

The code includes ten main provisions:

- No advertising of breastmilk substitutes.
- No free samples of breastmilk substitutes to mothers.
- No promotion of products through health care facilities.
- No company mothercraft nurses to advise mothers.
- No gifts or personal samples to health workers.
- No words or pictures idealizing artificial feeding, including pictures of infants, on the labels of the products.
- Information to health workers should be scientific and factual.
- All information on artificial feeding, including the labels, should explain the benefits of breastfeeding and the costs and hazards associated with artificial feeding.
- Unsuitable products, such as sweetened condensed milk, should not be promoted for babies.
- All products should be of a high quality and take account of the climatic and storage conditions of the country where they are used.

Source: https://snugabell.com/summary-code-including/ (accessed 9 May 2019)

acknowledged the difficulty in determining – if a breastfed infant was subsequently shown to be infected – the route of transmission of the virus; there was simply no way of knowing whether the baby had become infected before, during or after birth:

> *'Breast-feeding should continue to be promoted, supported and protected in both developing and developed countries. In individual situations where the mother is considered to be HIV-infected, and recognizing the difficulties inherent in assessing the infection status of the newborn, the known and potential benefits of breast-feeding would be compared to the theoretical, but apparently small, incremental risk to the infant of becoming infected through breast-feeding'.*[7]

Two years later, in 1989, the Convention on the Rights of the Child explicitly specified protection of a child's right to enjoyment of the highest attainable standard of health, making special note of the advantages of breastfeeding. In fact, breastfeeding as a risk factor for HIV transmission was not even mentioned.[8]

Innocenti Declaration

In August 1990 UNICEF convened a meeting for world health leaders, in Florence, Italy, resulting in the signing of the Innocenti Declaration on the Protection, Promotion and Support of Breastfeeding.[9] Over 30 prominent health officials from around the world attended this landmark event, including Zimbabwe's Minister of Health and Child Welfare, Dr Timothy Stamps. Along with other La Leche League representatives in Zimbabwe, I had lobbied Dr Stamps to attend. We knew that he was a big fan of breastfeeding. He was known to write his own speeches extolling its benefits, so it wasn't surprising that he was eager to be in Florence for the adoption of this potentially wide-reaching declaration. Innocenti recognised the importance of recreating a global breastfeeding culture with the need for protection of mothers from inappropriate marketing of breastmilk substitutes. Once again the possibility that HIV could be passed on to the breastfed baby was an important and deliberate omission.

The Innocenti meeting was followed in September 1990 by the United Nations World Summit for Children in New York. It was the largest gathering of heads of state and government in history.[10] A Plan of Action was agreed by 159 nations to try to end child deaths and malnutrition in the following decade. Respiratory infections and diarrhoea were recognised as the most common infant illnesses in almost every developing country and breastfeeding was singled out as a primary strategy to address young child malnutrition and death. The direction of the summit recommendations was clear and prescriptive:

> *'All mothers should know, and be helped to put into practice, five basic facts:*
> 1. *Breastmilk ALONE is the best possible food and drink in the first 4–6 months of life.*
> 2. *Virtually every mother can breastfeed her baby. Babies should start to breastfeed as soon as possible after birth.*
> 3. *Frequent sucking is needed to produce enough breastmilk for the baby's needs.*
> 4. *Bottle-feeding [formula] can lead to illness and death.*
> 5. *Breastfeeding should continue well into the second year of a child's life.'*

In May 1992 WHO/UNICEF held a second consultation on HIV transmission and breastfeeding. They subsequently issued an unambiguous Consensus Statement[11] endorsing continued breastfeeding in the face of HIV, and the risks of formula-feeding in resource-poor areas. Dr Ted Greiner, a long-time breastfeeding advocate, remembers that wording that he had previously suggested in 1987 was included in the statement coming out of the 1992 Consultation:

> *'Where infectious diseases and malnutrition are the main cause of infant deaths, breastfeeding should be the usual advice given to pregnant women, including those who are HIV infected because their baby's risk of HIV infection through breastmilk is likely to be lower than the risk of death from other causes if it is not breastfed.'*

UNICEF 1991 Baby Friendly Hospital Initiative

In 1991 UNICEF also began implementing a programme called the Baby Friendly Hospital Initiative (BFHI).[12] The BFHI was based on the UNICEF Ten Steps to Successful Breastfeeding[13] (see box). Brilliant in its conception, it was extremely effective in protecting and promoting hospital policies and practices that would ensure successful initiation and support for breastfeeding in the first few days after birth. All healthcare staff having any contact with mothers or babies were to receive 18 hours of training specifically focusing on how to help mothers breastfeed. Hospitals wishing to become Baby Friendly (meaning that they would support breastfeeding) underwent a thorough assessment process, which included random sampling and exhaustive cross-checking of hospital practices, staff skills and mother and baby wellbeing.

In 1993, I was recruited by the Zimbabwe Ministry of Health and Child Welfare as a BFHI Facilitator (trainer) and subsequently as a BFHI Assessor. Later I served on the national BFHI Task Force. Before policies casting doubt on the wisdom of promoting breastfeeding due to fears about HIV could really take hold, Zimbabwe had quickly succeeded in having one-quarter of its hospitals progress through the Baby Friendly process. Our Ministry of Health also issued directives stating that hospital practices would support breastfeeding even if institutions had not yet been through the formal BFHI accreditation. There was to be no formula-feeding for full-term healthy babies in any of the country's hospitals, public or private. No bottles, teats or dummies (pacifiers) were permitted in our maternity units for full-term healthy babies, nor in our neonatal units for premature or sick babies. New mothers were expected to breastfeed, and were helped to do so, and newborns were not discharged home until they were exclusively breastfeeding. Working as a new IBCLC in such an environment, to simply facilitate a policy that was already in place, was a joy.

In 1993, global support for breastfeeding continued with WHO and UNICEF jointly publishing an extremely comprehensive 40-hour Breastfeeding Counselling Course[14] reinforcing protocols to maximise child survival through optimal breastfeeding.

Ten Steps to Successful Breastfeeding

Every facility providing maternity services and care for newborn infants should:

1. Have a written breastfeeding policy that is routinely communicated to all health care staff.
2. Train all health care staff in skills necessary to implement this policy.
3. Inform all pregnant women about the benefits and management of breastfeeding.
4. Help mothers initiate breastfeeding within half an hour of birth.
5. Show mothers how to breastfeed, and how to maintain lactation even if they should be separated from their infants.
6. Give newborn infants no food or drink other than breast milk, unless medically indicated.
7. Practise rooming-in – that is, allow mothers and infants to remain together – 24 hours a day.
8. Encourage breastfeeding on demand.
9. Give no artificial teats or pacifiers (also called dummies or soothers) to breastfeeding infants.
10. Foster the establishment of breastfeeding support groups and refer mothers to them on discharge from the hospital or clinic.

The winds of change

In 1995, the United Nations established The Joint United Nations Programme on HIV/AIDS (UNAIDS) in Geneva (Switzerland) to deal with the AIDS crisis. This was an unprecedented collaboration that pooled the experience, efforts and resources of six United Nations organisations:

- UNICEF
- United Nations Development Programme (UNDP)
- United Nations Population Fund (UNFPA)
- United Nations Educational, Scientific and Cultural Organization (UNESCO)
- World Health Organization (WHO)
- World Bank

Then in 1997, UNAIDS dropped a bombshell in the form of a major policy change, which left the lactation community reeling. They issued a statement[15] saying:

> *'....When children born to HIV-infected women can be assured of uninterrupted access to nutritionally adequate breastmilk substitutes that are safely prepared and fed to them, they are at less risk of illness and death if they are not breastfed. However, when these conditions cannot be met – in particular in environments where infectious diseases and malnutrition are the primary causes of death during infancy – then artificial feeding substantially increases children's risk of illness and death. The policy objective must be to minimize all infant feeding risks and to urgently expand access to adequate alternatives so that HIV-infected women have a range of choices. The policy should also stipulate what measures are being taken to make breastmilk substitutes available and affordable; to teach the safest means of feeding them to infants; and to provide the conditions which will diminish the risks of using them.'*

Furthermore, because breastfeeding carried a risk of transmission of HIV, whereas 'replacement feeding' (a euphemism for formula-feeding) did not, an individual HIV-positive mother now had the right to choose how she wanted to feed her baby and should be 'empowered' to do so, while keeping the reasons secret:

> *'it is mothers who are in the best position to decide whether to breastfeed, particularly when they alone may know their HIV status and wish to exercise their right to keep that information confidential. It is therefore important that women be empowered to make fully informed decisions about infant feeding and that they be suitably supported in carrying them out'*

Thus the previous WHO/UNICEF population-based guidance for developing countries was formally changed to one based on stated individual human rights principles, particularly the right of maternal choice. UNICEF wrote in *SCN News* the following year that the policy 'upholds the fulfilment of women's rights as paramount.'[16]

While the previous policy acknowledged the dangers to infants of abandoning breastfeeding, the new one assumed the intrinsic safety of breastmilk substitutes, the need to minimise the risks and constraints to the use of formula, and to make 'replacement feeding' accessible, affordable and safe. Certain new initiatives needed to be introduced so that HIV-positive women's capacity to freely choose alternatives to breastfeeding could be maximised. In language often reminiscent of industry marketing, these measures seemed to stray into active promotion. The policy turnaround on such a pivotal issue, which posed potentially life-threatening consequences for vulnerable babies in developing countries, constituted a profound reversal of decades of breastfeeding support. Inexplicably, breastfeeding would be undermined in areas where it offered major protection against infant and young child mortality. Lactation experts wrote to the *Lancet* and other medical journals to express their serious concern.[17,18]

What could have caused such a reversal in the protection, promotion and support for breastfeeding? With the benefit of hindsight, it can be seen that these changes had been brewing for some time.

The Nairobi group

In 1986, the year after the report of the Australian baby infected with HIV through breastfeeding, a group of researchers from the University of Nairobi in Kenya began studying mother-to-child transmission (MTCT) of HIV in African women. Headed by Dr Ruth Nduati, the Nairobi group produced a large number of different research studies carried out on the same cohort of 300 or so local breastfeeding HIV-positive women which they published over the next decade.

Dr Nduati was a paediatrician who had had close ties to the University of Washington, Seattle, where she had studied for her Master's degree between 1991 and 1994 and met Dr Peter Piot, the first Director of UNAIDS. Between 1994 and 1998 Dr Nduati was an Advanced In-Country Scholar in the International AIDS Research and Training Program.

Dr Piot had been a Senior Fellow at the University of Washington. He had also held several professorships in microbiology and public health, including at the University of Nairobi. After spending a sabbatical year with WHO in 1992 he became Assistant Director of WHO's Global Programme on HIV/AIDS. In December 1994 he was appointed Executive Director of the Joint United Nations Programme on HIV/AIDS (UNAIDS), and Assistant-Secretary-General of the United Nations.

Starting in November 1992 the Nairobi group began a randomised controlled trial in which untreated Kenyan HIV-positive mothers were assigned to either formula-feed or breastfeed their babies. Breastfeeding lasted a median duration of 17 months.[19] The risk of HIV transmission through breastfeeding was found to be 16%, which was similar to the 14% risk attributed to breastfeeding in David Dunn's 1992 meta-analysis. The majority of infections occurred early during the breastfeeding period. Due to the design of the study, Dr Nduati was able to report that the use of formula prevented 44% of infant infections and led to significantly improved HIV-free survival. The study did not formally end until July 1998 and was not published in a peer-reviewed journal until 2000,[19] but the initial results from the trial must have been available to the World Health Organization, and no doubt exerted a profound influence on the change in

HIV and infant feeding policy. In 1998 it was Dr Nduati who wrote the *Review of the Evidence of Transmission of HIV through Breastfeeding* for the WHO. Her name appears as the author on an early edition of this document, though it has been removed from later versions. Curiously, this background evidence review (referenced WHO/FRH/NUT/CHD 98.3) appears to have been published *after* either of the tools which would actually implement the change of policy – the *Guidelines for Decision-makers* (WHO/FRH/NUT/CHD 98.1) or the *Guide for Health Care Managers and Supervisors* (WHO/FRH/NUT/CHD 98.2).

Ghent working group

In February 1992, an international group of researchers, the Ghent working group, was formed to look at mother-to-child transmission of HIV. The Ghent group appears to have been the brainchild of Dr François Dabis, a 34-year-old French medical doctor, who had interned with the CDC and developed a special interest in the public health challenges of HIV in general, and in vertical transmission in particular. A prodigious author, by 2015 he had published more than 600 papers and two leading textbooks in the field of epidemiology.[20] Other members of the group included upwards of 50 researchers, authors and statisticians in the field of MTCT of HIV and public health, many of whom would become well known in the AIDS community, as we began to call it: Marie-Louise Newell, Joseph Saba, Philippe Lepage, Valeriane Leroy, Nicolas Meda, Catherine Peckham, Ruth Nduati, Philippe Msellati, Isabelle de Vincenzi, Glenda Gray and Philippe van de Perre. The Ghent working group received the support of various very influential bodies: the WHO Global Programme on AIDS, the European Community AIDS Task Force, the Commission of European Communities, the Institute of Child Health in London, the University of Nottingham, the University of Nairobi, programme SIDA, and later UNAIDS. Members met over the course of the next three years, to establish the direction of future research.[21]

In the early 1990s the focus of the AIDS research community had turned to quantifying the risk of transmission of HIV through breastfeeding. In September 1992, five months after the second WHO/UNICEF consultation, the *Lancet* published a systematic review of published studies compiled by Dr David Dunn of the Institute of Child Health in London,[22] quantifying the risk of HIV transmission through breastfeeding. Several of Dr Dunn's co-authors were members of the Ghent working group and had also attended the WHO Consultation on HIV transmission and breastfeeding, held in Geneva at the end of April 1992.[23] The Dunn meta-analysis[24] looked at five studies showing that when a mother was infected prenatally, the additional risk of transmission through breastfeeding, over and above transmission *in utero* or during delivery, was 14%. Based on four studies in which mothers acquired HIV postnatally, the estimated risk of transmission to the baby when a mother was newly infected was 29%. Dr Dunn recommended that a reduction in the number of vertically infected children might be achieved by safe alternatives to breastfeeding. He was also clear that breastfeeding should still be recommended where infectious diseases were a common cause of death in childhood, despite the additional risk of HIV. So in September 1992 the Dunn findings did little to change global policy, which continued to promote breastfeeding for all babies in all settings for another five years. This could have been because at the time of publication in 1992, there was not enough certainty about whether the magnitude of transmission through breastfeeding was substantial enough to require a change in policy. However, by 1997, developments had conspired to ensure that it received a lot of traction. Even today, the Dunn meta-analysis is consistently invoked by organisations that advocate formula-feeding for HIV-infected mothers.

Ghent working group meetings, 1993–94

Meanwhile, the Ghent working group met again in 1993 and 1994 to iron out many of the technical difficulties which were beginning to emerge in collating or comparing research on HIV and breastfeeding. Many of the studies conducted in the previous eight years had faced problems in data collection and analysis, making comparison difficult. There had been 14 teams of investigators representing five studies from central Africa, three from eastern Africa, two from Europe, one from Haiti and three from the United States. A critical evaluation of the projects reported transmission rates ranging from 13–32% in industrialised countries and from 25–48% in developing countries, but methods of calculation differed from study to study. Nevertheless, a common methodology was developed and agreement was reached on definitions of HIV-related signs and symptoms, paediatric AIDS and HIV-related deaths.[25,26]

Participants discussed and set criteria for various ways of studying MTCT of HIV in developing countries. They determined what interventions were used, the design and conduct of trials, how to provide guidelines for research groups, inclusion and exclusion criteria, target populations, use of placebo, follow-up, definition of endpoints, formation of data and safety monitoring boards, ethical issues and the possible impact of trial results on public health policy.[25] Trials which included alternatives to breastfeeding in Kenya and South Africa were actually under way and the group noted that transmission of the virus through breastfeeding was now beyond doubt.

The Ghent working group formulated international standards for the development, implementation and analysis of intervention trials to reduce MTCT of HIV in developing countries. Affordable, sustainable and appropriate interventions with proven efficacy were urgently needed to decrease the burden of MTCT. International coordination would be necessary in order to share information from planned and ongoing trials. Sharing of data had implications for agencies like the Global Programme on AIDS (WHO) or the European Communities AIDS Task Force, and could make a major contribution towards the success of intervention trials.

The jury may still be out on whether the ambitions of the Ghent working group for ethical conduct of trials designed to reduce or prevent paediatric HIV infection in developing countries were realised. As it turned out, the prioritisation of breastfeeding avoidance rather than provision of antiretroviral therapy was put into effect within just a couple of years as the actual Prevention of Mother to Child Transmission (PMTCT) pilot projects got underway, and were subsequently scaled up and rolled out to hundreds of sites in developing countries. (See chapters 14, 15, 16.)

Developing country health budgets are always very stretched. The funding provided by international agencies or overseas universities provides such needed injections of cash, and job creation, that the balance of power between host country and research project can easily become skewed. For instance, the funding for one very large research project in Zimbabwe, supported by Johns Hopkins University, was said to exceed the annual budget of the entire Harare City Health Department.[27] The project offered such attractive salaries and working conditions compared to local employers that the team was able to easily headhunt healthcare personnel. Ethical concerns can become lost when considering the opportunities they provide for acquisition of foreign exchange, funding, employment and remuneration.

These factors may have formed the basis for the confusion that the lactation community felt about why so much subsequent research appeared to endorse the new policy developed by UNAIDS, WHO and UNICEF. Study after study attested to the feasibility and acceptability of 'replacement feeding', while failing to report on its safety and sustainability, i.e. how many babies were actually saved from HIV infection through breastfeeding avoidance, and how many babies died as a result of not being breastfed.

Early US and French research on antiretroviral therapy to prevent MTCT

The early nineties also saw the first attempts to reduce the risk of vertical transmission to babies through the use of antiretroviral drugs. The AIDS Clinical Trials Group conducted a randomised controlled clinical trial (called the ACTG 076 Protocol) in the USA and France, sponsored by the US National Institutes of Health, and the National Agency of Research on AIDS in France, which began in April 1991 and produced an interim analysis in December 1993.[28] HIV-positive women received either zidovudine or a placebo during the last 14–34 weeks of pregnancy. Treatment continued during labour and delivery, and the newborn babies received zidovudine prophylaxis for six weeks after birth. In the absence of breastfeeding, since HIV-positive mothers in Europe and the US were recommended to formula-feed, this regimen showed an important reduction in the rate of MTCT transmission, from 25.5% to 8.3%. The success of this trial was heralded as a major breakthrough which was to exert a considerable influence on the HIV and breastfeeding story.

Trials with simplified, shorter and standardised regimens of drug administration were recommended for developing countries, as were trials involving vitamin A supplementation. Once again, the Ghent working group took great care to monitor and coordinate all the criteria surrounding studies of ART. The group recommended that trials in developing countries should try to strengthen the national research capacity in shared responsibility with donor agencies, and should also be relevant to the population being studied. The possibility of confusion about study objectives was also acknowledged; would they be designed to increase knowledge, or to promote action? In other words, would they evaluate the efficacy of a treatment, or the effectiveness of a policy?

Several years later, Lynne Mofensen, a highly respected researcher, confirmed:

> *'Prevention of perinatal HIV-1 transmission became a reality in 1994, when the Pediatric AIDS Clinical Trials Group (PACTG) protocol 076 showed that a 6-week regimen of zidovudine, given to the mother during pregnancy and labour and then to the neonate for 6 weeks reduced transmission rates by nearly 70%.'*[29,30]

Following the success of the zidovudine trials in the US and France, the CDC and other organisations began collaborating on similar projects with ministries of health in Asia and Africa, initially in trials where breastfeeding would be suspended, and later where breastfeeding would be continued.

Thailand

At the Vancouver International Conference on AIDS in July 1996, Dr Nathan Shaffer, who had done research for the CDC for 10 years, and went on to eventually work for the WHO in their PMTCT division, reported that in Thailand 20,000 HIV-positive women became pregnant every year.[31] It was thought that a drug regimen similar to the ACTG 076 Protocol wouldn't be feasible in most developing countries, due to both complexity and cost. Annual national health budgets were often less than $10 per day and the cost of the drugs alone for the ACTG 076 regimen was at least eighty times that amount, whereas a 'short course' of zidovudine confined to the last four weeks of pregnancy and during labour would cost only $50.[32]

A trial was planned to provide ART and formula to mothers who agreed not to breastfeed. Between May 1996 and December 1997, pregnant women were randomly assigned placebo or zidovudine twice daily from 36 weeks' gestation and during labour. Notably, the Thailand trial also included a placebo arm, even though the ACTG 076 study had been terminated early due to ethical concerns and the standard treatment in the US was now to treat all pregnant HIV-positive mothers with zidovudine. Nevertheless, with a median duration of treatment of only 25 days, MTCT was reduced by 50%, with 55 of 392 babies testing positive, i.e. 9.4% on zidovudine and 19% on placebo. About 80% of the treatment effect was explained by lowered maternal viral concentrations at delivery. It was concluded that this regimen could prevent many HIV infections during late pregnancy and labour in less-developed countries unable to implement the full ACTG 076 regimen and if mothers didn't breastfeed.[33]

Côte d'Ivoire and Burkina Faso

Starting in September 1995, trials were planned for Côte d'Ivoire and Burkina Faso, where mothers continued breastfeeding. These studies were 'logistically simpler' and a lot cheaper, with shorter treatment regimens, and no treatment for newborns. Women who received ART received three doses of zidovudine over a treatment period of 25 days. At six months the HIV infection rate was 18.0% in the zidovudine group and 27.5% in the placebo group – a 38% reduction in the treatment arm despite breastfeeding.[34] A follow-up in Côte d'Ivoire [35] from April 1996 to February 1998 looked at the safety and efficacy of the shortened zidovudine regimen during the final four weeks of pregnancy and where all babies were breastfed. Transmission in the zidovudine group was again reduced compared to the placebo group.

Implications of research on ART and no breastfeeding

These early studies on the use of ART were hugely influential. They changed the possibility of MTCT of HIV from a situation of hopelessness to one where preventive care might be possible. There was an urgent need to begin to implement such interventions to combat MTCT of HIV. It was also seen as important to find ways to overcome the social and economic barriers that prevented HIV-infected women from utilising safe alternatives to breastfeeding.[36] Arjan de Wagt and David Clarke of UNICEF wrote later that it was the Thai study, showing that MTCT of HIV could be reduced by 50% when mothers were given a short course of zidovudine and then used commercial infant formula to feed their babies, that formed the model for the PMTCT pilot sites.[37] The general consensus was moving towards the possibility that an integrated prevention programme which combined the use of antiretroviral therapy and safe alternatives to breastfeeding would be effective in reducing mother to child transmission of HIV among breastfeeding populations.

Public pressure at the International AIDS Conference, Vancouver, 1996

The One World One Hope International AIDS Conference held in Vancouver, Canada, from 7–12 July 1996 brought together researchers, activists and community organisers from around the world. Up to now, there had been no effective treatment for AIDS, but in the months leading up to the conference, researchers were beginning to see the results of the promising new treatment provided by a three-drug combination antiretroviral therapy (ART),[38] as well as early results from short-course ART to reduce transmission of HIV from mothers to babies.

Julio Montaner, the Argentinean-Canadian physician, professor and researcher who was president of the International AIDS Society,[39] described how everything from the weather to the venue to the environment and, most importantly, the data, was such that it was the 'perfect storm' to revolutionise the history of the epidemic, and it was possible that no one even began to comprehend the magnitude of this breakthrough. David Ho and colleagues presented viral dynamics showing that the average person with HIV produced 10 billion virions per day, pointing to the need for antiviral treatment. Dr John Mellors presented data showing that HIV viral load, as well as CD4+ cell decline, predicted disease progression, and the HIV viral load test with a threshold of detection at 15–25 copies/ml was introduced. But the most important research presented was the studies of triple-drug therapy. These all converged to initiate a decade of progress that was truly extraordinary, in terms of the intensity of the effort and the progress achieved, against an important disease. Together they constituted what is often considered to be the beginning of the era of HAART (highly active antiretroviral therapy).

Speaking at the Conference, Dr Montaner said:

'We want this to be only the beginning of a truly unique, wonderful exercise. We want each one of you to go home and disseminate what you have learned here this week. So that we can say... Vancouver was truly a catalyst for change.' Looking back later, he said, 'From there, we dramatically increased our number of international collaborations, we dramatically increased our number of opportunities to collaborate with industry, and funding agencies, we substantially increased our ability to attract new talent... In medicine, I don't think we ever witnessed... such a single turnaround at a single point in

time that basically transformed the outcome of this epidemic globally. And we are not done yet. And I tell you, Vancouver is at the centre of it.'

Organisers had been mindful that at the previous conference the subjects of women with HIV, and HIV in the developing world, were foremost in the minds of delegates. HIV continued to spread unchecked, with 7,500 new infections per day, up 25% from the 6,000 cases per day two years previously. The conference attracted almost 15,000 participants from 125 countries, making it the largest-ever gathering of medical experts, healthcare workers, people living with HIV/AIDS (including 1,500 from the developing world), commercial exhibitors and news media. Due to prohibitions against HIV-positive individuals obtaining visas to the US, the Canadian conference was the first venue on the North American continent that could be attended by delegates with HIV. Funding of $2.4 million had come from Health Canada and the Canadian International Development Agency (CIDA) to bring people living with HIV and from the developing world to the conference.

There was hope and optimism about the new medical and scientific developments to finally overcome the HIV pandemic. But there was recognition that the doom and gloom of previous conferences would continue unless politicians and their governments began to show the necessary leadership. They needed to show a willingness to commit and sustain the necessary resources to act in concert with medical scientists, community activists and caregivers. Active participation of community groups, public and non-government representatives and, most significantly, people living with HIV/AIDS was essential to the success of the conference.

Major advances in the prevention of transmission of the virus from mother to baby, announced the previous year, were explored. Importantly, pressure was exerted on UN agencies by African delegates, who believed that while babies in Europe and North America were able to receive infant formula in order to protect them from postpartum HIV transmission, their babies were being allowed to die due to breastfeeding.

The *New York Times* later reported:[40]

'Research also indicates that exclusive bottle-feeding can play a key role in combating transmission of HIV. Last year, South African researchers reported the preliminary findings of a study in Soweto comparing HIV transmission rates between mothers who breast-fed with those who bottle-fed. The team, led by Dr. Glenda Gray, a pediatrician at the Perinatal HIV Research Unit at Baragwanath Hospital in Soweto, found that 46 percent of infants in the study group who were breast-fed became infected with the AIDS virus, compared with 18 percent of babies who were bottle-fed... "The relative risk for breast-feeding was about twofold," Dr. Gray said. Significantly, the study also found that the formula-fed infants in Soweto, which has both poor and middle-class neighborhoods, did not experience the potential negative effects of artificial feeding, such as higher rates of respiratory and gastrointestinal disease.'

Dr Glenda Gray had indeed reported on the preliminary findings of breast vs bottle-feeding at Baragwanath Hospital in Soweto outside Johannesburg.[41] Whether the 1997

New York Times report was entirely accurate, however, is open to challenge; when I met Dr Gray at a subsequent AIDS conference held in Toronto in 2006, she described to me how she had had to follow up the bottle-fed babies at Baragwanath Hospital as often as three times a day to keep them alive through the infections they were experiencing.[42]

Dr Peter Piot had been appointed as the new Director of the fledgling UNAIDS, launched in December 1995. By June 1996, UNAIDS staff had met with political, economic and social leaders in more than 50 countries to brief them on UNAIDS' mandate and work. Being past president of the International AIDS Society from 1991–94, Dr Piot was able to address a symposium at the July AIDS Conference in Vancouver about future plans.[43] Delegates heard that 'the pandemic has become immensely complex. It has become fragmented and is now a mosaic composed of a multitude of epidemics, which can be distinguished on the basis of: predominant modes of transmission; geographic focus; [HIV sub-types]; age, sex, socioeconomic or behavioural characteristics of populations most affected.' By mid-1996, UNAIDS estimated that women accounted for over 47% of nearly 21 million adults living with HIV. In Africa, young women with HIV outnumbered their male peers by a ratio of 2:1.

Naomi Baumslag, a long-time breastfeeding advocate, wrote an article in 2001 in which she retrospectively reviewed developments occurring in Vancouver in 1996:[44]

> *'Despite the incomplete and conflicting scientific evidence on the transmission of HIV through breastfeeding, the [infant formula manufacturing] corporations have seized on the HIV epidemic as an opportunity to push formula feeding to the third world. For the formula companies, AIDS is a window of opportunity that is exploited to the nth degree. They had used AIDS research presented at the AIDS International Meeting in Vancouver, 1996, and cited on the front page of the New York Times, to pressure UNICEF to endorse formula for babies born to HIV-positive mothers. The industry endorsed this research even though it had not been published in a peer-reviewed journal. The author of the New York Times article interviewed six 'breastfeeding experts' but never reported any of their views. He did, however, report the view of non-breastfeeding advocates such as Thad Jackson, an immunologist who formerly was a full-time employee of Nestlé and now works for them as a consultant. The report was very biased and accused WHO and UNICEF of dragging their feet and not looking out for third world infants. According to the Wall Street Journal, "UNICEF remains captive to a clutch of activists who have been leading boycotts and protests against the baby formula makers since the 1970s on the highly spurious grounds that the companies trying to supply better nutrition 'exploit' the poor... If the toll of African AIDS babies continues to rise, the credibility of one of the most beloved UN agencies may sink." This statement was on the front page, not in the editorial section!'*

1996 UNAIDS meetings on human rights

Very shortly after the Vancouver IAC meeting, UNAIDS and the UN Commission on Human Rights organised a Second International Consultation on AIDS and Human Rights in Geneva from 23 to 25 September 1996,[45] bringing together 35 experts, government officials and staff of national AIDS programmes. Importantly, participants also included people living with HIV, human rights activists, academics, representatives of regional and national networks on ethics, law, and human rights, as well as non-governmental organisations and AIDS service organisations. At the first human rights meeting, held in 1989, there was acknowledgement of the widespread abuse of human rights in the wake of the HIV/AIDS epidemic. Participants had discussed the possible elaboration of guidelines to assist policymakers and others in complying with international human rights standards regarding law, administrative practice and policy. At the second meeting in 1996 guidelines were adopted ensuring community consultation in all phases of HIV policy design, reviewing and reforming public health laws to ensure that they adequately addressed issues raised by HIV/AIDS and promoted a supportive and enabling environment for women, children and other vulnerable groups.

Also in September 1996, UNAIDS quietly released an interim statement on HIV and infant feeding in the WHO *Weekly Epidemiological Record*,[46] which set out the policy underpinning the announcement which received a lot more publicity in June the following year. This said that:

1. *as a general principle, in all populations, irrespective of HIV infection rates, breast-feeding should continue to be protected, promoted and supported... but ...preliminary studies indicate that more than one-third of infected infants are infected through breast-feeding. These studies suggest an average risk for HIV transmission through breast-feeding of 1 in 7 children born to, and breast-fed by, a woman living with HIV*
2. *there should be improved access to voluntary HIV counselling and testing*
3. *informed choice should be ensured... but 'When children born to women living with HIV can be ensured uninterrupted access to nutritionally adequate breast-milk substitutes that are safely prepared and fed to them, they are at less risk of illness and death if they are not breast-fed'.*
4. *commercial pressure for artificial feeding should be prevented* [i.e. it was necessary to support the Code].

In 1997 the press continued to exert pressure on the UN agencies to intervene to reduce the risk of HIV transmission through breastfeeding. In June 1997, the *New York Times* ran a special report under the heading 'In War Against AIDS, Battle Over Baby Formula Reignites'.[40] Since the UN had recently estimated that one-third of all infants with HIV acquired the virus through breastmilk, the accusation was that the AIDS pandemic should reverse the usual advice to new mothers in poor countries to breastfeed. While breastfeeding should be protected, pregnant women should also be tested for HIV and counselled about the risks and 'possible benefits' of bottle-feeding.

To breastfeeding advocates the implications were unthinkable – a product that was once blamed for killing one and a half million babies a year was now being portrayed as a panacea to reduce childhood deaths from AIDS. When told about the risks of breastfeeding, women in developing countries faced excruciating choices and societal taboos. But the *New York Times* went on:

> *'Others say... that it is imperative to find alternatives to breast-feeding, including ways to make safe, affordable formula widely available. Some advocates of breast-feeding are prepared to work with formula makers, their sworn enemies for decades, on combating the growing threat. Meanwhile, the United Nations has come under criticism from scientists who say that the group, in its zeal to promote breast-feeding, has not confronted the HIV issue.'*

The example of Thailand was held up as the developing country that had reacted earliest to the new worries about breastmilk. As early as 1993, government officials had begun a programme that now provided free one-year supplies of infant formula to HIV-infected mothers through health centres and community and provincial hospitals.[40] At Chulalongkorn Hospital in Bangkok, for example, HIV-positive women were enrolled in a programme that gave them both free formula and zidovudine to reduce prenatal transmission of the virus. Some research was showing poor results for breastfeeding compared to formula-feeding.[47] The UN agencies were clearly impressed by these results.

Several prominent researchers had become increasingly and openly critical of global policy which continued to support breastfeeding by HIV-positive mothers. Dr Angus Nicoll, a British government epidemiologist in London, was reported to have said: 'For years, they could say that "Breast is Best" full stop', referring to the slogan of advocates for breastfeeding. That mother's milk might also pose dangers, he said, 'is a difficult thing for them to take on board... The biggest conundrum is for countries like South Africa, Brazil and Thailand, they have a lot people infected with HIV as well as a substantial number of well-educated people able to deliver artificial feeding.'[40]

Joan Kreiss, a member of the Nairobi group, suggested that there was an urgent need to implement an integrated prevention programme which combined the use of the zidovudine regimen and safe alternatives to breastfeeding, and to find ways to overcome the social and economic barriers that prevented many HIV-infected women from utilising these alternatives.[36]

Dr Glenda Gray, the popular South African researcher and political activist, was reported to have said that even the United Nations' new stance was a 'cop-out'. It was not enough for the UN and governments to warn women about breastfeeding risks; they must help get formula to mothers who wanted it. Dr Gray said that her hospital had attempted to get short-term welfare grants for mothers who decided, after counselling, to bottle-feed. 'I'm not saying that we have to encourage formula, but if we are counselling them, we have a responsibility to help them to get formula, if that's the way they choose to go... It's like telling someone you are positive and you can transmit the virus through unsafe sex and then not providing condoms. That is exactly what we are doing with formula.' Dr Gray later revealed that she had been on an expert panel on HIV for Nestlé Nutrition Institute Africa that assessed interventions to prevent postnatal transmission of HIV.[48]

Botswana's Health Minister Sheila D. Tlou was also on record as angrily accusing policymakers of urging mothers with HIV in rich countries to use formula while telling those in poorer, less-developed ones to breastfeed. A *Washington Post* article reports Tlou as saying, 'We saw red! ...Why are you sentencing all of our children to death? And why are you sentencing all of us to psychological damage in knowing that we were the ones who infected them?'[49]

The lactation world was further stunned when an IBCLC published a well-researched book which apparently came down in favour of bottle-feeding to protect the babies of HIV-positive mothers from infection through breastmilk.[50] In 1997 the *New York Times* had reported that 'Edith White of Massachusetts, who has developed hospital training courses on breast-feeding, said that she recently became convinced that findings showing a substantial risk from breast-feeding were not getting out to women.' When former advocates of breastfeeding were prepared to endorse formula-feeding, an anathema for years, it felt as if the battle to protect breastfeeding was being lost.

Researchers from Zambia, also working on breastfeeding-associated transmission of HIV, observed later that an all-or-nothing approach and the shift away from breastfeeding dominated thinking in the field for several years, providing the impetus for a major pendulum swing in international infant feeding policy.[51] Dr Connie Osborne, a Zambian national, whose career had spanned a wide range of experience as a Senior Lecturer at the University of Zambia School of Medicine, working for UNAIDS in Ethiopia and Switzerland, UNICEF in Botswana, and WHO in China as the African Medical and Research Foundation Southern Regional Director covering South Africa, Mozambique and Malawi, commented that 'We have not learned enough about the risks and benefits of all infant feeding options for HIV positive women. While we need to redouble our efforts in learning more, we need not wait until we have all the answers.'

The *New York Times* article of 8 June 1997[40] reported that in previous meetings between breastfeeding advocates and industry officials one goal had been to develop a project to demonstrate that cheap, sanitary supplies of infant formula could be provided to HIV-infected women in places like Africa. Edith White had also reported in her book that in 1998 the Infant Food Manufacturers (IFM) had been asked to work with UNICEF to supply formula for 'a ten-country demonstration project'.[50] Rod Leonard, director of the Community Nutrition Institute, a non-profit group in Washington that was sponsoring the talks, suggested that such a plan might involve distribution of formula at hospitals and clinics where it could be mixed with clean water and bottled. Up to that time, formula makers, apparently wary of being accused of exploiting the AIDS crisis, had been reluctant to commit themselves to specific projects. But Carol Emerling, a spokeswoman for the Wyeth-Ayerst division of the American Home Products Corporation, said the company was 'actively exploring' participating in such a plan. Thad Jackson, an immunologist in Sterling, Virginia, and a consultant to Nestlé, acknowledged that for a programme to work, industry would very likely have to provide formula at or near cost. 'It has to be done as some sort of relief project,' Mr Jackson said. Niels Christiansen, spokesman for Nestlé in Vevey, Switzerland, who, 10 months later, would attend the April 1998 WHO/UNICEF/UNAIDS Technical Consultation on HIV and Infant Feeding, added that the company would need the cooperation of United Nations officials before agreeing to take part in such an effort.

Thus trapped between a rock and a hard place, the UN agencies bowed to pressure to provide guidance in the public health minefield of prevention of MTCT of HIV. A growing disregard for the dangers of abandoning breastfeeding had begun with the results of the Nairobi study, which seemed to show that formula-feeding saved lives, even though there was a lot of criticism of its methodology. Zambian researchers later wrote, 'It remains unclear why this study reported so few adverse outcomes of formula feeding. No study to date has been able to replicate such good outcomes with formula. All studies in subsequent years, many of them considerably larger and some of them randomised and with at least equivalent methodological rigor, have reported, at best, no benefit with shifts away from breastfeeding or, in program settings, worse HIV-free survival.'[51] And so it was that the UN agencies shifted towards provisional support for formula-feeding, allowing policymakers and implementers to be lulled into thinking that there were no real dangers of artificial feeding that could not be easily overcome.

The Ghent group convened a three-day workshop in Belgium, from 13–15 November 1997, to undertake a thorough review of current information on MTCT of HIV and its prevention with a view to proposing policy options for developing countries.[52] The thinking was that following the success of the first trials of the short regimen of zidovudine in Thailand, Côte d'Ivoire and Burkina Faso, postnatal transmission of HIV through breastfeeding was an essential component of the overall risk of transmission and must be taken into account when designing prevention strategies in developing countries.

Then in 1998, the UNAIDS Secretariat, UNICEF and WHO convened an Interagency Task Team (IATT) for the Prevention and Treatment of HIV Infection in Pregnant Women, Mothers and Children.[53] The IATT was a partnership of UN organisations, with donor agencies, non-governmental organisations and networks of people living with HIV (see box) that worked in collaboration to provide technical support for a 'Global Plan Towards the Elimination of New HIV Infections Among Children by 2015 and Keeping Their Mothers Alive'.

The IATT partners were 'committed to addressing issues related to policies, strategies, mobilizing and allocating resources, providing technical assistance to governments for accelerating the scaling up of programmes, and tracking the global progress of the prevention of mother-to-child transmission of HIV, and HIV care and treatment for children.'

Some of these private organisations and governmental agencies had provided funding for bringing activists to the Vancouver AIDS conference, which undoubtedly helped to eventually influence HIV and infant feeding policy. Were these activists bussed in by organisations and departments that might have had a special interest in promoting formula-feeding?

Writing retrospectively in their 2005 *Report Card*,[54] UNICEF acknowledged the pivotal role of the IATT in setting up the PMTCT pilot projects. Shortly after the release of findings of the Thai Zidovudine PMTCT Study, the IATT provided leadership and support for the implementation of the first pilot projects in 11 countries (Botswana, Burundi, Côte d'Ivoire, Honduras, Kenya, Malawi, Tanzania, Rwanda, Uganda, Zambia and Zimbabwe.)'

Dr Joseph Saba, a French Lebanese medical doctor specialising in infectious disease, health management and statistics, and known internationally for his expertise in the prevention of MTCT of HIV, who had joined the World Health Organization in 1993, revealed that UNAIDS, in cooperation with UNICEF, was preparing a guide for health workers in developing countries to use in counselling HIV-infected mothers, but it was unclear what specific advice would be offered. Dr Saba was reported to have said, 'We have to come from global thinking about this issue to a case-by-case thinking where we discuss this with the interested woman and let her make her choice.'[40] Where sanitary conditions permitted, training could be given to mothers on how to prepare homemade formulas, which were cheaper than commercial products. Alternatively, relatives might be encouraged to act as wet-nurses, but they too could have HIV. The primary goal of the integrated package supporting these interventions was to alleviate overall maternal and infant morbidity and mortality.

IATT member organizations

Academy for Educational Development (AED)
Baylor International Pediatric AIDS Foundation (BIPAI)
Canadian International Development Agency (CIDA)
Catholic Medical Mission Board (CMMB)
Centers for Disease Control and Prevention, USA (CDC)
Clinton Health Access Initiative (CHAI)
Elizabeth Glaser Pediatric AIDS Foundation (EGPAF)
Ensemble pour une Solidarité Thérapeutique Hospitalière en Réseau (ESTHER)
FHI360 (Family Health International)
Global Fund for AIDS, Tuberculosis and Malaria (GFATM)
Global Network of People Living with HIV (GNP+)
International Center for AIDS Care and Treatment Programs (ICAP) at Columbia University's Mailman School of Public Health
International Community of Women Living with HIV/AIDS (ICW)
International Planned Parenthood Federation (IPPF)
Joint United Nations Programme on HIV/AIDS (UNAIDS) Secretariat
Management Sciences for Health (MSH)
Mothers2Mothers (M2M)
U.S. Office of the Global AIDS Coordinator (OGAC)
Population Council
UK Department for International Development (DFID)
United Nations Children's Fund (UNICEF)
United Nations Population Fund (UNFPA)
United States Agency for International Development (USAID)
World Bank (WB)
World Health Organization (WHO)

UNAIDS workshop: how to promote and normalise formula-feeding, March 1998

In March 1998, UNAIDS convened a workshop to give effect to the 1997 change in global policy on HIV and breastfeeding.[55] Dr Peter Piot opened the workshop by outlining UNAIDS' ambitions:

1. promoting primary prevention among women during pregnancy and while breastfeeding;
2. ensuring access to voluntary counselling and testing as an entry point to access care and for interventions to prevent mother to child transmission
3. ensuring better access to antiretroviral therapy in the perinatal period; and
4. ensuring access to safe and affordable breast milk substitutes for HIV+ women.

Dr Kevin de Cock, another native of Belgium (like Peter Piot) who now supervised HIV-prevention programmes for the CDC in Kenya, subsequently spoke at length. Transmission of HIV could be prevented by avoiding the infant's exposure to breastmilk, a contentious issue since breastfeeding was widely recognised as being nutritious, economic and convenient, provided immunological protection, reduced infant exposure to pathogens, and prolonged birth spacing. However, he stressed the futility of promoting PMTCT interventions before and during birth only to witness children being infected after birth through breastmilk. As previously described in Chapter 4, this would become a recurring theme reiterated by the AIDS community. It was central to Dr de Cock's widely cited meta-analysis, subsequently published in 2000.[56]

Interventions to prevent breastfeeding could include

i. infant formula
ii. early weaning
iii. an HIV negative wet-nurse or donor milk
iv. pasteurisation of breastmilk

Limitations of availability, acceptability and cost were associated with each of these options. Additionally, women who did not breastfeed their infants might experience serious stigmatisation. The key components of an effective MTCT prevention programme would include:

- education, counselling and support for primary prevention interventions using zidovudine
- infant feeding counselling and support along with access to breastmilk substitutes

Preliminary evidence from Uganda suggested that few women were likely to give up breastfeeding even in circumstances where they knew the risks. Not breastfeeding was tantamount to public admission of HIV infection. Attention needed to be given to the distress many women would experience when not breastfeeding, especially in communities where it was expected. Future pilot projects should be conducted according to the highest ethical standards, emphasising the Western principles of autonomy, beneficence, non-maleficence and justice, while scaling up the use of these interventions – even if there remained some programmatic obstacles and scientific uncertainties.

Major challenges lay in promoting the acceptability of breastmilk substitutes in circumstances where breastfeeding was the norm. Counselling would not simply involve telling mothers not to breastfeed, but supporting women in finding breastmilk substitutes and sustaining their use. A learning-by-doing approach was advocated (i.e. operational research). The main issue was not *whether* interventions were to be implemented and scaled up, but *how*? UNICEF, WHO and UNAIDS were currently discussing how best to approach this.

Two documents (one for policymakers and another for healthcare managers) were being prepared. If a mother knew she was HIV-positive then she must receive counselling to explore alternatives to breastfeeding and where these existed they should be promoted. Decisions must be made in the light of individual circumstances. The role of animal or modified animal milks needed to be more thoroughly explored.

A wide range of technical and operational issues were discussed, e.g. the need for a national policy framework; a communication strategy for voluntary counselling and testing and adequate numbers of trained counsellors; a sustained supply of relevant drugs, test kits and breastmilk substitutes. The challenge, therefore, lay in identifying a set of guiding principles to inform international concerted action. These principles included enduring concern for the protection and promotion of human rights, including measures to reduce the stigmatisation of HIV-positive women and women who might choose not to breastfeed.

20–22 April, 1998: WHO Technical Consultation – implementation of guidelines (the formula solution)

The following month, a further WHO/UNICEF/UNAIDS Technical Consultation on HIV and infant feeding to discuss implementation was held in Geneva.[57] Participants included researchers, country representatives, members of UNAIDS, WHO and UNICEF, a member of La Leche League International, (the worldwide breastfeeding mother-support group) and IBFAN (the organisation which monitors and reports on violations of the International Code of Marketing of Breastmilk Substitutes). Surprisingly, two members of the Infant Formula Manufacturer's Association had been invited: Dr Andrée Bronner (Secretary, Infant Formula Manufacturers, Geneva, Switzerland) and Dr Niels Christiansen (Assistant Vice President, Food & Nutrition Issues, Nestlé SSA, Vevey, Switzerland).

The focus was global implementation of formula-feeding for the babies of HIV-positive mothers. Dr Peter Piot described how in 1997 more than 500,000 infants, mostly in Africa, were infected with HIV, whereas, thanks to zidovudine and avoidance of breastfeeding, perinatal transmission was rare in the developed world, where the recommendation was also to avoid postnatal transmission by avoiding breastfeeding. The ethical imperative therefore was to find ways to make breastmilk substitutes available for all mothers. The time to act was now. The overall objective was to provide national health authorities with clear guidance on HIV and infant feeding options and policies. A package of care, framed as a public health imperative based on human rights, needed to be integrated into national maternal and child health services. It should include:

- HIV testing
- short-course antiretroviral drugs for infected HIV-positive women
- alternatives to breastfeeding for HIV-exposed babies

For the 1998 meeting, UNAIDS, with UNICEF and WHO, had commissioned and published a set of three working documents for participants:

- *HIV and Infant Feeding: A review of Transmission of HIV Through Breastfeeding*[58,59]
- *HIV and Infant Feeding:Guidelines for Decision Makers*[60] and
- *HIV and Infant Feeding: A Guide for Health Care Managers and Supervisors*[61]

The first *Review of Transmission through Breastfeeding* was authored by Dr Ruth Nduati, who had been the first author of the randomised controlled trial from Nairobi. This trial, concluding that formula-feeding was safer than breastfeeding in the context of HIV, had been conducted between 1992 and 1998 but was only published in the *Journal of the American Medical Association* in 2000.[19] That this important evidence was only actually published two years later is intriguing. It's difficult to imagine that WHO would not have been aware of the results of Dr Nduati's research at the time that policy was being decided, nor that it had not exerted a major influence in the change of policy to favour formula-feeding. WHO's Randa Saadeh described how the *Review* presented the background scientific information about HIV and MTCT and provided the basis for decision-makers and health-care managers to advise mothers on sound infant feeding choices. Actually, the way that WHO catalogued this booklet (as the third in the series) indicates that it may have been published after, rather than before the guidance documents, i.e. it endorsed a *fait accompli* rather than underpinning it. Subsequent reprints of the *Review* omit Dr Nduati's role in writing it, and merely show that it was published by WHO, UNICEF and UNAIDS.

The Guidelines described a number of infant feeding options which women who were HIV-positive might consider:

- replacement feeding (formula-feeding),
- modified breastfeeding, (early cessation of breastfeeding, i.e. premature weaning, or expression and heat-treatment of a mother's own milk)
- breastmilk from other sources (banked or donor milk, or wet-nursing)

Dr Ruth Nduati spoke of the experience of counselling and informed consent that she had gained while conducting her randomised controlled trial, where women had been randomised to either formula-feeding or breastfeeding, 'Explaining scientific method is not easy. If one arm of a randomised controlled trial is known to produce a superior outcome, the trial should not be conducted. One particular difficulty lies in patients' mistrust of a researcher who admits to a balanced state of ignorance, which in fact is the rationale for the trial and an ethical condition for undertaking it. Such trials are ethically permissible only when the likely outcome it is not known.'

David Clarke, legal adviser to UNICEF, confirmed that respect for human rights was necessary for the effective implementation of public health measures, meaning that women should have a free and fully informed choice about how to feed their infants. The human rights principles which were particularly relevant in the situation of mother-to-child transmission of HIV/AIDS were:

- the right to life, and the highest attainable standard of physical and mental health; in the case of children, breastfeeding is an important component of the right to health, however, only the mother can decide whether to breastfeed her child or not;
- the right to privacy, including the obligation to seek informed consent to HIV testing and privacy of information, including the confidentiality of all information relating to a person's HIV status;

In order to provide a balanced view, Dr Felicity Savage of the WHO, who would later become chair of the Steering Committee of the World Alliance for Breastfeeding Action (WABA), discussed the risks of replacement feeding. Lida Lhotska of UNICEF, who later joined GIFA, the European branch of IBFAN, which monitors the Code, discussed the costs of various types of replacement feeding including the use of animal milks. Ironically, both women would, within a year, and in their capacities as representatives of WHO and UNICEF, be instructing healthcare providers how to implement the 1997 policy, specifically by teaching HIV-positive mothers how to choose, prepare and feed formula to their babies.

Participants at the workshop spent six hours in working groups discussing the need for operational research, monitoring, implementation and governmental responsibility. The meeting concluded that HIV-positive mothers should be enabled to make fully informed decisions about the best way to feed their infants in their particular circumstances. Whatever they decided, they should receive educational, psychosocial and material support to carry out their feeding decision as safely as possible, including having access to adequate breastmilk substitutes. Efforts would have to be made to make suitable alternatives available and affordable for these mothers, and to give them the guidance and support they needed to feed their children as safely as possible. It was no longer a question of if and when the world should act, but how. Governments in particular needed practical guidance to implement recommended policy and to educate community members about the importance of not discriminating against or stigmatising HIV-infected individuals so that they could understand and provide support to the women and children concerned. Whatever the infant feeding decision, support would need to be long-term, continuing until a child was at least two years old.

With these deliberations, participants arranged for implementation of plans to introduce replacement feeding as set out in the 1997 Policy Statement:

> *when replacement feeding is acceptable, feasible, affordable, sustainable and safe, avoidance of all breastfeeding by HIV-infected mothers is recommended.*
>
> *otherwise exclusive breastfeeding is recommended during the first months of life and should then be discontinued as soon as it is feasible.*
>
> *HIV-infected mothers should be supported in their choice, whether they choose*

breastfeeding or replacement feeding.

when children born to women living with HIV can be ensured uninterrupted access to nutritionally adequate breast-milk substitutes that are safely prepared and fed to them, they are at less risk of illness and death if they are not breastfed.

it is considered that milk in some form is essential, and replacement feeding options include commercial infant formula, and home prepared formula which can be made from animal milks, typically from cows, goats, buffaloes, sheep or camels.

Replacement feeding

Providing a child who receives no breast-milk with a diet that contains all the nutrients that the child needs throughout the period for which breast-milk is recommended, that is for at least the first two years of life.

From birth to six months of age, milk is essential, and can be given in the form of commercially produced infant formula; or home-prepared formula made by modifying fresh or processed animal milk, which should be accompanied by micronutrient supplements

From six months to two years, replacement feeds should consist of appropriately prepared nutrient-enriched family foods given three times a day if commercial or home-prepared formula continues to be available, or five times a day if neither formula is available...

Announcing the UN PMTCT Pilot programmes

The *New York Times* of 30 June 1998 carried the report that the United Nations would be starting a PMTCT (Prevention of Mother to Child Transmission) of HIV pilot programme in 11 countries, mainly in Africa, where HIV was rapidly spreading.[61] The UN would provide voluntary counselling and testing of pregnant women to identify 30,000 HIV-infected mothers, followed by treatment with antiretroviral therapy and provision of free formula to their babies. The priority was to demonstrate the feasibility and acceptability of these measures in resource-poor settings. The initial projects would be set in Ivory Coast, Tanzania, Thailand and Uganda and in Botswana, Burkina Faso, Cambodia, Honduras, Rwanda, Zambia and Zimbabwe.[37] In selecting the pilot sites, the UN had targeted areas where women of childbearing age had high HIV infection rates and where local health systems were strong enough to deliver the measures needed to reduce MTCT of the virus.

12th World AIDS Conference, 28 June–3 July 1998

The announcement about the PMTCT pilot projects was made at the 12th World AIDS Conference in Geneva which was held from 28 June to 3 July 1998, and attended by more than 12,000 scientists, health workers, policymakers, activists, journalists and people with HIV and AIDS from all over the world. Country-by-country estimates of HIV infection and AIDS deaths underscored the devastating impact of the epidemic. Each year an estimated two million HIV-infected women worldwide became pregnant. About 680,000 babies were born with AIDS in the previous year, thrusting mother-to-child transmission to centre stage.

Protestors attacked the proposed plans as unethical, saying the programme would provide treatment to women only during pregnancy and not afterwards. They also criticised the failure to address the fate of the children who would be born uninfected, since approximately 1.6 million children worldwide lost their mothers to the disease in 1997. As we saw earlier, the first Asian and African antiretroviral studies had been criticised for giving placebos to a control group of women when the drug's efficacy had already been confirmed in industrialised countries.[62] Questions were raised about the ethics of giving an infected mother a short-course therapy that only benefited her baby, and of testing treatments in developing countries that were not likely to be affordable and widely available after the end of the trial. The dramatic results of the Thai study had not only raised the possibility that something could be done to reduce how many babies were being infected, but also the need to assure access to breastmilk substitutes, or to make breastfeeding safer, in order to reduce breastfeeding-associated transmission.

Dr Peter Piot of UNAIDS strongly defended the proposed PMTCT projects, citing budget constraints for full treatment of all HIV-infected pregnant women and the need to act now even if the programme created some orphans in the face of what Dr Piot called a 'runaway epidemic'. Pregnant women would be offered testing and infected mothers would receive free zidovudine starting at the 36th week of pregnancy and during labour. The AIDS programme had negotiated with zidovudine manufacturer, Glaxo Wellcome, for 'a substantial reduction in the cost of the drug: $50 for the course of zidovudine and $20 for testing'. Programme officials still needed to address the spread of the virus through breastfeeding, but mothers who did not breastfeed would receive counselling.

A month later, on 26 July 1998, the *New York Times* reported on the new initiative, with the headline, 'AIDS brings a shift on breastfeeding'.[63] The *Times* reported from Geneva:

> *'countering decades of promoting "breast is best" the United Nations is issuing recommendations intended to discourage women infected with the AIDS virus from breast-feeding. It is advising governments to consider bulk purchases of formula and other milk substitutes and to dispense them mainly through prescriptions. The compelling reason for the action is the soaring HIV infection rates in much of the world. In recent surveys, as many as 70% of women at a prenatal clinic in one city in Zimbabwe and 30% of women in major urban areas in six African countries were found to be infected.'*

The *New York Times* article continued that it was unethical to deliberately, consciously breastfeed an infant with milk that you know has HIV in it. The United Nations was reported as responding that in affected areas, some anxious women and families were beginning to demand that their governments provide information about alternatives. The epidemic had altered population demographics in some African countries. The rights of children to be born uninfected were also being invoked for personal and public health reasons; an overwhelming majority of infected children and adults in developing countries were doomed to die from the lack of anti-HIV drugs and standard healthcare. The new policy had emerged after years of internal debate that had sometimes been as emotional as it was scientific. Even now, the guidelines were cause for some dispute within the three United Nations agencies that put them out: UNAIDS, UNICEF and WHO. Dr Peter Piot, the executive director of UNAIDS, the agency that had pushed hardest to discourage infected mothers from breastfeeding, said he was deeply concerned about sending to third world countries a 'double message' that told some women breastfeeding is best for their babies, but told others that breastfeeding could kill. But 'we urgently need to find solutions to the AIDS epidemic and those recommendations were part of that', Dr Piot said.

The *New York Times* reported that the use of drugs to prevent MTCT had been hailed as one of the rare triumphs in the war against AIDS. However, concern was growing that it could become a hollow victory. The very same babies spared HIV infection during pregnancy and delivery could, just a few months later, become infected through breastfeeding. 'That's the elephant in the room', said Dr Kevin De Cock, in a telephone interview. The United Nations' directive represented a significant change in policy. For large agencies that had worked hard and long promoting breastfeeding, 'to say that women with HIV should avoid it, if possible, has been a very difficult policy pill to swallow', he said.

Dr Dorothy Odhiambo of Nairobi, Kenya, a representative of African non-governmental organisations, and another of the Nairobi group of researchers who had conducted the trial showing that formula was safer than breastfeeding, had said at the recent 12th World AIDS Conference in Geneva that 'it becomes unethical to continue not to do anything about it knowing very well that children are getting infected daily'.

Why some babies breastfed by infected mothers did *not* get infected was not known. Dr Philippe Van de Perre of Bobo-Diolassa, Burkina Faso, who had been among the first scientists to recognise the hazards of HIV and breastfeeding, said that a partial answer was that a baby's risk of becoming infected rises significantly if a woman became infected during pregnancy or breastfeeding or had advanced AIDS. Dr Van de Perre had been among leading experts who had developed HIV and infant feeding guidelines for the UN after they met at WHO the previous year, the first the United Nations had prepared for dealing with breastfeeding and HIV, and they were being sent to all governments. The guidelines spelled out the need for training in the nitty-gritty of providing alternatives to breastmilk. If commercial formula was not available, the guidelines described how to prepare cows' milk to make it safe for babies to drink and how to avoid mistakes that would endanger a baby. Emphasis was on practical advice, like the need to prepare a new batch every time an infant was fed. For women using formula, the guidelines explained the need to boil water and then not keep the mixed formula in the hot sun for hours.

For infected mothers who chose not to breastfeed, the United Nations recommended that all countries make safe, affordable infant-feeding alternatives available, including

- commercial infant formula;
- home-prepared formula made from fresh or processed cows' or goats' milk that was diluted with sugar water,
- HIV-negative wet-nurses,
- breastmilk banks, and
- mother's milk that had been heated to kill HIV – a solution still under study.

Success would 'depend on the political will' of the United Nations and affected countries, said Dr Isabelle De Vincenzi, a UNAIDS epidemiologist. It was anticipated that costs would be heavy. 'The cost of providing breast milk substitutes to all women needing them in Tanzania, for example, dwarfs the present health budget and dwarfs all of UNICEF's funds in Tanzania for the next two years', David Alnwick, a UNICEF official in New York city, said in an interview. He and other officials acknowledged that the recommendations would not immediately save many lives. Dr James Tulloch, a WHO official, said the United Nations viewed its directive as part of a package intended to have longer-term benefits. The hope was that as more women learned they were infected and talked to others in the community, the HIV problem would become more visible and lead to political action to raise the quality of maternal health services.

The guidelines also spelled out the risks of not breastfeeding, which were particularly great for women in communities where having many children was considered both a duty and a status symbol. But many women in Africa and elsewhere had been thrown out of their homes when families had learned that they carried HIV. Thus, a grave concern was the stigmatisation of an infected mother who did not breastfeed and was seen using bottles or cups to feed an infant. Dr Felicity Savage, for WHO, expressed extreme caution about the new guidelines, citing the risk of contamination of breastmilk alternatives in areas that lacked clean water and loss of nutrients if a woman mixed water and formula inaccurately. Such hazards could 'endanger a lot of lives that would otherwise not have been at risk at all, and could produce more deaths among those receiving replacement feedings than AIDS among those breast-fed by infected women'.

Dr Holck, another WHO expert, said she was 'struck by how much denial there was around the evidence we had that HIV could be transmitted through breast-feeding'. Much of the denial, Dr Holck said, 'undoubtedly was fed by people who had invested so much in promoting breast-feeding and feared what confirmation of that transmission might do to the gains that were made in breast-feeding.' She was also 'struck by the lack of information on the risk of not breastfeeding, and that is still the case.'

UNAIDS gave this further information on provision of formula in their October 1998 update.[64]

> *Given the vital importance of breast milk for child health, and the proven risk of HIV transmission through breastfeeding, it is now crucial that governments and public health authorities develop policies on HIV infection and infant feeding... Decision-makers need to consider the following: ...If the government offers free or subsidized breast-milk substitutes to some or all HIV-positive mothers who choose not to breastfeed, these mothers must be assured of breast-milk substitutes for at least 6 months. Additional costs include micronutrient supplements and extra health care costs for non-breastfed children. Against this can be set reduced costs of treating fewer children with AIDS. ...The risk of giving replacement feeds must be less than the risk of HIV transmission through breastfeeding, or there is no point in using them. ...Women choosing not to breastfeed will need extra support and counselling. ...If free or subsidized breast-milk substitutes are to be offered, they need to be distributed efficiently to the mothers who are eligible for them, but controlled to prevent spillover to mothers who are HIV negative or of unknown status.*

Discussions with industry about obtaining formula

The discovery that HIV could be passed through breastfeeding was a heaven-sent opportunity for legitimate promotion of infant formula in parts of the world where its use had been almost unknown. There were deep concerns in the breastfeeding community about collaboration between the UN agencies and industry. It emerged that Peter Piot, of UNAIDS, who had incidentally been a co-author of one of the first papers published by the Nairobi group in 1994, giving the risk of transmission of HIV through breastfeeding as 32%, had had a paper published the previous year in *Annales Nestlé*, the journal of the Nestlé Nutrition Institute, about the impact of HIV on women's health.[65] It was troubling too to learn that industry representatives had been invited to deliberations of WHO, UNICEF and UNAIDS where replacement feeding policy was being developed.

Reporting retrospectively in 2000 on developments over that time, the *Wall Street Journal*[66] noted that the issue of whether and how infant formula should be made available to poor African mothers had become mired in an incendiary debate that appeared to be driven more by politics and ideology than science. On one side was UNICEF, charged with protecting the interests of children. On the other was the $3 billion infant formula industry. Within months of the announcement of the UNAIDS/UNICEF/WHO change in policy to endorse replacement feeding in October 1997,[15] Nestlé's chief executive, Peter Brabeck, flew to New York from Switzerland to meet UNICEF CEO Carol Bellamy. When Ms Bellamy was appointed in 1995 by UN Secretary General Kofi Annan, both she and the infant formula industry had hoped to mend a rift between them which had existed since before the 1981 World Health Assembly adopted the International Code of Marketing of Breastmilk Substitutes. Her predecessor, the late James Grant, had held meetings with the formula makers that had degenerated into mutual accusations, and a public boycott of Nestlé had been in place for many years. Ms Bellamy told the industry's trade association she wanted to avoid this, and invited the companies to come to New York and detail how they marketed infant formula around the world. But the October meeting degenerated into an impasse. Nestlé said it had received 'desperate' requests for free formula from some African hospitals. But if it made donations, UNICEF would view its action as a violation of the Code, generating bad publicity and possibly fuelling renewed boycott efforts. A testy exchange of letters followed. A month later, Ms Bellamy wrote to Mr Brabeck, citing a number of 'not reconcilable' differences over the International Code and concluding that future contact would not be useful. Mr Brabeck, clearly offended, wrote to Ms Bellamy and then to Secretary General Kofi Annan. Mr Annan replied that he hoped 'for a continued dialogue in a constructive spirit' between Nestlé and the UN. The standoff was to persist for nearly two years.

It was perfectly true that industry was wary of providing unsolicited donations in developing countries. The Zimbabwean legislation giving effect to the International Code, which was passed through parliament in 1998, required that any formula donation be preceded by an official written request on behalf of an individually named baby, from either the Nutrition Department of the Ministry of Health and Child Welfare, or the Chief Nutritionist of the Harare City Health Department. Nestlé (the only local manufacturer) took this responsibility seriously. It would never give away free formula and such requests were rarely made; in my experience only the birth of triplets would qualify. Furthermore, if Nestlé responded to such a request, they were required to donate sufficient formula to feed the individually named baby for the whole time that a breastmilk substitute was needed – usually for two years.

Meanwhile, in New York Nestlé tried a new tactic. It retained Ms Ferraro, a former vice presidential candidate, as a business consultant, at an undisclosed fee. Ms Ferraro and Carol Bellamy had been close friends since 1978. The two women lunched in the UN delegates' dining room and later, Ms Ferraro lugged to UNICEF headquarters a shopping bag containing a lengthy Nestlé analysis of how its overseas sales force had been trained in Code compliance. In spite of this, talks broke down due to UNICEF's continued concern about Code violations.

As the contretemps between Nestlé and UNICEF dragged on, the *Wall Street Journal* reported that another formula maker had quietly begun putting out feelers to the agency. Wyeth, a unit of American Home Products Corporation that sells formula under the brand names SMA and Nursoy, caught wind that UNICEF was planning to launch a pilot program to try to reduce MTCT at some African hospitals. To conform with the new 'informed choice' policy, formula would likely be offered as an option to participants. Wyeth sensed an opportunity, but the objective of saving babies' lives was soon overtaken by a dispute over public relations.

In November 1998, Daniel Spiegel, a Washington attorney for Wyeth, who had been the United States Permanent Representative to the European Office of the UN in Geneva from 1993 to 1996,[67] had begun conducting some very quiet conversations with top officials at UNAIDS. Mr Spiegel told UNAIDS that Wyeth wanted to donate formula to HIV-infected women in Africa. The company believed it could make such a donation because of an exception in the International Code that allows formula giveaways to babies 'who have to be fed on breast-milk substitutes'. The company assumed this could include 'AIDS babies', and that a programme administered by UNICEF itself would use the formula safely, thereby averting the potential for bad publicity. UNAIDS began acting as a broker between Wyeth and UNICEF to put the precedent-setting deal in motion. 'This was very new ground for everyone', recalls Jim Sherry, a UNAIDS official involved in the talks. 'Because of AIDS, the public-health community was in a turnaround situation: formula had been like tobacco and suddenly it wasn't.'

On 26 March 1999, after lengthy negotiations, Wyeth and UNICEF representatives finally met face-to-face at the company's Philadelphia headquarters. UNICEF, worried that Wyeth would try to exploit its donation for marketing purposes, insisted the free formula could carry no brand name. Wyeth agreed. The company also said it was prepared to provide free formula for six months to 100,000 infants, a figure based on UNICEF's initial estimates of what its pilot programme would require, and was willing to give more later. (The original pilot programme had been designed to recruit only 30,000 HIV-infected mothers.) At UNICEF's request, about a week later Wyeth sent in a draft proposal of its offer. But the *Wall Street Journal* reported that, unknown to the company, the deal was fast unravelling. A month later, on 28 April, Mr Lewis, Ms Bellamy's aide, received an email from UNICEF's lawyer Peter Mason saying that Wyeth had suggested getting UNICEF to commit to a thank-you letter. According to the email, Wyeth's Mr Spiegel expressed 'outrage and shock' when told that UNICEF might not agree to a letter, but said that the company might settle for a meeting with UNICEF officials. Wyeth also requested a jointly issued press release and a photo opportunity with Ms Bellamy and Wyeth executives, which could have led to a misunderstanding of the UNICEF-Wyeth relationship. Wyeth maintained that it made suggestions about recognition only after UNICEF itself brought up the subject, and that these weren't conditions of the donation; all they wanted was an appropriate acknowledgment for a multi-million-dollar donation. Their only demand was that they would not be attacked by UNICEF for past Code violations if they made it. In the end, UNICEF rejected the proposed Wyeth donation without giving any explanation, and the talks ended there.

UNAIDS was also contacted by Nestlé again. Nestlé had learned of Wyeth's overture and didn't want to be left out. At two meetings in Switzerland in March 1999, Nestlé said it favoured an all-industry approach, implemented by the industry's trade association, according to Nestlé vice president of public affairs, Niels Christiansen, who attended both sessions. But after the Wyeth deal faded away, UNAIDS heard nothing further from Nestlé.

Having rejected Wyeth's offer, UNICEF still needed to line up a supply of formula for its pilot programme. The agency's options were limited, since it considered most of the major formula makers to be Code violators. UNICEF's $1.1 billion annual budget comes entirely from government and individual donations, but it initially anticipated it could afford to pay for the relatively small amount of formula required by the programme. Before soliciting bids, UNICEF checked with a group of pro-breastfeeding advocates that coordinated the continuing Nestlé boycott, and who had written a 1997 report called 'Cracking the Code'[68] outlining Code violations such as formula giveaways and other promotional activities aimed at mothers around the world.

In late 1998, in an article written in *SCN News*, UNICEF had summarised the UN PMTCT initiative and their support for implementation of the pilot projects.[69] They specified that the primary beneficiaries of the project were the infants of HIV-positive women in the pilot sites, up to one-half more of whom would be born and remain uninfected as a result of the interventions. In addition, all pregnant women in the pilot sites would benefit from improved antenatal and maternity services and voluntary and confidential counselling and testing. Monitoring and evaluation was stressed (bold emphasis mine):

> *Recent research has enabled a drastic reduction in the cost of the drug intervention that prevents mother-to-child HIV transmission by* ***shortening the duration of treatment while maintaining a good level of effectiveness.***
>
> *UNICEF, in close collaboration with the UNAIDS Secretariat, has been able to obtain a donation from the Glaxo Wellcome Company, the producer of AZT, for 30,000 pregnant women. It is likely that the total cost of reducing the risk of transmission of HIV from a mother to her child will be reduced to about $200 per treated HIV infected mother...*
>
> *The overall goal of this UN initiative is to assess the* ***feasibility*** *of prevention of mother-to-child transmission (MTCT) of HIV in a variety of situations in some of the worst-affected countries in Africa and South East Asia, thus reducing the infection rate in infants and young children.*

Specific objectives:

- *To make available good quality voluntary confidential counselling and testing to 10,000 pregnant women and their partners* ***in each pilot country.*** *The comprehensive package will include voluntary and confidential counselling and testing, provision of AZT to HIV+ women, modified delivery practices, provision of information on infant feeding options, and where necessary, a supply of breastmilk substitutes.*
- ***To carefully monitor implementation and document experiences*** *in order to facilitate replication in other facilities within countries and to other affected countries.*

Two major outcomes are expected:

- *Through a better understanding... governments and the donor community will* ***expand*** *efforts to reach more HIV-infected mothers.*
- *Voluntary and confidential counselling and testing for HIV will become more acceptable and accessible*
- *Reduced number of infected infants born to HIV positive mothers.*

Monitoring and Evaluation

The monitoring and evaluation arrangements for this project are critical, because it is aimed at establishing the feasibility of the intervention... Close monitoring will be necessary in order to modify site specific approaches if problems are identified and/or a particular strategy is shown to be successful and warrants adaptation in other areas.

Data from the countries will be periodically reviewed at this level, and site visits undertaken as and when necessary. At the onset of the project in each country, ***a monitoring and evaluation plan*** *will be agreed ...The results of the evaluation will be presented as case studies in various international fora,*

Lusaka 1999 Africa Regional Conference and
Durban 2000 XIII International AIDS Conference.

UNICEF and the UNAIDS Secretariat are supporting HIV networks in Eastern Africa and South East Asia which will be used to disseminate the information among the countries.

Finally, as this intervention is part of a combined effort of the UNAIDS Secretariat, WHO, UNFPA and UNICEF, the results and lessons learned will be compiled and disseminated as part of the UNAIDS best practice collection of materials.

In 2000 and 2001, controversy about provision of formula to HIV-exposed babies in developing countries escalated. WHO was accused of being too pally with formula manufacturers,[70] and UNICEF was accused of planning to let HIV-exposed babies die. In January 2001, Gavin Yamey wrote in the *British Medical Journal:*[71]

'After years of being hated by advocates of breastfeeding, Nestlé and the rest of the baby food industry must have wept with delight at articles in the Wall Street Journal last month. Their early Christmas present came in the form of a front page, lead news story (5

December) and an accompanying editorial in the European edition (6 December), which painted the baby food manufacturers as heroes poised to save African children from certain death. What was the nature of their heroism? "One major formula maker," said the article, "Wyeth-Ayerst Laboratories Inc, says it stands ready to donate tons of free formula to HIV-infected women. No.1-ranked Nestlé SA says it too would donate, if asked." Such donations, argued the reporters, would stop the transmission of HIV from mothers to their children via infected breast milk, halting the spread of AIDS through sub-Saharan Africa. All heroic tales need a villain, and this one was no exception. "Unicef," said the paper, "refuses to greenlight the gifts, because it doesn't want to endorse an industry it has long accused of abusive practices in the Third World." If there was any doubt in readers' minds about the goodies and baddies in this epic struggle for infant health, the headline hit the message home: "African Babies Fall Ill as Unicef Fights Formula Makers." The editorial went further still, blaming Unicef's "feud against the industry" for "killing millions of children." Formula fever soon spread west across the US, reaching the pages of the Houston Chronicle (December 10). Michelle Malkin, a nationally syndicated columnist, cited the Wall Street Journal report and accused Unicef's "breast feeding crusade" of "killing the children it's supposed to protect." She also offered her advice to the agency: "There is a very simple solution: feed the babies formula."'

In six days, the American dailies had taken a highly contentious health issue – the merits of breast and bottle-feeding in the era of AIDS – and turned it into a simple battle between the benevolent corporations and a seemingly malicious international health agency. Headlines read 'African babies fall ill as UNICEF fights formula makers. Conflict with Nestlé, Others, allows AIDS to spread' and 'African babies sicken amid UNICEF battle'.

The *BMJ* article continued:

'accepting donations from the formula industry seems to be tearing apart the UN health agencies, adding fuel to the paper's condemnation of Unicef. "Even some UN officials," said the Wall Street Journal reporters, "contend that Unicef's decades-old distrust of the formula industry should yield to a moral imperative to get formula to destitute, HIV-infected mothers." Who were these officials? None other than Peter Piot, executive director of UNAIDS, the Joint UN Programme on HIV/AIDS, who is quoted as saying that Unicef is "having difficulty accepting that the world has changed." Perhaps the papers, then, were merely reflecting a growing polarisation of opinion within the UN itself. ...Julia Cleves, chief at Dr Piot's office, said that Dr Piot's comments were taken out of context, and that the quotation was an oversimplification. "Peter made these comments," she said, "about those in Unicef who pursue a hard line on baby milk, the so-called 'lactation police.' The point is, it wasn't a comment on Unicef as an institution." But I then spoke to Dr Piot himself, who stood by his attack and expressed frustration that it was taking "too long to find practical solutions" to the HIV crisis. "The solution," he said, "will have to involve both industry and breastfeeding activists." The old mantra of 'breast is best,' he said, was no longer appropriate. He admitted that "there is a divide across organisations about what is right and wrong, and there are strong feelings."'

But the *BMJ* also quoted a letter, dated 14 December 2000, sent to the *Wall Street Journal* by UNICEF Executive Director Carol Bellamy, which stated: 'You fail to acknowledge that UNICEF is leading the way in addressing mother to child transmission, and you fail to explain fully why UNICEF so strongly supports breastfeeding.' Research showed, she said, that formula-fed infants were four to six times more likely to die of disease than breastfed infants, and 'exclusive breastfeeding can save lives, as many as 1.5 million a year. A rush to promote formula feeding,' she explained, 'could lead to the spread of other infectious diseases. UNICEF's view is that if formula is to be used, it needs to be done in a targeted manner. The organisation is currently piloting projects in 11 countries to offer women HIV testing and counselling, offering formula to those who then choose to use it.'

Purchasing formula while abiding by the Code

Eventually, based on an exhaustive pre-qualification process of suppliers and competitive bidding, UNICEF decided to buy the formula required for its pilot projects from a French dairy cooperative, Jammet Dietetique Nouvelle SA,[37,66] whose brands include Jammet generic formula and whose parent company makes Yoplait yogurt.[72] UNICEF officials were reported to have said that they settled on a no-name product in a deliberately unattractive box to discourage healthy women from wanting to use it. However, Helen Armstrong, a UNICEF employee who came to Harare in March 1999 as one of the officials tasked with field-testing the WHO-UNICEF HIV Counselling Course, outlined in the following chapter, told me that their final decision was based on the fact that the company had never been recorded as a Code violator.[73] The commercial infant formula was distributed in carton boxes with an inner foil wrapping containing 500 grams of powdered formula suitable from birth.[37] Carton boxes were used because they were cheaper than tins and weighed less. Larger packages were considered unsuitable because of the risk of contamination and deterioration after opening.

A label for the boxes was developed which was in accordance with the conditions of the International Code of Marketing of Breastmilk Substitutes. (This label was made available in French, Spanish and English). Given that the International Code requires infant formula to be labelled in an appropriate language, UNICEF country offices were required to provide text for labels in local languages where necessary. It was acknowledged that the mother might not have appropriate measuring utensils, so the cartons also contained two scoops, a larger one for measuring 30ml of boiled water and a smaller one for measuring the correct amount of formula for each 30ml of water.

Nevertheless, mistakes happen. Some time later, a large consignment of UNICEF generic formula was seized by the Zimbabwe Customs department at the Chirundu border post with Zambia. Officials noted that the boxes did not comply with labelling requirements of the Zimbabwe Code; they were in French, not one of the official languages. After some time they were sent back through the border. We heard eventually that Uganda took them, although they don't speak French there either.

Refining the strategy

In February 2000, the findings of a WHO commissioned Collaborative Study to assess the effect of not breastfeeding on the risk of death due to infectious diseases, were published in the *Lancet.*[74] Data from studies conducted in Brazil, the Gambia, Ghana, Pakistan, the Philippines and Senegal was pooled. The odds of infant death due to not breastfeeding were highest in the early months and declined as the baby got older, with the relative risks being:

Relative risk according to age of infant	
5.8	<2 months
2.6	4–5 months
1.8	6–8 months
1.4	9–11 months

The findings of the Collaborative Study, especially showing that the risk of formula-feeding decreased as the baby grew older, underpinned continued work by the UN agencies to move the PMTCT agenda forward.

The October 2000 WHO Technical Consultation

WHO convened another Technical Consultation in October 2000. The proceedings were published in January 2001.[75] Updated recommendations to reduce MTCT of HIV focused on a stepwise prevention strategy:

1. primary prevention of HIV infection among parents to be,
2. prevention of unwanted pregnancies in HIV-infected women, and
3. prevention of HIV transmission from HIV-infected women to their infants.

Some experience had been obtained with pilot intervention projects, many initiated by UNICEF under the umbrella of the UN Inter-Agency Task Team (IATT) on MTCT. The entry point to the interventions was voluntary counselling and testing (VCT) for HIV, followed by zidovudine from 36 weeks and during labour to mothers who were HIV-positive, and counselling on infant feeding options. Recent clinical trials had shown that short-course antiretroviral regimens using zidovudine alone or in combination with lamivudine and nevirapine, were effective in reducing transmission. Consequently there was now no justification for restricting their use to pilot projects or research settings: they should now be recommended for general use and PMTCT should be part of the minimum standard package of care for HIV-positive women and their infants. In revised guidance emanating from the 2000 Technical Consultation there was an ambiguous mix of support for a mothers' own infant-feeding decision combined with a greater emphasis on the risks of breastfeeding and facilitation of formula-feeding to create a measure of subtle coercion favouring the latter. It seems clear that the findings of the WHO Collaborative Study facilitated this approach:

- *When replacement feeding is acceptable, feasible, affordable, sustainable and safe [which subsequently came to be known as the AFASS conditions] avoidance of all breastfeeding by HIV-infected mothers is recommended.*
- *Otherwise, exclusive breastfeeding is recommended during the first months of life.*
- *The risk of MTCT of HIV through breastfeeding appears to be greatest during the first months of infant life but persists as long as breastfeeding continues.*
- *Half of the breastfeeding-related infections may occur after 6 months with continued breastfeeding into the second year of life...* ***To minimize HIV transmission risk, breastfeeding should be discontinued as soon as feasible,*** *taking into account local circumstances, the individual woman's situation and the risks of replacement feeding (including infections other than HIV and malnutrition).*
- *When HIV-infected mothers choose not to breastfeed from birth or stop breastfeeding later, they should be provided with specific guidance and support for at least the first 2 years of the child's life to ensure adequate replacement feeding. Programmes should strive to improve conditions that will make replacement feeding safer for HIV-infected mothers and families.*

The previous recommendation that HIV-infected mothers avoid all breastfeeding when replacement feeding was feasible was retained, but an added condition now qualified that advice, saying, 'otherwise, exclusive breastfeeding is recommended during the first months of life'. Another addition was the specific recommendation that mothers who lacked an AFASS alternative and initiated breastfeeding should discontinue breastfeeding 'as soon as feasible'. It was hoped that this guidance would provide an optimal compromise, maximising breastfeeding benefit while minimising HIV transmission risk.

New recommendations were added aimed at reducing the changeover time during which mixed feeding might occur as a result of premature weaning:

- *There are concerns about the possible increased risk of HIV transmission with mixed feeding during the transition period between exclusive breastfeeding and complete cessation of breastfeeding. Indirect evidence ...suggests that keeping the period of transition as short as possible may reduce the risk. ...The best duration for this transition is not known and may vary according to the age of the infant and/or the environment.*
- *HIV-infected mothers who breastfeed should be provided with specific guidance and support when they cease breastfeeding to avoid harmful nutritional and psychological consequences and to maintain breast health.*

There was further guidance concerning infant feeding counselling:

- *All HIV-infected mothers should receive counselling, which includes provision of general information about the risks and benefits of various infant feeding options, and specific guidance in selecting the option most likely to be suitable for their situation. Whatever a mother decides,* ***she should be supported in her choice.***

- *Assessments should be conducted locally to identify the range of feeding options that are acceptable, feasible, affordable, sustainable and safe in a particular context.*
- *Information and education on mother-to-child transmission of HIV should be urgently directed to the general public, affected communities and families.*
- *Adequate numbers of people who can counsel HIV-infected women on infant feeding should be trained, deployed, supervised and supported. Such support should include updated training as new information and recommendations emerge.*

In the year 2001 alone, 800,000 children became infected with HIV.[76] In June 2001, a General Assembly of the UN was held at which a declaration of commitment was made to reduce HIV infection in children by 50% 'by ensuring that 80% of pregnant women accessing antenatal care have information, counselling and other HIV-prevention services...including voluntary counselling and testing... and especially antiretroviral therapy and... breastmilk substitutes.'[77]

The WHO Global Strategy on Infant and Young Child Feeding

Around this time, WHO had been simultaneously beginning work to tie up all the loose ends in breastfeeding policy and to include HIV and infant feeding within various other aspects of their work with children. In March 2000, WHO invited technical and programme experts from all regions to Geneva to begin work on development of what was to become an over-arching Global Strategy on Infant and Young Child Feeding. This was a brilliant and timely concept, aiming to improve the feeding of infants based on evidence of the importance of the first years of a child's life for growth and development. It sought to tie into a cohesive whole the targets and goals of the International Code of Marketing of Breastmilk Substitutes, the Innocenti Declaration, and the Baby Friendly Hospital Initiative, together with efforts to empower working women, guidelines for HIV and infant feeding, and feeding children in emergencies and exceptionally difficult circumstances.

The Global Strategy was intended as a guide for action, emphasising support for mothers and defining the obligations and responsibilities of governments, international organisations and other concerned parties. However, it envisaged promotion of formula-feeding to HIV-positive mothers and drafted various sections accordingly, e.g. 'training health workers who care for mothers, children and families with regard to counselling and assistance skills needed for HIV and infant feeding and, when necessary, feeding with a breast-milk substitute.'[78]

During 2000 and 2001 the draft strategy was considered at country consultations in Brazil, China, the Philippines, Scotland, Sri Lanka, Thailand and Zimbabwe. In collaboration with the Zimbabwe Ministry of Health, WHO had organised the preliminary field test of the Global Strategy for September 2000 in Harare. Our National Breastfeeding Co-ordinator told me that WHO 'liked' Zimbabwe – if something could pass Zimbabwe it could be used anywhere! Felicity Savage, consultant to WHO, arrived to conduct the field test at the Harare Holiday Inn. I was invited to the workshop – surprisingly since I had made little effort to hide my concerns about the content of the HIV Counselling Course when that had been field-tested by WHO and UNICEF in

Zimbabwe in March the previous year (See Chapter 13).

In June 2001 I was invited in my capacity as the African representative for my professional association, the International Lactation Consultant Association (ILCA), to attend a further WHO Regional Consultation on the Global Strategy on Infant and Young Child Feeding, to be held at the Sheraton Hotel, Harare, from 26–28 June. Participants also included two friends, our National Breastfeeding Co-ordinator, Rufaro Madzima, and the IBFAN Africa representative, Pauline Kisanga. On the eve of the consultation, I collected three of the WHO Geneva organisers from the airport: James Akre, Randa Saadeh and Jelka Zupan, and brought them to dinner at my home. We had an enjoyable evening talking breastfeeding. Joining us was another friend, Gill Browne, the La Leche League Leader who lived on a tea estate in southern Zimbabwe and had hosted Kiersten Israel Ballard when she was conducting her focus group discussions on flash-heated breastmilk (see Chapter 11). Gill had done a lot of work with HIV-positive mothers and babies, and with grandmothers who were looking after AIDS orphans. Jim had kindly brought a whole suitcase of clothes for Gill to distribute to the orphans.

The Regional Consultation was really a microcosm of what was happening in breastfeeding in Africa at the time.[79] It was attended by approximately 30 Ministry of Health or UNICEF representatives from all corners of sub-Saharan Africa: Angola, Burkina Faso, Burundi, Côte d'Ivoire, Democratic Republic of Congo, Ethiopia, Ghana, Kenya, Mauritius, Mozambique, Nigeria, South Africa, Swaziland, Tanzania, Togo, Uganda, Zambia and Zimbabwe. IBFAN and ILCA were the only non-governmental organisations represented. It was a great pleasure to have the opportunity to meet and brainstorm with such a diverse group of African experts on such vital topics as the health, nutrition and feeding of babies and young children. There was considerable agreement among the delegates. Many expressed unease about the way that the international community was responding to their concerns. Reporting back to ILCA after the Consultation, I wrote, 'The global strategy will no doubt set breastfeeding policy, and thus the ways in which breastfeeding is to be promoted and practised, for the next decade'. As it happens, it remains unaltered in 2021.

It was clear then that a vast amount of work had already gone into the preparation of the document, now up to Draft 21B, before it was presented in Harare in 2001. We were tasked with identifying the specific needs of Africa and making further recommendations.

The country reports outlined the shocking situation on our continent and the urgent challenge facing governments and policymakers. Malnutrition contributed to 49% of all the 10.7 million deaths worldwide which occurred in children under five years of age in 1999. Most Africans lived on less than US$2 per day and in Zambia 80% of the population were living in abject poverty. Angola had been at war for 35 years, and we heard that there was no industry and very little agriculture, and the country survived mainly on contributions. Throughout Africa trends in child nutrition over the last 20 years had shown limited improvement. Underweight rose from 12–36 months. Stunting occurred in 32.5% of all African children, rising to 43% in Tanzanian under-fives. There was vitamin A deficiency in over 100 countries and anaemia affected two out of every five young children. Breastfeeding was universally practised throughout Africa and the average age of weaning was 21 months. But although only a tiny percentage of babies were never breastfed at all, only 18.4% of those under six months were exclusively breastfed. In Burkina Faso in west Africa, only 50% of neonates were still exclusively breastfed by 12 days of age, and the policymaker in the African household was often the grandmother or the father, not the mother. Africa was home to 1.1 million of the 1.4 million children under 15 living with AIDS at the end of the year 2000.

Presentations were followed by plenary sessions and group work. WHO representatives and members of the different countries spoke about the current nutritional status of young children in each region. Additional topics included low birth weight and the potential for poor health outcomes, complementary feeding, advocacy in infant feeding matters, legislation to give effect to the Code and human rights, as well as several sessions on HIV and infant feeding.

While there was discussion of the recently announced deliberations regarding exclusive breastfeeding for six months, I felt that this could have received a more enthusiastic plug. Concerns were expressed that starting complementary foods too late was as bad as starting too early. A doctor from Uganda questioned whether it was physically possible for women to exclusively breastfeed for that long, and his scepticism was echoed by someone from the Mozambique Health Ministry who said that they were continuing to advise mothers to breastfeed exclusively for a maximum of four months only, notwithstanding the new evidence from the expert consultation. There was universal acknowledgement of the cultural constraints to promotion of really exclusive breastfeeding, and of the need to educate mothers and other family members about the benefits, but there were few concrete recommendations within the document about the information mothers might need to have, or the practical measures which mothers could take, in order to make exclusive breastfeeding a successful reality. This was in contrast to the many alternatives to breastfeeding that mothers could employ if they chose not to breastfeed in order to reduce the risk of transmission of HIV through breastmilk.

The general impression I received at the meeting was that HIV and infant feeding was the most burning current issue for African governments and healthcare workers. This was not surprising, since this same concern had been urgently and repeatedly expressed by all healthcare personnel I had worked with in Zimbabwe over the previous five years. These fears were well illustrated during the first plenary by a participant from Swaziland who wanted to know whether breastfeeding should be stopped at two, three, four or five months in order to best reduce the risk of infection. High rates of HIV infection among the general population, and fear of transmission of HIV to babies through breastfeeding, were causing an extremely negative down-scaling of breastfeeding promotion efforts, in particular affecting the Baby Friendly Hospital Initiative and implementation of the Code. Health workers from every region were becoming less and less eager to promote breastfeeding because of the apparent risk of acquiring HIV through breastmilk, and they seemed to be genuinely unsure about how to juggle the risk of infant mortality from HIV infection against mortality from replacement feeding.

Participants were asked to sign up to the group session topic which most interested them and in which they had the most expertise, for example education about breastfeeding, the duration of exclusive breastfeeding, or HIV and breastfeeding. Pauline Kisanga of

IBFAN and I were keen to join the HIV group, but found that we had been assigned to two other separate groups, and we believed that this was a way to divide and silence us, since we had both spoken out about our concerns in previous plenary sessions. Pauline made a very clear call for information to be made known about the UNICEF MTCT pilot projects, especially before they were scaled up and rolled out to additional sites. I had queried the quantification of HIV transmission through breastmilk, based on the figures given in the Nduati and the Dunn research (14–29% risk of transmission through breastmilk)[19,22] and was told by one of the WHO personnel who had sat at my dining table, 'A *lot* of people have done a *lot* of work and spent a *lot* of time and money on this, and you are only one.'

But our concerns were real. Although international guidelines recommend that only those mothers who know that they are infected should be 'counselled' about 'infant feeding choices', the practical application of this recommendation presented a dilemma. For example, anonymous sentinel surveillance testing provided evidence for high rates of infection in antenatal mothers (20%–40% in southern Africa) yet only a minute fraction of pregnant women knew, or wanted to know, their HIV status. (Few women actually received the promised ART – see Chapter 13 – so there was no benefit to this knowledge in the absence of treatment). Was it right to promote breastfeeding to these women? There were additional concerns that even mothers uninfected at the time of delivery risked becoming infected later during the course of breastfeeding, thus placing the nursing infant at high risk. The result was that breastfeeding itself was being perceived as dangerous even in the absence of known individual HIV status. Early cessation, or replacement feeding, was being seen as a solution to reduce that risk. This fear was not alleviated by the wording in the draft Global Strategy (sections 5.5, and 5.6):

> *'Globally, the risk of mother-to-child HIV transmission through breastfeeding is between about 10% and 20% if the infant breastfeeds for two years. ... Therefore, mothers who are tested HIV-positive... need counselling to enable them to make a choice that is appropriate to their specific circumstances. This should consist of a discussion of the risks and costs of a range of feeding options, which may include exclusive breastfeeding with early cessation to reduce the risk of HIV transmission; heat-treatment of expressed breast milk; wet-nursing by an HIV-negative woman; and replacement feeding with commercial formula (whether bearing a proprietary brand or generic label) or home-prepared formula...'*

Since individual testing was for the most part unavailable and/or unwanted in Africa, and since treatment was unaffordable and difficult to implement, then the only route left by which attempts could be made to reduce transmission seemed to be complete avoidance of breastfeeding, or breastfeeding for the shortest possible time. If only replacement feeding could be made safer for African babies then this would be the most appropriate response. The estimated absolute rates of MTCT by timing of transmission, in the absence of peri-partum interventions, with 25–35% attributable to breastfeeding, as computed in the recent Kevin de Cock analysis[56] were highlighted as evidence of the way in which the industrialised world had responded by advising 'no breastfeeding', compared to the way in which Africa had failed to respond, with consequent apparent high transmission rates.

Exclusive breastfeeding for six months was not promoted by anyone present (except me) as a method of reducing transmission, the rationale being that the Coutsoudis research[80,81] had only noted the protective effect of three months' exclusive breastfeeding, and thus early cessation of breastfeeding from three to six months was generally agreed as the safest course for HIV-positive mothers who chose to breastfeed at all.

Pilot projects (more fully described in chapters 14, 15 and 16) were being conducted in several developing countries to assess the feasibility of replacement feeding. Expansion of the existing South African pilot projects was being planned to 18 additional new sites. Data about HIV transmission and child mortality was supposed to be obtained, but it seemed that the situation was fairly chaotic; formula was being provided, but with little guidance. Some of the mothers were using bottles, rather than cup-feeding which was recommended as much safer; they often moved away from the project site and could not be traced; and health workers involved in the Khayelitsha and Chris Hani Baragwanath projects in South Africa did not always have the chance to follow up adequately. It was also possible that recruitment into the PMTCT projects, where the mothers and babies received nevirapine, was conditional upon mothers agreeing to use formula-feeding for their babies. Of course, there were concerns about mixed feeding, or about mothers starting with formula and then abandoning it because it was too difficult. With Pauline Kisanga, I also repeatedly asked during the plenary sessions, and privately, if data from the existing MTCT projects could be made public, but whether this information was actually available to UNICEF or WHO was unclear.

Two of the groups at first contained participants who spoke either English or French. In the interests of communication, participants were reshuffled into anglophone and francophone groups, and the differences in attitude and practice between these groupings of countries were subsequently obvious when they reported back to the plenary sessions. Those from English-speaking countries were more knowledgeable about and more in favour of breastfeeding than those from the francophone or lusophone (Portuguese-speaking) countries. Similar findings had been reflected in the early research on MTCT of HIV from west and central Africa compared to reports coming from east and southern Africa. The group work was lively but there was never enough time. Many questions went unanswered.

The WHO team returned to Geneva with the recommendations of the African region and with the task of sifting the information and incorporating their suggestions. The next regional meeting was to be held in the Philippines, and the document was to be finalised before the end of the year. Poverty, food insecurity and emergencies including HIV/AIDS and their socio-economic consequences were global concerns, but with an intensity and urgency in Africa that exceeded other continents. It was hoped that these overriding environmental constraints would help to define the magnitude and urgency of consequent resolutions.

The Global Strategy was endorsed, by consensus, on 18 May 2002 by the 55th World Health Assembly, and on 16 September 2002 by the UNICEF Executive Board. Finally, concluding several years of consultations and deliberations designed to integrate a comprehensive approach to appropriate feeding for the world's children, the Global

Strategy was published in 2003.[82] It renewed commitment to continuing joint action consistent with the Baby Friendly Hospital Initiative, the International Code of Marketing of Breastmilk Substitutes, and the Innocenti Declaration on the Protection, Promotion and Support of Breastfeeding. It recorded that:

> *Breastfeeding is an unequalled way of providing ideal food for the healthy growth and development of infants; it is also an integral part of the reproductive process with important implications for the health of mothers. As a global public health recommendation, infants should be exclusively breastfed for the first six months of life to achieve optimal growth, development and health. Thereafter to meet their evolving nutritional requirements, infants should receive nutritionally adequate and safe complementary foods while breastfeeding continues for up to two years of age or beyond. Exclusive breastfeeding from birth is possible except for a few medical conditions, and unrestricted exclusive breastfeeding results in ample milk production.*

However, on HIV the Global Strategy made an exception, saying:

> *The HIV pandemic and the risk of mother-to-child transmission of HIV through breastfeeding pose unique challenges to the promotion of breastfeeding, even among unaffected families… An estimated 1.6 million children are born to HIV-infected women each year, mainly in low-income countries. The absolute risk of HIV transmission through breastfeeding for more than one year – globally between 10% and 20% – needs to be balanced against the increased risk of morbidity and mortality when infants are not breastfed. All HIV-infected mothers should receive counselling, which includes provision of general information about meeting their own nutritional requirements and about the risks and benefits of various feeding options, and specific guidance in selecting the option most likely to be suitable for their situation. Adequate replacement feeding is needed for infants born to HIV-positive mothers who choose not to breastfeed. It requires a suitable breast-milk substitute, for example an infant formula prepared in accordance with applicable Codex Alimentarius standards, or a home-prepared formula with micronutrient supplements. Heat-treated breast milk, or breast milk provided by an HIV-negative donor mother, may be an option in some cases. To reduce the risk of interfering with the promotion of breastfeeding for the great majority, providing a breastmilk substitute for these infants should be consistent with the principles and aim of the International Code of Marketing of Breastmilk Substitutes. For mothers who test negative for HIV, or who are untested, exclusive breastfeeding remains the recommended feeding option.*

Meanwhile, in March 2002, WHO convened another meeting in Switzerland to discuss various programme approaches to preventing HIV infection in infants in different epidemiological situations.[83] Importantly, participants recommended that, in addition to the three-pronged strategy then supported by the UN agencies (outlined below), a fourth component (in bold) should be added in recognition that on humanitarian grounds, it is difficult to defend providing a short course of antiretroviral drugs to save a child but deny basic care and, when indicated, antiretroviral treatment to the mother.

- primary prevention of HIV infection;
- preventing unintended pregnancies among HIV-infected women;
- preventing HIV transmission from HIV-infected women to their children;
- providing care for HIV-infected mothers

A Framework for Priority Action on HIV and Infant Feeding

In 2003, the HIV and Infant Feeding Framework for Priority Action was published,[84,85] with recommendations for key actions by governments to scale up interventions to reduce HIV transmission through breastfeeding:

- *Expand access to, and demand for, quality antenatal care for women who currently do not use such services.*
- *Expand access to, and demand for, HIV testing and counselling, before and during pregnancy and lactation, to enable women and their partners to know their HIV status, know how to prevent HIV/sexually transmitted infections and be supported in decisions related to their own behaviours and their children's health.*
- *Implement other measures aimed at prevention of HIV infection in infants and young children, including provision of antiretroviral drugs during pregnancy, labour and delivery and/or to the infant and safer delivery practices.*
- *Support the orientation of health care managers and capacity-building and pre-service training of counsellors (including lay counsellors) and health workers on breastfeeding counselling, as well as primary prevention of HIV and infant feeding counselling, including the need for respect and support for mothers' feeding choices.*
- *Improve follow-up, supervision and support of health workers to sustain their skills and the quality of counselling, and to prevent 'burn-out'.*
- *Integrate adequate HIV and infant feeding counselling and support into maternal and child health services, and simplify counselling to increase its comprehensibility and enhance the feasibility of increasing coverage levels.*
- *Carry out relevant formative research, and develop and implement a comprehensive communication strategy on appropriate infant and young child feeding practices within the context of HIV.*

These documents were followed, in 2004, by updated versions of the original 1998 trilogy of *HIV and Infant Feeding Guidelines for Decision Makers,*[86] for *Health-care Managers and Supervisors,*[87] and a *Review of HIV through Breastfeeding.*[88] These newer revisions did not materially change previous guidance, they simply refined it, and made information about replacement feeding easier to teach and disseminate. The main changes were outlined as follows:

- *incorporate recommendations from a WHO Technical Consultation on prevention of mother-to-child transmission of HIV, held in October 2000 (ie 3 years previously)*
- *take account of the Global Strategy for Infant and Young Child Feeding jointly*

developed by WHO and UNICEF
- *list the actions recommended in the HIV and Infant Feeding Framework for Priority Action*
- *incorporate programmatic experience since 1998*
- *give more guidance for countries considering providing free or subsidized infant formula*
- *reduce the volume of information on prevention of HIV infection in infants and young children in general*
- *include new research findings.*

The emphasis on individual maternal infant feeding choice remained and was expanded:

- *Counselling of HIV-positive mothers should include information about the risks and benefits of various infant-feeding options... and guidance in selecting the most suitable option in their circumstances.*
- *On the basis of local assessments and formative research, some of the options in this document may be excluded as not locally suitable. Local options, however, should never be narrowed to one blanket recommendation for all HIV-positive women, since specific circumstances will vary even within seemingly homogeneous settings, and women have the right to make an individual choice.*
- *Whatever a mother chooses, she should be supported in her decision. The exact support that might be provided will depend on the policy, capacity and socioeconomic conditions of the country, but would always include information, counselling and monitoring of the growth and health of her child.*
- *Postnatal support for women, regardless of their infant-feeding choice, is often inadequate. In most countries, policy must cover a range of socioeconomic conditions; its aim must be to promote, protect and support breastfeeding for most mothers and infants; at the same time it must provide for women who are HIV-positive to receive suitable information on alternative feeding options, enabling them to decide what, in the circumstances, is best for them and their babies, and to receive support to carry out their choice.*
- *The information must be free from commercial pressures and counsellor bias, and the support should include helping a woman to reduce the social risks of acting on her choice.*

In 2003, then, it can be seen that problems with ethical promotion of maternal choice remained. Wording on the assumption of safety of formula-feeding and the exaggerated risk of transmission of the virus through 'breastfeeding' remained in this guidance. Information stressing the importance of *exclusive* breastfeeding to reduce the specific risk of HIV transmission to HIV-exposed babies had not yet been taken on board by the international policymakers, on the rationale that more research was needed. The guidelines merely said:

'There is evidence from one study that exclusive breastfeeding in the first 3 months of life may carry a lower risk of HIV transmission than mixed feeding.'

What information, then, were mothers being given with which to make a choice? Choice is usually only promoted when the outcome is unknown. In fact this may be the only ethical way that choice can be promoted. When the risks of a certain course of action in any other medical setting are known, they are communicated to the patient and there is an ethical obligation to provide a clear recommendation about the healthiest way forward. Counsellors in resource-poor settings experienced great difficulty in understanding themselves, and then explaining to their HIV-positive clients, that they were giving clients information about a feeding method they were not necessarily expected to follow. This confusion was never understood in the West and will be explored more fully in chapters 13 and 29.

By 2004, WHO/UNAIDS/UNICEF recommended several variations of replacement feeding or breastfeeding for infants of HIV-infected mothers[86–88] in order of preference, as follows:

- ***Commercial infant formula:*** *specially formulated milk made specifically for infants and sold in shops or provided through programmes designed to prevent HIV transmission to infants*
- ***Home-modified animal milk:*** *fresh or processed animal milk that is modified by adding water, sugar and micronutrient supplements*
- ***Exclusive breastfeeding:*** *giving only breast milk and prescribed medicine but no water, other liquids, or food to the infants for the first months of life*
- ***Wet-nursing:*** *having another woman breastfeed an infant; in this case, ensuring that the woman is HIV negative*
- ***Expressing and heat-treating breast milk:*** *removing the milk from the breasts manually or with a pump, then heating it to kill HIV*
- ***Breast-milk banks:*** *centres where donor milk is pasteurized and made available for infants*

To help counsellors, an expanded definition of the pre-conditions for formula-feeding (known as the AFASS conditions) was also included.

Counselling tools

In 2005, in recognition that counselling and support for HIV-positive women was the most demanding aspect of PMTCT programs,[89] a set of Counselling Tools was developed and issued separately, to help clarify what steps needed to be taken during a counselling session.[90] Still, in spite of little evidence to underpin the safety of formula-feeding, the Counselling Tools emphasised how to counsel HIV-positive mothers about feeding breastmilk substitutes, if not from birth, then at the latest from six months. More guidance was given on what was termed 'early cessation of breastfeeding'. Infant feeding counselling for HIV-positive women had three objectives:

- *To* ***provide women with information*** *about the risks and benefits of various infant feeding options;*
- *To* ***guide them to choose*** *the one that is most likely to be suitable for their situation;*

AFASS CONDITIONS FOR REPLACEMENT FEEDING

Acceptable: The mother perceives no barrier to replacement feeding. Barriers may include cultural or social reasons or be caused by fear of stigma or discrimination. According to this concept, the mother is under no social or culture pressure not to use replacement feeding, and she is supported by family and community in opting for replacement feeding, or she will be able to cope with pressure from family and friends to breastfeed, and she can deal with any stigma attached to being seen with replacement food.

Feasible: The mother (or family) has adequate time, knowledge, skills and other resources to prepare the replacement food and feed the infant up to 12 times in 24 hours. According to this concept, the mother can understand and follow the instructions for preparing replacement feeds and with support from the family can prepare enough replacement fees correctly every day and at night, despite disruptions to preparation of family food or other work.

Affordable: The mother and family with community or health system support if necessary, can pay for the cost of purchasing/producing, preparing and using replacement feeding, including all ingredients, fuel, clean water, soap and equipment, without compromising the health and nutrition of the family. This concept also includes access to medical care as necessary for diarrhoea, pneumonia and other illnesses and the cost of such care.

Sustainable: The mother or other care-giver has available a continuous and uninterrupted supply and dependable system of distribution for all ingredients and products needed for safe replacement feeding for as long as the infant needs it, up to one year or age or longer. According to this concept, there is little risk that the replacement food will ever be unavailable or inaccessible. It also means that another person, who can prepare and give replacement feeds, will always be available to feed the child in the mother's absence.

Safe: Replacement foods are correctly and hygienically prepared and stored and fed in nutritionally adequate quantities with clean hands and clean utensils, preferably by cup. This concept means that the mother or caregiver:

- Has access to a reliable supply of safe water (from a piped or protected well source).
- Can prepare replacement feeds that are nutritionally sound and free of pathogens.
- Is able to wash hands and utensils thoroughly with soap and to regularly boil utensils to sterilise them.
- Can boil water for at least 10 minutes to prepare each of the baby's feeds, and
- Can store unprepared feeds in clean, covered containers and protect them from rodents, insects and other animals.

- *To **support them** in implementing the method that they have chosen by **helping them carry it out safely and effectively**.*

There was also a flow chart which counsellors could use as they explored various feeding options with HIV-positive mothers:

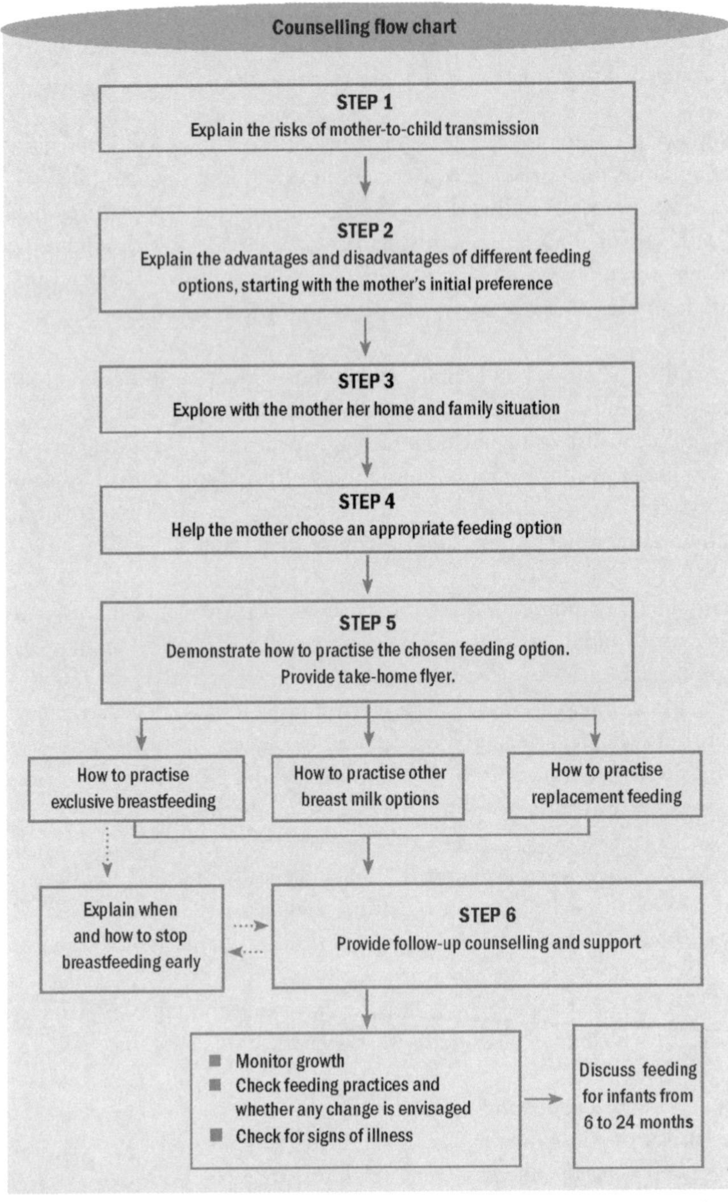

Source: WHO 2005 HIV and Infant Feeding Counselling Tools, ISBN 92 4 159301 6

Summary

Decisions by the UN agencies responsible for child health during 1996 and 1997 had ushered in a dark period during which breastfeeding in the context of HIV became hugely problematic, with consequences for breastfeeding protection and promotion. Furthermore, it must have seemed like an undreamed of opportunity for the infant formula industry, opening up, as it did, the first legitimate chink in the international public health recommendations. A company representative who asked to see me in Harare to discuss the provisions of the very stringent, newly gazetted Zimbabwean version of the 1998 Code of Marketing of Breastmilk Substitutes[91] told me with confidence, and even some pride, that he was advising doctors that the risk of transmission of HIV through breastfeeding was 60%. That breastfeeding could transmit HIV constituted the one incontrovertible rationale justifying the legitimate promotion of breastmilk substitutes to millions of women as a safer infant feeding alternative – especially through the healthcare system.

It's important to remember that when the 1996-97 guidance was developed, research on HIV and breastfeeding was beset by several difficulties, as set out in Chapter 4, including lack of accurate definitions of 'breastfed', the impossibility of determining the route of transmission to the infected baby, and specifically the risk percentage that could be attributed to breastfeeding. There were also problems in interpretation of research due to variations in the length of, or complete lack of, follow-up. Differences in methods used to account for missing data, deaths, and children of different ages and of indeterminate infection status plagued documentation of risk. Most importantly, there had been no research to compare the risk of death due to HIV transmission during breastfeeding versus the risk of death from no breastfeeding at all. Thus, while announcements between 1996 and 1998 appeared to support the HIV-positive mother's right to choose her own infant-feeding method under the guise of supporting her human rights, it is clear that an HIV-positive mother could not make an informed choice due to little or no data on which to base such a vital decision. There simply was no existing evidence to show that withholding breastfeeding would enhance overall child survival. The major flaw was the assumption that HIV transmission through breastfeeding would make formula-feeding any safer in resource-poor settings than it ever had been.

In a major article entitled 'From the Bottle to the Grave',[92] Barry Meier and Miriam Labbok wrote:

> *'With millions dying each year from a lack of optimal feeding in the developing world, breastfeeding – the optimal form of infant and young child feeding – holds the potential to save more lives than any other public health intervention. Yet despite this unrivaled lifesaving potential, achievable at a comparatively minimal cost, international law has been unable to develop the global policies necessary to ensure the protection, promotion, and support of breastfeeding. As international law has faltered, human rights advocacy has been conspicuously absent in debates on this pressing public health issue.'*

This observation highlights how differently human rights advocacy has been interpreted in the global north compared to the global south. Maternal rights to choose an individual preferred infant feeding method were invoked to facilitate formula-feeding as a key element of HIV and infant feeding policy, rather than promotion of breastfeeding for all as a proven public health measure to combat infant mortality. That the concept of replacing mother's milk with formula was sold to an unsuspecting continent on a platform of human rights holds a certain irony. It's hard to believe that decades of research on the life-saving properties of breastmilk could be dismissed so easily by so few studies of such questionable rigour. Was it public pressure which persuaded policymakers to accept results exaggerating the risks of of HIV transmission through breastfeeding, while minimising the risks of formula-feeding? Or was it the few studies on antiretroviral drugs cutting MTCT by between one-third and one-half in non-breastfeeding mothers that proved persuasive enough to ask mothers to sacrifice breastfeeding? Did it seem wasteful to 'save' babies from HIV transmission during pregnancy and birth, only to expose them to the risk again through breastfeeding? Was it necessary to stop breastfeeding at any cost? How could these plans not have been seen as a formula for disaster?

CHAPTER 13

Implementing the policy through the HIV and Infant Feeding Counselling Course

'Reversing the decline of breastfeeding in the developing world could save the lives of an estimated 1.5 million infants every year. Bottle-fed babies … are several times more likely to die in infancy. Breast milk is the complete nourishment, safe, hygienic, inexpensive and helps fight common infections …In the industrialized world, after a steep decline, there is today a pronounced trend back towards breastfeeding. A similar decline in the developing world, where bottle feeding entails much greater risks, would lead to millions of infant deaths.'

UNICEF, *The State of the World's Children 1991*,
reporting on the Year 2000 goal of the World Summit for Children.

After the Technical Consultation in Geneva in 1998, where it was agreed that as part of the global facilitation of formula-feeding for the babies of HIV-positive mothers health workers would be trained using the 16-hour HIV and Infant Feeding Counselling Course (HIVC), WHO and UNICEF once again chose Harare as the location for field-testing of the new course. In March 1999 Dr Felicity Savage of WHO, Lida Llotska and Helen Armstrong of UNICEF, and Genevieve Becker, an Irish IBCLC who had authored the course, arrived to begin the training of local healthcare personnel.

Course participants were high-level nursing staff and policymakers from Zimbabwe, and senior nursing staff who had travelled down from Zambia. As an IBCLC, with a special interest in HIV and breastfeeding, and because I was a member of the Breastfeeding Committee convened by the National Breastfeeding Coordinator at the Ministry of Health and Child Welfare, I was also invited to participate.

A Training of Trainers course was held first, to train the most senior staff, and then both the overseas trainers and the newly trained local personnel shared the teaching of the HIVC Course to the remaining 28 participants. This tiered teaching followed protocols I had seen used before by WHO, UNICEF and other NGOs, such as during the first influential Breastfeeding Counselling course for senior Zimbabwean healthcare personnel held in 1989, during a training course I had attended on Code Monitoring, and again during the early stages of the Baby Friendly Hospital Initiative training in 1992.

It was specifically recommended that participants who undertook the HIVC training should have already undergone lactation management training provided in the WHO 1993 40-hour Breastfeeding Counselling Course.[71] However, this requirement was not enforced. While I knew that many of the Zimbawean participants had undergone training in breastfeeding, others had not, and this shortcoming among both Zimbabwean and Zambian participants became obvious during later group discussions.

That we were not all on the same page, as it were, was not surprising. Due to the risk of HIV breastfeeding was receiving very bad press. Ministries of health, desperate to prevent the spread of the disease to the next generation, were reluctant to spend time and resources educating their healthcare personnel about how to facilitate a known route of transmission – they preferred to just go straight to the HIV and infant feeding training designed to avoid breastfeeding altogether. Unfortunately, WHO and UNICEF, who no doubt knew that this was the case, but were also eager to reduce postnatal transmission of HIV through breastfeeding, did not insist, and simply looked the other way. Ironically, this was obvious right from the very beginning of the first field-testing, starting in Harare.

Illustrations from the covers of the 1993 *Breastfeeding Counselling Course* and the 2000 *HIV and Infant Feeding Counselling Course* reveal the differences in focus. The former depicts a nurse providing hands-on help to a mother to breastfeed her baby. The latter shows a nurse giving instruction to a mother before the birth of her child, with the mother appearing to ask whether the information being imparted is really for her.

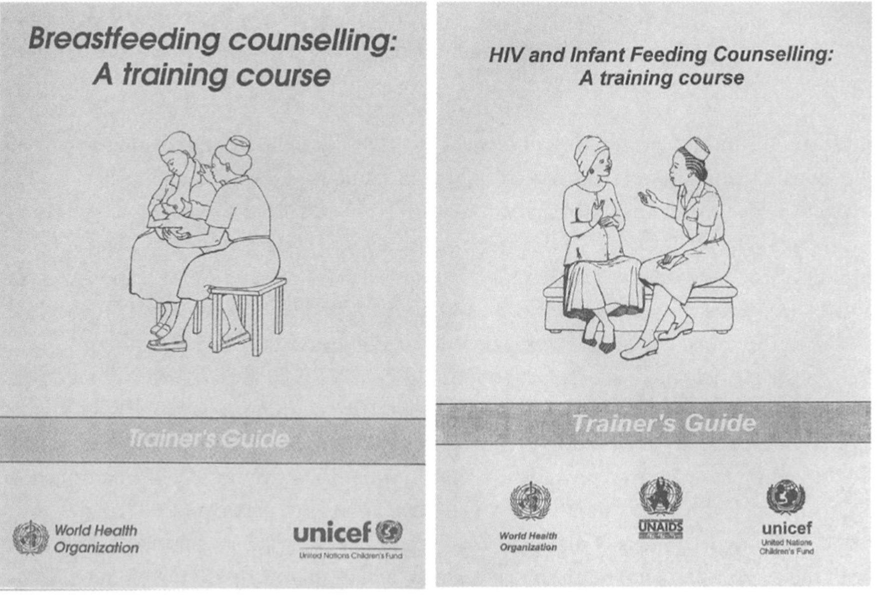

Breastfeeding Counselling Course, Trainers' Guide, World Health Organisation 1993
HIV and Infant Feeding Counselling Course, Trainers' Guide, World Health Organisation 2000

The training was held at the large and sprawling Harari Hospital[1] south of Harare city. Harari was a teaching hospital with a large maternity section serving the city centre and taking referrals from 13 small clinics in the suburbs, at one time delivering 90 babies per day. Harari had labour, postnatal and caesarean surgical wards, and impressive neonatal, preterm and kangaroo care units. Practical sessions of the Baby Friendly Hospital Training course were held at Harari. My paediatrician mentor also sometimes asked me to see mothers who were experiencing unusual breastfeeding difficulties at this hospital, so I was familiar with the different wards and units, and with its very breastfeeding-friendly policies. In accordance with government policy all babies were breastfed, and there was no formula-feeding at all for full-term healthy babies. Bottles and teats were never used. Babies didn't just room-in with their mothers, they bedded-in. In the Prem Unit, premature or sick babies might be fed very tiny quantities of formula for the first day or two of life until the mother was able to express enough milk for their needs, but then they were fed exclusively on their own mother's milk. The tiny ones (who might be housed two to an incubator) would be fed expressed breastmilk by naso-gastric tube, then by cup, and finally they would graduate to breastfeeding direct. Milk intake was individually tailored to the weight, gestational age, health and competence of each baby. Human milk fortifier for prem babies was unknown, but babies who were well might be fed up to 300ml/kg/day of their mother's milk to fatten them up so they could go home. Mothers sat together on wooden benches to express their milk into metal bowls, encouraging and supporting each other. Breast pumps were also unknown and all mothers were taught to hand express. They quickly became very skilled: I have seen a mother express 120ml in 10 minutes, raising froth in the milk from the strength of the jets of milk she could direct into the bowl. The mothers were very patient while teaching their babies how to breastfeed; breastfeeding was a life-skill and it was unthinkable that they wouldn't eventually be able to breastfeed well. Mothers of pre-term infants stayed in a hostel on the hospital premises so they could be close to their babies in the prem unit. The babies were discharged home when they reached 1,800g or 34 weeks corrected gestational age, and could breastfeed well.

This, then, was the environment into which WHO-UNICEF-UNAIDS introduced and field-tested their HIV and Infant Feeding Counselling training. The theoretical sessions were held in a classroom within the hospital and the practical session was held in a 'banda' in the hospital grounds; a building with a roof, a concrete floor and open sides, without running water or electricity. The banda was chosen as being representative of conditions experienced by most urban poor or rural African mothers in their own little one-roomed corrugated iron houses or mud huts.

The aim of the Course was to teach participants how to provide counselling on HIV and infant feeding, which included assisting individual mothers to make their own infant feeding choices, and then teaching them how to prepare different kinds of replacement feeds correctly. Participants learned that there was a 15% to 20% risk of early postpartum transmission of HIV due to breastfeeding. Major emphasis was placed on how healthcare workers could teach replacement feeding to HIV-infected mothers to avoid that risk. There was almost no course content on how to support breastfeeding, and nothing on exclusive breastfeeding.[2] Introducing the course to the Zambian and

Zimbabwean participants, WHO's Dr Savage commented that 'We didn't start this epidemic, we're just responding to it.' Asked about whether it would be safe to not breastfeed she responded, 'We can't wait for the research to be in, we have to act now!'

The HIVC Course was brilliantly developed, presented and written. The extremely user-friendly materials made it possible for trainers with limited experience and in fact no medical training whatsoever to teach HIV and infant feeding counselling to health workers in maternity facilities, hospitals, and clinics. The trainer's guide was 230 pages long. Training materials included overheads (both in the form of slides and in ring-binders), worksheets, checklists, and demonstration instructions. Feeding option cards showed illustrations, diagrams, and text. There were diagrams for teaching aids. Easy-to-follow modules outlined objectives, content, and summaries using participatory learning, group work, discussion, role play, reading, and exercises. While most of the course was theoretical, a practical sesssion lasting two hours would focus on participant preparation of milk feeds, so that counsellors would have practical experience to share with mothers. Text and line-drawings made it clear the course had been developed for third-world countries, especially those in sub-Saharan Africa.

Dr Genevieve Becker told me that she had been asked by Dr Felicity Savage of WHO to write the course. Dr Savage had at one time been the International Delegate for the International Lactation Consultant Association (ILCA) and Genevieve had succeeded her in that role. Felicity and Genevieve had shared a room at an ILCA conference, and it was there that she had been asked to help. Genevieve was a dietitian/nutritionist, an educator and IBCLC who had worked in maternal, infant and young child feeding, particularly in breastfeeding, having served as a volunteer counsellor with a mother-to-mother support group for several years. Genevieve continues to be involved in training of health workers nationally and internationally, for agencies such as WHO and UNICEF.[3] Clearly, she was a very experienced IBCLC and educator, but I was shocked to learn that this was the first time she had set foot in Africa. What did she know about breastfeeding in African societies? Did she have any experience or insight into the value that African women and indeed African communities placed on breastfeeding? On the other hand Felicity had lived and worked as a paediatrician in developing countries for a total of 18 years; in Zambia (1966–72), Indonesia (1972–78) and Kenya (1979–84), so she knew about the likely consequences of formula-feeding for African babies.

Course content

Seventeen sections provided clear and detailed ways to teach counselling for infant feeding decisions, breastmilk options, different replacement feeding methods up to and beyond the first six months (see box), preparation of milk feeds, how to engage community support, and composition of UNICEF micronutrient supplements. Participants were enabled to build a thorough knowledge of which milks could be used as breastmilk substitutes, and how much to feed. There was information on availability, how to calculate costs, and how to encourage practical community support for replacement feeding to reduce stigma.

A total of 180 minutes of practical work familiarised participants with:

1. how to make their own utensils, including containers from cut-off plastic bottles, home-made scales from rubbers and rulers.
2. boiling water and milk for feeds on wood, charcoal, or paraffin stoves,
3. measuring quantities (e.g. 8g sugar, 40ml milk and how to prepare milk feeds).

UNAIDS REPLACEMENT FEEDING OPTIONS

BIRTH TO SIX MONTHS

1. Commercial infant formula
2. Home-prepared formula

· fresh/pasteurised animal milk	cow/goat/	100 ml milk
· dried milk powder	camel	50 ml boiled water
		10g sugar
· evaporated milk		micronutrients*
	sheep/	50 ml milk
	buffalo	50 ml boiled water
		5 g sugar
		micronutrients*

3. Unmodified cow's milk (offer extra boiled water after feeds) and micronutrients*
4. Modified breastfeeding
   - Early cessation of breastfeeding (optimum duration unknown, as soon mother is able to prepare and give replacement feeds)
   - Heat-treated expressed breastmilk
     - pasteurized
     - boiled
   - Banked human milk
   - Wet-nursing

*micronutrients, type and quantity not specified

SIX MONTHS TO TWO YEARS

1. Replacement feeds (if available) and home-prepared family foods 3 x daily
2. If replacement feeds unavailable give home-prepared family foods 5 x daily.

Source: WHO/FRH/NUT/CHD/98.2, UNAIDS/98.4, UNICEF/PD/NUT(J)98-2 HIV and Infant Feeding: A Guide for health care managers and supervisors

Measuring quantities for different milks

Before the practical session, participants received classroom instruction on how to prepare four different kinds of replacement feed using evaporated milk, powdered milk, liquid animal milks or infant formula. To make home-prepared formula it was necessary to add extra water and sugar to either liquid milk, evaporated milk or milk powder. Mothers were unlikely to own the infant-feeding equipment so easily available in western societies, and would have to make do with other materials, so these sessions were particularly difficult. Infant-feeding bottles for actually feeding babies were not recommended because it was hard to keep them clean, so measuring quantities of water and other ingredients would be problematic. It was suggested that mothers could use the increments shown on the side of a feeding bottle to measure the quantities of milk and water they would need, by cutting off the top of the bottle and keeping the bottom.

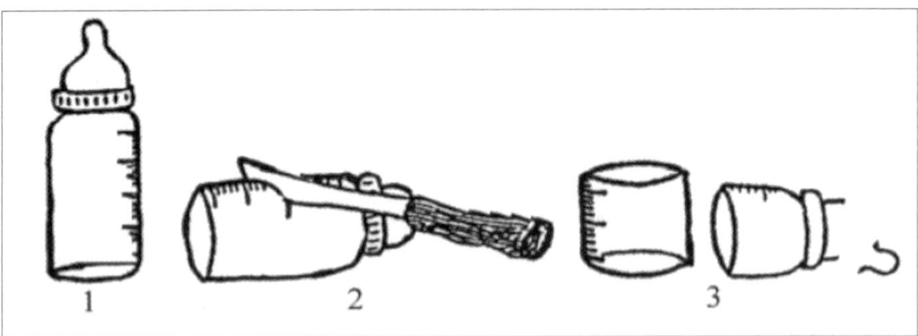

Measuring liquids in a cut-off baby bottle[4]

Mothers whose cultural norm was breastfeeding would not own bottles. So as an alternative, the Zimbabwe participants were recommended to use cut-off plastic drinks bottles. Since these did not have graded measurements, the counsellor was to 'help the mother to mark the level that the [required amount] of water reaches' and to make another mark for the level that an extra amount of milk reaches if home-prepared formula was being prepared.

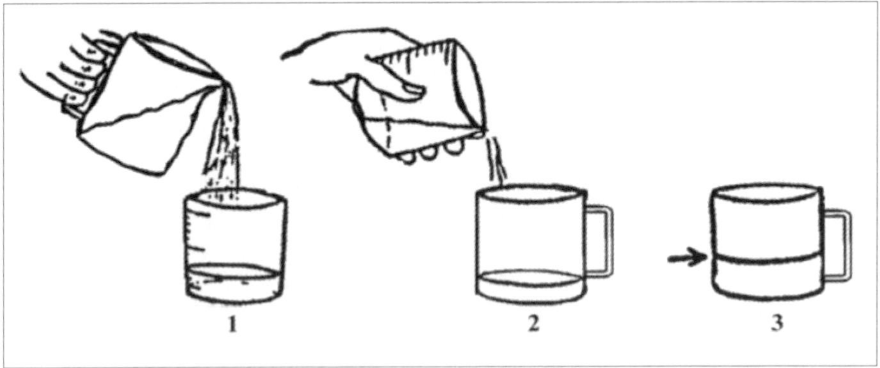

Measuring liquids in a cut-off drink bottle[4]

It was advised to weigh quantities on scales at a pharmacy or a post office. If a mother could not access scales, then there was another alternative – a home-made scale using a ruler and a rubber and plastic lids from aerosol sprays:[5]

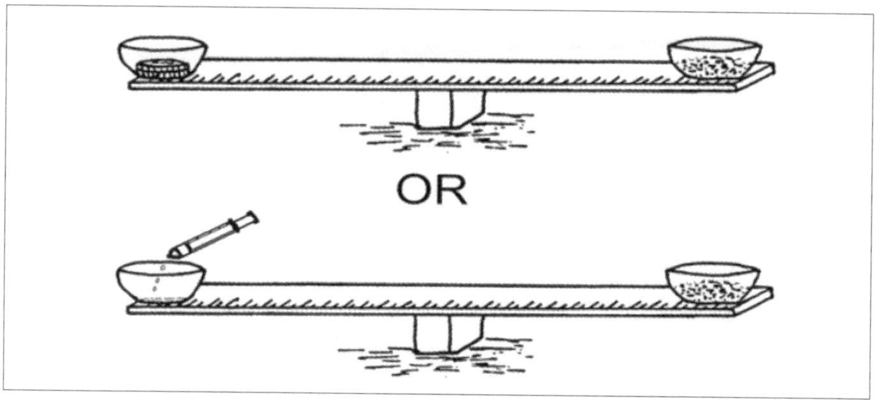

Step 1: Stand an eraser on its side, and make the ruler balance on it. The eraser should be in the middle of the ruler.
Step 2: Take two equal sized light cups (or plastic lids) and put them one each end of the ruler. They should be exactly at the ends of the ruler. Make sure that the ruler balances with them on.
Step 3: Put the 8g weight into one of the cups (your 2 x 4g coins, or the 8 ml of water – not the syringe itself) That end of the ruler will go down.
Step 4: Put the sugar into the empty cup on the other end of the ruler.
Step 5: Show all the participants the sugar in the cup, and point out that this is what 8g of sugar looks like.

Making a simple balance, p151 Trainer's guide[6]

The course explains how to teach measuring sugar[7]

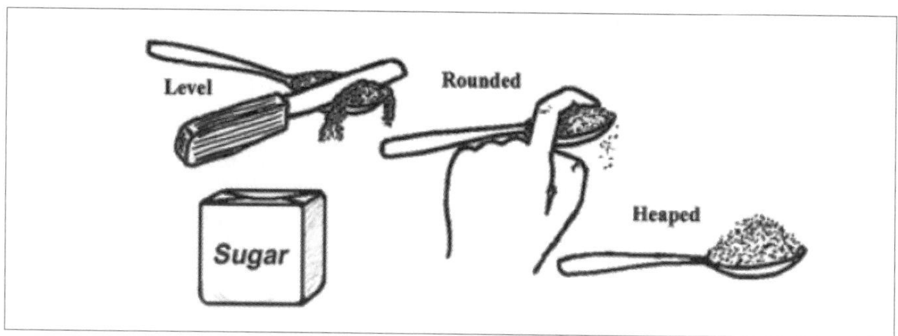

Ask: Is a mother going to balance her sugar this way each time she makes up a feed?

No. You can show her how much sugar to put into her spoon to make up the 8g (or the amount she needs for one feed.)

Demonstrate and explain how you will show mothers how to measure 8g sugar with a spoon. Your bag or bowl of sugar should be on the demonstration table...

Ask one participant from each group in turn to tip the 8g of sugar on the balance into her spoon to see how full it makes it. Then she can use her spoon and practise measuring

8g and checking the weight by using the balance. She may need to use a level, rounded, heaped spoonful or two spoonfuls depending on the size of her spoon.

Ask the participant to keep the spoon that she used, and to remember how she measured 8g with it. Her group will use the spoon to measure sugar later [i.e. at the practical session].

Measuring a spoon of sugar, p156 Trainer's guide[14]

Exclusive breastfeeding shown to have no increased risk vs replacement feeding

By a small twist of fate, while I was attending the March 1999 field-test of the HIV and Infant Feeding Counselling Course, and a full four months before its publication in the August 1999 *Lancet*, I received a pre-publication copy of Anna Coutsoudis' paper showing that exclusive breastfeeding carried no higher risk of postpartum transmission of HIV than exclusive formula-feeding. The double-spaced draft had been anonymously hand-delivered to my home postbox in Harare. It arrived inside a large brown envelope addressed to me, bearing a handwritten caution that the results were not to be shared before publication. I never did find out who sent it. But it was heartbreaking and not a little frustrating to have knowledge of the study results even as the HIV and Infant Feeding Course facilitators were teaching future counsellors that breastfeeding was risky and that formula-feeding was safe. There was no benefit to replacement feeding. Babies would die in vain.

My dismay at what was being taught in the HIV Counselling Course, which would go on to be imparted to HIV-positive mothers in resource-poor countries from the Cape to Cairo, was expressed in a message to an overseas friend, when I wrote:

'The paraphernalia for formula feeding can be any container, it can be bottle-caps for measuring quantities, or sawn-off plastic drink bottles, or almost anything. The sugar is the thing that grabs me – 8g to mix with 120ml home-made formula (that's two parts cow's milk and one part water, boiled up together). You can measure this on scales at the post office, or at a pharmacist's. Or you can make a home-made scale out of a rubber and a ruler, with two plastic bottle-tops at each end. You measure 8ml of water in a syringe and squirt it into one of the cups, and then you put enough sugar in the other cup to balance the scale. Then you tip that into a spoon, see if it's flat, rounded (with your curved finger!) or heaped, and voila – there you have it, 8g of sugar to mix in every time you feed the baby! Of course, once a day you have to mix in the 2g sachet of micronutrients available from UNICEF, or you can sprinkle a bit in to several feeds – you're the mom, you get to choose!'

Eventually, one of the overseas trainers called me aside to say that my questions and comments were upsetting the trainers. Responding to a question posed in class about which method of replacement feeding might be 'best' I had answered that none of them were, and that only breastfeeding could be considered a healthy way of feeding a baby. I went to my friend the city health nutritionist to say I was sorry if I was upsetting them. She said I certainly wasn't. When I gave this feedback to the visiting trainer, she said that if I wasn't upsetting the trainers, then I was upsetting the other participants. Clearly the UN teachers did not welcome criticism.

The practical session and materials needed

Course participants were divided into groups for the practical session, so that each group would have the opportunity to see how a different type of replacement feed should be prepared. We were given an advance shopping list of items to bring from home. The idea was to mimic, as far as possible, conditions that would be experienced by African women feeding their babies, i.e. among the majority of the population in Zimbabwe, the urban and rural poor, over 50% of whom were unemployed, and reeling from an economic crisis that had caused the cost of food to double in the past year.

I needed to either buy or bring from home all the items that would enable me to safely prepare one commercially manufactured or home-prepared formula feed. I had to bring to the workshop one tin of formula which, had I been a rural woman, would have cost over 10% of my husband's monthly salary. And we were about to learn that it takes 80 x 500g tins of powdered infant formula to feed one baby for one year.[8] I had never prepared formula in my life, so this would be a real learning experience. I also needed matches, wood for my fire, and an assortment of spoons, measuring cups and containers, and soap to wash my hands and feeding utensils.

From my time working with the Baby Friendly Hospital Assessments and the stories that my nursing friends had told me, I already knew that many Zimbabwean mothers do not even own a teaspoon. In the banda, there was no running water, no electricity and no refrigerator. Since rural women usually have to carry water on their head from a river or communal borehole to their homes, participants were asked to bring from home a 5-litre container of water. Effective hand-washing is impossible without running water or another person to help. Another of the group participants poured out water for me so that I could wash my hands. How would a woman manage this alone? We washed our feeding cups, mixing spoons and water containers in a bowl of the water taken from our bottle. There were no instructions for rinsing in clean water. If this had been water collected from the river, would it be clean, or would we need to boil it first? We boiled the water for the various replacement feeds on a wood fire. It took about 30 minutes for the water heated in this manner to reach a rolling boil.

It was not so easy to apply lessons learned in a classroom to conditions that would be experienced in a little rural dwelling. It was very difficult in these conditions, kneeling on the floor and spreading your feeding equipment out on newspaper, to mix powder, water and sugar together and then to wash and dry all the utensils and keep everything clean. Suddenly we realised that in the time that it had taken us to set up, prepare and cool our 'replacement feed' and then wash up our equipment, two hours had passed. In real life, the baby would need feeding again very soon. Without storage facilities, each feed had to be prepared just before it was needed. How would it be possible for an ordinary African mother to freshly prepare eight replacement feeds for her baby in each 24 hours in these conditions? How would she manage in the middle of the night? How would she be able to comfort her baby without breastfeeding? At this point we really began to question the practicalities, as well as the health implications of these plans.

Towards the end of the course, our National Breastfeeding Co-ordinator whispered fiercely to me, 'We're *not* changing our breastfeeding policy!' This influential lady was a Wellstart graduate, and had also been a student of Professor Ted Greiner, the eminent international breastfeeding advocate who had himself been a student of Michael Latham, who had in turn been a student of Derrick Jelliffe. The baton had been passed from hand to hand down the generations, and the enthusiasm and dedication of all of these people in keeping breastfeeding on the international map had been inestimable. She was aware of the issues.

Implications of replacement feeding

Several unanswered questions arose as a consequence of the new policy, particularly once the HIV Course exposed the practical problems inherent in formula-feeding in conditions of poverty. In Zimbabwe the Ministry of Health had recorded that close to 100% of women successfully breastfeed their babies up to one year of age. Most continued well beyond a year. What were the implications of disturbing the customs and traditions of a whole country, or of a whole continent like Africa, where breastfeeding was the cultural norm? Would HIV-infected women, the urban and rural poor, pitifully short of economic resources, be able to safely provide replacement feeding for their babies? Since it seemed that representatives of the infant formula industry had been included in deliberations leading to the new HIV and infant feeding policy, how would offers by industry to make their products available affect implementation and enforcement of the provisions of our new Zimbabwean Code legislation, passed through parliament in 1998?[9] Why were options to feed home-prepared formula using animal milks included when such mixtures were considered to be nutritionally inadequate and harmful for long-term feeding of infants in industrialised countries?[10,11] (This is explored more fully in Chapter 19). Would cash-strapped third-world governments see the use of animal milks as an attractive feeding option because difficulties with cost, supply and distribution could be avoided if they were passed on to individual families and communities? How many families would realistically have access to camel or buffalo milk?

Did the HIV Counselling Course also manage to neatly bypass any reservations there might have been about suspension of strict observance of provisions of the International Code of Marketing of Breastmilk Substitutes?[12] The Code prohibited promotion of infant formula through healthcare facilities, did not allow idealisation of artificial feeding and set out that information on formula needed to explain the benefits of breastfeeding and the costs and hazards associated with artificial feeding. The HIV Course skated pretty close to abandoning these criteria, through characterisation of breastfeeding as a hazard, and formula as a safer alternative which would be needed on medical grounds. Policy statements also promoted acceptance of formula-feeding by communities and urged reduction of stigmatisation of mothers who formula-fed.

At the time of the field-testing of the HIV and Infant Feeding Counselling Course in March 1999, breastfeeding was universally practised in sub-Saharan Africa. In fact, Africa was probably the last continent where breastmilk substitutes had not made much of an impact. As well as being the cultural norm, involving many traditional beliefs and customs, breastfeeding was truly a cornerstone of child survival.

Why had international agencies elected to assist and fund formula-feeding in pilot studies in developing countries, rather than directing research towards ascertaining the feasibility and safety of the most logical alternative to breastfeeding – mothers' own expressed, stored and/or heat-treated breastmilk? Would interrupting breastfeeding lead to malnutrition, increased birth rates, reduced maternal health and higher morbidity and mortality in children? Would the reduction in the number of HIV-infected children achieved by cessation of breastfeeding in HIV-positive mothers be balanced against the increased mortality among their uninfected children?[13]

The latest Zimbabwe Sentinel Surveillance data indicated that up to 40 % of pregnant women in Harare were HIV-positive.[14] Feeding replacement milks to such a high percentage of the nation's babies would require a major outlay in funds. Would scarce resources for replacement feeding not be better spent on the provision of healthcare, nutrition, housing and sanitation for the healthy majority?[10] Or antiretroviral drugs?

Zimbabwe was in a fairly unique position regarding official endorsement of a return to breastfeeding, which received extremely strong support from national and local government personnel. Following independence in 1980, and due to its cultural importance, the Ministry of Health and Child Welfare had easily managed to revive the popularity of breastfeeding in hospitals and maternity units countrywide. My first baby, born in 1977, had been formula-fed on his first day of life in a hospital nursery; my twins, born after independence, had been exclusively breastfed and roomed in with me.

Senior health and nursing personnel had attended the important breastfeeding training course, organised by UNICEF and La Leche League in 1989. As a La Leche League Leader at that time, I had helped with some of the background work of organising this event, including offering hospitality to the overseas trainers, Elizabeth Hormann and Helen Armstrong, who came to teach the course. In fact it was Elizabeth Hormann's description of her wonderful job as an IBCLC that had inspired me to explore the possibility of this new profession as a career. Thus the most senior and influential personnel in the country had been exposed to up-to-date, evidence-based training on lactation and breastfeeding from world experts – and, coming as it did in the post-independence era when Zimbabwe was setting new policies and receiving input from many international agencies, e.g. WHO on the rational use of drugs, the ILO on up to date maternity legislation and UNICEF on vaccine programmes, the Zimbabwe policymakers took the ball of breastfeeding promotion, which was after all in line with their cultural norms, and ran with it.

Two four-member teams of key personnel from the Ministry of Health and the City Health department had attended the Wellstart Lactation Management Education Program in San Diego, California.[15] Wellstart education courses ran from 1983 to 1998, with the purpose of developing cadres of skilled and knowledgeable leaders for medical, nursing and nutrition education programmes as well as policymakers in lactation management and breastfeeding promotion. The eight Zimbabwean Wellstart graduates did indeed go on to profoundly influence the breastfeeding climate in Zimbabwe, ensuring that breastfeeding and lactation management was taught to nursing staff, trainee doctors and allied healthcare personnel at the University of Zimbabwe Medical School, issuing directives about and enforcing breastfeeding promotion and support in our maternity units and hospitals, working to give effect to Code legislation, later organising Code monitoring, initiating and implementing the Baby Friendly Hospital Initiative, educating high-school children about breastfeeding, supporting maternity legislation for working mothers, supporting and celebrating countrywide activities during World Breastfeeding Week, starting the Zimbabwe Infant Nutrition Network for local nursing staff, organising workshops for the Zimbabwe media on the importance of accurate journalism on breastfeeding as a health matter, and generally protecting, promoting and supporting breastfeeding at every level of society.

So much of the HIV Course content was devoted to teaching women how to feed replacements for breastmilk, while so little focused on breastfeeding, that there was no mistaking the message that replacement feeding was considered to be safer. Furthermore it seemed much more likely that 'good' mothers would perceive the teaching as not only informational, but also motivational.

It seemed that in the haste to prevent the babies of HIV-infected women from acquiring a fatal disease through mother's milk, the likelihood of infection via breastfeeding was being exaggerated, while the risks of alternatives to breastfeeding were being downplayed. The major concern was to ensure the health and survival of the greatest number of children, but this focus seemed to have been missed. Placing 100% of babies born into an under-privileged environment at higher risk for morbidity and mortality from replacement feeding in order to prevent approximately 15% of them acquiring HIV from breastmilk made no sense. Those of us who worked with mothers and babies on a day-to-day basis wondered how it was possible, with the current state of research, to give the individual mother who was looking for information about the best way to ensure the wellbeing and survival of her child, any true answers about whether her baby had already been infected at birth, whether the baby would or would not sero-convert at any time in the future (even if breastmilk was withheld), and whether she should or should not breastfeed. There were too many questions and too few answers.

Of particular concern was the information passed on to me by my friend at UNICEF in Harare that there was no intention by the international agencies to monitor the health outcomes of babies included in the PMTCT pilot projects. I could hardly believe it! There were plans to monitor the feasibility of replacement feeding, to see whether it was possible for women living in resource-poor settings to feed replacements for breastmilk, and to see whether the alternatives would be acceptable to them. But astonishingly, there were no plans to monitor the safety or sustainability of formula-feeding – to record health outcomes including the number of babies who would be protected from postnatal transmission of HIV due to replacement feeding, nor – crucially – to record morbidity and mortality or cause of death of babies who were not breastfed. Thus it would not be possible to know which method of infant feeding would result in the greatest number of babies surviving overall. If a formula-fed baby sickened and died, would there simply be an assumption that they were already infected and that death was due to HIV transmission *in utero* or at birth? Would the overall prevalence of MTCT of HIV be lower as a result of the PMTCT pilot interventions? Would rates of diarrhoea and malnutrition increase as a result of formula-feeding? In other words, would more babies be 'saved' by HIV-laced breastmilk than would die from formula-feeding (due to not being breastfed?) How would anyone know which feeding method would be 'best' before the original pilot sites were scaled up and rolled out to include even more mothers and babies? In encouraging HIV-positive mothers to choose the best infant feeding method for themselves and their babies, there was no information with which to make an informed choice.

Utility of the HIV Course

UNAIDS rhetoric characterised HIV transmission through breastfeeding as an emergency situation that could not wait. After field-testing in Harare in March 1999, the final version of the HIV Course was published in 2000. In the following years it has been taught extensively to health workers up and down Africa. It is still available on the WHO website. While the stated objective of counselling was to assess the mother's personal circumstances in order to help her select the best feeding option for herself and her baby,[16] the major emphasis was on how health workers could teach HIV-infected mothers to feed their babies replacements for breastmilk (formula). Little attention was paid to the vital importance of exclusive breastfeeding to reduce postnatal HIV transmission, as had been recently shown in the research coming from South Africa.[2,17,18] Without conveying to the mother the risks of *not* breastfeeding, nor the comparative survival benefits for HIV-exposed babies between breastfeeding and formula-feeding, it was not possible for her to make an informed choice.

The approach used by the UN agencies, to characterise infant formula as a replacement which could side-step HIV infection through breastfeeding, and which mothers could 'choose' to use, i.e. on a platform of human rights, is especially interesting. A wise woman I sat next to at a conference once told me that if you want to facilitate behaviour change on a population basis, you need to frame it as a human right. She cited an example. A country in South America had been selected for an infant vaccination programme, but there was considerable suspicion and resistance. Nothing anyone said could persuade the mothers to take their babies to be vaccinated – until finally the authorities hit on the idea of telling the mothers that it was their right to have their babies immunised. This changed the whole perception of the programme – suddenly mothers were clamouring for the vaccine.

When I asked Genevieve Becker, the author of the HIV Course, how African mothers living in mud huts in rural areas would be able to comply with the very difficult ways of preparing commercially manufactured or home-prepared formula that had been demonstrated, she answered that because formula-feeding seemed so difficult, perhaps they would opt to breastfeed. This naivety reflected an astonishing ignorance about how HIV-positive African mothers would view the information they would receive through HIV and infant feeding counselling. There seemed to be no recognition of how African people accepted healthcare. The overseas trainers seemed not to be aware that the concept of infant feeding 'choice' was alien in Africa; it would be inconceivable to an ordinary African mother to be offered information on infant feeding as an option that she could select if she wished, but that she was not necessarily expected to follow.

In my experience working with African women it is very clear that they do not expect to make choices about something as important as how to feed their babies. Fertility is so important that it is a prerequisite to marriage – a potential husband will not offer *lobola* (bride-price) for a woman unless she has become pregnant with his child. Becoming a mother elevates a woman's position in society. Breastfeeding is seen as both a duty and a privilege – a mother who has many children and is seen to breastfeed them signals to her friends and neighbours not only that she is a fertile woman, but also that she is a good wife; if her baby was to refuse the breast her neighbours would think that she had been unfaithful to her husband. So African women, certainly in eastern, central and southern Africa, the areas of highest HIV-prevalence, expect to breastfeed. A nurse in a white uniform presenting a novel infant feeding method – a gift of formula in a tin, being prepared in a special way – would be thought of as a teacher showing a mother how to keep her baby safe. It would seem as if the nursing sister was *recommending* replacement feeding – otherwise why would she take the time and trouble in her busy list of duties to bother? The South African researcher on women's experience with HIV and infant feeding, Tanya Doherty, also confirms that in developing countries and especially in health settings, the relationship between healthcare staff and clients is often heirarchical.[19] Health workers have authority over infant feeding choices. The mother thinks she is receiving a *recommendation* to formula-feed, in the same way that her friend or sister or cousin received a recommendation to breastfeed last year. She certainly doesn't hear the nursing sister's words as a choice that she can adopt or not. What the overseas experts failed to factor in was that the difficulties in feeding babies with breastmilk substitutes could just as easily have been seen as the lengths to which a conscientious mother would have to go to protect her baby from a terrible outcome – and the more difficult the task, and perhaps the more elaborate the ritual surrounding it, the greater the protection, or even the magic, that would be attributed to it.

But as an early form of virtue-signalling, the UN agencies had framed replacement feeding as the right of a mother to choose – reflecting societal norms in the global north, where standards are set for what is and what isn't a human right. But it was never seen like that when this solution was exported in 1999 to the African societies hit so hard by HIV – it was, in fact, a formula for disaster.

As a participant at the field-testing of the HIV and Infant Feeding Counselling Course in Harare in 1999, I realised that what was being taught sounded the death-knell for breastfeeding promotion as we had known it. PMTCT pilot projects providing counselling suggesting that infant formula was safe and that breastfeeding was not would be rolled out all over the developing world. The countries that most needed breastfeeding to combat high infant and young child mortality were often the very ones with high numbers of HIV-positive mothers. The HIV Course taught health workers how to teach mothers to formula-feed. By channelling this information through healthcare providers breastmilk substitutes received official endorsement from respected health authorities. UNICEF and then governments provided free starter supplies. They satisfied the two conditions for formula-feeding to be possible; that it should be acceptable and accessible. This has created a terrible legacy. We are still experiencing the fall-out, or the 'spillover', today. A friend who has just defended her thesis on infant feeding trends in South Africa describes how 25% of today's mothers in her country never put their babies to the breast at all.[20] They now cite mental health difficulties or single motherhood as reasons why they cannot breastfeed. It is uncertain whether the casual normality of breastfeeding that Africa enjoyed before HIV and infant feeding counselling was introduced will ever be recovered. This is a tragedy.

'Those who make claims about infant formula that intentionally undermine women's confidence in breastfeeding are not to be regarded as clever entrepreneurs just doing their job but as human rights violators of the worst kind.'

Stephen Lewis, 1999, former UNICEF Deputy-Executive Director

CHAPTER 14

Outcomes from the first PMTCT pilot sites

'Breastfeeding is the most precious gift a mother can give her infant. If there is illness or infection it may be a life-saving gift. If there is poverty it may be the only gift.'

Ruth A. Lawrence, M.D., FABM

The formal global initiative to reduce postnatal transmission of HIV from one generation to the next began to take shape with the 1996 and 1997 change in policy. UNAIDS announced that when formula feeding was safely provided and fed to HIV-exposed babies, then they would be at less risk of HIV-infection than if they were breastfed. Planning for the Prevention of Mother to Child Transmission (PMTCT) pilot projects began in 1998.

As set out in Chapter 12, in 1998, shortly after the release of the findings of the Thai Zidovudine PMTCT Study, the UNAIDS Secretariat, UNFPA, UNICEF, and WHO had established the Inter Agency Task Team (IATT) on Prevention of MTCT. The IATT provided leadership and support for the implementation of the first pilot projects in 11 countries.[1]

The initial standard PMTCT programme package for sub-Saharan settings was to be exclusively preventive.[2] Pregnant women would be offered HIV-testing and counselling, and those who tested positive would receive antiretroviral prophylaxis and free breastmilk substitutes. Infant feeding options included exclusive replacement feeding with infant formula or modified cow's milk.

Additional guidance based on what became known as the AFASS criteria was introduced in 2001.[3,4] A mother needed counselling to determine whether formula feeding would be Acceptable, Feasible, Affordable, Sustainable, and Safe (AFASS) in her individual circumstances. If the AFASS criteria couldn't be fulfilled, then infants should be exclusively breastfed 'for the first months of life' and mothers should discontinue breastfeeding as soon as possible. The time at which exclusive or any breastfeeding should cease was not specified. Worryingly, of the AFASS criteria *sustainability* and *safety* are the last conditions listed, but no matter how acceptable, feasible, and affordable a particular method of artificial feeding may be for the mother, unless it is safe for the baby, and in the context of HIV whether it is *safer* than breastfeeding, and whether, once breastfeeding has been abandoned, continued and sufficient supplies of breastmilk substitutes can be sustained, then ethical questions could be raised about offering it to a mother as an intervention intended to maximise the wellbeing of her baby.

Health workers would receive training by means of the HIV and Infant Feeding Counselling Course, developed in 1998, field-tested in 1999 and finalised in 2000. Both the motivation and the means were in place to reduce the rate of HIV transmission in areas where 90% of paediatric infection occurred, while coincidentally also reducing breastfeeding on the last continent where it was almost universally practised, and which depended on it for child survival.

How did these plans turn out? What happened as the pilot sites were set up and then rolled out? The answers are far from clear.

Initially UNICEF provided support to 11 countries to pilot the feasibility of PMTCT services. My friend Arjan de Wagt, who had worked for the UNICEF Harare office, wrote an analysis in 2000 intended to guide the UNICEF Eastern and Southern Africa regional office in ongoing PMTCT programme development.[5] Various studies had assessed the outcomes of possible feeding alternatives, but while the results had been shared at internal meetings, they had not been widely published. This was not surprising. Arjan had told me before they even began that UNICEF intended that the first pilot sites would test only the *feasibility* of artificial feeding in resource-poor settings, i.e. whether mothers from a breastfeeding culture would find formula-feeding easy and doable, but UNICEF never intended to explore the *safety* of such a plan.

This was a concerning development. Without any monitoring of the early pilot projects, we would never know how safe or sustainable formula-feeding might be in places where it had never been tried before. Why would UNICEF not want to learn about what happened to the babies served by the pilot sites? After all, isn't this what pilots are for: to make preliminary assessments with a small cohort about whether an intervention is safe and effective, before scaling it up to a wider population? Since WHO and UNICEF were the world health agencies with access to data collected over several decades about poor health outcomes for non-breastfed babies in developing countries, it was worrying that they wouldn't want to test such an initiative on an initial cohort of babies before rolling it out more widely.

Julie Patricia Smith, the Australian expert on the economic value of breastfeeding, who comments on the costs of not breastfeeding in the industrialised world, has observed that, 'Data is a constraint on what researchers can do. If governments don't bother collecting the data... then research cannot be done. High-income countries have particularly poor data...'.[6] This is perfectly true. There are large grey areas where stats on primary health indicators should be on tables and maps from first world countries: reports of infant morbidity and mortality, type of feeding and duration of breastfeeding are simply missing. Gaps are most likely where formula is the predominant mode of infant feeding. It's often easier to find breastfeeding stats for Bangladesh or Uganda than it is for Brisbane or the US.

Giving infant formula to new mothers in the industrialised global north is recognised as one of the most effective marketing tactics that can be employed. Formula donations undermine breastfeeding. For this reason manufacturers are expressly prohibited from making donations in terms of the International Code of Marketing of Breastmilk Substitutes.[7] However, it is common practice for hospitals in the UK to distribute formula to mothers who request it, and this is not seen as violating the Code so long as the hospitals pay for the supplies. Similarly, when formula was freely distributed on a vast scale by international agencies or research institutions involved in PMTCT programmes, it appeared to fall under the radar. This is curious because while there are acceptable medical reasons for the use of breastmilk substitutes, and maternal HIV infection is one of them,[8] the formula for mothers in the PMTCT programmes was not provided on prescription. It was donated to enable an HIV-positive mother to formula-feed if she had *chosen* to do so, but couldn't otherwise afford to pay for it herself.

It is inconceivable that the international health agencies would have *unknowingly* worked to undermine an existing infant feeding method – breastfeeding – which was well known to protect babies against death and disease. Could they have been unable to see the harm in promoting formula-feeding, where the requisites for its safe use – clean water, sterile equipment, doctors, antibiotics and hospitals – were known to be largely inaccessible to the poor (those most affected by HIV)? Or did they plan that there would be no records kept of illness and death due to formula-feeding, nor paediatric HIV transmission rates, no data to guide future health planning by governments, local health authorities or indeed by mothers themselves? It's chilling to contemplate that international health agencies with head offices in New York and Geneva would have been able to donate formula to new mothers and fail to record the outcomes; that the maps of mortality according to feeding method for the PMTCT programmes in under-developed countries would also remain grey. Was it intended that there would be no evidence on which to pin blame years into the future should things go wrong with such an experiment? Why else would the international health agencies embark on the PMTCT pilot projects in such a way that no record would exist of the results?

Without such data, research could not be done. But ultimately, even without it WHO, UNICEF and UNAIDS *should have known* that formula-feeding in resource-poor settings would be unsafe and unsustainable. They would have had to ignore both previous and current research in order to justify their support for replacement feeding. They certainly should have been guided by the preliminary results coming out of several early, informal assessments which are described here, some of which they themselves commissioned, but then did not publish.

Unheeded warnings

In October 2000, at the request of the East African Regional UNICEF office in Nairobi, Michael Latham, Professor of International Nutrition at Cornell University and Pauline Kisanga, Regional Coordinator of IBFAN Africa, conducted a four-country review of HIV and infant feeding in Kenya, Uganda, Botswana and Namibia.[9] Their report, completed in 2001, provides a rare glimpse into what happened in the early years of the PMTCT pilot projects.

I had met Michael at a meeting at the Nutrition Unit of the Zimbabwe Ministry of Health and Child Welfare, in Harare, to which we'd both been invited by the National Breastfeeding Coordinator, Mrs Rufaro Madzima. Michael seemed very self-effacing and quiet, and I knew he was a visitor to Zimbabwe, so I invited him to lunch. I had no idea he was so famous. He was Professor of International Nutrition at Cornell University,[10] had been a student of the late, great Derrick Jelliffe,[11] a founding member of the World Alliance for Breastfeeding Action (WABA), and he had been a major actor in the breastfeeding movement for all of his professional life.[12] I was fascinated to learn that Michael had been born, raised and worked in Tanzania and spoke, and even lectured in perfect 'safi' (clean/pure) Kiswahili, a more rudimentary version of which I had learned to speak myself as a child living in Kenya. I had first met Pauline, another Tanzanian, through my friend Clare Zunguza, the Senior Nutritionist responsible for successfully promoting breastfeeding within the Harare City Health Department. Pauline was head of IBFAN Africa, based in Swaziland. We met many times subsequently, while travelling to and attending WABA events, and most notably had shared the dubiously enlightening experience of being effectively silenced at the WHO Global Strategy meeting in Harare, when attempting to speak for breastfeeding in the face of HIV. Pauline was always a welcome ally.

Those of us in the breastfeeding community knew that Michael and Pauline's compilation of the early problems of the PMTCT pilot sites[9] was a document put together by people steeped in breastfeeding expertise, who would know what to look for. As it happened, having commissioned the work, UNICEF never formally published the report, but it provides an important account of the difficulties experienced by both healthcare workers and HIV-positive mothers in the early years of the PMTCT programme.

In 2002 the Quality Assurance Project, comprising several experts in the field, including Peggy Koniz Booher, Arjan de Wagt, Peter Iliff and Juana Willumsen, was commissioned by UNICEF, with USAID funding, to compile a report which was published in 2004.[13,14] The goal was to inform those working in HIV and infant feeding about the experiences of the PMTCT programmes from 1998. The investigators collected and reviewed over 100 documents from more than 17 countries, mainly previously unpublished material, programme evaluations and field assessments. This 'grey literature' may be especially valuable precisely because it had not been formally published. The compilation found, summarised, and analysed individual reports on a wide variety of relevant PMTCT programmes. The experiences of the individual authors ranged from small community research projects to national programmes. What happened before and during the rolling out and scaling up of the PMTCT projects underscored the similarities and differences between projects implemented in different social, economic and cultural settings. The compilation also laid out the main questions that the projects addressed (or failed to address), such as the difficulties experienced in operationalising the necessary counselling and community support for informed infant-feeding choice, and the far reaching effects of stigma that women faced.

Another useful resource has been an extensive report of UNICEF's support for free infant formula for African HIV-positive mothers, put together in 2004 by Arjan de Wagt and David Clarke of UNICEF.[15] David Clarke was the UNICEF legal guru on the International Code of Marketing of Breastmilk Substitutes. I had the pleasure of meeting him in Arusha, Tanzania, at the 2002 WABA-UNICEF Symposium on HIV and Breastfeeding. Arjan had joined the UNICEF office in Harare after having previously worked on Code monitoring in Malawi. He'd called me with a view to seeing how we could work together. He was a great ally, alerting me to industry opposition to the Code and suggesting ways that I could help advocate for breastfeeding while we worked together on preparations for the Code legislation passed through the Zimbabwean parliament in 1998. I was sad when Arjan was posted to the UNICEF Regional office in Nairobi, Kenya. He later moved on to south-east Asia, and then New York, where his experience in HIV and breastfeeding in developing countries would have been invaluable. The de Wagt and Clarke report outlines details of the procurement, distribution and use of free formula in the PMTCT programmes.

Putting the plan into effect: the initial PMTCT programmes

In 1998 the UN agencies had considered the feasibility and suitability of various interventions to reduce postnatal transmission of HIV.[16] The new PMTCT sites were modelled after a 1994 study from Thailand where vertical transmission of HIV had been reduced by 50% when mothers received a short course of zidovudine and did not breastfeed. This compared favourably with the 10–20% infection rate for all HIV-exposed babies when they were breastfed for two years.[17]

The situation was seen by many to be so urgent that action needed to be taken immediately to stop more babies becoming infected. The original plan had been to provide 30,000 HIV-infected mothers at 18 pilot sites in 11 developing countries with a package of services which included voluntary counselling and testing for HIV, and, for those testing HIV-positive, antiretroviral prophylaxis, and replacements for breastfeeding. The full range of infant feeding options included:

- Exclusive replacement feeding, i.e. complete avoidance of breastfeeding from birth.
- Exclusive breastfeeding.
- Early cessation of breastfeeding at 3–6 months to reduce the length of time that the infant is exposed to the virus in breastmilk.
- Gradual cessation (weaning) to avoid increasing transmission during this period.
- Heat-treating mother's own expressed breastmilk to inactivate HIV.
- Use of pasteurised human milk from a milk bank.

Commercially manufactured formula was considered to be the most feasible option, but more affordable home-prepared alternatives were possible, for example formula made from animal milks.[18] Any effort to reduce the cost of using commercial alternatives to breastmilk needed to conform to the International Code of Marketing of Breastmilk Substitutes and subsequent World Health Assembly resolutions. However, this still allowed considerable flexibility in price negotiations, bulk buying and distribution programmes.

Between 1999 and 2002 the governments of eight countries in Africa (Benin, Burundi, Côte d'Ivoire, Kenya, Nigeria, Rwanda, Uganda and Zambia) requested and received support from UNICEF for the provision of free formula.[15] UNICEF distributed a total of 365,351 packs of formula at about US $2.25 per kg, for a total cost of US

$412,077. Some governments decided not to distribute free formula at all, and the Botswana and South African governments decided to use their own resources to buy infant formula on the local market.

Counselling leading to testing

Ambition exceeded outcome in the PMTCT programmes. On average, 30% of women who visited the PMTCT sites for antenatal care (ANC) were not counselled. Of those women who did receive counselling, 30% were not tested for HIV.[19]

From January 2000 to June 2002, pilot sites counselled more than 385,000 women and gave HIV tests to 270,000.[20] However, while 64–83% of women accepted HIV testing, many did not; and of those who accepted testing, not all wished to know their results. Reasons included women having been persuaded by health workers to have the test when they didn't really want it, not wanting to be tested without a husband's knowledge, fear of stigma if the result turned out to be positive, not being sure of any benefit to the test, test results being delayed, and women not returning to the clinic for the results due to lack of transport.

A 2004 UNICEF survey reporting on progress in provision of PMTCT services in 58 countries found that over 81 million pregnant women gave birth every year.[1] In that year alone, over 8 million (11% of all pregnancies) received counselling through the PMTCT programmes as part of a package of maternal and child health services. Of those who received counselling, 90% were tested for HIV, a doubling of the rate from three years previously. Overall, almost 10% of pregnant women had an HIV test done during antenatal, delivery or postnatal care. However, there were regional variations, with the lowest HIV testing rates in west Africa (2%), Asia (4%) and east and southern Africa (11%) when compared with higher rates in Latin America and the Caribbean (39%) and eastern Europe (64%).

To understand the reasons for the very low uptake of HIV testing and PMTCT drugs in Botswana, in 2003 Dr Tracy Creek polled 500 women and 50 health workers. Dr Molly Smit, Medical Officer at the BOTUSA (joint Botswana/USA government) PMTCT Operational Research site in Francistown, commented on the survey results:

> *'Many didn't want to test because of fear... We knew fear was there, but we didn't know to what extent. They were afraid to know [their] status, and they were asked a lot of personal questions before testing, which they weren't used to. Usually [in Botswana], a doctor does things and explains after. So the mentality had to change. HIV testing gets into your personal life and Batswana are not used to talking about personal problems. They didn't feel comfortable with that, except they were more comfortable talking to a doctor because they were used to that. There was a lot of emphasis on pre-test counseling and that may have made it worse for them. [It] reinforced stigma because the process for counseling was so different than a normal visit to a doctor.'*[21]

Providing antiretroviral drugs

One measure of the effectiveness of PMTCT programmes was the proportion of all

HIV-positive pregnant women attending antenatal clinics who received antiretroviral therapy (ART) or antiretroviral prophylaxis (ARVs). In most countries of high HIV prevalence, ARV prophylaxis comprised a short course of zidovudine for mothers started during the last weeks of pregnancy, or a single dose of nevirapine given at the start of labour.[1] To increase use of ARVs, programmes began relying more heavily on single-dose nevirapine, which required less planning. Women would be given nevirapine to take home with them and ingest at the onset of labour.[19]

It was as difficult to provide ARVs to mothers as it was to provide them with HIV testing. In nine of 11 pilot countries, less than half the number of women who had tested positive (nearly 12,000) obtained ART.[20] In most countries, 25% or fewer ultimately received even a short course of ARVs.[19] In Botswana, only 8–10% of eligible mother/infant pairs received them.[22] By 2004, about two-thirds of HIV-positive pregnant women identified through PMTCT programmes received ARV prophylaxis.[1] However, comparison in different regions showed that fewer than 20% of mothers in west and central African countries vs 60% of mothers in Central and Eastern Europe received ARVs.

ARV prophylaxis for children

The situation for HIV-exposed babies was even more alarming. It was known that mortality among HIV-infected children was extremely high, with half of them not making it to their second birthday. In 2004, 2.2 million children were living with HIV/AIDS, 640,000 children were newly infected and 510,000 died because of AIDS.[1] Yet UNICEF reported that ARV prophylaxis to infants had been challenging, with only 25% of babies born to positive women in PMTCT programmes receiving any ARV prophylaxis, necessary to protect them from any virus acquired during labour or birth.

Reducing transmission through breastfeeding

So there were missed opportunities at each step along the way: in pre-test counselling, HIV testing, post-test counselling and results, and in the provision of ARVs to mother or baby and of course in monitoring the effectiveness of each intervention.

With testing rates being so low, and provision of ART to infected women being even lower, it became apparent that the major focus and funding of the PMTCT programme in Africa was on provision of infant feeding counselling and provision of formula. The HIV and Infant Feeding Counselling Course, released in its final form in 2000, provided the means by which the feeding of substitutes for breastmilk could be implemented. The stated rationale was '*.... When children born to HIV-infected women can be assured of uninterrupted access to nutritionally adequate breastmilk substitutes that are safely prepared and fed to them, they are at less risk of illness and death if they are not breastfed.*'[23]

Making breastmilk substitutes affordable

A UNICEF survey had shown that most mothers in resource-poor settings could not afford to purchase formula themselves.[15] An infant needs about 20kg of powdered infant formula during the first six months of life and a further 20kg during the following six months. In Zimbabwe, India and Nicaragua this would mean that the cost of formula to feed one baby for one year would equate to 139%, 34% and 64% of GNP per capita respectively. In Kenya the cost would equate to 84% of the minimum urban wage, in Brazil to 22%. This meant that unless there were free supplies mothers struggled with affordability.[24] Formula was thus to be provided free to those mothers who, after counselling, decided that they wanted to formula-feed.

Anna Coutsoudis and colleagues argued that free and reasoned choice on infant feeding, according to the social and economic circumstances of HIV-positive mothers, could be compromised by subsidies. A woman could be subtly induced into making an inappropriate decision as the risks associated with exclusive replacement feeding vs exclusive breastfeeding were simply unknown.[25] Furthermore, the very families who met the UN criteria for safe replacement feeding were the ones most likely to be relatively advantaged compared to the rest of the population, and therefore the least likely to need free handouts.

The cost of providing formula was enormous, amounting to between 25% to 60% of PMTCT budgets depending on whether individual programmes also provided ARVs to mother and/or baby. For example, where PMTCT programmes offered short-course zidovudine, the cost of providing free formula could amount to 25% of the programme budget, and where programmes offered nevirapine, formula could account for 50% of the budget.[26–28] The major costs in South Africa's PMTCT project were drugs (30%), staff salaries (29%), and infant formula (24%). A model simulation of the cost-effectiveness of PMTCT interventions[29] revealed that 'the appropriateness of formula feeding was highly cost effective only in settings with high sero-prevalence and reasonable levels of child survival, and dangerous where infant mortality was high or the protective effect of breastfeeding substantial.' Planners did not factor in that a combination of high HIV-prevalence *and* low child mortality did not exist anywhere: the reality was that in poverty-stricken areas of high HIV-prevalence, infant mortality was also high and child survival depended on breastfeeding.

Mothers recruited into the ZVITAMBO study in Zimbabwe inadvertently provided one of the most intriguing ironies of the HIV and infant feeding story. During antenatal education sessions, pregnant women received various forms of basic information about infant feeding in the context of HIV.[30] Key messages included these facts:

- only some (not all) babies of HIV-positive mothers become infected themselves;
- exclusive breastfeeding was recommended for all mothers, i.e. those of unknown or negative status, as well as HIV-positive mothers who chose to breastfeed.

Mothers who chose not to learn their HIV status were educated in 'safer breastfeeding', consisting of four practices:

- Exclusive breastfeeding to six months
- Proper infant positioning and attachment to the breast to minimise breast pathology
- Seeking medical care quickly for breast problems
- Practising safe sex, especially during the breastfeeding period

HIV-positive mothers who chose to learn their HIV status received HIV and infant feeding counselling integrated into their post-test counselling. This included a full discussion of the risks, benefits, and costs of the various feeding options:

1. 'safer breastfeeding', as described;
2. heat-treated expressed breastmilk;
3. replacement feeding with commercial formula;
4. replacement feeding with homemade formula;
5. initiation of exclusive breastfeeding followed by early and rapid cessation of breastfeeding at six months and then feeding with locally available foods.

As well as counselling, the mothers received or were exposed to educational materials developed by ZVITAMBO personnel, including two videos, three pamphlets, counselling tools describing the costs, advantages and disadvantages of each feeding option, and take-home factsheets providing step-by-step instructions for implementing each feeding option safely.

The unique aspect of the ZVITAMBO study was that mothers *could* learn their HIV test results at any time during the study with appropriate pre- and post-test counselling. But they were not *required* to do so. Intriguingly, only 15.5% chose to learn their HIV status at any time and only a tiny percentage – 7.1% – chose to do so before 3 months. A halving of breastfeeding-associated HIV transmission and mortality was achieved for the 93% of the mothers who did not receive the anticipatory special individualised 'HIV and infant feeding counselling'. It turned out that 32% of the mothers had been HIV-positive, but breastfeeding rates of 99.1% and 94% at six and 12 months were achieved and only a tiny 1.3% of the babies of the ZVITAMBO mothers who exclusively breastfed for three months became infected through breastfeeding.[31]

The mothers' decision to breastfeed exclusively was independent of knowledge of HIV status in this study. But exposure to information about the value of exclusive breastfeeding through both group and individual contacts was important. The more exposures a mother had, the more likely she was to exclusively breastfeed. Just over a quarter of mothers reported five or more exposures to the programme.[32] Those who received repeated exposure to the messages in the programme were between two and five times more likely to exclusively breastfeed compared to mothers with no programme exposure. It seems clear that these good results were achieved because the value of exclusive breastfeeding was stressed regardless of maternal HIV status, *and no information about replacement feeding was received.* The ZVITAMBO results sealed the deal on the value of exclusive breastfeeding as a way to achieve low postpartum transmission rates *and* very low infant mortality; in fact it was ZVITAMBO which confirmed that counselling on the importance of exclusive breastfeeding would result in the greatest HIV-free survival (see Chapter 10). Sadly, however, it would be another five years before the international agencies would provide formal recognition of the significance of this finding.

Summary

In the decade between 1999 and 2009 HIV-positive mothers included in the PMTCT pilot sites were asked to choose their own infant feeding method, breastfeeding or formula-feeding, even as each mother's ability to make an educated assessment about which infant feeding method would pose the least risk to her baby was simply not possible.

The HIV transmission and infant mortality results from the initial PMTCT pilot projects involving the first 30,000 mothers and babies have never been publicly disseminated. In 2002 UNICEF estimated that 1.8 million HIV-positive women became pregnant every year and 200,000–350,000 of their babies would become infected with HIV through breastfeeding. Replacement feeding was the only way to avoid those infections and so the intention was to counsel women not to breastfeed.[33] In 2007 Dr Hoosen Coovadia of South Africa, commenting on the risk of mortality from acquisition of HIV through breastfeeding compared to no breastfeeding at all, wrote, 'If you choose breastfeeding, you would of course have HIV infection. You would have about 300,000 per year in the world. But if you avoided breastfeeding, the mortality would be about 1.5 million per year. So on the balance of probabilities for poor women in the developing world, there is no other choice than to breastfeed their infants. You shouldn't devise policies for the rich few... the majority of HIV-infected women are poor.'[34]

Before the Botswana floods in 2006 exposed the scale of what was happening in the PMTCT sites, remarkably few published papers were available giving infant mortality results according to feeding method. This meant that early national HIV and infant feeding policies were formulated on the basis of inadequate information.[35] The status quo was maintained by lack of monitoring and evaluation. National policymakers looked to the international agencies for guidance; health workers and infant-feeding counsellors were guided by national directives. Mothers were counselled accordingly. But there was simply no safety information to go on. Was the intention to deliberately keep policymakers, health workers and counsellors in ignorance about health outcomes? Would this enable them to more easily encourage mothers to make their own infant feeding choice – and at the same time absolve health workers of accountability if a mother made a poor choice? Continuing the narrative of maternal empowerment, further PMTCT sites were rolled out to encourage formula-feeding for hundreds of thousands – perhaps millions – of babies.

Clearly, limiting paediatric HIV by limiting breastfeeding must have seemed like a solution when it was believed that maternal drug therapy would be wasted if babies faced continued exposure to the virus in breastmilk. But few realise that breastfeeding avoidance was often the *only* intervention on offer. The fate of the babies from the early PMTCT sites will likely never be known because whether they lived or died was not monitored or recorded.

The feasibility of formula-feeding by mothers in developing countries of high HIV prevalence was facilitated through a special educational course for healthcare staff developed by UNAIDS, WHO and UNICEF. It was so well crafted that formula-feeding seemed to be feasible and desirable even in the poorest conditions. It was made acceptable because it was provided for free. The legacy of this initial promotion is still being felt today and we still have work to do to put things right.

Looking back, Stephen Lewis, former UN envoy on HIV-AIDS, had it right when he observed in July 2009, barely four months before the UN agencies were finally persuaded to alter their stance on promotion of replacement feeding:

> *'....Prevention of mother to child transmission should have been the easiest intervention of all, instead we've had a panorama of unnecessary death for both the mothers and their children. So-called PMTCT has been a colossal failure, subjected to twisted linguistics, lousy science, governmental chicanery, and astonishing delinquency on the part of United Nations agencies. Only now is the political establishment coming to its senses. But it needs your help so that it never goes off the rails again.'* [36]

CHAPTER 15

Problems with counselling, but scaling up anyway

'In my humble view health workers who provide counseling on infant feeding must be trained on lactation management before going into a discussion of replacement feeding otherwise infant feeding counseling is a formula for disaster where there will be a simple promotion of bottle feeding.' Ruth Nduati

Following expected norms in the industrialised world, but against every tradition and cultural belief in most of Africa, the guiding principle of the infant feeding component of the PMTCT programme was that every HIV-positive mother should be supported to make her own informed decision about how best to feed her infant. This positioned the counsellor as an informed and kindly expert possessing the knowledge and authority to enable individual mothers to decide which infant-feeding method seemed most suitable to her.[1]

Those of us working with breastfeeding mothers and babies in developing countries watched the developments taking place in the PMTCT sites with mounting dread. It became clear that 'HIV and infant feeding counselling' – which really meant teaching mothers how to formula-feed – was by far the most important aspect of the PMTCT programme.

The 2000 WHO HIV and Infant Feeding Counselling Course[2,3] provided detailed and comprehensive training on how to counsel HIV-infected mothers using a rights-based approach. Every opportunity was taken to teach participants the principles of listening carefully to the mother, reflecting back her feelings, drawing out her concerns and helping her to make her own decision. But counsellors also learned how to outline the risk of HIV transmission through breastfeeding and provide extensive instruction on how to prepare and feed breastmilk substitutes so as to eliminate the risk of postnatal transmission of the virus through breastfeeding. Counsellors were usually nurse-midwives, employed in hospitals, clinics and other health institutions, or they may have been infant-feeding or lactation counsellors. They could also be untrained community volunteers with no specialised medical training.[4] Importantly, the decision about whether or not to breastfeed was to be made by the mother, not the counsellor, based on full information about the options available.

But there was a problem – which was just not seen by those who had developed policy for the countries so badly affected by HIV. As well as being tied to strong cultural beliefs and traditions, breastfeeding was seen as the normal way to feed a baby. Breastfeeding was universally practised; it was never framed as optional. Furthermore, the concept of choice in health matters was alien to African healthcare systems. Ministries of health, having the expertise and knowledge of healthcare matters, set policy, nursing staff carried it out, and the knowledge and authority of nurses was never questioned by patients.

The take-home HIV and infant feeding message promoting formula-feeding was not only understood by mothers. Reading between the lines, counsellors themselves understood that the 16 hours training they had received really meant that formula-feeding for HIV-positive mothers was being recommended. Why else would their ministries of health want to spend so much time and funding on it? National health authorities were, in turn, persuaded by the time and effort spent on HIV and infant feeding by WHO, UNICEF and UNAIDS.

The box below outlines how counselling may have evolved and been understood by the global north before being exported to the global south. Unfortunately, counselling for informed infant-feeding choice was regrettably not perceived in quite the same way by African healthcare staff, nor by the HIV-positive mothers themselves.

What is counselling?

Adapted from An Introduction to Counselling, *McGraw-Hill Education http://highered.mcgraw-hill.com/sites/dl/free/0335211895/135446/Chap01.pdf accessed 24 January 2022*

Counselling is an activity that emerged within Western industrial society in the twentieth century. Counselling has for many people largely taken over the role in society once filled by religion and community life. In a mass urban society, counselling offers a way of being known and being heard. The task of counselling is to give the client an opportunity to explore, discover and clarify ways of living more satisfyingly and resourcefully. Counselling denotes a professional relationship between a trained counsellor and a client. This relationship is usually person-to-person. It is designed to help clients to understand and clarify their views of their lifespace, and to learn to reach their self-determined goals through meaningful, well-informed choices and through resolution of problems of an emotional or interpersonal nature.

Counselling is a principled relationship characterised by the application of one or more psychological theories and a recognised set of communication skills, modified by experience, intuition and other interpersonal factors, with a focus on clients' intimate concerns, problems or aspirations. Its predominant ethos is one of facilitation rather than of advice-giving or coercion. It may be of very brief or long duration, take place in an organisational or private practice setting and may or may not overlap with practical, medical and other matters of personal welfare. It is both a distinctive activity undertaken by people agreeing to occupy the roles of counsellor and client... and an emerging profession... It is a service sought by people in distress or in some degree of confusion who wish to discuss and resolve these in a relationship which is more disciplined and confidential than friendship, and perhaps less stigmatising than helping relationships offered in traditional medical or psychiatric settings.

One of the essential common features of all counselling is that it can only happen if the person seeking help, the client, wants it to happen. Counselling takes place when someone who is troubled invites and allows another person to enter into a particular kind of relationship with them. If a person is not ready to extend this invitation, they may be exposed to the best efforts of expert counsellors for long periods of time, but what will happen will not be counselling... Counselling must also be understood within its social and cultural context: counsellor and client are social roles, and the ways in which participants make sense of the aims and work of counselling are shaped by the culture within which they live. ...In many ways, counselling is a product of late twentieth-century modernity. A person seeks such a relationship when they encounter a problem in living that they have not been able to resolve through their everyday resources, and that has resulted in their exclusion from some aspect of full participation in social life. The person seeking counselling invites another person to provide him or her with time and space characterized by the presence of a number of features that are not readily available in everyday life: permission to speak, respect for difference, confidentiality and affirmation.

Permission to speak. This is a place where the person can tell their story, where they are given every encouragement to give voice to aspects of their experience that have previously been silenced, in their own time and their own way, including the expression of feeling and emotion.

Respect for difference. The counsellor sets aside, as far as they are able, their own position on the issues brought by the client, and his or her needs in the moment, in order to focus as completely as possible on helping the client to articulate and act on his or her personal values and desires.

Confidentiality. Whatever is discussed is confidential: the counsellor undertakes to refrain from passing on what they have learned from the person to any others in the person's life world.

Affirmation. The counsellor enacts a relationship that is an expression of a set of core values: honesty, integrity, care, belief in the worth and value of individual persons, commitment to dialogue and collaboration, reflexivity, the interdependence of persons, a sense of the common good...

The potential outcomes of counselling can be understood as falling into three broad categories:

1. Resolution of the original problem in living. Resolution can include: achieving an understanding or perspective on the problem, arriving at a personal acceptance of the problem or dilemma and taking action to change

the situation in which the problem arose.
2. Learning. Engagement with counselling may enable the person to acquire new understandings, skills and strategies that make them better able to handle similar problems in future.
3. Social inclusion. Counselling stimulates the energy and capacity of the person as someone who can contribute to the well-being of others and the social good.

Fragmentation of counsellor training

A UNICEF evaluation from 2003[5] recorded that infant feeding was the most challenging component of PMTCT programmes. Although the very user-friendly HIV and Infant Feeding Course had standardised teaching methods, UNICEF considered that each country needed to develop or adapt policy guidelines based on local conditions. This opened the door to fragmentation of care and the justification for gaps in provision of counselling and antiretroviral drugs to mothers. Programmes used a variety of personnel for infant-feeding counselling; most used nurse-midwives, some used specialised counsellors, and one programme in Rwanda had separate nutrition centres. Despite training, staff knowledge and counselling abilities remained weak. Counsellors frequently steered a woman towards an infant-feeding method based solely on her HIV status rather than a comprehensive assessment of her social and economic ability to implement various feeding options. Once babies were born, very few programmes provided ongoing support for women to carry out the infant-feeding method that had been decided upon antenatally.

Five of 11 original pilot countries – Côte d'Ivoire, Tanzania, Uganda, Zambia and Zimbabwe – offered separate HIV and infant-feeding training, while six other countries integrated infant-feeding counselling into PMTCT training. Training was therefore often inadequate or non-existent.

Many counsellors felt under-trained. This may have been partly due to understaffing and lack of time, as well as a lack of printed materials and little knowledge of national HIV and infant feeding guidelines.

In 42 observations at UNICEF-supported PMTCT sites counsellors provided information about the advantages and disadvantages of the various infant feeding options, but in the majority of cases little or no time was spent discussing the mother's circumstances and living conditions.[6] There was often a lack of understanding of the advantages and disadvantages of various feeding methods, and counsellor bias, usually in favour of formula feeding, due to incorrect information or ambiguous training, was common.[7–12] In Botswana the knowledge of many staff was poor,[7,13] only half were satisfied with the training they had received, and others reported that they felt uncomfortable when counselling about infant-feeding practices.[6] In Zambia less than half of counsellors had attended a separate course on infant feeding.[6,14] In Rwanda only a minority of PMTCT programme staff (four of 17 at two sites) had been trained.[6] At a third Rwandan site, although all staff had either attended a formal PMTCT course, or received training from a fellow staff member, their knowledge was poor; for example, they described seeing mothers with formula and breastfeeding difficulties which had not been addressed in their training.[15] There were few clear protocols or guidelines,[16] resulting in poor knowledge of the advantages and disadvantages of different feeding options. There was a tendency for counsellors to actually recommend formula to all mothers,[5] despite the fact that only 41% of the population had access to a good water supply and 8% to good sanitation.

In South Africa health workers would have liked additional training. Only one in 11 could define 'exclusive breastfeeding' correctly and knowledge of other feeding methods was limited. While some health workers were willing to change their advice to take into account the findings of the Coutsoudis study showing that exclusive breastfeeding might reduce the risk of HIV transmission,[17] others said they wouldn't, either because they didn't believe the results, or because they thought that the information would confuse mothers. Opinion was divided about the use of heat-treated expressed breastmilk. About 70% of counsellors showed a clear preference for a certain infant feeding option, in most cases formula. They sometimes pressured mothers to choose formula by telling them that if they were HIV-positive they shouldn't breastfeed.[6] And although they were happy to provide mothers with free supplies for six to 12 months, they gave inadequate information on safe preparation.[18]

The burden on counsellors

Sebalda Leshabari, whom I'd met at a WABA-UNICEF symposium in Arusha, looked at the challenges faced by nurse-counsellors in four PMTCT sites in the Kilimanjaro region of northern Tanzania.[19] The nurses experienced a high level of stress and frustration when they felt unable to give qualified and relevant infant feeding advice to HIV-positive women. They were confused about the appropriateness of the feeding options they were expected to provide, since they thought that both exclusive breastfeeding and exclusive replacement feeding were culturally and socially unsuitable. In general the nurses were not comfortable in their newly gained role as counsellors and felt that the authority and trust traditionally vested in nursing as a knowledgeable and caring profession was being undermined. Sebalda's findings illuminated the immense burden placed on nurses. She concluded that organisation of counselling services should take more notice of the local working realities of nurses.

When I worked for the World Alliance for Breastfeeding Action, both health workers and mothers made many requests for clarification of ambiguous guidelines and recommendations. Participants at the La Leche League International/WABA Symposium on HIV and Breastfeeding held in Washington DC in July 2005 voted 'counselling' as the major problem to be addressed.[8] Conscientious and experienced counsellors in poverty-stricken areas continued to be extremely troubled by directives which undermined decades of effort to rebuild local cultural breastfeeding norms following the departure of Western colonial administrations. They were acutely conscious of the differences between promotion of 'breastfeeding' vs the euphemistic 'infant feeding' which they were well aware meant replacement feeding (formula-feeding). Generally speaking, peer PMTCT support programmes operated in a context fraught with tension and fear,[1] as peer counsellors were left with the challenge of convincing HIV-positive mothers that either of two particular exclusive feeding options were a safe and feasible way to feed a baby to reduce the risk of HIV transmission. A paper from South Africa described how counsellors struggled to 'sell their service' to a sceptical group of potential recipients through a continuous negotiation of their own credibility.[20]

Counsellors' knowledge of MTCT

The HIV and Infant Feeding Counselling Course was so thorough and user-friendly that prior medical knowledge was not needed as a prerequisite to either teach it or to undergo training.[21] Botswana had taken advantage of this in 2004 when voluntary counselling and HIV testing for expectant mothers in their PMTCT programme was task-shifted away from nurses and midwives to lay counsellors.[22] However, even by 2000, Arjan de Wagt's review of independent research studies of the PMTCT sites had already uncovered some serious concerns.[23] Counsellors' knowledge about the risk of MTCT was inadequate; only 51% of those interviewed were aware that HIV transmission to infants was preventable. Some, including traditional birth attendants, thought that all HIV-positive mothers would pass on the virus through breastfeeding, while still others simply did not know.

There seemed to be few clear protocols and inadequate knowledge of national HIV and infant feeding guidelines.[7,24] Most providers were not familiar with ways to reduce HIV transmission through different types of breastfeeding, e.g. exclusive breastfeeding for six months, wet nursing, donated milk obtained from milk banks, or expressed and heat-treated breastmilk. Nor could most providers cite all the strategies (for example correct positioning, and feeding on demand) that would optimise exclusive breastfeeding and minimise the risk of transmitting HIV. The large number of PMTCT providers needing training, and high staff turnover and rotation, meant that programmes struggled with avoiding gaps in knowledge.[7]

Counsellor confusion

Counsellor bias, usually in favour of formula feeding, due to a counsellor's own lack of understanding or ambiguous training, was problematic. Many staff who had been through the WHO training understood that the intention was for HIV-positive mothers to formula-feed. Counselling often promoted one feeding method over others.

Confusion about infant feeding choice led to deterioration of support for breastfeeding in many settings.[5] Reports were received from Honduras, Rwanda, South Africa, Tanzania and Zambia that counsellors simply did not help mothers to make an informed choice, or attempt to assess the feasibility of different options based on the client's circumstances.[10,12,18,25–27] In Rwanda, providers believed that the PMTCT programme recommended replacement feeding over exclusive breastfeeding.[25] When asked 'What are your opinions about HIV-positive women who do not breastfeed?' 28 Zambian providers said the woman is doing the 'right thing'; only one had a negative opinion, and seven were neutral. When asked whether they thought there was one best infant feeding method, 21 counsellors replied formula, one replied exclusive breastfeeding for six months, and 10 said there was no best method – each had advantages and disadvantages. The responses were unrelated to whether the health worker had received training.[7]

On balance, most counsellors in northern Tanzania[1] believed that formula-feeding was the best option for preventing MTCT and generally recommended this feeding method, even if they didn't think it was feasible. The major barrier to commercial formula-feeding was cost. Very few referred to gender or other contextual issues such as a woman's poor decision-making power, fear of disclosure, or social pressure to breastfeed. Neither were literacy and access to clean water and fuel needed for safe formula-feeding mentioned as conditions affecting which feeding method to recommend.

Mothers' understanding

In PMTCT sites in Soweto and Khayelitsha in South Africa HIV-positive mothers indicated that they chose to formula-feed because they were advised to do so by their nurse/counsellor, because of their HIV status and health, or as an interim measure until they disclosed their status to their families.[28]

A 2002 UNICEF report about PMTCT sites in India found a counselling bias toward artificial feeding since such a high proportion of women chose it.[29] Although a woman's informed decision was promoted, counsellors had actually understood that artificial feeding was the preferred alternative. This was further confirmed when women reported that they had been given this advice, that 81% had chosen artificial feeding, and family members tended to support their decision. Health workers who indicated it was possible for women to stop breastfeeding at six months based their responses on the mother's HIV status and her concern for her infant's health. One nurse said, 'If the mothers are told good reasons for stopping, they will listen and follow what they are advised.' Similarly, a medical assistant mentioned that fear might influence infant feeding behaviour: 'HIV-positive mothers with a fear of transmitting HIV to their child could stop breastfeeding at 6 months.'[30]

In Thailand, the government PMTCT programme actively endorsed formula-feeding by all women. This was generally acceptable everywhere and in 2001/02 the uptake of formula-feeding was over 80%.[28] In research sites, almost 100% of HIV-infected women were formula-feeding; only 6% were reported to have ever breastfed vs >95% in the HIV-uninfected population. Among the HIV-positive women, 62% were concerned about not breastfeeding and 70% acknowledged that other family members and friends were concerned. About half had found it hard to explain to other people in the community why they were not breastfeeding. Although high compliance with exclusive formula-feeding could be successfully achieved in both research and government PMTCT programmes, no morbidity or mortality data were available from these sites.

In Abidjan, Côte d'Ivoire, there was no support offered in the postnatal wards to help initiate breastfeeding or to sustain exclusive breastfeeding in the first days, nor was there specific counselling at the antenatal clinics preparing women for initiating and sustaining exclusive breastfeeding. Those taking part in the PMTCT project who elected to breastfeed were followed up and specifically counselled on how they might *stop* breastfeeding and when stopping would be appropriate and possible in their circumstances.[28] This could be any time up to six months postpartum. Counselling included practical demonstrations on how to use a cup for giving replacement feeds, workshops on preparing complementary feeds and mothers were given free formula for nine months after stopping.

Counsellor bias

In some sites in India and South Africa counsellors showed a bias in favour of exclusive breastfeeding and were against replacement feeding.[31,32] In one Indian report, all of the counsellors believed that exclusive breastfeeding was the best choice for all women, regardless of HIV status. The low socioeconomic status of women using public sector services in part influenced this view.[7] Modified cow or buffalo milk was the only replacement feed that programmes discussed as an option. Officials were reluctant to promote or offer formula to poor, uneducated women and only discussed formula with those women specifically requesting it and who appeared to be able to afford it.

Observation of services in Honduras, India, Rwanda, and Zambia found that programme staff generally only mentioned a few kinds of replacement feeds (formula, modified animal milk, and heat-treated expressed milk). In other places, counsellors rarely discussed other choices such as heat-treating expressed breastmilk or wet-nursing.[7] Bias against abrupt cessation of breastfeeding was also reported as an issue in studies in Nigeria and Tanzania.[7,27,33]

Mothers' experiences with counselling

For African women who tested positive, the decision about whether or not to breastfeed was regarded as complicated and difficult. Information about exclusive breastfeeding was perceived as contradictory and only one-third of HIV-positive mothers would be willing to try it. Firstly, most women did not believe that a baby could thrive on breastmilk alone, and the older the baby, the more the doubt increased. Secondly, since breastmilk could transfer the virus, it seemed counter-intuitive to most women that exclusive breastfeeding could be more protective than mixed feeding, since reducing the quantity of breastmilk that the baby received should logically mean reduced risk. Information about the protective effect of a short period of exclusive breastfeeding followed by abrupt weaning was also received with some scepticism, since mothers thought that the baby would be infected during the first few months anyway.[6]

Mothers harboured many misconceptions. They saw little distinction between HIV and AIDS. They thought that mosquitoes could transmit the virus or that the risk of HIV transmission was 100%. It was not commonly known that HIV could be transmitted during labour and birth, although nearly half of women knew that HIV could be transmitted through breastfeeding. No women knew that the risk was higher if they became newly infected during the breastfeeding period, but when husbands understood this point, they often saw for the first time a reason for knowing their own status.

Ethiopian HIV-positive mothers were reported to have faced confusion and fear when trying to adhere to the advice given by their nurse-counsellors.[34] Fear about transmitting HIV to the infants dominated the messages of the PMTCT counsellors, who commonly ended up recommending that breastfeeding should be avoided if at all possible. The intense experience among many mothers of having 'poisonous milk' led to desperate attempts to secure infant formula, even knowing they were too poor to buy enough. Many of the women eventually resorted to breastfeeding when they ran out of cash, leading to experiences of guilt and deep regret – as well as mixed breast and formula-feeding, the most risky feeding method of all.

At PMTCT sites assessed between January and June 2002, 30% of antenatal mothers received no counselling at all.[5] Those who did received mixed messages due to lack of standard protocols. In counselling designed to help HIV-positive women make informed infant-feeding decisions, there were several inherent difficulties:

- Informed choice was selectively confined to developing country settings since industrialised countries employed a clear recommendation to formula feed.
- The content rather than the process exerted the most influence, e.g. increasing exclusive breastfeeding rates to 70% in Bangladesh,[35] or achieving 100% formula-feeding in breastfeeding populations in South Africa.[7,32]
- The unknown HIV status of the individual newborn always precluded truly informed decision-making.
- Mothers' lack of autonomy about infant feeding led to an increased risk of mixed feeding; many HIV-infected mothers compromised by artificially feeding their babies at home, and breastfeeding in public, thus increasing the risk of HIV transmission through mixed feeding.[36–38]
- Exploitation of mothers' fear about HIV in their milk allowed promotion of formula feeding.[7,39]
- African mothers often perceived infant-feeding counselling as prescriptive, favouring formula feeding.[35,38] Communities often took the recommendations of health providers as the final word, even when their information was poor.
- In the absence of antiretroviral therapy, infant-feeding counselling may have been the only therapy available to HIV-infected mothers who agreed to be tested.
- Most babies were lost to follow-up and an extremely small percentage were finally tested to determine whether prevention strategies achieved overall HIV-free survival.

Frequency of counselling

Researchers in Zambia found that more frequent counselling was more effective than one-off sessions in enabling mothers to be more successful with their chosen feeding method.[28] Single counselling sessions were not sufficient to prepare mothers for exclusive breastfeeding – they needed more steps.[40] Better results were achieved when counselling began antenatally, breastfeeding initiation was supported by midwives after delivery, postnatal counselling included both a home- and clinic-based component, and women randomly allocated to abrupt cessation of all breastfeeding at four months received an additional counselling intervention.

The number of exposures to counselling significantly influenced exclusive breastfeeding rates in the ZVITAMBO study in Zimbabwe. The more times that mothers were exposed to information about the benefits of exclusive breastfeeding, the better they were able to exclusively breastfeed. Adherence to feeding intention and reduced spillover of suboptimal feeding practices (i.e. formula-feeding) to HIV-negative women was also minimal.[41] Other health workers elsewhere had also been able to increase rates of exclusive breastfeeding with increased frequency of counselling,[35,42,43] suggesting that failure of mothers' ability to practise exclusive breastfeeding was due to inadequate counselling rather than anything else.

The PROMISE-EBF trial in sub-Saharan Africa conducted from 2006 to 2008 assessed the effect of individual breastfeeding counselling by peer-counsellors compared to control groups who received no extra visits.[44] Exclusive breastfeeding rates at 12 weeks of age for mothers who received five home visits from peer supporters, antenatally and continuing until 10-16 weeks after birth, compared to no extra counselling, increased in Burkina Faso (83% vs 36%), Uganda (87% vs 49%) and South Africa (11% vs 7%).

Dr Ruth Bland and colleagues in Durban, South Africa, examined infant feeding intentions of both HIV-positive and HIV-negative mothers and the appropriateness of their choices depending on the resources they enjoyed during the first week postpartum (clean water, adequate fuel, access to a fridge and regular maternal income).[45] Exclusive breastfeeding was more socially acceptable than replacement feeding and mothers who chose this option were able to stick to their feeding choice more easily than those who chose to formula-feed. Conversely, of 60 mothers interviewed at three other purposively selected PMTCT sites across South Africa, only two HIV-positive mothers were asked about essential conditions for safe formula-feeding before a feeding decision was made. None of the 12 mothers choosing to breastfeed were shown how to position the baby correctly at the breast or asked whether they thought exclusive breastfeeding was feasible. Fewer than a quarter of them expressed confidence in their choice. It was concluded that the poor quality of counselling in the PMTCT programmes would reduce their effectiveness.

Uptake of formula

The uptake of free formula by mothers varied between and within countries as shown in the box below.[6] Involvement of male partners in making decisions about infant feeding seemed to be a key factor in increasing the acceptability of formula.[37] Facilitating acceptability and feasibility of formula-feeding, while ensuring its accessibility and affordability, led to successful demand-creation. Even as provision of antiretroviral therapy was low, there was high uptake of formula.[5,7,13,28,32] and in the research sites, almost 100% of HIV-infected women were formula-feeding.[28]

Thailand	80%–100%
Botswana	~ 89%
Rwanda	~ 87%
South Africa	40%–100%
Zambia	~ 60%
Nigeria	~ 50%
Uganda	30%–50%

Percentage of HIV-positive mothers formula-feeding in HIV-affected countries

A study in Abidjan used for planning purposes before implementation of PMTCT programmes had found that although all but two children were breastfed, exclusive breastfeeding was not practised, and the use of formula was relatively common from an early age.[46] In a later study 53% of antenatal mothers chose formula-feeding, although in fact 41% were temporarily practising mixed-feeding by the second day of life because of social stigma or poor health of the newborn.[47,48] In Nigeria, antenatal counselling increased acceptance of HIV-testing, antiretroviral therapy and avoidance of breastfeeding.[49]

Sustainability

In a situation of poverty, where there is a lack of adequate water and poor sanitation, exclusive breastfeeding for the first six months serves to ensure to some extent the safety and good health of the infant. Shortages of formula supplies placed the food security of non-breastfed babies at risk in South Africa.[18,45,50] Most mothers who were receiving PMTCT services said that the quantities of formula received were insufficient. Strategies used by mothers who ran out of formula included: going to the clinic earlier than scheduled to get a new supply,[13] buying an alternative milk or formula, giving sugar and water or fruit drinks between formula feeds, giving fewer feeds per day, or over-diluting the formula.[18] When mothers could not afford to buy their own supplies it often led to mixed feeding as they returned to breastfeeding. It's important to note that it was not always an inadequate supply system that was to blame for mothers running out of formula. In the first year of the programme with passive follow-up, only 50% of women initially receiving infant formula returned for a new supply at six weeks.

Uganda had enjoyed a robust breastfeeding culture when pilot PMTCT sites introduced free generic UNICEF formula in five hospitals in three districts in 2000. At Mulago Hospital in Kampala, a six-month supply was provided to women who decided not to breastfeed. Staff used an infant-feeding checklist to help determine whether formula would be a safe option. Among 870 HIV-positive mothers, 43% chose to formula-feed. Problems encountered included difficulties in follow-up, lack of storage space, expiration of the formula, contamination, stealing, and supply interruptions.[7] The former national PMTCT coordinator in Uganda said that mothers who were really in need of infant formula did not get it and that the logistics were 'a nightmare'.

In Botswana the infant formula programme struggled to maintain a consistent formula supply.[51] Mothers were given 10 tins per month, but data from 2006, 2007 and 2008 indicated that infants were getting an average of only 60% of the formula they needed over the course of their first year.[52] Some infants who lacked additional sources of food needed more than the 'average' amount that national PMTCT guidelines suggested for each child based on age. Families without access to refrigeration tended to waste it, as any mixed formula that was not consumed by the infant had to be discarded.

Safety

A report from Côte d'Ivoire found there were no differences in risks of diarrhoea, respiratory infection, malnutrition, hospitalisation or death in breastfed versus formula-fed infants of HIV-positive women. The authors said that offering safer conditions (clean water, free formula) and a more supportive environment (replacement feeding counselling and education) were elements that reduced the potential threat of mortality among formula-fed infants. These findings were sustained after a two-year follow-up period.[53]

This was not the general finding of Koniz-Booher and colleagues.[7] Although replacement feeding was only recommended under AFASS conditions, they had concluded, 'In general, the studies we reviewed suggest that it is difficult to meet all of the conditions necessary for safe replacement feeding.' There was no well-defined definition of what 'safe' meant in the context of mothers living in resource-poor settings. The 2005 World Health Organization guidance[54] specified that 'water should be boiled vigorously for 1 to 2 seconds to prepare the formula.' Bacterial contamination of infant formula can occur through mixing with dirty water, but what is less often recognised is that the powder itself can contain disease-causing bacteria which damages and kills babies.[55] This is more fully explored in Chapter 20.

It is difficult for women to prepare formula hygienically in resource-poor settings. Mothers who chose formula feeding were not always supported in preparing and feeding it safely. Mothers in Khayelitsha, South Africa, received little information on safety issues and consequently most formula feeds were prepared incorrectly.[18] In Botswana[13] at least 35% of HIV-positive mothers did not clean the feeding container before every use. Only 27% of HIV-positive mothers living in urban areas in Botswana had a refrigerator, meaning that most would have had to prepare all feeds separately. In fact 70% of those that had a refrigerator were storing the prepared formula at room temperature anyway.

Data on bacteriological contamination and nutrient concentration of prepared free formula feeds from Durban, South Africa,[56] showed that 70% of mothers attending a PMTCT clinic had received free formula with extensive counselling on hygiene and milk preparation. However, two-thirds of milk samples collected from the mothers at the clinic contained *E.coli* and one-quarter contained *Enterococci*. While boiling water separately for every feed significantly reduced the risk of contamination compared to boiling and storing water for several feeds, the risk of preparing contaminated milk during the night was higher if each feed was prepared separately. Between 28% and 44% of the collected samples were also over-diluted. Another study from Kwa-Zulu Natal in 2007 showed that approximately 80% of formula-feeds prepared at home after instruction from counsellors were contaminated with faecal bacteria. Approximately 20% of the samples that the counsellors prepared at the clinic while showing the mothers how to do everything correctly were also contaminated.[57]

De Wagt and Clarke found that information on safe preparation of formula was frequently contradictory, even when provided by formula manufacturers themselves, and the experiences of mothers pointed to serious concerns.[6] They outlined the often conflicting safety guidance provided by several formula manufacturers:

'First of all bottles and utensils need to be sterilized by boiling them for 5 to 10 minutes' (Nutricia, 2003; Abbott Industries, 2003; Nestlé, 2003).

'Then the water for the formula also needs to be boiled for 10 minutes before the formula powder can be added' (Nutricia, 2001)

'Prepared formula can be kept in the fridge for up to 24 hours' (Nutricia, 2003; International Association of Infant Food Manufacturers, 2003) 'and outside the refrigerator at room temperature for two hours' (Mead Johnson, 2003; Nestlé, 2003).

'Prepared formula that has not been consumed by the baby should be thrown away' (Nutricia, 2003; Nestlé, 2003).

'Opened cans of powdered formulas need to be stored in a cool, dry place and need to be used within one month after opening the can' (Abbott Industries, 2003).

Water quality

In 2000 only 50% of the population in sub-Saharan Africa had access to safe water, and only 45% had adequate sanitation.[58] Hygienic replacement feeding was difficult under such circumstances, and most of these populations were reliant on breastmilk to nourish young children well into their second year of life and beyond. Thus for most women in Africa, breastmilk substitutes were costly and had been seldom used before the PMTCT programmes began introducing them.

In Abidjan, Côte d'Ivoire, one study on water safety showed that even though municipal water was widely available and of good quality, it was often stored improperly in the home, resulting in many of the samples containing *E.coli*.[59] If replacement feeding was going to be more widely used, interventions were needed to make the stored water safer. There were also concerns about storage of pasteurised cow's milk when there was no access to refrigeration.

Only half of Zambian households interviewed used boiled water, a third added chlorine and the rest took no precautions at all.[60] In Myanmar, women were reluctant to boil water at all, and domestic hygiene, including handwashing, was poor.[7]

The risks of formula feeding

The De Wagt and Clark review concluded:[6]

'The review of experiences from the field has shown that inclusion of free formula as part of the PMTCT package has addressed the affordability component of these conditions. However in many cases it has left mothers struggling with issues around feasibility, safety, and acceptability, increasing the risk of mixed feeding and consequently increased risk of morbidity and mortality due to diarrhea, respiratory infections and MTCT. There is also a real risk of negatively influencing infant feeding practices by HIV-negative mothers and mothers of unknown HIV-status. Experience has shown that in many cases mothers who cannot prepare formula safely and for whom the use of formula was not safe did receive and try to use free commercial infant formula. The ironic thing is that it is really only the better off women, those with better incomes, access to safe water and higher levels of

education, who can safely use free formula. PMTCT interventions providing free formula therefore mainly support these better off women, often ignoring the needs of the poorer women who do not have any alternative to breastfeeding, at least for some months.'

Taken together, several factors contributed to the conclusion that formula was feasible only for educated women living mostly in urban areas: inadequate knowledge about how to prepare, store, or give replacement feeds in a cup; having no clean water, and having no refrigerator. The *safety* of formula feeding received least attention until severe flooding occurred in Botswana (see Chapter 17) when it became very clear how unsafe it was in most African settings. After the Botswana experience, it seemed that the floodgates on notification were opened; suddenly many researchers reported the risks that had been experienced in other countries too, and many more journal editors now seemed willing to publish their findings.

In an eye-opening paper on the perils faced by poverty-stricken populations who abandoned breastfeeding, and citing a respected UNICEF annual publication[61] and a Human Development Report,[62] Anna Coutsoudis wrote:[63]

'There is a global "water crisis", with sub-Saharan Africa bearing the brunt. Lack of clean water kills five times more children than HIV/AIDS and curtails economic growth; sub-Saharan Africa loses 5% of its GDP every year, more than it obtains through aid, due to lack of access to water and sanitation. And, central to this discussion, more than 1.1 billion people do not have proper access to clean water and 2.6 billion lack access to sanitation. There are dismal comparisons between the situation in sub-Saharan Africa as compared to the rest of the world in terms of improved drinking water, adequate sanitation, primary health care services and gross national income. The under-five and infant mortality rates are twice as high in sub-Saharan Africa as compared to the rest of the world; life expectancy at birth is 46 years compared to 68 years. ...the current "water crisis" is not only caused by shortages of physical supplies but is deeply rooted in "poverty, inequality and unequal power relationships"... equity, fairness and the reversal of poverty are not likely to be reached in the near future. We therefore need to engage in two parallel processes: (1) developing safer infant-feeding options for infants of HIV-infected women; and (2) development and poverty-alleviation programmes. The one cannot wait for the other; they need to occur as two simultaneous and interlinked processes. ... We face a replay of the events during the last quarter of the past century, when the global health community opposed the unethical promotion of formula by food manufacturers among impoverished populations. At the time, it was noticed that in developing countries replacement of breastfeeding with formula and other milks and foods was attended by increased mortality and weak growth and development.'

Mixed feeding

The risk of any infection was known to be increased with mixed feeding – when breastfed infants under six months received other foods and liquids besides breastmilk – and unsurprisingly, HIV proved to be no exception. In their 2001 report, Latham and Kisanga confirmed that feeding both formula and breastmilk leads to a higher risk of infection for the infant. The first research showing that this was indeed the case in the context of HIV too had been published in the *Lancet* in August 1999,[17] coincidentally just as the finishing touches were being made to the HIV Infant Feeding Counselling Course, although this important finding was not included on the grounds that it was a single study, and the study itself had been done to look at whether vitamin A would reduce the risk of transmission (it didn't). The physiology behind this phenomenon is described in Chapter 9.

In several studies, even with a good deal of counselling, and with free regular supplies of formula, it had been reported that many mothers did not exclusively formula feed, and therefore added a much higher risk of transmission due to mixed feeding. Reasons for these difficulties varied. To avoid stigmatisation associated with formula-feeding, some mothers might breastfeed when neighbours visited, or in public. Or perhaps a mother would sleep with her baby who then breastfed at night. Practical difficulties in preparing formula at night vs the ease of breastfeeding resulted in mixed feeding.[37] In three African countries where PMTCT pilot projects were being started, it was reported that many mothers came irregularly for their supplies of infant formula, and were breastfeeding when supplies ran out, meaning that they were mixed feeding. In Tanzania 50% of the women who originally decided not to breastfeed switched back to breastfeeding later because of the non-affordability of alternatives and pressure from their husband or family – which would have meant that their babies had received mixed feeding.[6]

Sharing and misuse of formula

Anecdotally, we heard stories of mothers accepting formula from the PMTCT sites, and then selling it on or feeding it to older children while they continued breastfeeding the baby. Nurses in South Africa also reported that women were feeding some of the free formula to siblings and other family members, or that some had been sold in the community.[6] The physiology of lactation makes it impossible to practice a stop-start pattern of breastfeeding; the breasts need to be well drained to go on producing milk, and it takes many weeks to relactate after producing no milk at all. Thus reports indicating that mothers restarted breastfeeding after a long interval are likely mistaken; much more likely is that they never stopped. In this, as in other situations, the lactation community could have been used as a resource to clarify or expose what was really happening.

UNICEF stops providing free formula

In 2002 UNICEF made plans to end the procurement and distribution of free formula.[6] There had been criticism of its misuse, including theft and mixed feeding, elevating the risk of HIV transmission.[64] One of the arguments was that women might be induced into choosing it inappropriately.[65,66] UNICEF planned to direct its support instead to development of national HIV and infant feeding policy and 'give support to the counselling of HIV-positive mothers and helping them carry out whatever feeding option they choose, breastfeeding or replacement feeding, as safely as possible'.[6]

Where governments were interested and had resources to provide free or subsidised formula, UNICEF would support them to conduct assessments of the feasibility, safety, acceptability and sustainability of its use. UNICEF would also provide support to ensure that the necessary conditions were in place to make the distribution of free or subsidised formula as safe and sustainable as possible. Thus, although UNICEF pulled back from actually paying for, providing and distributing free formula to the PMTCT projects, and in fact never did any monitoring or evaluation of their own pilot projects, they offered to help governments to do so.

The 2003 revised guidelines on HIV and infant feeding suggested that several conditions needed to be in place before free or subsidised formula was provided:[67]

- Formula should only be made available to HIV-positive women and their infants under AFASS conditions.
- Implementation and enforcement of the Code should be ensured.
- Counsellors trained in breastfeeding, complementary feeding and HIV and infant feeding should be available for all mothers. Staff should know which HIV-positive women would receive formula, when and for how long.
- Strategies that reduce stigma surrounding formula-feeding among the general population should be in place.
- Health outcomes of formula-fed infants should be monitored.
- Once started, formula should continue to be supplied to infants for at least the first six months of age and preferably up to two years. Formula or milk should also be available for infants of mothers who practice early weaning.
- Countries that provide free or subsidised infant formula for HIV-positive women should consider some type of support to those who breastfeed.
- Supply management should be arranged in the planning phase of programming. Supplies should be monitored to ensure that infants who need them always had them, but that there was no spillover to others. Formula should be procured through the normal channels.

Foreign influence and conflicting views

The infant feeding dilemma had confused many health workers and led to the deterioration of support for breastfeeding in many settings.[5] Developers of the HIV and Infant Feeding Course may have lacked knowledge of local infant feeding norms, though of the personnel who had come to Harare to field-test the course in 1999, one had lived and worked as a paediatrician in three developing countries (two in Africa) for a total of 18 years, and another who represented UNICEF had lived and worked in Kenya, including in breastfeeding support, for over a decade.

Latham and Kisanga had reported that an influx of donor agencies and outside researchers had arrived in Kenya eager to help with the HIV and infant feeding problem.[68] The country had no national PMTCT policy and it was not clear whether suggestions for policy formulation were well balanced or acceptable, nor whether those making them were familiar with local conditions and with breastfeeding. The Kenya UNICEF representative, Dr Nicholas Alipui, had strongly expressed concern that actions to reduce

MTCT of HIV were undermining breastfeeding, creating the possibility of a spillover effect. Most Kenyan health workers had correct knowledge of the importance of early initiation, exclusivity, frequency and normal duration of breastfeeding. However, different government departments, local NGOs, and many external donor-supported large pilot trials showed some confusion, which had filtered down to frontline health workers so that they, in turn, became unsure about what to advise their patients. Many personnel interviewed by Latham and Kisanga stated that until the pilot projects provided strong evidence, breastfeeding as usual was what they would recommend and promote.

Scaling up

There had been a huge disparate effort by scientists (local and foreign) to conduct PMTCT projects beyond the sites supported by UNICEF. Each of the many new sites had different protocols and regimens, and most seemed to have the sole aim of addressing only HIV transmission through breastfeeding. Not one had a central focus to look at the possible negative impacts of formula feeding on malnutrition, morbidity and mortality due to diarrhoea, pneumonia, and other infections, family economics and birth spacing. External forces, including research scientists and even UN agencies, unfamiliar with average living conditions for the poor, added to the confusion, and were unwilling to slow down and consider the real outcome of the actions they recommended or introduced, before moving to much wider implementation.

The initial plan was to provide counselling and testing to 30,000 mothers at 18 sites in 11 developing countries. Two of the pilots took place in Honduras and India so that it could be seen how the introduction and scaling up of programs might differ in relatively low prevalence settings outside Africa.

In Zimbabwe there were initially two PMTCT pilot sites, and in South Africa there were four. In Uganda the PMTCT program was initiated at three sites in Kampala and in four other districts.[69] But in spite of much uncertainty, the initial pilot projects were scaled up to reach ever-increasing numbers of pregnant women. By 2001 over 80,000 women had been seen in the UN-sponsored PMTCT programme. While 19% had tested HIV-positive, only one-third of these had received treatment.[70] The Elizabeth Glaser Pediatric AIDS Foundation was supporting 70 sites worldwide through its Call to Action programme.

Three years after South Africa began implementing its programme attempts had been made to scale it up across all provinces under routine health service conditions. A study was conducted to collect data from all 18 pilot sites for January to December 2002. During this period, 84,406 women received antenatal care and 58% of HIV-positive women, almost 49,000, expressed an intention to exclusively formula feed, but fewer than 1,000 infants were tested for HIV infection at 12 months. What was the fate of the other 48,000 babies? The conclusion was that programme effectiveness was limited by the low rate of HIV test acceptance, poor delivery of nevirapine to mothers and inability to track mother-infant pairs postnatally. However, infant feeding intentions of mothers suggested inadequate counselling and possible negative effects of the provision of free formula milk.[71]

By December 2002 UNICEF reported having supported the planning and/or implementation of PMTCT in 54 countries.[6] However, by June that year, while the number of sites was expanding, the care they provided was questionable; 30% of women who had visited the PMTCT sites had received no counselling. Of those who did, 30% did not receive testing. Of those who tested positive, <50% received ARVs.[5] In 2003 UNICEF recommended:

> *'PMTCT programs must not only expand to new sites but enlarge the scope of activities within existing sites to reach more women and to provide a comprehensive package of HIV prevention and care. This requires human resources and expertise, coordination and collaboration between partners, a well functioning supply system and resource mobilization. Strong leadership and good coordination of the many institutions and individuals involved is critical to successful scaling up. The pilot experience has shown that introducing PMTCT programs into antenatal care in a wide variety of settings is feasible and acceptable to a significant proportion of antenatal care clients who have a demand for HIV information, counseling, and testing. In many aspects, however, programs can be strengthened. As they go to scale, PMTCT programs have much to learn from the pilot phase, during which they successfully reached hundreds of thousands of clients. Hopefully, they can translate this knowledge into better services for many more women, children, and families.'*

As the PMTCT programme was scaled up, the numbers of mothers and babies served became eye-watering. By 2003 it was reported that 205 sites were offering PMTCT services in 10 of the original 11 pilot countries on three continents.[5] Botswana had scaled up its programme to the national level.

By the end of 2004, 48 UNICEF-supported countries had expanded beyond the original pilot sites. By December 2005 UNICEF were supporting PMTCT sites in 79 countries and >100 countries had national coverage.[72] In India alone there were about 300 facilities providing PMTCT services, with a goal to expand that to 780.[73] The PEPFAR programme estimated that 2 million women in 2,200 sites in 15 countries of high HIV prevalence had received PMTCT services. The AXIOS group reported donations of rapid HIV testing and antiretroviral prophylaxis to >600 000 mothers at 7,477 PMTCT sites, mainly in Africa.[74]

Nevertheless, WHO reported that global coverage of PMTCT services was still low; in 2005, only about 11% of pregnant women living with HIV gained access to HIV testing and antiretroviral prophylaxis interventions during pregnancy. Most national programmes had paid little attention to primary prevention of HIV in women of childbearing age: preventing unintended pregnancies among women living with HIV and access to antiretroviral therapy for women and children.[48]

By 2005, UNICEF reported that awareness about PMTCT had been created; national governments' commitment had been demonstrated through the establishment of PMTCT programmes in over 100 countries, of which 13 had achieved national coverage.[69] Over 8.5 million women in countries which accounted for 90% of all paediatric infections had received counselling on prevention of mother-to-child transmission, while 7.8 million had received HIV testing. About two-thirds of HIV-positive pregnant women identified through PMTCT programmes received ARV prophylaxis, which, in most countries, comprised a short course of zidovudine started during the last weeks of pregnancy, or a single dose of nevirapine given at the start of labour. Only 25% of babies in the PMTCT programmes received ARV prophylaxis.

At the end of 2006, 71 countries were implementing PMTCT programmes, and 45% of them had developed national scale-up plans.[75] By 2007, UNICEF supported PMTCT programs in more than 90 countries. In a letter to *The Washington Post* during the 2007 World Breastfeeding Week, UNICEF confirmed that they sustained efforts to ensure that women knew their HIV status, and were given the advice they needed to make informed decisions about infant feeding and the backup to implement their personal decisions.[76] By December 2007 South Africa had plans to increase its PMTCT coverage from 80% to reach all 3,663 primary healthcare facilities.[77]

By 2008, as shown in the following WHO 2010 table,[78] an estimated 105,700,000 HIV-positive pregnant women needing PMTCT services were living in low and middle-income countries of the highest HIV prevalence. All but one of the countries (India) were in sub-Saharan Africa. It was in these countries that WHO estimated that it could have the greatest impact on 'infections averted and lives saved'. WHO planned to focus PMTCT global efforts in the next few years on the 10 countries with the highest number of pregnant women with HIV.

1.	Nigeria	210,000	11.	Ethiopia	36,000
2.	South Africa	200,000	12.	Cameroon	36,000
3.	Mozambique	110,000	13.	Congo (DRC)	32,000
4.	Kenya	110,000	14.	Côte d'Ivoire	22,000
5.	Tanzania	100,000	15.	Burundi	16,000
6.	Uganda	82,000	16.	Angola	16,000
7.	Zambia	70,000	17.	Chad	15,000
8.	Malawi	73,000	18.	Lesotho	14,000
9.	Zimbabwe	53,000	19.	Ghana	13,000
10.	India	49,000	20.	Botswana	12,000

PMTCT need, Estimated number of HIV+ pregnant women in 2008

Source: WHO 2010, PMTCT strategic vision 2010-2015, Preventing mother-to-child transmission of HIV to reach the UNGASS and Millennium Development Goals https://www.who.int/hiv/pub/mtct/strategic_vision/en/ (accessed 2 May 2020)

What was the point?

Latham & Kisanga[69] had written in 2001:

'If the only consideration is to reduce transmission of HIV through breastfeeding then mothers should not breastfeed if they are HIV positive. But if the objective of advice

> *and policy is to do the most good or do the least harm, then the broad range of risks for mothers who opt not to breastfeed their infant from the day of birth, need to be very carefully considered. The pilot PMTCT projects now being undertaken ...are large African experiments using human subjects. They need to be independently evaluated. It surely will be unethical to expand these interventions without a proper evaluation of the outcomes in terms of human wellbeing... Our visits ...revealed strikingly wide differences in the national policies directed at PMTCT. Yet [all the countries] have a relatively high prevalence of pregnant women who are HIV sero- positive, have strong breastfeeding cultures with extremely high prevalence of breastfeeding in early infancy, have access to the same scientific literature on risks of HIV transmission, and on the risks of not breastfeeding. An important question is why have countries responded so differently. Some countries do not have a clear national policy on PMTCT, but in all there are government agencies moving ahead with advice, or there are draft policies, or there have been parliamentary statements, and in three countries there are pilot projects on PMTCT...'*

Failure to record and evaluate the effect of different infant feeding methods on HIV transmission and infant mortality began with the first 11 countries selected for the pilot projects. This omission resulted in loss of data which could have been used to inform locally appropriate, evidence-based HIV and infant-feeding recommendations to guide mothers and health departments alike. As PMTCT projects were quickly scaled up and rolled out, the compounded loss of information on which to inform future decisions and future policy was incalculable.

CHAPTER 16

What we don't know about the outcomes from the PMTCT sites

Before 1996, the international health agencies had heavily promoted breastfeeding, particularly in developing countries, as a natural, cost-effective means of providing optimal nutrition and protection against disease. After 1997, however, the response to the HIV/AIDS crisis succeeded in turning protection, promotion and support for breastfeeding on its head. UNAIDS, UNICEF and WHO now took another tack, invoking maternal rights *not* to breastfeed, asserting, 'It is mothers who are in the best position to decide whether to breast-feed, particularly when they alone may know their HIV status and wish to exercise their right to keep that information confidential. It is therefore important that women be empowered to make fully informed decisions about infant feeding, and that they be suitably supported in carrying them out.'[1]

But making a choice about how to feed their babies proved to be a much more difficult dilemma for HIV-positive mothers in areas of high HIV prevalence than UNAIDS had ever anticipated. The cost of infant formula, along with the clean water and fuel needed to prepare it, was recognised as being beyond the means of poor families in developing countries. The extra medical care required by formula-fed babies would also be burdensome for cash-strapped governments in resource-poor areas. When incorrectly used, or mixed with dirty water, or if instructions were not followed, feeding with infant formula was known to lead to severe malnutrition and fatal infectious diseases. Even in safe conditions, formula could not compete with breastmilk. Use of formula could also lead to stigma and rejection for women who found they were infected with HIV.

Little thought was given to the broader cultural, social, psychological and physiological impact of disrupting breastfeeding. Among Western health experts who worked in the field of HIV/AIDS there was little appreciation of the very high value attached to breastfeeding throughout most of Africa, nor of the political significance attached to the return to traditional infant feeding norms following majority rule in the newly independent African states. Health workers in Zimbabwe had wholeheartedly embraced a return to breastfeeding promotion following a UNICEF training course held in 1989. In 1990, as a newly certified lactation consultant whose ambition was to work with mothers in Harare, in a brand-new profession that doctors and nursing staff had never heard about ('You're a what?'), I quickly realised that breastfeeding was an idea whose time had come. Unlike my overseas colleagues who struggled so hard to get recognition for their skills, I was seen as a practitioner enabling mothers to breastfeed, someone to refer on to, to preserve breastfeeding if there was a difficult problem, to further national policy. There was high social approval of breastfeeding. I didn't need to persuade or advocate at all. Mothers could be seen breastfeeding on street corners, outside banks, inside hospital waiting rooms, everywhere. Local maternity units did not permit the use of formula at all for healthy newborns. Local norms in eastern and central Africa were well illustrated by the traditional perception of breasts as primarily functional, that is, producing milk for the infant, since the Kiswahili word for milk and breast, *maziwa*, is the same.[2]

Sera Young and colleagues had written in 2011[3] that much of the research on postnatal PMTCT had been confined to the biomedical consequences. Yet there had been a range of unintended and often unmeasured psychosocial ramifications. These included physical abuse, rejection by partners, ostracisation by families and abandonment of infants.

Researchers in Malawi described how the PMTCT programme discouraging breastfeeding had been named 'the divorce programme', vividly expressing the local dynamics at work.[4] Interviews in Malawi revealed that a mother's commitment to breastfeed and the husband's commitment to provide for the family were intertwined. Not breastfeeding a newborn was seen as dangerous and unacceptable, except in cases of maternal illness. Men argued that not breastfeeding could entail sanctions by kin or in court. In focus group discussions where men were active participants, they communicated how breastfeeding had a deep-seated cultural significance. In Uganda, breastfeeding was seen as the only culturally appropriate way to feed an infant.[5]

These views were not only confined to rural people, but to well-educated nursing staff in the cities too. Kiersten Israel Ballard,[6] who had come to Zimbabwe to research the acceptability of heat-treated expressed breastmilk as a replacement feed, described how a midwife from Harare placed this stigmatisation within a broad cultural and community context: 'In the African societies, [an issue around] the family, you know is not an individual decision. Although the final decision lies with me, because I decide to do whatever I want to do. But culturally, it's not acceptable. I might have given birth to that baby, but that baby does not belong to me alone. It belongs to the clan'. Corroborating this opinion, one grandmother from Chipinge noted, 'Everyone is affected when the child is not breastfed.' Discussion around community pressures in turn elicited discussion around forms of social control and witchcraft, which surfaced even among urban participants. Participants agreed that using formula, or other breastmilk substitutes, as well as expressing breastmilk, could identify a mother as HIV-positive and thus target her for stigma in the community. 'They will say you have been attacked by AIDS', concluded one mother. The extent to which people framed this stigma as socially alienating was significant. As a father noted: 'You'll be saying to people: I'm infected.'

After listening to the chatter in online discussions among overseas colleagues about how mothers should be supported to freely make their own infant feeding choice, I asked the nurses in the maternity unit at the Avenues Clinic in Harare, where I often provided lactation consults, what they thought about the matter. Should mothers breastfeed, or should they be supported to bottle-feed if that was their choice? The good nurses were shocked by the question. They assured me that mothers had an absolute duty to breastfeed their babies.

In Zimbabwe and in other eastern, southern and central African countries, mothers whose babies were not breastfeeding experienced stigma, ostracism, abandonment or violence, with accusations of being promiscuous, unfaithful, a bad mother, a witch, or a prostitute.[7–9] A project in Zambia found that if a woman did not breastfeed, people would wonder why and suspect that she was engaging in promiscuous behaviour, or was ill (usually with HIV). The decision not to breastfeed might anger other family members and in some cases it might lead to violence from her husband.[10] It would be difficult or impossible for such women to safely offer replacement foods to newborn babies. People could not afford infant formula, and the time needed to boil water and clean utensils would be too great. Community members would suspect they had HIV/AIDS, shun them, think they were crazy, and gossip. Counsellors needed to be careful not to force women into decisions that would cause them or their babies additional physical and psychological harm.

Breastfeeding as an indicator of maternal fidelity

According to Craig Timberg and Daniel Halperin in their riveting book *Tinderbox: how the west sparked the AIDS epidemic and how the world can finally overcome it*, concurrent sexual relationships in eastern and southern Africa had been recognised as one of the main drivers of the spread of heterosexual transmission of HIV. However, there was an unspoken assumption that any singling out of sexual behaviour would be viewed as being 'radioactive' by researchers worried about voicing any moral judgement on African customs.[11] Nevertheless, a report published by WHO in 1995[12] pointed to a fundamental difference in sexual behaviour between Africa and the rest of the world; what was striking were the percentages of men – and women – who reported having more than one regular sex partner at a time, e.g. a wife and a girlfriend, or a husband and a boyfriend. These were an order of magnitude greater than anywhere else and were an accepted part of the culture. Although less has been written about women's concurrent relationships, in Lusaka 11% of women said they maintained more than one regular sexual relationship. And in Lesotho, which went on to have the world's third highest HIV rate, 39% of women did so. The numbers of concurrent relationships in other parts of the world paled in comparison to those in Africa: in Sri Lanka, Thailand and even in Rio de Janeiro in Brazil, fewer than 1% of women had more than one. Several subsequent studies confirmed the WHO findings. The differences were described as 'spectacular'. In Rakai in Uganda, one of the most heavily affected parts of the country, a majority of men and women over the age of 30 reported having had at least one concurrent relationship, more than 90% of which had a period of overlap averaging more than two years. In effect these relationships were a modern variation of polygamy and the speed and pervasive spread of HIV in these populations has been attributed to the network structure created by this pattern of partnerships.

What does this have to do with breastfeeding? The existence of concurrent sexual relationships has profound effects on infant feeding norms in a community, because of the widespread belief that by going to the breast a baby signals to the family that a woman's husband *is* his father – if a baby refuses the breast, the mother is believed to have been unfaithful to her husband. A non-breastfeeding baby can disrupt families and cause women to be abandoned or ostracised, or even murdered. Thus public breastfeeding was and still is not only seen as quite normal, but also to be eagerly desired, since by having a baby at the breast, a mother is able to simultaneously demonstrate not only that she is a good mother, but also that she is a faithful wife.

When I was assisting a client to provide expressed breastmilk for her premature baby in the neonatal unit at the Avenues Clinic, I observed the critical reaction of her in-laws on discovering that the baby was not yet breastfeeding. The mother, on maternity leave from a very prestigious and high-powered job, became very worried. I carefully explained to the grandparents that of course the baby was receiving his mother's expressed breastmilk, and little premature babies always needed some extra time to learn to breastfeed; their tiny grandson would certainly breastfeed well when he grew bigger. But to no avail. Several months later her husband divorced her.

A crying child is not tolerated in African societies and everyone within earshot will urge a mother to comfort an unhappy little one at the breast – something that is not possible unless the baby or child is breastfed. Most African infants are breastfed whenever they cry or are in need of comfort. In most traditional African cultures near-constant mother-baby contact was the norm. Rural mothers often kept their infants with them as they worked in their fields during the day – for example, tying them to their backs and shifting them to the front for breastfeeding. Most infants slept with their mothers during the night and were given free access to the breast. They continued to breastfeed at night well into their second year of life.

Breastfeeding was valued so highly that other feeding methods were simply unknown. During Baby Friendly Hospital Initiative Assessments in Zimbawe, BFHI assessors observed that mothers seemed to be confused by the question about whether their infants had ever received bottles or pacifiers during their hospital stay. The hospitals always scored 100% on this question because artificial milk, teats and dummies were simply not permitted in the maternity units. Assessors were concerned that mothers might assume from the question that they were being neglectful if their babies didn't have these items. There was serious discussion about whether the question should be removed from the assessment forms altogether.

Formula-feeding as an aberration

Almost all studies reported that not breastfeeding attracted strong social stigma and almost counted as 'forced disclosure' of HIV status. Since breastfeeding had always been practised, formula feeding was not seen in the same way as it is in the West – as an exercise of a woman's autonomy – but as an aberration. In Zambia and Kenya poorer mothers in particular faced very strong social pressures to breastfeed. They were afraid to be seen formula-feeding, believing that people would not only suspect that they were ill with HIV, but that they might also be prostitutes, promiscuous, have stolen their babies, or be pregnant again.[13] Breastfeeding during a subsequent pregnancy was traditionally perceived as taboo, since it was believed that the milk became poisonous, requiring immediate weaning. Formula-feeding mothers were also seen to be arrogant, irresponsible or unfaithful to their husbands. Very few mothers thought their relatives and friends would accept them not breastfeeding. Asked about this, mothers responded by saying, 'They will say the mother wants to play', or 'not be happy', or 'want to know why (I'm) not breastfeeding' and 'think the mother has an illness which is transmitted in breastmilk'. Most mothers said they would lie about the reason for not breastfeeding if found to be HIV-positive, and about two-thirds responded that they would definitely not show in public that they practised replacement feeding.[14] In Tanzania, researchers found that strongly held beliefs about the benefits of breastfeeding for the baby and perceived social norms induced deep tensions in HIV-infected mothers who received counselling about breastmilk alternatives.[8]

Although several studies reported that HIV-positive mothers found formula-feeding to be *acceptable* and *feasible*,[15,16] and it was often free, only half of mothers who were offered formula in the Zambian PMTCT projects actually chose it. Family issues were particularly difficult for younger, newly married Zambian women to manage.[17] In Botswana[18] the father and grandmothers of the baby had considerable influence on the choice of infant-feeding method.

Tanya Doherty's empathetic article written for the *Bulletin of the World Health Organisation* in February 2006, entitled, 'Effect of the HIV epidemic on infant feeding in South Africa; When they see me coming with the tins, they laugh at me' asserted that HIV-positive mothers, predominantly young, single and unemployed, struggled to protect their autonomy.[9] Uncertainty about the safety of breastfeeding increased the power and influence of health workers who acted as gatekeepers not only to new knowledge, but also to essential resources such as formula milk. Fear of disclosure of HIV status and stigma weakened mothers' ability to resist entrenched family and community norms that encouraged early introduction of fluids and foods, and that questioned non-breastfeeding. Women who chose to exclusively formula-feed had difficulty accessing formula milk because of inflexible policies and a lack of supplies at clinics. Limited postpartum support led to social isolation and undermined mothers' ability to care for their children.

Although HIV-positive mothers in the PMTCT projects might start out formula-feeding, researchers reported that they often later changed to breastfeeding (or mixed feeding) due to pressure from friends or neighbours, and gave the free formula to older children.[19] However, this would have been physiologically difficult, since once a baby stops draining breastmilk from the breasts, milk production gradually dwindles and stops. Relactation is possible, but difficult; what is more likely is that these women practised mixed feeding from the beginning and then abandoned formula-feeding altogether due to stigma. Thus the success of exclusive formula-feeding depended very much on whether HIV-positive mothers were able to deal with the stigma, and in modifying its cultural acceptability.

In a heart-wrenching study written as a thesis in 2010, Modipadi R. Mugivhi identified the challenges and coping strategies adopted by HIV-positive mothers living in a resource-constrained area who opted for replacement feeding, going against established norms[20] and resulting from the advice, recommendations or even preferences of an infant-feeding counsellor. In certain cases, participants were effectively forced by health care workers to give formula and its use demonstrated the power hierarchy that existed between participants and health care workers, as had been confirmed by others. Mothers known to have formula milk tins from the clinic were easily identified. These tins carried a government stamp and looked different from the tins bought in shops. Mothers often breastfed their babies in public in an attempt to avoid stigma attached to formula-feeding, even when they understood that this could result in a high chance of MTCT of HIV due to mixed feeding. The plain packaging of the formula provided by UNICEF at the PMTCT sites, designed to be Code friendly since it could in no way 'advertise' a brand, nor 'idealise' a product, instead served to identify the recipient as being infected with HIV.[21] If they could afford to, mothers would work around this by buying commercially produced formula and then decanting the UNICEF product into tins bearing company packaging complete with logos, teddy-bears and chubby white babies.

In an attempt to avoid criticism, South African mothers, encouraged by counsellors, used a variety of excuses to explain why they were not breastfeeding.[14] They would say that formula was recommended by the doctor, that their breastmilk was insufficient, or that they had TB, were ill, had breast sores or poison in the breast. Mickey Chopra concluded that dealing with stigma needed to be a fundamental aspect of the counselling of mothers.[7] However, these strategies have had important effects in facilitating later spillover of formula-feeding to the general population.

Disclosure of HIV status to assist formula-feeding

In Nigeria 93% of HIV-positive mothers enrolled in a PMTCT programme in Ibadan were formula-feeding at six weeks after birth. One of the most enabling factors was disclosure of HIV status to the family. The main motivation was 'the desire to reduce the risk of transmission'. The most important influence in maintaining the chosen infant-feeding option was the support of the spouse to address how best HIV-positive mothers could handle or overcome criticisms and stigmatisation by others.[22]

WHO's answer to reducing stigma towards formula-feeding in the community was to suggest in 2004 that managers should ensure that 'HIV-positive women who choose not to breastfeed are not discriminated against, and that they receive help to deal with possible stigma, especially in communities where breastfeeding is the norm. To prevent discrimination, staff may need special training, and certain procedures may have to be adopted or strengthened'.[23] This directive was a little short on specifics, but the intention was clear.

Monitoring and evaluation

There had been no intention to monitor infant health outcomes in the PMTCT pilot projects. Several reports had outlined unforeseen problems such as incomplete, inadequate or erroneous recording of data at PMTCT clinics.[7,24–28]

The pilot sites aimed to test the feasibility and sustainability of carrying out PMTCT programmes in resource-constrained countries, to measure impact, and to guide expansion of successful programmes to other countries.[29] Policymakers omitted important indicators such as HIV testing of infants at birth, and at 4–6 weeks. Indicators for infant morbidity and mortality, and the ability to tie that data to infant-feeding choice, could have informed future infant-feeding policy. Whether formula-feeding saved lives in the context of HIV compared to breastfeeding remained a grey area until 2006. The nursing sisters at the City Health Department in Harare told me that their Zambian colleagues were reporting that formula-fed babies there were 'dying like flies', but there was no data.

In 2003 a UNICEF evaluation of United Nations-supported pilot projects for the prevention of MTCT of HIV[30] recommended:

'PMTCT programs should establish national infant feeding guidelines which include recommendations for HIV-infected women, based on an assessment of local feasibility, acceptability, affordability, safety and sustainability of various feeding options. Also needed are postnatal follow-up protocols including outreach and support groups to help mothers safely apply their infant feeding decision, encourage good maternal nutrition, and address infant feeding after six months. Pilot sites have forged many successful partnerships between the PMTCT program and NGO care and support groups, and scaled-up programs should replicate similar partnerships at all sites...... New measurement tools and systems should be developed through field trials, and expanded programs will require monitoring and evaluation staff.'

Peggy Koniz Booher and colleagues pointed to the importance of documenting experiences.[25] In 2002, when the international scientific community called for an update of the 1998 HIV and infant feeding guidelines, there was interest in reviewing not only the new scientific and medical evidence, but also recent programmatic experience. Specific studies were conducted or were currently in progress to assess various recommended feeding options for HIV-positive mothers and inform programme development. However, much of this experience had not been formally documented. The results of programme evaluations were often shared only internally or with donor agencies. Much of the research had only been presented to select audiences at professional meetings, which were inaccessible or unaffordable to policymakers. The majority of reports had never been published in any systematic or useful way to the global community, making access to this information difficult.

Peggy and colleagues' worldwide search for documents had revealed that systematic evaluations of HIV and infant-feeding programmes were rare. Efforts should have been made to encourage evaluations, more effective documentation and dissemination of experiences by individual programmes. Then there needed to be support and continued efforts to identify and creatively share this information. Koniz Booher and colleagues not only made available their 2004 compilation of evidence in original source documents (the grey literature), but they also provided contact information for editors, researchers, authors, and organisations of the source materials. Their rationale was to encourage future communication, continuing dialogue, and the sharing of materials, ideas, and lessons learned between projects, countries, and regions of the world.

In 2004 Ellen Piwoz also developed a manual for WHO, designed to provide basic guidance to PMTCT personnel about how to conduct local assessments and formative research.[31] Building on previous experience, this document was extremely thorough. She described how findings from local assessments could be used to develop national policies and guidelines for health workers, materials for training of counsellors and behaviour change communications strategies to support safe PMTCT programmes.

Later in 2004 WHO published a guidance document on monitoring and evaluating to inform future planning.[32] Its stated purpose was to determine the success of the programmes, to identify areas where further support was required for scaling-up strategies. Core indicators should include women completing testing and counselling, antiretroviral prophylaxis, HIV-infected infants born to HIV-positive mothers, reported feeding choices at delivery (percentage of women who planned to either exclusively breastfeed or exclusively use replacement feeding) and women receiving counselling on infant feeding at their first infant follow-up visit. So intention was well covered, but, astonishingly, no further indicators were suggested for feeding outcomes or later infant HIV testing.

By December 2004, only 29 countries had a national PMTCT monitoring system, and over half did not have a national PMTCT database. Indicators to monitor and evaluate the programmes were inadequate, with most children being lost to follow-up.[33] Thus the evidence-base from which to gather infant feeding data was never made available, and may not even have existed.

In 2007 UNICEF described how they had been working together with UNAIDS and national governments and partners to develop a core set of coverage- and survey-based indicators that could be used to track progress on the number of HIV-infected pregnant women, the number of pregnant women counselled on PMTCT services and the number who received antiretrovirals to prevent MTCT of HIV. But still there seemed to be little appetite for assessing the effects of replacement feeding.[34]

Wendy Holmes and Felicity Savage wrote in the *Lancet* in 2007, 'Counsellors need training, management, support, and supervision, and health-care services need strengthening to provide this intervention. Health workers should be adequately informed and able to give mothers appropriate help—currently they are not.'[35] There is more than a little irony to this observation. Felicity Savage had not only been involved in the preparation of the text of the HIV and Infant Feeding Counselling Course, but she had also been the WHO representative in charge of its field-testing in Harare in March 1999 and continued to be a consultant to WHO. So she knew that it was simply not true that the mechanism to train, manage and supervise PMTCT project staff was not yet in place. It was, but WHO and UNICEF were simply looking the other way, rather than lending their support to full implementation of the training. Importantly, had previous guidance on HIV and infant feeding been appropriately applied – and in particular if replacement feeding had *only* been used in situations where it was acceptable, feasible, affordable, sustainable and safe – then the best chance of HIV-free survival of all infants from birth would have been assured.

Looking back in 2009, WHO wrote:[36]

'The programmatic effects of interventions aimed at preventing mother-to-child transmission in sub-Saharan Africa have seldom been systematically evaluated. ...The

actual measured impact of scaled up programmes and service delivery, including on HIV infections averted and on maternal and child survival, is not well documented in many low- and middle-income countries except from specific settings or research sites. Most routine data collected on preventing mother-to-child transmission provide information about the processes that deliver these interventions rather than their effect. Assessing how many infants of pregnant women living with HIV ever become infected is difficult for at least two reasons. First, not all pregnant women living with HIV are identified during antenatal care (or women become infected during pregnancy or postpartum breastfeeding), and the infants of these women are therefore not usually tested after birth. Second, in many settings, even when mothers do know their status and have even received an antiretroviral intervention to prevent HIV transmission to their child, relatively few bring their children for testing at follow-up clinics, and tests for infants are not always available.'

Not knowing that formula-feeding was of no benefit and in fact increased morbidity, malnutrition and mortality, meant that policymakers could continue to encourage mothers to exercise their choice to use it without violating any ethical principles.

Loss to follow-up

Information about what happened in the PMTCT sites was additionally hampered by a large number of mothers and babies being lost to follow-up. Between 19% and 89% of infants in the PMTCT programmes in sub-Saharan Africa were not followed up.[37] This meant that the HIV status of most exposed babies could not be known and the effectiveness of PMTCT services generally in sub-Saharan Africa was overestimated. Dr Nigel Rollins also noted that PMTCT surveillance failed to quantify numbers of infant HIV infections averted, often because of poor postnatal follow-up.[38] Most studies had focused on individual aspects of the programme, such as the adequacy of counselling and so on. 'But what we are really interested in preventing is death in children and the number of transmissions', said Dr Rollins.[39] While standard PMTCT surveillance usually involved HIV testing at the antenatal clinic, most children were lost to follow-up shortly after delivery.

Only 19% of Malawian women recruited into a PMTCT program in a rural district hospital in 2005 were followed up at six months. At least nine out of every 10 mothers attending antenatal services accepted voluntary counselling and testing, approximately a quarter tested HIV-positive and were included in the PMTCT programme, but researchers wrote that 'the progressive loss to follow-up of more than three-quarters of this cohort by the 6-month postnatal visit demands a "different way of acting" if PMTCT is to be scaled up in our setting.'[40]

On a global scale, 10% of all infections were in infants and young children, and over 90% occurred through mother-to-child transmission.[41] UNICEF reported in 2003 that most PMTCT programmes planned to follow-up children for the first 18 months of life to monitor sickness and death and to measure HIV transmission rates. However, this had not happened except in research settings.[30] In fact the PMTCT projects often failed to test infants in order to assess whether their strategies were working.

A 2007 systematic review of African ART programmes found that up to 40% of all patients receiving anti-HIV drugs in sub-Saharan Africa were known to have died and 56% had been 'lost to follow-up'.[42] This phrase covered many different interpretations. Those running ART treatment programmes faced very practical difficulties in ascertaining the precise reasons why so many patients did not return for further care, and the authors argued that 'better information on those who are lost to follow-up is urgently needed'.

Susan Burger, a lactation consultant colleague with experience working in developing countries, describes a phenomenon called 'drop-out bias'.[43]

> *'Researchers assume that because things get better after we intervene that it was a result of our intervention. This assumption is subject to drop-out bias. There is the "get better or die" phenomenon seen in nutrition programs. If you track a cohort of children (that means children of a certain age) over time (the same children as they age) then they will always appear to have better nutrition. This is because as they age, the children who are not getting better will get worse and eventually die. Because the dead children drop out, the remaining children are healthier. So, it looks like the program is effective.'*

Issues that complicate comparisons between studies include variations in the length of follow-up and differences in methods used to account for missing data, deaths, and children of indeterminate infection status.[44] Studies that estimate transmission due to breastfeeding require repeated follow-up HIV testing over time. Mothers need to bring infants back at frequent and regular intervals and invariably some mothers are unable to comply. To complicate matters, not all researchers clearly indicate how they handle missing data, losses in their analyses and estimations of transmission rates. In some cases, studies only report their findings on infants who have survived into the second year of life. The length of the follow-up period, as well as the ways that investigators handle infants with uncertain diagnoses, can affect population estimates of MTCT rates by as much as 40%.[45] A Malawian study found that breastfed babies who returned to the clinic for testing had significantly lower perinatal HIV transmission,[46] suggesting that perhaps more formula-fed babies had already died. Thus, the high loss to follow-up in the PMTCT sites could have had a more sinister aetiology. The most likely reason for a mother not to return for follow-up could well have been death of the baby, but this was almost never reported.

A small study from BOTUSA in Francistown, Botswana,[47] had documented poor infant follow-up after the Botswana flooding and how lack of monitoring had hidden what happened, more fully discussed in the next chapter. Of 78 infants diagnosed with HIV, 19 were alive and on ART; 25 had died (13 before starting treatment and 12 while on treatment); 10 were referred for ART but never appeared in the clinic and 24 could not be located. The lack of a medical record system meant there was no way to track HIV-exposed infants over time to document mortality rates. Consequently, it was difficult to estimate the country's MTCT rate accurately. Dr Tracy Creek of the CDC, who investigated what happened, estimated a much higher MTCT rate than the previously reported 4%, which applied only to women who brought their infants for a six-week test. These women were largely those who received good PMTCT care or

ART. Combining the 'known' HIV cases and the incident HIV cases, Creek estimated a 7.8% MTCT rate in 2007. In light of the 2006 diarrhoea outbreak, it was clear that simply providing clean water for formula could not make formula-feeding safe. Infants contracted diarrhoea from other sources. Creek wrote that the goal, or success point, of the PMTCT programme should be 18 to 24 months of HIV-free survival for infants. 'Just an HIV test at six weeks is not sufficient to prove that your program has succeeded. We want better monitoring of HIV-free survival at 18 or 24 months, that means the child is HIV negative and alive. It is not hard to report how many babies test or how many babies are HIV-positive. Reporting the number of babies alive is much more difficult because no one goes back to the clinic and informs someone that their baby has died.'

A 2017 paper described how HIV-infected pregnant and breastfeeding women were offered lifelong antiretroviral therapy (ART) in Malawi. Their HIV-exposed children were enrolled in the national PMTCT programme, but many were lost to follow-up. The researchers estimated the cumulative incidence of vertical HIV transmission between 2011 and 2014 taking loss to follow-up into account. A total of 9,285 children were born to women who initiated ART during pregnancy. At age 30 months, close to 60% were lost to follow-up. Only 2.2% remained in the programme.[48]

Morbidity and mortality

Of course, the risks of not breastfeeding were well known. A 1999 study in the *British Medical Journal* had reported that infants in Brazil[49] who were not receiving breastmilk were 17 times more likely to present with pneumonia at hospital than those receiving breastmilk but no artificial milk. This pointed to the anti-infective properties of breastmilk since, unlike diarrhoea, pneumonia was not related to bacterial contamination of water or infant formula.

Data on the number of infections and deaths according to feeding method was stated to be difficult to obtain. For example, in the Thai government PMTCT research sites, where almost 100% of HIV-positive mothers formula-fed their babies, no morbidity or mortality data were available.[50] This was not the experience of WABA delegates who visited a central African health centre in 2004, who were told by the nurses that it was a great tragedy that free formula had been withdrawn 'because now the mothers have no [infant feeding] choice.' The nurses had apparently only seen one problem with diarrhoea 'when the mother had died and the grandmother didn't know how to prepare the formula'. Yet when the visitors looked at the records they found that 27% of the formula-fed babies had died. Of babies abruptly weaned 10% had died. There were no deaths among those who were exclusively breastfed. Of those who had reached 18 months and survived to be tested, 5% of the formula-fed babies were infected compared to 15% of those who were breastfed. The cause of death for orphaned babies was listed as 'lack of care'. The visitors were able to easily record this data in 15 minutes, but they were told that results from this PMTCT site were never formally reported due to lack of time and money.[51]

Michael Latham and Pauline Kisanga had very strongly urged reconsideration of the use of free infant formula, especially for poor families, and provided economic benefits for only one group of mothers.[52] They had said, 'Without a proper independent evaluation of all benefits and risks, the expansion beyond pilot sites would be dangerous' and concluded:

> *'In general, there is an exaggerated belief in the risk of viral transmission through breastfeeding and a very much unappreciated knowledge of the high risks in formula feeding from birth in poor families. It seems vital that persons involved at all levels have a reasonable knowledge of these relative risks. This lack of knowledge was extremely widespread and included highly placed officials in Ministries of Health; persons responsible for national AIDS policy; programme officers in UNICEF, WHO and UNAIDS; front line health workers; and not unexpectedly ordinary citizens... Based on our findings, and the views of many professionals who really understand current conditions for most poor families... "going to scale" with formula feeding seems unsupportable. To do this without an independent thorough evaluation of the relative risks cannot be justified. Pilot sites are not truly "pilot sites," if they are not very thoroughly evaluated. ...we were not made aware of plans for any adequate evaluation of the relative risks for infants, mothers and families where the option was taken not to breastfeed in poor communities.*
>
> *The facts are we do not have good data to know what the morbidity or mortality rates will be if large numbers of infants from poor families in sub-Saharan Africa are formula fed from the day of birth. But data from better off countries suggest that both morbidity and mortality rates would be very, very high. And sick children need good medical care, which is not widely available in many African countries.*
>
> *It needs to be recognised that, although important, only a relatively small proportion of women attending ANC's will transmit HIV to their infants through breastfeeding. This can be illustrated for 100 women attending an ANC in an urban setting with 12% sero-positive and 33% MTCT.*
>
> | *Of 100 women* | |
> |---|---|
> | *Number sero-positive* | *12* |
> | *Number of infants with MTCT (all methods of transmission)* | *4* |
> | *Number of infants infected through breastfeeding* | *1.3* |
>
> *So only 1 or 2 infants out of 100 mothers attending antenatal clinics in urban areas are likely to become infected through breastfeeding. In rural areas with a sero-prevalence of 5% only about 1 infant out of 200 would be infected through breastfeeding. If 30% of pregnant women were HIV positive about three infants would be infected through breastfeeding.'*
>
> Latham & Kisanga, 2001

Full implementation of the PMTCT sites was undertaken without access to any evaluation of the infant-feeding component of the initial PMTCT programmes. There had been no mechanism built in to record either the number of infant HIV infections averted through formula-feeding, nor the growth, morbidity and mortality of formula-fed vs breastfed children in the poor and unhygienic environments most likely to be found in developing countries.

The UN agencies should have known that interrupting breastfeeding would lead to increased risks of malnutrition, morbidity and mortality for babies in the resource-poor countries which also had the highest HIV prevalence. Subsequent informal reports and data from the research sites show that actually they did know. It's inexplicable that from 1997 to 2009 no UN agencies were formally monitoring the health outcomes of the PMTCT initiative. It seems hardly credible to contemplate that the intention was only to test acceptability and feasibility of formula-feeding, while attempting to ignore its safety and sustainability. This omission enabled the status quo to continue.

The band played on in the PMTCT sites, and nothing changed until 2009 when, rumour has it, attendees at the 2009 WHO Technical Consultation in Geneva threatened to go to the press if WHO didn't backtrack on its anti-breastfeeding stance, and once again endorse breastfeeding as the cornerstone of child survival that it had always been.

CHAPTER 17

Botswana, poster child of the PMTCT programme

Set in the Kalahari, Botswana is a large land-locked country, bounded by South Africa, Namibia, the Caprivi Strip and Zimbabwe. I've only visited Botswana once, crossing from South Africa to drive the very long, dusty, dry, featureless murram road through parched desert terrain, from Lobatse in the south, to Francistown in the east before crossing the border into Zimbabwe at Plumtree.

Botswana is actually a comparatively well-off country, with a population of only 1.8 million in 2005, and home to the largest diamond-mining industry in the world, accounting for 22% of global output, but there is a wide divide between the rich and poor. A letter to *Pediatrics* in 2009 alleged that Botswana had the worst income distribution in the world. The top 10% of the population earned 77 times the wages of the bottom 10%. Half of Botswana's people were living on less than US $2 a day.[1] Almost a quarter of the population were unemployed, while the diamond-mining industry employed only 4%. Food security was problematic due to the government's focus on diamonds and because of Botswana's desert location. A large percentage of Botswana's children were stunted. But Botswana was also almost unique in Africa for being stable and peaceful – you never heard anything about it.

The country was hit very hard by HIV. The first case was recorded in 1984. By 2000 WHO estimated that 85% of 15-year-olds would eventually die of AIDS-related illnesses. In 2002, life expectancy due to HIV/AIDS had plummeted to 36. By 2003, 37% of women were infected. This was the second highest rate in the world, exceeded only by Swaziland and just ahead of Zimbabwe.[2]

Of interest to the lactation community, Botswana is home to the highest population of !Kung San hunter-gatherers, one of the very few peoples left on the planet reputed to breastfeed their babies in the way that nature intended. !Kung babies enjoy truly unlimited access to the breast whenever they're awake, and suckle for short times roughly every 15 minutes. Breastfeeding duration is 3–4 years, leading to natural birth spacing of about four years.[3]

Botswana's PMTCT programme

After establishing a National AIDS Coordinating Agency (NACA) Botswana introduced the first PMTCT programme in Africa in 1999, with initial pilot sites in Francistown followed by the capital, Gaborone, in 2000.[2,4] After the advent of the national ART program in 2002, women testing positive for HIV during pregnancy had access to ART after they gave birth.[2] WHO recommended formula-feeding only if the AFASS criteria were fulfilled, and advocated for individual counselling so women could make an informed choice about infant feeding. However, Botswana's government decided that formula-feeding was best because its citizens had universal access to clean water and could prepare infant formula safely. So lay counsellors and midwives advised all HIV-positive mothers to formula feed. Little consideration was given to hygienic practices and conditions or to access to refrigeration and electricity. Joe Makhema, co-director of a Botswana-Harvard Partnership, established in 1996 to focus on locally relevant HIV research, noted that 'Culturally, breast has always been "best", but the risk of [HIV] transmission basically deterred the policy from advocating, in any way, breastfeeding. And therefore, we went with formula feeding. So with PMTCT… we took the protocols initially from the West'.

Botswana had initially been the only one of the 11 pilot countries to decline free formula from UNICEF. It was extremely proud of its ability to provide 10 tins of formula per month free of charge to every HIV-positive mother until the baby's first birthday. A study in 2001–02 concluded that Botswana met all the UNAIDS conditions for safe formula preparation (an uninterrupted formula supply for at least six months; access to safe drinking water; and the means to boil water for preparing formula and sterilising utensils).[5] However, in 2002 the Ministry of Health and a UNICEF team published a study identifying problems with the quality of counselling and patient education and found that mothers were not using formula correctly.[2]

In 2004, the MASHI study showed that formula-feeding protected infants against HIV infection, but was associated with higher mortality in the first six months of life than the combination of breastfeeding and infant zidovudine. Zidovudine alone was not effective at preventing breastfeeding-related MTCT and did not provide an encouraging alternative to formula-feeding.[6] Despite these results, having made bulk purchases of the three drug combinations needed to treat HIV, the MOH decided to stick with the formula-feeding strategy and work on improving patient education.[2] Botswana thus became the first country in southern Africa to provide free treatment to its citizens, and the PMTCT program was rolled out across the entire country by 2002.

Botswana as an example to the rest of Africa

In April 2001, Botswana's PMTCT program received high acclaim from African leaders meeting at the first African Summit on HIV/AIDS, Tuberculosis and Other Infectious Diseases in Abuja, Nigeria. By the end of 2004, of the 11 countries where pilot projects had been initiated by the Interagency Task Team to demonstrate the feasibility of PMTCT, only Botswana had achieved national coverage with at least 50% of HIV-positive pregnant women receiving services.[7] Botswana became the PMTCT poster child, with its policies and practices held up as an example for the rest of Africa to follow.

By 2005, HIV prevalence among pregnant women in Botswana was 33.4%. The national PMTCT programme continued to provide free infant formula and advised HIV-infected women not to breastfeed. Unfortunately, HIV-negative women also began bottle-feeding their infants, so that an estimated 35% of *all* infants under the age of six months were not breastfeeding.[8] The government was by now spending roughly 6% of its total domestic budget on HIV/AIDS, or about US $100 per capita. But the Botswana PMTCT programme had achieved an 80% reduction in transmission to infants, with an overall rate of only ~7%,[9] and it received high praise from the international community for its approach. William Jimbo, a PMTCT advisor, encapsulated the acclaim when he was reported to have said, 'I think Botswana is different from many other countries because the government put a big chunk of its own money in the budget of HIV/AIDS. And I think at one point they were funding almost 60% of the AIDS budget, which I don't think any other [low-income] country has done. So I don't think that the political will or commitment is demonstrated by just words. They are walking the talk.'[2]

The flood

Then disaster struck. Unusually heavy rains from November 2005 to February 2006 caused major flooding.[5] By January 2006, there was an increase in infant diarrhoea and mortality. The situation was so severe that by February the number of cases and deaths were overwhelming hospitals throughout the country. The Botswana government asked the US Centers for Disease Control and Prevention to investigate. The CDC reported 35,000 cases of diarrhoea resulting in 532 infant deaths in the first quarter of 2006, compared to 9,166 cases and 21 deaths in the same period in 2005.[10] It was found that of the patients hospitalised, 97% had piped water in their homes; this was a situation with a clear sufficiency of basic resources. What went wrong?

Early in the outbreak, health facilities reported anecdotally that most of the seriously ill babies were bottle-fed.[11] Joining the dots, the CDC found widespread water contamination in 26 villages in four northern districts of the country. A variety of pathogens were identified, including *Cryptosporidium*, *Salmonella*, *Shigella* and *E.coli*. Risk factors for bottle-fed babies included contaminated standing water near homes, overflowing latrines, unsafe methods of storing drinking water and poor hand-washing by caregivers. But the most significant risk factor was lack of breastfeeding.[5] Closer evaluation of 154 children, with a median age of nine months, hospitalised for diarrhoea, found that 93% were not breastfeeding. Twenty percent of mothers had stopped breastfeeding before their babies were six months old. Surprisingly, there was no connection between HIV infection and diarrhoeal infection among affected hospitalised children. While 65% of the mothers were known to be HIV-positive (94% had been tested), in fact 82% of the infants were uninfected. The hospitals became overwhelmed by the number of diarrhoeal infections. Among the hospitalised infants, illness was prolonged, with 43% being discharged and then readmitted at least once.

More than half of the babies (51%) developed severe acute malnutrition. It was revealed that most had been growing poorly even before falling prey to diarrhoea, and 21% of them died. HIV status, socioeconomic status, water source, urban vs rural residence and pathogen were not associated with risk of death, but there was a strong correlation between lack of breastfeeding and kwashiorkor or marasmus. Mothers had often run out of formula. Of the babies who had died, mothers had received only half the formula that their babies had needed and 60% had not gained any weight in the three months before they became ill.[8] Dr Creek reported, 'In many cases, mothers returned to clinics multiple times per month but still were not given adequate formula.'

The true extent of infant mortality due to the diarrhoea outbreak remained unknown, since many infants died outside of the health facilities, but according to the CDC estimates, it appeared to be far beyond what was reported above, with 547 excess deaths in three districts alone. Not breastfeeding led to a 50-fold higher risk of diarrhoea and an 8-fold higher risk of dying from diarrhoeal illness. In a presentation at the CROI conference the following year, Dr Creek reported, 'One village we visited lost 30% of their formula-fed babies (and no other babies) during the outbreak.'[8]

An additional irony was that the disaster had happened in Botswana. Botswana had been the continent's flagship HIV control programme, active since 1999, and by 2006 had been providing free PMTCT services to 85% of pregnant mothers with HIV, a much higher percentage than any other country.[5] Formula-feeding among HIV-positive women was virtually universal in Botswana, with 98% of babies in the PMTCT sites being bottle-fed. Promotion of formula had been so successful that even many HIV-negative women were using it, showing that the practice had 'spilled over' to the uninfected population.[12] While there was a low rate of paediatric HIV transmission, Botswana's infant mortality rate was nevertheless increasing, showing that something wasn't working.

Craig Timberg, co-author with HIV expert Daniel Halperin of *Tinderbox*, the book which outlined the successes, failures and missed opportunities in the battle against HIV, wrote in the *Washington Post*[13] that the findings joined a growing body of research suggesting that supplying formula to mothers with HIV – an effort led by global health groups such as UNICEF – had cost at least as many lives as it had saved. 'The nutrition and antibodies that breast milk provide are so crucial to young children that they outweigh the small risk of transmitting HIV, which researchers calculate at about 1 percent per month of breast-feeding'. Hoosen Coovadia, a University of KwaZulu-Natal paediatrician and author of a recent study on formula-feeding, was reported as commenting from Durban, South Africa, 'Everyone who has tried formula feeding... found that those who formula feed [babies] for the first six months really have problems. They get diarrhea. They get pneumonia. They get malnutrition. And they die.' A study by Coovadia and other South African researchers published in the *Lancet* in August 1999 found that breastmilk alone, when not mixed with other foods, was no more likely to infect children than formula.

Timberg's article described how the vast diamond reserves in the landlocked southern African nation had allowed Botswana's government to build a safety net unmatched on the continent, offering its 1.8 million citizens cradle-to-grave support for education and healthcare. And though it had one of the world's highest rates of HIV, with one in four adults infected, it had some of Africa's most celebrated programmes to combat AIDS, including effective measures to prevent mothers from infecting their children during pregnancy and birth.

'The country was also a pioneer in the international drive to protect babies at risk of becoming infected through breast-feeding. In 1997, the United Nations began urging new mothers with HIV to use formula wherever supplies could be provided safely and reliably. Botswana, with an extensive public water system, good roads and a legacy of competent governance, joined the UNICEF-led effort and agreed to pay for the program as a standard service to new mothers... There were skeptics. Some international public health experts, including Coovadia, cautioned that few Africans had the means to prepare formula in a sanitary manner – a process that requires access to clean water, utensils, formula powder and heat for sterilization. And even for those who could make formula safely, some experts warned, breast-feeding's other health benefits could not easily be replaced.'

A grandmother from Botswana in Timberg's article was quoted. 'Since I was a girl, I can't remember a time when we lost so many kids.'

The CDC investigators concluded that the formula programme for HIV-positive women was expensive, complex, and that data from the outbreak indicated that it was not saving lives; Botswana needed to consider whether alternative infant-feeding strategies could achieve higher child survival. Dr Creek believed that one of the first things that Botswana needed to do was promote breastfeeding, especially as 'early weaning is common even among HIV-negative women'. In addition, the example of Botswana had important implications for other programmes.[10,5] The WHO policy had stated that HIV-positive mothers should be given information about both the risks and benefits of various infant-feeding options based on *local assessments* and guidance in selecting the most suitable option for their situation. The problem was that few countries had such data available – and a number of settings were probably encouraging mothers to formula-feed based on an overly optimistic assessment of whether they truly met AFASS criteria. 'Safety cannot be assumed,' said Dr Creek. 'New programmes should verify that formula saves lives in their context *before* widespread implementation.'

The tragedy of Botswana, however, achieved something nothing else had managed to do. Since 2002, nursing sisters in Zimbabwe had been hearing worrying rumours about the fate of dying babies in PMTCT programmes in other countries, but they were only hearsay. The news from Botswana, carefully documented by Tracy Creek of the CDC, finally opened the floodgates to revelations of what had been happening elsewhere. At last, editors of the prominent medical journals seemed willing to publish papers about other countries' experiences. Results from PMTCT sites in Malawi, Zambia, Zimbabwe, South Africa and other African countries soon followed as the importance of HIV-free survival was acknowledged. These findings will be more fully set out in Chapter 21.

In 2008, Anna Coutsoudis and colleagues summarised what happened during the Botswana disaster.[12] They wrote in the *Bulletin of the World Health Organization*:

'Efforts to reduce mother to child transmission (MTCT) of HIV by the use of antiretroviral drugs, caesarean section and formula milks have been extremely successful in industrialized countries and some middle-income countries. These experiences have resulted in implementation of programmes that promote the use of formula feeds in poor populations. There is no doubt that there are small groups in resource-constrained countries with basic

and essential services that allow the hygienic preparation of formula milks. However, for the child population as a whole the unrestrained promotion of formula is generally harmful. Many of these programmes ignore the biological, cultural, social, economic and political contexts in which breastfeeding is embedded.'

The importance of the Botswana experience

In so many ways Botswana is a microcosm of the story of HIV and infant feeding. Before the advent of the HIV pandemic, Botswana was home to an ancient people, one of only two societies left in the world who breastfed in ways almost unchanged since the Stone Age. Then it embraced formula-feeding so enthusiastically that its response was held up to the world as a shining example of the PMTCT programme. This led directly to infant mortality on an almost unimaginable scale, forcing a rethink of global policy. Finally, it was a study in Botswana that demonstrated to the rest of the world that the use of antiretroviral drugs combined with exclusive breastfeeding could reduce the risk of HIV transmission through breastfeeding to virtually nil, allowing breastfeeding to continue when mothers received the treatment they needed for their own health. Looking back, it's hard to believe that all these developments took place in the space of a decade.

There is no doubt that what happened in Botswana exposed the risks of formula-feeding in a way that nothing else had done. It triggered a full investigation, and opened the door for publication of other studies documenting the risks of formula-feeding by HIV-positive mothers in other developing countries. The tragic deaths of the Botswana babies may have saved the lives of many thousands more.

CHAPTER 18

Early cessation of breastfeeding

For HIV-infected mothers who were unable to formula-feed from birth, the next best idea might be to breastfeed for a short time and then to wean as soon as possible. This would permit breastfeeding in the early weeks, when non-breastfed babies were most at risk for other infections such as pneumonia or diarrhoea, but shorten the overall length of time that the baby would be exposed to the HIV virus in breastmilk. In theory this might perhaps achieve the best of both worlds.

The first suggestion that early cessation of breastfeeding might provide an advantage in reducing transmission through breastfeeding was received from Rene Ekpini in 1997.[1] He found that while more than a quarter of mixed-breastfed, HIV-exposed children became infected, breastfeeding longer than six months increased the risk by an additional 9%. The estimated rate of 'late postnatal transmission' was 12%.

However, a short duration of breastfeeding remained an untested strategy. When the idea was first floated, researcher Philippe Van de Perre wrote that it should be regarded with caution.[2] He asked:

> *'What would be the effect of early weaning on growth, morbidity and mortality, if such a policy were adopted by mothers with known HIV-1 infection?... the choice of 6 months to withdraw breastfeeding in order to reduce HIV-1 transmission is arbitrary. The benefits of breastfeeding beyond 6 months in terms of infant morbidity and mortality are well known... The worst case would be to expose infants to the highest risk of postnatal transmission during the first 6 months of breastfeeding and to deprive them of the benefits of breastfeeding when the risk of HIV-transmission is less important. Indeed... although late transmission exists, transmission before 6 months is predominant and accounts for 70% of postnatal transmission. We need to know more about the timing of transmission of HIV and the advantages and risks of prolonged breastfeeding.'*

Early weaning and mortality

The WHO-commissioned study of babies in six countries, published in 2000,[3] had found that the risk of dying of ordinary childhood infections such as diarrhoea and pneumonia declined the older the baby. The protective effects of breastfeeding seemed to be less important for an older baby. This provided the rationale for early weaning. The only problem was that until the HIV pandemic, breastfeeding was so universally practised, that no populations of non-breastfed African babies could be found to study. It was known that the risk of infectious disease was highest in countries with the highest HIV prevalence, especially in neonates (babies aged 0–27 days).[4]

Since 1998 the PMTCT sites had reported on the acceptability and feasibility of formula-feeding by HIV-positive mothers, but had not reported on mortality rates for formula-fed babies.[5–7] A large body of research was available from the late eighties and early nineties in developing countries, showing that extended breastfeeding was protective against under-5 morbidity and mortality. In particular, the 6–24 month period had been recognised as a time of major risk for morbidity, mortality and malnutrition, stunting and wasting even in young children who were still partially breastfed. These interconnected risks were due to:

- Increased episodes of infection due to exposure to pathogens in other foods and liquids
- Inadequate nutrition when other foods and liquids displaced breastmilk
- Reduced food security
- Loss of emotional security provided by breastfeeding

Nevertheless, the plan to promote 'early cessation of breastfeeding' went ahead. The 2005 HIV and Infant Feeding Counselling Tools[8] included the following recommendation:

> *'HIV-positive women who breastfeed their babies are encouraged to breastfeed exclusively and to stop as soon as their individual situation allows it. The decision about exactly when to stop should take into account the affordability of breastmilk substitutes, the woman's available time to prepare them, the pressure she may experience to continue breastfeeding, her own health, and the child's health and development.'*

The same document (page 56 onwards) also contained information for *mothers*:

- Even if you remain healthy, it is best to stop breastfeeding as soon as you can afford to safely feed your baby another way.
- When your baby is under 6 months of age, he/she will need 4–8 500g-tins of commercial formula per month or 9–18 litres of animal milk per month until he/she is 6 months old. The amount of milk needed increases as the baby gets older. This will cost about _______ per month (insert local costs.)
- Once your baby is over 6 months of age, he/she can drink regular animal milk. This still may require some preparation though, depending on the type of milk.
- Another option is to express and heat-treat your breast milk once your baby is a few months old and you feel you can handle it.
- To stop breastfeeding, your baby should be in good health. If he/she is under 6 months of age, he/she should learn how to cup-feed. If he/she is 6 months old or

older, he/she should already be eating other foods.
- Once you stop breastfeeding, you will lose your natural protection against pregnancy. Therefore, you will need another family-planning method.

Once again, the lactation community viewed this latest recommendation with trepidation. Breastfeeding counsellors know that the benefits of breastfeeding into the second or third years of life or beyond are three-fold: nutritional, immunological and emotional. Guidelines on replacement feeding for infants of HIV-infected women tended to focus on the first, pay less attention to the second and completely disregard the third.

Nutritional benefits of extended breastfeeding

Among healthcare workers there was obvious confusion about the ideal time that breastfeeding should actually end. Programme managers expressed concern about how to facilitate early cessation of breastfeeding. Reports were received of PMTCT support staff justifying the recommendation because they believed erroneously that there was little nutritional value in breastmilk after six months. However, the *WHO Guidance for Healthcare Managers and Supervisors* of 2003, on page 63, clearly set out the proportion of the baby's diet which could be met by breastmilk:[9]

'Breast milk is the best food for infants. It provides:
- *an infant's **complete** nutritional needs usually up to the age of **6 months**,*
- *up to **half** of nutritional requirements between **6 and 12 months**, and*
- *up to **one third** between **12 and 24** months....'*

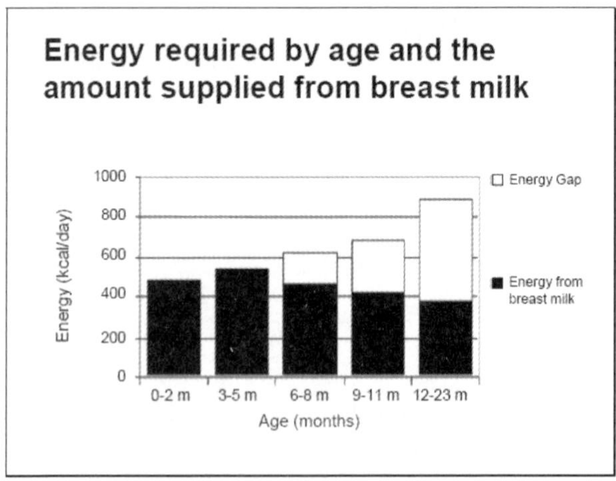

Source: WHO 2006 IYCF integrated course, participants' manual [10]

Continued breastfeeding fulfilled a large part of the young child's energy and protein requirements, which could not be met elsewhere. In their 2001 report on the negative impact that PMTCT policies were having on breastfeeding in African countries,[11]

Michael Latham and Pauline Kisanga had written:

> *'Increasingly we see that a "compromise" is being recommended – a compromise between those advocating only formula from birth, and those supporting breastfeeding as usual. This alternative is short-duration exclusive breastfeeding, and then abrupt cessation, with introduction either of alternatives, or family food. It is important to recognise that in developing countries this also is an almost untested strategy that has its own problems, and its own serious risks. Currently breastmilk even in the second year of life of an African infant provides around 55% of total energy, and a high percent of protein, fat and most micronutrients. How will this be replaced? Will early cessation of breastfeeding not lead to poor growth, and even severe malnutrition? Rutishauser in Uganda in 1975 showed that infants not breastfed in the second year of life had a 28% energy deficit, even though fed on a diet of matoke (plantain), legumes, some animal milk, plus fruits and vegetables.*
>
> *Some MTCT projects (including in Uganda) are suggesting exclusive breastfeeding, and then rapid cessation when the infants are three months of age... It is not even certain that this is feasible, or what problems will arise, or result. We doubt that untested "policies" should be widely promulgated. We recommend these new regimens be carefully evaluated in true-life situations, without subsidisation or free formula, and only in small pilot studies.*
>
> *In the MTCT pilot projects in Botswana, Uganda and Kenya a similar problem might exist for those provided with free infant formula for six months. What in the family diet will be used to replace that after six months of age – an age when in most infants 60-80 percent of energy usually comes from milk, mostly breastmilk in Africa? Some would suggest that animal milks be used to replace breastmilk or infant formula. But in many parts of Africa this is expensive for poor families, and may not always be available. And animal milks as infant foods can produce many of the same risks as infant formula.'*

Immunological protection

As normal weaning progresses, the immunological components in a lower volume of breastmilk became more concentrated than in higher volume early milk.[12] Extended breastfeeding beyond a year provides important protection against many diseases for a young child at a time when he grows more sociable and adventurous and is thus increasingly exposed to new infections. The immunological components in even a small quantity of breastmilk every day provided important protection against disease.[13–16]

Emotional benefits and cultural attitudes towards breastfeeding an older baby

As the nutritional importance of breastmilk dwindles as the child grows older, so the emotional benefits of breastfeeding assume greater importance. In initiatives to promote early weaning for HIV-exposed babies, the emotional benefits of extended breastfeeding for both mother and baby had been overlooked. A mother whose workload was high due to caring for other family members, generating income or growing food for her family, valued the convenience of being able to calm and comfort a curious, active, yet still-vulnerable toddler at the breast.

Cultural practices borrowed from western countries where extended breastfeeding is unusual were set out in the 2005 HIV and Infant Feeding Counselling Tool. While prolonged breastfeeding and mother-baby co-sleeping was almost universally practised in sub-Saharan Africa, particularly in rural areas,[17,18] these 'tips' demonstrated an astonishing under-appreciation of the value placed on breastfeeding in settings where it was regarded as normal, and of the living conditions of most African women. Furthermore, in practical terms, preparation of formula for night-feeding in resource-poor areas, as shown previously, was extremely difficult.

- Women may also wish to find ways to prevent night-time crying, which could disturb other family members. If the woman is worried about these problems, these tips can help her baby sleep through the night.
- Teaching your baby to sleep through the night may make it easier for you to stop breastfeeding completely.
- Getting more sleep may also help you to stay rested and healthy.
- You can start teaching your baby to sleep through the night by following these steps:
  - Breastfeed your baby late at night, before going to bed;
  - Reduce the number of night feedings gradually so that by the time you want to stop breastfeeding, your baby is not waking often to feed;
  - Avoid breastfeeding your baby to sleep; instead, lay the baby down and pat his/her back gently and rhythmically to help him/her fall asleep.
  - Help your baby to learn the difference between day and night: follow the same bathing, cuddling and feeding ritual every night, and don't over-stimulate your baby with loud noise or play before bedtime.
  - If your baby cries at night, see if he/she is cold or uncomfortable or has a wet diaper and rock him/her back to sleep. Babies cry for many reasons, not only because of hunger, so carefully check these things before feeding your baby during the night.
  - If you must feed the baby at night, give him/her expressed breast milk.
  - If possible, avoid sleeping with the baby when you are teaching him/her to sleep through the night. Sleeping together may make it more diffcult to teach him/her not to want to breastfeed upon waking up.

The implications of premature weaning on women

Policymakers and health workers experienced significant difficulties helping women weigh the risks and benefits of various options, including recommendations for premature weaning.[19] In Malawi researchers found that many women were not able to stop breastfeeding as early as the health workers wanted them to. Breastfeeding was the cultural norm, and was not regarded as a mother's personal choice. If the mother's HIV status became known due to early weaning she faced the same risks as if she had formula-fed from birth. Should recommendations for early weaning have been viewed with some concern? Did they attempt to introduce into developing country societies,

Western childcare practices that trivialised both the need for attachment parenting and the convenience of breastfeeding in little one-roomed dwellings?[20,21] Did they suggest that the physiological needs of babies and young children for food and comfort should be ignored? Should babies have been 'trained' not to need their mothers, undermining the enjoyment that each party in the mother-baby relationship gained from the other?

In African societies public breastfeeding received high social approval. A baby's crying was not tolerated and it was normal for a mother to comfort an unhappy toddler at the breast in order to keep him quiet and happy wherever she happened to be. A young child crying in a supermarket would attract hisses and suggestions from other shoppers, both men and women, to offer the breast. A mother would place strong reliance on sleeping with her baby at night to keep him close and safe, and to use the breast as a means to keep her baby content and quiet, so that she and other family members could sleep.

Ellen Piwoz and colleagues summed up the physical and emotional consequences of early weaning for the HIV-infected mother thus; 'Risks for the mother include engorgement, mastitis, an early return to fertility and loss of the wonderful and satisfying power associated with the ability to comfort, calm and nourish an infant in a way no other family member can, predisposing to grief, depression and stigmatization.'[11,22] Should the nurturing role of women have been undermined in this way unless there was clear evidence that there was a benefit? The HIV-infected mother with an already compromised immune system was at greater risk than her uninfected counterpart for mastitis and breast abscess following the breast engorgement and milk stasis that followed precipitous weaning. A sharp reduction in prolactin levels occurring with abrupt weaning would not only negatively affect a mother's emotional state, leading to grief and depression, but would also physiologically guarantee the premature return of her fertility.[23]

The consequences of premature weaning on the breastfed baby

While Western societies have a particularly callous attitude to early weaning and the distress that it can cause, there is evidence that early trauma can have long-term negative effects on immune function[24] and that attachment insecurity leaves individuals more susceptible to disease,[25] meaning that children who are under emotional stress may be more vulnerable to infection.[26,27]

Some experts noted that it was irrational to promote early weaning for an infant who had escaped HIV transmission during the time of greatest risk – birth and during the early months of breastfeeding – only to expose him to an even greater hazard to his survival later through formula feeding. Others suggested that if a mother lived in conditions where replacements for breastmilk were not likely to be acceptable, feasible, affordable, sustainable or safe from birth, they were unlikely to be any safer when the baby was older.

Breastfeeding experts had shown that an extended period of breastfeeding is a species-specific adaptation of the human mammal which spreads women's reproductive load between pregnancy and lactation to assure the survival and optimal development of the especially vulnerable and late-maturing human baby.[28] Research indicated that the physiological period of breastfeeding for our species is at least 2.5 years and may be as long as seven. Unless there was compelling evidence to demonstrate that early cessation of breastfeeding would provide a child survival benefit in areas of high HIV-prevalence, coincidentally the same areas where long-term breastfeeding was still routinely practised and sorely needed to protect against the major killers of young children, the conservative course would be not to disturb it.

Mortality and early weaning

Sera Young and colleagues, in their excellent review of knowledge and research on infant feeding in the context of HIV,[29] noted that multiple studies in low-income settings had documented increased morbidity and mortality associated with early cessation of breastfeeding. In Uganda, breastfeeding for only four vs nine months or in Malawi for six vs 9–12 months, led to more severe gastroenteritis; in Zambia there was low weight gain at 4–16 months, and inadequate diets in Zimbabwe for prematurely weaned babies. The 2006 flooding in Botswana exposed the risk of gastrointestinal disease for babies weaned too soon. In summary, not breastfeeding increases morbidity and mortality in HIV-exposed and unexposed children in developing and industrialised countries.

Other researchers and reviewers also raised questions about the advisability of recommendations for early abrupt cessation of breastfeeding and some concluded that the option of exclusive breastfeeding with premature weaning was not considered feasible.[30–34] In a very thorough review paper, Louise Kuhn and Grace Aldrovandi[35] described disconcerting findings uncovered by researchers who initially theorised that shifts away from breastfeeding simply to avoid HIV would not result in adverse health outcomes.[36] They observed substantial elevations in mortality in babies of women who elected not to breastfeed.[37] There were consistently worse outcomes or at best no benefit to artificial feeding in several other programmes, even after other treatments to prevent MTCT had been taken into account.[38–41] Kuhn and Aldrovandi also wrote that four separate cohorts (two in Malawi, one in Kenya, and one in Uganda), had reported elevated morbidity and mortality due to diarrhoeal disease at the time of weaning.[42–45] All of these studies had included education and counselling, close monitoring and follow-up designed to make early weaning safe. But as it happened, the situation was so bad that two of the studies were interrupted by their data safety and monitoring boards, which noticed the elevations in morbidity after weaning.[43,45] Subsequent comparisons with historical cohorts at the same sites revealed even worse outcomes in spite of access to antiretroviral therapy and prophylaxis and improvements in services for children. Significantly, all four groups of researchers had revealed their findings in early February 2007 at the 14th Conference on Retroviruses in Los Angeles. This had been within just a few months of publication of Tracy Creek's shocking results from the year before which had first blown the lid on the very high death rate for formula-fed babies in the PMTCT programmes.[46] News of this disaster had first been presented at the Durban PEPFAR meeting in August 2006, but now Dr Creek had re-presented her findings at the Los Angeles conference.[47]

Difficulties in implementing early cessation of breastfeeding

A 1988 paper had shown the importance of extended breastfeeding, and of breastmilk itself as a weaning food resource.[13] In a very comprehensive paper on 'Issues Risks and Challenges of early breastfeeding cessation to reduce postnatal transmission of HIV in Africa',[22] Ellen Piwoz and colleagues gave the opinion that implementation of early breastfeeding cessation might prove difficult. Breastfeeding in all countries studied typically lasted a minimum of 18 months, and the use of bottles in eastern, central or southern Africa was very infrequent. Frequent day and night time feedings and the unavailability of other means to comfort infants accustomed to suckling at the breast represented additional obstacles to success.

A study published in 1998 had followed mothers of infants aged 12–24 months to assess breastfeeding practices around the time of weaning.[48] The median age at the first weaning attempt was 17.5 months. Just over a quarter of women had tried and failed to wean their infants by 12 months of age, and almost two-thirds had attempted to wean but relactated. The weaning-relactation cycle was found to occur as early as three months and as often as four times during the first two years of life. Two-thirds of those who relactated did so because the child cried excessively and 16% because the child would not eat. Mothers were especially reluctant to wean because their poverty left them with few foods to use to entice reluctant or picky toddlers to eat, while breastmilk provided an excellent source of nutrition.

Early cessation following exclusive breastfeeding

By 2005 no results had been published to support early weaning. Nor had there been any research to show the extent of HIV transmission during continued partial breastfeeding after six months of age for infants who had been exclusively breastfed for the first six months (i.e. for those whose immature intestinal mucosa had not been damaged by too-early mixed feeding). Instead, the guidance was misunderstood by counsellors and mothers alike. All experienced severe difficulty in trying to make formula-feeding safe and sustainable in conditions where it should never have been considered.

Professor Ted Greiner had organised a satellite session on breastfeeding at the Toronto International AIDS Conference in 2006. A wealth of information on the experiences of early weaning was presented at this event. Healthcare staff were generally confused about how to counsel HIV-positive mothers and they felt especially distressed by working with HIV-positive women to help them fulfil the early weaning part of the new WHO guidance.[49]

- A Zimbabwean study on the feasibility of early breastfeeding cessation at around six months was presented by Naume Tavengwa, a Zimbabwean nurse I had known in Harare, who now worked for the ZVITAMBO project.[50] Eleven of 12 mothers stopped breastfeeding after receiving their infant's HIV-negative test result at six months. Most weaned very rapidly – six within two days and five within one week. 'Mothers had difficulty accessing replacement milks and nutritious foods due to economic constraints and food insecurity'. Eight of the 12 mothers who planned on weaning at six months said that they could not afford milk, and 10 said it was hard to get the variety of foods for a balanced infant diet.

- Dr Nigel Rollins , who had worked on HIV and infant feeding projects in Kwa-Zulu Natal, and now works for WHO, reported on a South African study comparing HIV-positive and HIV-negative women counselled antenatally on infant feeding according to the WHO recommendations. 'We interviewed women before, during and after cessation of breastfeeding about their experiences, and it was very humbling. It really is hanging out our dirty washing because even though we thought that we had a reasonable support network, the women find [abrupt weaning] uniformly awful, isolating and very, very stressful... There's obviously the nutritional needs that need to be met, but one of the main messages from our side was that crying was the major driver of mothers' responses and in a way, *crying is the new risk factor for mother-to-child transmission*. Because it is crying and the behaviour of the child that drives mixed feeding. The staff were very clear on the fact that exclusive breastfeeding was protective and that with the introduction of other feeds the risk increases, but it is the crying of the baby in public that really drives mothers' behaviours in many situations… the counsellors have the very same [stressful] experience [as the mothers]. They didn't know where to go, they didn't know what to do, and it said that we have to have a much more structured set of counselling tools and awareness around this whole process.'
- A researcher from Tanzania said that the likelihood of feeding difficulties after partial weaning was high, because many mothers hadn't formed a clear plan of how they would feed the infant once it was weaned.[51]
- Describing the difficulties mothers face in Burkina Faso, Dr Alfieri described how in the first couple of days after weaning, 'many mothers start a "quest for food" that ends with various feeding patterns,' and when no suitable alternative food can be found, it must be difficult to stick to weaning – especially when the baby is hungry and crying.[52]
- In another presentation from Tanzania, which was published the following year,[53] Sebalda Leshabari also noted that counsellors lacked confidence and had high levels of stress and frustration. She said that there was 'an urgent need of updated training on HIV and infant feeding, review of pre-service curriculum and provision of tangible tools (quick reference) to be used during counselling.' Counsellors didn't know how to assess women´s individual situations in order to advise mothers about which infant feeding options were best for them. But a grave finding was that the counsellors simply didn't agree with the programme recommendations – exclusive breastfeeding or exclusive formula feeding – 'since both violated cultural norms... and they expressed reluctance in promoting those options perceived to be culturally unacceptable.'
- Another study at four sites in South Africa, Namibia and Swaziland,[54] reported that clients as well as counsellors described encounters as disempowering. 'Counsellors experience burn-out and clients report feeling judged, blamed and stigmatised... MTCT Infant Feeding Counselling, because of its nature, is drawn into the "minefield around motherhood and sexuality". With such an emotionally charged issue, the results can be disastrous when counsellors are biased against one or the other infant feeding practice. It is a very common occurrence for healthcare workers

to push mothers with HIV to formula feed to avoid HIV-infection, even without determining whether replacement feeding is safe or available.'

- Kagoda and Bakaki noted in their study[55] that criteria for determining whether formula feeding is truly AFASS before six months had been extensively discussed. However, counsellors and mothers needed similar training for determining whether adequate replacement foods are available to provide an infant upon weaning. 'Several infants suffered from diarrhoea, malnutrition or even death following cessation of breastfeeding. This appears to be relatively common when quality replacement foods are either not available or not adequate – and when mothers are unprepared for what they will do after weaning.'
- Some studies and programmes provided HIV-positive mothers with free or low-cost food supplements, such as Plumpy'Nut, previously used to treat severely malnourished children in Malawi. A sub-study of the BAN trial reported fairly good experiences using a locally produced spread made up of peanut butter, milk, oil, sugar, and micronutrients as a high-energy breastmilk replacement for infants.[56] Other studies used fortified flours which could be cooked up and served as gruel. As part of the Kesho Bora study of ART in breastfeeding mothers in Burkina Faso, a local flour producer and French food technologists (NUTRIFASO) collaborated to develop a locally produced AFASS baby food for weaned infants.[57] Feeding the baby about two to three cups of the gruel (made from half a cup of dry flour) and two cups of milk a day was estimated to meet his or her nutritional needs.
- The PMTCT programme in Haiti pioneered the addition of a nutritional and educational support programme for infants over nine months of age (when formula supplies ended). Mothers were given monthly food rations and money (~US $4) with which to buy provisions as children were weaned. According to Dr Ralph Ternier and colleagues, the programme was 'universally praised by the mothers... and was a relatively inexpensive addition to the program.'[58]

No survival benefit to early weaning

Dr Louise Kuhn, a researcher on HIV and infant feeding in Zambia, who became a champion of maintaining breastfeeding in the face of HIV, gave a disarmingly honest account of her research on early cessation of breastfeeding:[59]

> *'To our knowledge, no randomized study of how to support exclusive breastfeeding among HIV-infected women has yet been undertaken – a serious missed opportunity for operational prevention research. An even more serious confusion that arose out of discussions of the observations that exclusive breastfeeding reduces HIV transmission was the conclusion that all breastfeeding should stop when breastfeeding is no longer exclusive. WHO in an attempt to be responsive to new scientific findings issued a specific recommendation about the importance of supporting exclusive breastfeeding for HIV-infected women who elected to breastfeed. For reasons that remain unclear, almost everyone understood these recommendations to mean that exclusive breastfeeding should be supported for* ***no longer than*** *6 months and then women should be encouraged to stop all breastfeeding abruptly. We stand accused as one of the teams of investigators who*

thought that it was so plausible that a short period of exclusive breastfeeding followed by abrupt cessation of breastfeeding was the optimal strategy to preserve HIV-free survival that we designed a randomized trial to test just that. ***Unfortunately, we were dead wrong!***

As we published our results showing that early weaning neither improved HIV free survival nor was safe in terms of protecting survival of exposed-uninfected and infected infants,[60] we found ourselves up against a community who had already begun implementing this approach thinking it was the recommendation of the WHO!

As part of our trial, 958 HIV-infected women in Lusaka, Zambia were randomized to either stop breastfeeding abruptly at 4 months or to continue breastfeeding for their own preferred duration. ...Despite our best educational efforts, early weaning was not well-accepted by the study population. Thus, it became essential, in the interpretation of our results, to analyze the data based on actual feeding behaviors. What we observed was that infants born to women who adhered to their assignment and weaned early as instructed, had worse outcomes than those whose mothers ignored their random assignment and continued breastfeeding; as did infants born to women who refused to adhere to their assignment to the control group and weaned early.[61] Benefits of breastfeeding on infant and young child survival persisted into the second year of life to around 18 months.[62] Benefits of continued breastfeeding were also observed for child growth[63] and for diarrheal morbidity and mortality.[64]

The emotional consequences of abrupt weaning

Piwoz and colleagues[22] gave a harrowing account of what can happen during premature weaning. Early and rapid cessation of breastfeeding can cause physical and emotional trauma for both members of the breastfeeding dyad. Infants may experience dehydration, refusal to eat, malnutrition, cognitive and social deficits associated with disruption of the mother-child bond, and a higher risk of abuse and neglect. Citing previous research, Piwoz's team described how rapid cessation of breastfeeding causes trauma for the infant, manifested by intense crying. Alternatively some infants may also become silent and withdrawn, especially if they are becoming malnourished. Young infants who are not accustomed to other foods can quickly lose weight when taken off the breast. Additional short-term negative consequences demonstrate the grief a baby can feel. These may include a reversal in motor and language development, emotional disturbances (intense sorrow, resentment, crying, temper tantrums), learning difficulties and physical problems (illness, weight loss, loss of appetite, and loss of sleep).

For an infant, breastfeeding confers a special claim to the mother's care and attention, which cannot be assigned to others. When breastfeeding stops, infants lose this special claim, and they can be – and often are by tradition – 'handed-off' to grandmothers or siblings. For young infants, if rapid cessation of breastfeeding results in consistent physical or emotional distance from the mother, the attachment process will be drastically interrupted, and the impact can be severe, pervasive and long-lasting. Insecure, ambivalent, or disorganised attachments are associated with multiple effects on children, including increased stress reactivity, anorexia, non-organic failure to thrive, limited exploratory competence, and later behaviour problems in preschool, elementary school, and high school as well as psychopathology in adolescence. The list goes on. Research had shown that attachment problems were also associated with limited competence in the domains of peer relations, conduct, school, work, and social activities. Proximity, physical contact and responsive caregiving all play a major role in attachment formation. All three would be threatened by physical or emotional separation during early cessation of breastfeeding.

When they are removed from the breast, infants lose their main opportunity for suckling and skin-to-skin contact, major sources of comfort and warmth that come with breastfeeding. Being deprived of both breastmilk and comfort can make infants angry, frustrated, hungry, and sad, and they are likely to become fussy and cry. Turkana mothers in Kenya, like mothers in many other African societies, abruptly stop breastfeeding when they become pregnant, and this is a 'traumatic event for both mothers and children'. Children respond with 'frequent tantrums, loss of appetite and refusal to eat'.[65]

I had experience of the negative effects of sudden weaning in Harare when my housekeeper's wife weaned their 18-month old daughter abruptly on discovering that she was pregnant again. The family lived in the little *kaya* (Shona for house) on my property. I'd been alerted to a problem by hearing the little girl crying. I'd done my best to persuade my cook that the baby wouldn't be harmed by continued breastfeeding during a superimposed pregnancy, in spite of the traditional belief that the milk turned 'poisonous', but his wife was not persuaded and refused to return the baby to the breast. A month or so later, my cook told me the little one was was sick and not eating. She had also stopped talking and was no longer walking. Her face and legs were puffy, and she was sad and listless. The local clinic diagnosed kwashiorkor, the extreme protein deficiency first described by Cicely Williams in 1935, which leads to oedema and severe malnutrition.[66] My shame and distress that this had happened on my property, under my nose, was profound. We fed the little girl up with extra little protein-rich meals and she recovered, but knowledge of the consequences of premature weaning has stayed with me since.

The effects of premature weaning are not only borne by the baby. For the mother, weaning grief is an unrecognised but nonetheless real phenomenon.[67] In practical and hormonal terms, her body behaves as if the baby has died. Children of mothers who suffer long-term depression are at higher risk of maternal neglect and abuse. Mothers who are depressed and have low levels of social support and/or high levels of stress are significantly more likely to maltreat their children. Recent evidence indicates that childhood neglect is associated with reduced brain volume, failure to thrive and personality disorders during early adulthood. Ellen Piwoz wrote that HIV-positive mothers who are considering abrupt cessation of breastfeeding may already face a lack of traditional support networks and enormous added stress associated with their HIV status.[22]

Elevated viral load

Anthropological studies report that even mothers of toddlers frequently suffer swollen and painful breasts during abrupt cessation of breastfeeding and that has certainly been my own clinical experience. Mothers thinking about weaning often don't realise that they may still be producing 500–750ml of breastmilk in each 24 hours. Abrupt weaning can cause a cascade of physical problems, which can be exacerbated in an in immuno-compromised HIV-positive mother – engorgement, plugged ducts and mastitis, which can lead to breast abscess.

HIV concentrations in breastmilk during abrupt weaning are higher than usual. The viral load in the milk can become elevated with engorgement, whether it occurs at the beginning of lactation, during mastitis, or during suppression of lactation, and the mechanisms are discussed in Chapter 8. Data from Zambia showed that elevated viral load in breastmilk occurring during weaning entirely explained the higher-than-expected transmission rates in those who stopped breastfeeding early.[68]

The futility of early weaning

Early breastfeeding cessation had seemed like a viable approach to reduce postnatal transmission of HIV by shortening the duration of breastfeeding. But this plan was not well thought-out. It ran counter to traditional practices, and posed serious risks to mother and nursling. In another 2010 article Kuhn and Aldrovandi[69] wrote:

> *'The older the child when all breastfeeding ends, the less there is to gain. In essence, the horse is already out of the barn. Because there is less to gain by early weaning, the risks take on greater weight. Even a small increase in mortality can offset a small benefit of HIV prevented. ... analysis of the actual practices of [their own study population in Zambia] revealed that the magnitude of benefit (i.e., the amount of HIV prevented) was almost the same as the magnitude of the harm (i.e., the numbers of deaths caused in the population overall). Overall in the study population, women who stopped breastfeeding by 5 months added an HIV transmission rate of 1.1% after 4 months and a mortality rate in the uninfected children of 17.4%. Women who continued breastfeeding for 18 months added a transmission rate of 11.2% of late postnatal transmission and a mortality rate of 9.7% . These data are in the absence of either maternal antiretroviral treatment or extended antiretroviral regimens that continue during breastfeeding. Because these interventions reduce postnatal transmission considerably, it can be extrapolated from these results that the magnitude of mortality caused by artificial feeding will be larger than the magnitude of HIV transmission prevented.'*

In 2013, Philippe Van de Perre, the French expert who had been involved in HIV and breastfeeding research since the very beginning, asked how evidence-based public health policies for PMTCT were. 'The benefit of abrupt weaning for HIV exposed infants and their mothers was based only on "best guess" opinions of experts and on extrapolations of the risks and benefits of various durations of exposure.'[70] Abrupt weaning at six months postpartum was perhaps not such a good idea after all.

CHAPTER 19

Animal milks: errors, omissions and experiments

The WHO Technical Consultation of April 1998 affirmed the use of home-prepared, as well as commercially manufactured, breastmilk substitutes as a means to reduce the risk of mother-to-child transmission of HIV.[1] WHO specified that:

> *'From birth to six months of age, milk is essential, and can be given in the form of commercially produced infant formula; or home-prepared formula made by modifying fresh or processed animal milk, which should be accompanied by micronutrient supplements.*
>
> *Families need careful instruction about the preparation of adequate and safe replacement feeds, including accurate mixing, cleaning and sterilising of utensils, and the use of cups to feed infants instead of bottles.'*

Home-prepared formulas could be made from various powdered or full-cream animal milks (cow, sheep, goat, camel, buffalo) with added water, sugar and micronutrients. Exhaustive recipes were included in the WHO 2000 HIV and Infant Feeding Counselling Course.[2] Because of concerns about inadequate vitamins and mineral content, extra sachets of micronutrients were to be provided by UNICEF. The WHO 2006 Integrated Course on Infant and Young Child Feeding[3] also provided recipes for the preparation of various types of animal milks as home-prepared replacements for breastfeeding.

Home-prepared formula was defined as 'A breast-milk substitute prepared at home from fresh or processed animal milks, suitably diluted with water and with the addition of sugar and micronutrients.'

Powdered or full-cream milks

In 2004, C. Papathakis and Nigel Rollins from the Africa Centre for Health and Population Studies, Mtubatuba, Kwa-Zulu Natal, asked whether WHO/UNAIDS/UNICEF homemade formulas made from powdered milk or full-cream liquid milk were appropriate feeds for South African babies.[4] Preparation was time-consuming. Babies needed to be fed 6–8 times a day and it took nearly half an hour to optimally

Recipes for Home-Prepared Formula

Fresh cow's, goat's or camel's milk

40 ml milk	+ 20 ml water +	4g sugar =	60 ml prepared formula
60 ml milk	+ 30 ml water +	6g sugar =	90 ml prepared formula
80 ml milk	+ 40 ml water +	8g sugar =	120 ml prepared formula
100 ml milk	+ 50 ml water +	10g sugar =	150 ml prepared formula

Sheep and buffalo milk

30 ml milk	+ 30 ml water +	3g sugar =	60 ml prepared formula
45 ml milk	+ 45 ml water +	5g sugar =	90 ml prepared formula
60 ml milk	+ 60 ml water +	6g sugar =	120 ml prepared formula
75 ml milk	+ 75 ml water +	8g sugar =	150 ml prepared formula

Evaporated milk

Reconstitute with cooled, boiled water according to the label to the strength of fresh milk. Then modify as fresh milk by dilution and adding sugar. Check with specific brand. A typical recipe is:
32 ml evaporated milk + 48 ml water to make 80 ml full strength milk
plus 40 ml water + 8 g sugar = 120 ml prepared formula

Powdered full-cream milk

Reconstitute with cooled, boiled water according to the label to the strength of fresh milk. Then modify as fresh milk by dilution and adding sugar. Check with specific brand. A typical recipe is:
10 g powdered milk + 80 ml water to make 80 ml full strength milk
plus 40 ml water + 8 g sugar = 120 ml prepared formula

If mothers will use powdered full-cream milk or evaporated milk, provide a recipe specific to that brand. State the total amount of water to add both to reconstitute to the strength of milk and to dilute to make formula.

Micronutrient supplements should be given with all these kinds of home-prepared infant formula.

Source: page 130, WHO Infant and Young Child Feeding Counselling: An Integrated Course. Participant's Manual

prepare 120ml of replacement feed from powdered milk or commercial infant formula and 30–35 minutes to prepare a formula from fresh milk. Home-prepared formula cost approximately 20% of a family's monthly income averaged over the first six months of life. When mixed with water, sugar, and UNICEF micronutrient supplements, these milks provided inadequate quantities of vitamins and minerals. No home-prepared replacement milks in South Africa met all estimated micronutrient and essential fatty acid requirements of infants aged <6 months. Commercial infant formula was the only replacement milk that met all nutritional needs. Papathakis and Rollins were specific about the shortcomings in various components, and recommended a revision of the WHO/UNICEF/UNAIDS guidance.

Different preferences

Opinion was divided. In the Indian PMTCT programme, because formula was considered to be too expensive, the only recommended alternative to breastfeeding was modified cow or buffalo milk.[5] Mothers in Kenya and Tanzania[6] thought that cows' milk was an acceptable option for HIV-positive mothers to use if the family owned a cow.[7] However, mothers in Myanmar thought that animal milk was too expensive and too complicated to prepare several times a day.[8]

Subsequent research asked whether home-prepared formulas using animal milks were suitable for feeding infants in the long term.[9] Even with the addition of micronutrients, there were some serious inadequacies. At the WHO HIV and Infant Feeding Technical Consultation held in Geneva in October 2006, André Briend presented a review of evidence on the adequacy of home-modified animal milk for replacement feeding in the first six months of life. Dr Briend had been retained by WHO as a consultant on severe acute malnutrition. He was coincidentally the co-inventor of Plumpy'Nut, the nutritional supplement used then and today to treat severe acute malnutrition in young children. Dr Briend described how modifying animal milk for feeding infants <6 months raised difficult technical challenges. Firstly, the currently recommended recipe would need to have an increased essential fatty acid content, e.g. by adding daily small amounts of vegetable oil in quantities that would need to be adjusted according to their essential fatty acid composition and the weight of the child. The feasibility of this approach had never been tested in the field. Secondly, the present recommendation for adding a mineral and vitamin mix to the recipe had not proved feasible to implement in practice, even on a pilot scale. Giving a mineral and vitamin supplement once a day to the child as a drug or mixed with a feed might be possible, although the safety of this approach would be a concern if the supplement contained iron. Dr Briend described high rates of hospitalisation in India among young infants receiving home-modified animal milk. In addition, he also discussed the South African study which had found that no home-prepared animal milks met all estimated micronutrient requirements. Other major concerns were bacterial contamination and the difficulty mothers experienced trying to prepare correct dilutions. *No* examples of successful use of home-modified animal milk in the first six months of life had been demonstrated on a large scale. Dr Briend concluded that in view of the technical difficulties, home-modified animal milk should *not* be recommended as a feasible and safe long-term replacement feeding option in the first six months of infancy. Only in situations where access to commercial infant formula had been temporarily interrupted should home-modified animal milk be considered for short-term feeding of non-breastfed infants <6 months of age.

Ready-to-feed infant formula

Ready-to-feed infant formula, a breastmilk substitute which has been available for babies in resource-rich settings since 1960,[10] appears never to have been considered for babies in resource-poor settings. Powdered infant formulas are not sterile. The powder itself may contain low levels of *Salmonella*[11] or other contaminants,[12,13] raising the potential for outbreaks of diarrhoea, even in industrialised countries. This means that the choice of replacement feeding in any population should not be undertaken lightly.

Midwife Sue Jarman described to me how as a staff midwife in 1973 her hospital in England provided ready-to-feed formula to all newborns until the mother's milk came in on day three after birth.[14] Although preparation was difficult early on, since the mixture needed to be sterilised, later ready-to-feed preparations became available in cartons, obviating the need for any form of preparation, heating or sterilisation. This would have made it the obvious solution for circumventing the many difficulties inherent in ensuring safe feeding with artificial baby milks in resource-poor settings.

The extra risks of powdered infant formula for the youngest babies had been known for several years. The United States Federal Drug Administration (FDA) bans powdered infant formula in all newborn nurseries.[15] First Steps Nutrition Trust is a UK organisation that advises healthcare personnel and parents on the safety of breastmilk substitutes. Citing other experts, they described in a 2013 publication that powdered infant formulas may contain harmful bacteria[16,17] or be contaminated with *Salmonella* and *Enterobacter sakazakii*. In healthy infants, consuming small numbers of bacteria in powdered infant formula milks does not lead to illness. However, younger or pre-term or low birthweight infants are more susceptible. Infants of HIV-positive mothers are also at risk because they may be immunocompromised.

Enterobacter sakazakii was first described as a new bacterial species in 1980. It is a Gram-negative rod-shaped bacterium classified in the family *Enterobacteriaceae*, and over a hundred scientific papers have been written about it.[18] From 1980 to 2007 it was known as *Enterobacter sakazakii*, but in 2007 there was a proposal to reclassify it into a new genus, *Cronobacter sakazakii*. The prognosis for those infected is poor. Multiplication of *Enterobacter sakazakii* in prepared formula feeds can cause devastating sepsis, particularly in the first two months of life. In approximately 50 published case reports of severe infection, there were high rates of meningitis, brain abscesses and necrotising enterocolitis, with an overall mortality ranging from 33%–80%.

The European Society for Paediatric Gastroenterology, Hepatology and Nutrition (ESPGHAN), reporting on the topic, wrote in 2004, 'Milk products are excellent media for bacterial proliferation.[19] Powdered infant formulae are not sterile and may contain pathogenic bacteria'. Experts from the Food and Agriculture Organization of the United Nations (FAO) and WHO met in 2004 to summarise information and develop international guidelines and educational messages regarding *E. sakazakii*. In 2006, WHO confirmed that current manufacturing processes cannot achieve the production of sterile powdered infant formula.[20] Contamination with *E. sakazakii* and *Salmonella* can occur intrinsically during manufacture – from the environment, or from raw ingredients – with 3–14% of samples potentially being affected. WHO recommended that for non-breastfed infants, infant formula should be selected based on the medical needs of the infant. However, for neonates and those <2 months of age, sterile liquid ready-to-feed formula should be used.

Ready-to-feed infant formula was never suggested as a replacement feed for HIV-exposed babies in resource-poor settings. Why not? Perhaps storage conditions would have been difficult in tropical climates. Or perhaps this was an option which would have cost too much. Perhaps ready-to-feed cartons would have been too bulky or too heavy to transport easily. Yet sterile, ready-to-feed breastmilk substitutes would have been much safer. Was safety not a concern for African babies?

Cup-feeding and deprivation of sucking

Babies have a strong need to suck. Babies orphaned due to AIDS in the Harare Children's Home were cup-fed. Bottles or dummies were recognised to be difficult to clean, and their use violated local infant feeding recommendations so they were never used. The distressing consequence was that orphaned babies would often suck their fists raw, and would often need their hands to be bandaged so they could heal.[21]

Orphaned older babies aged 6–12 months, who were being cared for and cup-fed by their grandmothers, and had no access to sucking, often appeared to be 'sad and flat' to a colleague who described to me developmental delay and other problems in the babies she came across in the rural areas of Zimbabwe.[22] The babies were not reaching developmental milestones at the expected age. Both their demeanour and motor development quickly improved once the grandmothers were provided with bottles and taught how to keep them clean so that the babies were able to receive sucking opportunities during feeding.

Premature weaning and loss of sucking leads to traumatic nutritional, psychological, developmental and health risks to the infant.[23] Ellen Piwoz writes movingly about the consequences for babies who are weaned too early so that their mothers can comply with recommendations for 'early cessation' of breastfeeding. Sucking helps regulate an infant's emotional and physical state and reduces stress. Sucking induces calm, reduces heart and metabolic rates, and elevates the pain threshold in rats and humans. Even non-nutritive sucking (on a pacifier or fingers) improves heart rate, oxygenation and pain behaviour, the frequency of sleep and calm alert states, and nutrition and growth. Unless replaced, the loss of sucking caused by an abrupt cessation of breastfeeding may leave the infant less able to cope with everyday stresses and cause prolonged crying, which in turn may add to a mother's or carer's stress, eroding their relationship with the baby.

I was so concerned about sucking deprivation for babies who were to receive only cup replacement feeding that I wrote to several people about my concerns. Sometimes people replied and sometimes they didn't. One who did was Dr Nils Bergman, a public health physician who was raised in Zimbabwe and began working on his special area of expertise, kangaroo mother care, in the rural areas of the country before moving to South Africa. Nils was such a great advocate for the needs of tiny babies. He was working on setting up one of the South African PMTCT sites and was researching the risks and benefits of cup and bottle-feeding milks to babies who would not be breastfed when I wrote to him towards the end of 2000:

> *'I would be worried about babies who were not to be breastfed and who were not to have any sucking at all. Babies love to suck, it calms them, it organizes them, it makes them digest their food more efficiently, it helps with pain. With all your wonderful knowledge of the contact and other things that babies need and receive with Kangaroo Mother Care then I'm sure you're very au fait with these things, from a technical point of view and so I am probably preaching to the choir!*
>
> *Of course, I worry about all the replacement feeding, all aspects of it – not just the bottles. My own very personal view is that really, really exclusive breastfeeding will*

probably turn out to result in the lowest rates of morbidity/mortality for the babies of HIV+ mothers in Africa – in spite of the risk of transmission in breastmilk, which may cause less deaths than other diseases if the babies are ***not*** *breastfed, doesn't disturb the culture, doesn't stigmatize the mother, maximizes the mother-baby thing, costs nothing, is compatible with the Baby Friendly Hospital Initiative, leads to lower rates of malnutrition, wasting, stunting etc. from 6–24 mos – all sorts of advantages. And makes the cup/bottle question academic.'*

Finally I bent the ear of my friend Arjan de Wagt at UNICEF, in a personal email in 2000:

'From the baby's emotional and physical point of view, the baby needs milk in some form. As you know I have serious concerns about the suitability/nutritional content of animal milks for human babies (with or without micronutrients) so this should be formula. The baby needs to suck!! I know WHO and UNICEF are dead against bottles, but how else are you going to comfort the baby?? Breastfeeding is more than just providing food, it is the biggest mothering tool – used to feed and comfort the baby anywhere any time – how are you going to do this by cup-feeding formula??

*I have just written to a doctor in South Africa about their plans to feed formula (one of the pilot projects I think) – there's lots of UNICEF and WHO stuff on cup-feeding, but none on the baby's need to suck. I think this bit has been missed out. I know that it is considered more risky to bottle-feed a baby in an impoverished environment ...I should mention that I recently heard from Dr Nils Bergman, on this very question. I had met Dr Bergman at the LLL conference in Port Elizabeth in July and subsequently sent him a copy of my Breastfeeding Review papers. So he had some queries, and wanted refs for the risks/benefits of cup-feeding. I copied out excerpts in support of cup-feeding from various publications I have – mostly from UNICEF and WHO who come out *strongly* in favour of cup-feeding because of concerns about the ability of mothers to keep bottles clean in impoverished environments or emergency situations. This obviously reflects the belief that cup-feeding would lead to lower rates of diarrhoea/malnutrition/mortality. I have to say that I agree with this, but I think that this stops short of addressing the whole issue.*

Most of these WHO/UNICEF utterances were actually developed in circumstances where the individual mother would eventually be breastfeeding – in cases of re-lactation, and prematurity of the baby, and possibly emergency situations. One of the other reasons for promoting cups over bottles was that the babies should not become 'nipple-confused', so that breast-feeding could eventually be resumed.

But – and I think this is a factor that we haven't thought enough about – the babies of HIV-infected mothers who are to receive 'replacement feeding' (formula) will never be breastfed. And if they are cup-fed, they will never suck. In practical terms we all know how babies love to suck, how it calms them, organizes them, de-stresses them, helps with pain, allows them to suck strongly when hungry and more and more gently to drift off to sleep. In working with cup-feeding mothers and babies I have several observations:

- *many of the mothers will cup-feed for a short time, but after a while they find it messy, (sometimes the milk squirts out of the sides of the baby's mouth as he closes it to swallow ... then it gets in the creases of the neck, and the ears, etc). They may also find it unsatisfying for themselves and the baby so they resort to bottles and then feel guilty, but because it's so much easier they carry on with the bottles.*

- *incidentally I am beginning to believe that 'nipple-confusion' is a condition that is being misnamed. I see 'breast confusion' a lot; this is what happens when babies cannot latch, but bottle-feeding is frequently a response to that difficulty, and is not limited to being the cause. In practice I find that, once the original problem has been addressed, most mothers and babies can breastfeed after bottle-feeding.*
- *that mothers may be afraid of cup-feeding (I transition them by showing them how to spoon-feed first, then how to cup-feed when they become confident).*
- *that nursing staff are not afraid of cup-feeding, but they may pour the milk down the baby's throat to get him/her to take the milk, or to take all of the required amount. I see babies choking during cup-feeding. If the feed is EBM, a physiologic liquid containing antibodies and human components which will not irritate the lungs/cause infection, you simply tip the baby over, pound the little back, he/she splutters, stops breathing, re-organizes himself and then you see the little chest going up and down again. (I always HATE this!) But what if the feed is formula, based on cow's milk, a dead liquid, containing bacteria, "foreign" proteins and other ingredients?? Is there more risk of pneumonia etc. I'm not well-read on this, but I have seen concerns expressed about "silent aspiration", and it worries me. In short, my observation leads me to believe that swallowing is easier for a baby when there is sucking involved, than when there is no sucking, as when feeding from a cup.*
- *has anyone, anywhere, done any studies to show what happens to social/emotional/speech/palatal/dental development if a baby *never* sucks?*
- *I have seen somewhere, in the HIV Counselling course I think, the suggestion that a baby can suck on the mother's arm – i.e. it stresses don't use a dummy, don't use a bottle. Is this a suitable substitute for the breast??*

*Before everyone comes to the conclusion that I am trying to promote the use of bottles, I'm not! I find it interesting that *formula* can be promoted in this way, as long as the container for the formula is not a bottle. Obviously the formula manufacturers were fortunate enough to be able to provide input into the HIV and infant feeding guidelines, but bottle-makers were overlooked!*

My thinking is that if it is thought that an environment is safe enough to feed a baby formula – i.e. ***not*** *to breastfeed – then it should be a* ***very*** *safe environment. If it's only safe enough to use cups, but not bottles, then maybe it's not safe* ***enough****? If a mother living in such an environment does* ***not*** *have access to bottle-brushes, clean water, squeezy liquid, sterilizing fluid, or a nice electric or gas stove to boil her bottles and mixing-water for twenty full minutes, and doctors and nursing staff and antibiotics and IV drips for when the baby develops the pneumonias and diarrhoeas that s/he surely will if breastfeeding is withheld, then maybe it really isn't safe enough??? And maybe BREASTFEEDING – exclusive breastfeeding – should continue to be promoted????*

Just my .02.'

Peanut paste, another breastmilk substitute?

In an effort to combat malnutrition experienced by prematurely weaned infants, the BAN study in Malawi experimented with giving infants older than six months a 'lipid based nutritional supplement', as a breastmilk substitute.[24] This was basically Plumpy'Nut, a product manufactured by the private French company Nutriset, and invented by researcher André Briend, mentioned earlier, who subsequently became a consultant to WHO on severe acute malnutrition.[25] Plumpy'Nut is frequently advertised on British TV by UNICEF and Save the Children seeking donations to treat severe acute malnutrition in refugee children, particularly in resource-poor settings.[26,27] But HIV-positive children and HIV-negative children of mothers participating in the BAN study in Malawi who were weaned at six months and fed ready-to-use supplementary foods until 12 months were found to have dietary deficiencies 4–6 months later.[28] The BAN study had experienced many stops and starts and had at one time been halted due to poor results. For this intervention it was found that children consumed adequate energy, protein and carbohydrates, but inadequate quantities of fat and reduced micronutrient intake, e.g. of vitamins A, B6 and C, as well as iron and zinc. Early weaning was associated with dietary deficiencies and girls especially experienced reduced growth velocity. The conclusion was that in resource-poor settings, HIV prevention programmes must ensure that breastfeeding stops only once a nutritionally adequate and safe diet without breastmilk can be provided.

Cotrimoxazole prophylaxis

From 2006, WHO had recommended cotrimoxazole prophylaxis for HIV-exposed infants starting at 4–6 weeks of age, to be continued until HIV infection could be excluded by HIV testing of toddlers older than 18 months – or at least six weeks after all breastfeeding had ended (whichever was the later.)

Cotrimoxazole is an antibiotic, a combination of trimethoprim and sulfamethoxazole in a class of medications called sulfonamides. It works by stopping the growth of bacteria[29] and is used to treat infections such as pneumonia, bronchitis, and infections of the urinary tract, ears, and intestines. Sulfonamides transfer into breastmilk. Cotrimoxazole may cause liver problems, anaemia, and other unwanted effects in nursing babies, especially those with glucose-6-phosphate dehydrogenase (G6PD) deficiency.[30] In the literature for lactation consultants, this medicine is not recommended for use during breastfeeding, particularly for mothers nursing newborns, because sulfonamides may cause prolonged jaundice in the newborn.

Nevertheless, in 2007 UNICEF endorsed the use of this broad-spectrum antibiotic as the best way to protect all children born to HIV-positive mothers against opportunistic infections from six weeks of age.[31] Cotrimoxazole had been shown to reduce mortality in children living with HIV and AIDS by more than 40%, primarily by reducing the risk of pneumonia. It was also able to postpone the need for antiretroviral treatment. Priced as low as three cents a day, cotrimoxazole was proposed as an intervention that could make a real difference to children living with HIV/AIDS. It was widely used, cheap, and now on the essential drugs list in many countries. 2005 estimates put the number of children in need of this drug at about four million. Conveniently, it largely remained under the radar of the lactation community, since WHO permitted 'drops or syrups consisting of vitamins, mineral supplements, or drugs' within the definition of exclusive breastfeeding.

The widespread use of cotrimoxazole for HIV-exposed babies did however gain the attention of Anna Coutsoudis and colleagues, who in 2005 had looked at the influence of cotrimoxazole at two hospitals in Durban, South Africa.[32] HIV-infected infants who received cotrimoxazole prophylaxis had fewer respiratory infections, but an increased risk of diarrhoea. The authors suggested that because of this risk the HIV status of infants should be determined as early as possible in order to assess the need for this drug, and they suggested further research.

Throughout the years the lactation community has been aware that researchers on HIV transmission needed our input. This was one such instance. It was known that antibiotics caused diarrhoea in breastfed infants, and that diarrhoea was in itself a marker for damage to the intestinal mucosa, often causing secondary lactase deficiency.[33] Since HIV transmission is more likely where there is intestinal damage, questions needed to be asked about whether cotrimoxazole would in itself pose a risk for increased HIV transmission to the breastfed infant.

Anna Coutsoudis raised concerns over the use of cotrimoxazole again in 2011. In a research letter in the advance online edition of *AIDS*,[34,35] she reported that optimal use of cotrimoxazole prophylaxis in breastfed HIV-exposed negative infants in a community programme in Durban, South Africa, was associated with an increased risk of diarrhoea. She was concerned that this drug continued to be used in HIV-exposed breastfed infants while breastmilk itself provided immune protection against diarrhoea and pneumonia. Breastfed infants had a strong gastrointestinal system, but continued use of antibiotics would destroy the normal (healthy) gut bacteria, allowing disease-forming bacteria to proliferate.

Athena Kourtis and colleagues from the BAN study in Malawi discussed how increased intestinal permeability may be one of the mechanisms of transmission of HIV to infants through breastfeeding and looked at how this phenomenon could be measured. The use of antibiotic prophylaxis was associated with increased disruption of mucosal integrity which would be likely to facilitate HIV entry through the intestine.[36]

After reviewing research since 2006, WHO issued new guidance in 2014. They considered that cotrimoxazole prophylaxis should be started for all HIV-exposed infants, but not be once HIV-exposed uninfected infants had stopped breastfeeding.[37]

Shahin Lockman and colleagues in Botswana found in 2017 that prophylactic cotrimoxazole didn't improve 18-month survival among HIV-exposed uninfected children in a non-malarial area. She thought that where there was no malaria, and for children with a low risk of HIV-transmission, prolonged cotrimoxazole might not be required.[38] A recent commentary in the WHO *Bulletin* also questioned the necessity of cotrimoxazole prophylaxis for HIV-exposed negative infants who were already protected from infections through breastmilk, and called for a re-examination of the guidelines.[39]

In 2019, as the rationale for more research, Daniels and Coutsoudis again conducted a thorough review.[40] They noted that before ART was available, when HIV rates among children were high, cotrimoxazole prophylaxis was originally shown to be beneficial.

However, since then there had been much progress in diagnosing and treating HIV-positive children with ART. Between 2003 and 2012, MTCT of HIV in South Africa decreased from 23.2% to 2.4%. Given the increased data showing possible immune disruption and damage caused by interference with the microbiome, it was possible that cotrimoxazole prophylaxis might be harmful to the immune systems of HIV-exposed uninfected infants. Given the global rise in antibiotic resistance, overuse of this antibiotic could also cause bacterial resistance to cotrimoxazole, ampicillin, chloramphenicol and ciprofloxacin in infants and adults. In a randomixed controlled non-inferiority trial, from October 2013 to May 2018, half of the babies received cotrimoxazole and half did not. Although cotrimoxazole appears to confer a reduction in malarial morbidity, there was inadequate evidence to support any benefit for breastfed HIV-exposed uninfected infants, in terms of overall morbidity and mortality. Keeping these infants on prophylaxis without any clear health benefits, while potentially affecting their microbiome, immune development and overall health, was questionable. They therefore recommended that the WHO cotrimoxazole guidelines for breastfed HIV-exposed, uninfected infants in countries unaffected by malaria should be revised.

HIV-exposed babies have continued to be the subject of unresearched experiments, the victims of the errors and omissions of policymakers who often seemed to have little understanding of lactation and breastfeeding. African babies were most at risk and their mothers the unwitting collaborators, having been persuaded that almost any other milk, fed in any other way but at the breast, would protect their babies. We can learn from these experiences, to ensure that similar situations are not repeated in the future.

CHAPTER 20

Already HIV-infected infants and babies who escape infection

In the absence of antiretroviral treatment or prophylaxis, approximately 20% of babies of untreated HIV-positive mothers will be born already infected[1] – a larger percentage than will become infected through breastfeeding.

An immuno-compromised baby is likely to suffer an increased risk of acquiring many opportunistic infections, against which breastfeeding would be protective. HIV tends to behave aggressively in infected babies, and continued breastfeeding provides important ongoing protection from other infections. HIV-infected children have double the risk of diarrhoea, which is more likely to be persistent, as well as pneumonia – often in association with other infections – compared to uninfected children. They also suffer higher rates of failure-to-thrive, placing a heavy burden on healthcare facilities and on families.

A 2006 study showed that nearly half of all untreated HIV-infected babies died by six months of age.[2] Infants who acquired HIV in the first two months of life, either *in utero*, intrapartum, or through early breastfeeding, had significantly higher HIV RNA levels than either infants who were infected after two months of age[3] through late breastmilk transmission, or adults who were infected through heterosexual transmission.[4] A newly infected infant will have a higher viral load than a newly infected adult and levels reached at approximately four months post-infection were highly predictive of disease progression. Babies infected early *in utero* have a rapid increase in viral load and early progression to symptomatic disease within 3–12 weeks of age, leading more rapidly to the immune dysfunction of AIDS and to death. Untreated perinatally infected children may have mortality rates of over 80% in the first three years of life.[5] Those with late *in utero* or intrapartum transmission survived 10–31 months.[6]

In a 2002 article, three British HIV clinicians wrote, 'There are two principal categories of infected children. One-fifth of children infected perinatally develop rapidly progressive symptomatic disease, typically presenting with *Pneumocystis carinii* pneumonia around 10–14 weeks of age, or developmental delay or regression in the first year of life. The other four-fifths of perinatally infected children have a median survival without treatment of around nine years, and a proportion do not present until the second decade of life. Such children may have been born abroad, in high

HIV-seroprevalence areas such as sub-Saharan Africa, South East Asia, and increasingly India, Eastern Europe, the Caribbean, Latin America, and China. Infected individuals present with lymphadenopathy, hepatosplenomegaly, persistent parotid enlargement, shingles, extensive molluscum, thrombocytopenia, recurrent infections, failure-to-thrive, or unexplained organ disease.'[7] It is probable that these HIV-positive children who have survived babyhood to late childhood and adolescence in countries of high HIV prevalence have done so because they were breastfed.

In two separate papers, Louise Kuhn put forward the logical argument that it's not practical to have mothers make infant-feeding decisions during pregnancy, because the infant's HIV status cannot be known.[8,9] In the ZEBS study in Zambia breastfed HIV-positive babies older than four months had improved survival rates compared to prematurely weaned babies.[10] In the second trial mortality at 24 months was 55% among already infected babies randomised to continued breastfeeding compared to 74% among those who stopped breastfeeding early.[11] In a study in Botswana that randomised HIV-exposed infants to either breastfeed or receive infant formula, among infants that were already HIV infected mortality at six months of age was 7.5% in those who breastfed compared to 33% in those randomised to receive infant formula only.[12]

WHO concluded that these studies indicate that HIV-infected infants fare better when breastfed. The relatively high morbidity and mortality rates associated with the feeding of formula showed a need to carefully assess the local management of childhood illnesses in a given context before implementation of a formula-feeding strategy. Breastfeeding mothers of infants and young children who were known to be HIV-infected should be strongly encouraged to continue breastfeeding.[13]

Louise Kuhn concedes that 'To its credit, the WHO has clearly stated that known HIV-infected children should breastfeed without any equivocation about duration or AFASS. As HIV-infected children can progress rapidly[14] breastfeeding is essential for these infants to survive long enough to access pediatric HIV care and treatment programs offering antiretroviral therapy.'

In untreated populations, around two-thirds of MTCT occurred around the time of delivery. The question arises about the fate of babies of HIV-positive mothers in the early PMTCT programmes who were persuaded not to breastfeed. It was known almost from the beginning that HIV-positive babies survived longer if they were breastfed. In an Italian retrospective study conducted in 1990 to determine the interplay of breastfeeding with the development of AIDS in vertically infected children, the median incubation time for developing AIDS for bottle-fed children was 9.7 months, while for breastfed children it was 19 months.[15] Dr Rose Kambarami, a paediatrician who worked with HIV-infected babies at Harare Hospital in Zimbabwe, found that the odds of good nutrition if an HIV-infected infant was exclusively breastfed was almost three times higher than if the baby received other foods and liquids, and that mixed feeding started too early (from 1–4 months) was associated with poor nutrition. Exclusive breastfeeding was beneficial because malnutrition further compromised a baby's immune status.[16]

Incorrect information about the theoretical risk of 'superinfection' and drug resistance or toxicity was sometimes used to discourage women with newly identified infected children from breastfeeding. The risk of infecting a child who was uninfected past the newborn stage was also sometimes used to encourage early cessation of breastfeeding. When early weaning was first recommended, it was unlikely that HIV-testing of infants under 15 months was available in most settings. Thus it would not have been possible to establish whether it was justified. However, at a meeting of PMTCT staff that I attended in Harare, the point was made by well-known paediatrician Greg Powell[17] that HIV-infected infants could be identified by six months of age on clinical signs alone, for example by symptoms of lymphadenopathy and splenomegaly, and that even medical residents could be trained to identify these babies as a way to avoid inappropriate and harmful premature weaning from the breast.

One of the major problems with placing a blanket ban on breastfeeding by HIV-positive mothers in the global north is that there is still no way of distinguishing the infected from the uninfected baby at birth. If the decision is made not to breastfeed, reversing that decision later is difficult or impossible. HIV testing of infants even at birth may not identify an infected baby for several weeks because of the limitations in testing techniques. An infected baby can test negative because it takes time for sufficient virus to show up on a test. It is difficult to maintain lactation long enough for accurate test results to be available.

HIV-positive children who are formula-fed or who are weaned off breastmilk early are at high risk of dying prematurely. Thus, any means of slowing the progression of HIV infection is particularly important for HIV-infected infants if they are to benefit from antiretroviral therapy.[18,19] If there are major logistic challenges and delays in entering paediatric HIV care and treatment programmes, rapid progression of HIV infection in infants means that delays in identifying children and delays in starting therapy can lead to death.[14] Breastfeeding can buy a little time.

HIV-exposed babies who escape infection

The number of pregnant women living with HIV has remained unchanged at 1.3 million globally every year since 2000.[20] Their babies are described as 'HIV-exposed'. It's hard to be definite about how many HIV-exposed but uninfected infants there are because, astonishingly, UNAIDS only recorded their numbers for the first time in 2018.[21] But a group of researchers from Cape Town and Gabarone estimated their number using data from children aged 0–14 years generated by a UNAIDS module to estimate key HIV epidemic indicators from mathematical models. They also estimated the percentage change in the global population of HIV-exposed uninfected children between 2000 and 2018.[22]

Over the years we've come a long way in protecting babies from becoming infected with HIV. By 2019 a US government website reported that 85% of pregnant HIV-positive women received ART for their own health and to prevent transmission of HIV to their babies during pregnancy and childbirth.[23] As an increasing number of HIV-positive mothers are able to receive treatment, greater numbers of babies remain uninfected. In 2018, an estimated 14.8 million children globally were HIV-exposed, but uninfected. This population more than doubled from 6.7 million in 2000. Ninety percent (13.2 million) of these children live in sub-Saharan Africa and half of them come from just five countries, where at least one in every 5 children is HIV-exposed and uninfected – South Africa, Uganda, Mozambique, Tanzania and Nigeria. South Africa alone accounts for 3.5 million.[20] Five percent (760,000) live in the Asia and Pacific region.

In the past, HIV-exposed, uninfected infants have been found to have more health problems than babies of uninfected mothers, partly because children in many of the countries hardest hit by HIV also suffer from high rates of other infectious diseases, food insecurity and other serious problems. A family affected by HIV continues to experience ongoing difficult social, economic and health impacts of the disease. Babies may be at risk of long-term adverse effects of antiretroviral drugs and at higher risk during their childhood for acquiring HIV-related infections through ongoing exposure and malnutrition, particularly to diseases like measles and tuberculosis.

There is evidence that early exposure to HIV has health effects lasting beyond the transmission period.[24,25] The effects of exposure to HIV itself must be considered as well as the impact of environmental factors related to birth into an HIV-affected household, including orphanhood, stigma, discrimination and extreme poverty. A pooled analysis of seven trials found that risk factors for death among HIV-exposed infants included maternal death, lower maternal CD4 cell counts[26] and early weaning.[6] Though maternal ART adherence is effective in reducing under-five mortality,[27] further studies continue to link an increased risk of child mortality with poor maternal health and HIV exposure. Children born to HIV-infected mothers with high viral load who escape perinatal or early breastfeeding-related HIV infection are nonetheless at high risk of mortality and morbidity during the first few months of life.[28]

The immune system is underdeveloped at birth and as a result infants and young children may be thought of as immune-compromised regardless of previous HIV exposure.[29] Growth stunting is associated with pre-term or low birth weight, both of which occur more commonly in infants born to HIV-infected mothers.[30] Additionally, growth stunting is associated with discontinuation or reduction in breastfeeding, which significantly affects a child's health and cognitive development.[6] Shortening breastfeeding duration for uninfected children born to HIV-infected mothers living in low-resource settings is associated with significant increases in mortality extending into the second year of life.

Without breastfeeding and maternal ART, HIV-exposed uninfected infants experience more infections than HIV-unexposed infants. Researchers at Gugulethu Midwife Obstetrics Unit in Cape Town prospectively studied a cohort of HIV-positive pregnant women initiating ART, and a parallel group of HIV-negative pregnant women, starting from their first antenatal care visit.[31] They looked at the effect of HIV exposure on hospitalisation and diarrhoea and presumed lower respiratory tract infection. Despite ART in pregnancy, the breastfed HIV-exposed but uninfected infants had transiently increased infectious morbidity risks in early infancy. The differences in health outcomes were driven by factors potentially amenable to intervention, including delayed diagnosis and ART initiation in HIV-positive mothers, and suboptimal breastfeeding and vaccination of their infants. The babies of mothers who started ART with viral loads below 10,000, and before 24 weeks of pregnancy, were not significantly more likely to be hospitalised than babies of HIV-negative mothers. Of more influence was whether the babies received all their vaccinations, and whether they were optimally breastfed for the first three months. Both of these things needed to happen to reduce the relative risk of hospitalisation to zero. The babies born to HIV-positive mothers who were given timely ART, and who did not acquire HIV themselves, were at most time points as healthy as the children of HIV-negative mothers. There was no difference in mortality. Dr Le Roux commented: 'The increased risk of dying due to pneumonia or diarrhoea in the absence of breastfeeding outweighs the risks of breastmilk associated HIV transmission in most resource-limited settings, including South Africa – as our data shows.'[32] She pointed out that HIV incidence in the breastfed babies was below 2%, compared with 15% in babies breastfed by mothers not receiving ART.

Suzanne Filteau, in a very thorough 2009 review article,[33] writes 'The most important modifiable factor affecting health of HIV-exposed, uninfected children is infant feeding practice... Reduced breastfeeding by HIV-infected mothers could account for increased morbidity and mortality, increased exposure to dietary pathogens, altered immune functions and growth and potentially slower development in HIV-exposed, uninfected infants compared to unexposed infants... Unfortunately, confusion about infant feeding messages may lead HIV-infected women to stop breastfeeding early even when they lack AFASS alternatives. Less breastfeeding may explain some of the association between sick or dead mothers and higher risk of infant mortality.'

Contributors to sub-optimal health outcomes for HIV exposed uninfected babies

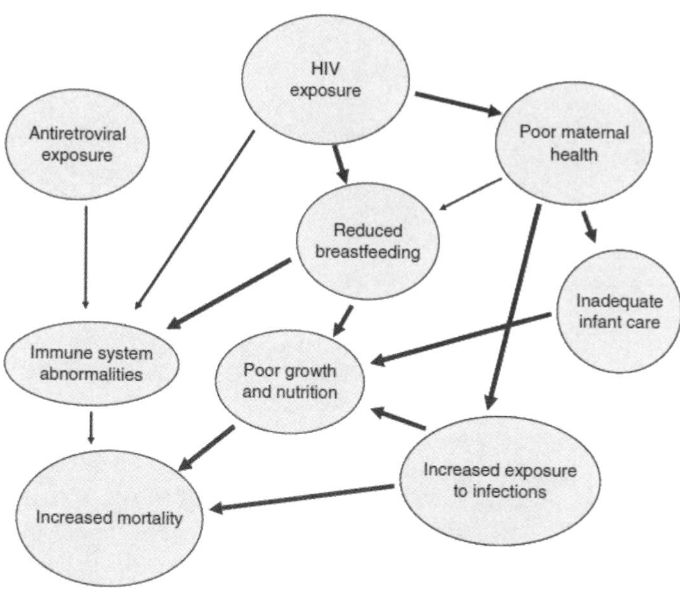

Source: Filteau S. The HIV-exposed uninfected African child. Trop Med Int Health 2009; 14:276–287.

Finally, in a recent large study in South Africa, which recruited over 1,200 mothers, one-third of whom had HIV, and not all were on ART,[34] researchers found that despite growing up with more indicators of social disadvantage, the HIV-uninfected children of HIV-positive mothers generally did just as well as the children of HIV-negative mothers in terms of weight, height, health and mental development at age five. A strength of this study was the long-term follow-up. The research followed 1,150 of the children up to the age of eight. The researchers described their findings as 'unexpected', and given that improvements to child health seem to have accelerated, particularly in the last three to five years, they interpret this as being possibly due to the improved health of mothers living with HIV. Could it also have been due to breastfeeding?

CHAPTER 21

HIV-free survival

'In sub-Saharan Africa today, few threats to infants' health are as unnerving as potential and actual shifts away from breastfeeding' Louise Kuhn, 2004

One of the omissions in the early phase of PMTCT programme planning was the failure to monitor whether PMTCT interventions such as breastfeeding avoidance, or caesarean section to avoid perinatal transmission of HIV, were actually saving lives. In the dilemma of competing risks, there was no information available to counsellors, or mothers themselves, about the number of children infected through HIV-laced breastmilk compared to the number of uninfected children who might have died because breastmilk had been withheld from them.[1,2]

The absence of information from the early PMTCT pilot sites about HIV-free survival of babies according to feeding method kept both health workers and mothers in ignorance. However, as it gradually became clear that suspending breastfeeding altogether, either from birth, or later with so-called 'early cessation' of breastfeeding, led to high rates of morbidity and mortality, questions began to be asked about the wisdom of this course. Were more babies dying from formula-feeding than would have died from transmission of HIV through breastfeeding?

Promotion of replacement feeding as a way to reduce postpartum transmission of HIV had been successful largely due to the stated futility of saving babies from transmission of HIV during pregnancy and birth by means of short-course maternal antiretroviral prophylaxis, only to have them infected immediately afterwards through breastfeeding. But in time the futility of saving babies from HIV in breastmilk only to have them die of pneumonia or diarrhoea due to not having been breastfed gradually became even more obvious. The public tragedy which had befallen Botswana in 2006, where so many formula-fed babies had died, drew attention to the risks of formula-feeding in resource-poor settings in a way that hadn't been acknowledged before. Understanding began to emerge that that there was a balance of risks to be considered. Experts began talking about the importance of 'HIV-free survival' as a more accurate measure of PMTCT outcomes.

What is HIV-free survival?

HIV-free survival is a public health indicator – a particular point in time, defined by the absence of either infant HIV infection or infant death, that is the net number of HIV-exposed uninfected children who managed to reach a particular age, usually 18–24 months, and survive. Research in the context of HIV-free survival began to question whether formula-feeding by HIV-infected mothers in areas of high HIV-prevalence saved more lives than continued breastfeeding.

The debate led to the development of several simulation models that attempted to assess the risks and benefits of breastfeeding. In order to obtain some real-life data, in 2000 WHO had commissioned a large collaborative study[3] to assess the effect of not breastfeeding on the risk of death due to infectious diseases in infants from developing countries, which found that it would be hard to safely feed formula to babies in under-developed countries.

2003 saw publication of the WHO blueprint for breastfeeding, the Global Strategy on Infant and Young Child Feeding,[4] which warned that 'Malnutrition has been responsible, directly or indirectly, for 60% of the 10.9 million deaths annually among children under five. Well over two-thirds of these deaths, which are often associated with inappropriate feeding practices, occur during the first year of life'.

Even as the PMTCT sites were continuing to be rolled out and scaled up, promoting replacement feeding for HIV-exposed babies, the *Lancet* had also published, in 2003, a set of chilling papers outlining the causes of worldwide infant malnutrition, morbidity and mortality.[5] More than 10 million children were dying each year from causes against which breastfeeding was protective, and almost all lived in poor countries. The series had used data from 2000, the year that the PMTCT pilots took off, as being the most complete, and little had changed in the interim. Breastfeeding alone was responsible for saving more lives than any other single intervention, including mass vaccination against common diseases. Not breastfeeding led to malnutrition, morbidity and mortality. Continued breastfeeding for an older child could provide needed calories and micronutrients in bad times to combat the malnutrition which was so often a contributing factor to mortality when combined with other infections.

Six countries accounted for 50% of worldwide deaths in children younger than five years, and 42 countries for 90%. Just over 40% of those deaths occurred in sub-Saharan Africa, the epicentre of HIV/AIDS, and 34% occurred in Asia,[6] coincidentally the very countries where breastfeeding prevalence was highest and the PMTCT programmes were most active. The tragedy in Africa was not only stark compared to the industrialised countries where formula-feeding was seen as normal, but it was getting worse. In 1990, there were 180 deaths per 1,000 live births in sub-Saharan Africa and only nine per 1,000 in industrialised countries—a 20-fold difference. A decade later, this gap had increased by 50%, to 29-fold, with mortality rates of 175 and six per 1,000 children in sub-Saharan Africa and the industrialised countries respectively. Inadequate availability and/or unsafe water for drinking or hygiene, and lack of access to sanitation contributed to about 1.5 million child deaths, 88% of which were due to diarrhoea. Infants aged 0–5 months who were not breastfed at all (as was being recommended for the babies of HIV-positive mothers) had a seven-fold increased risk of death from diarrhoea, and a five-fold increased risk of death from pneumonia compared with infants who were exclusively breastfed. At the same age, non-exclusive rather than exclusive breastfeeding more than doubled the mortality risk of diarrhoea or pneumonia. Even 6–11-month-old infants who were not breastfed had an increased risk of such deaths. WHO's global recommendation was that breastfeeding should continue for 'up to two years or beyond'.

Global infant mortality rates increased dramatically in the 15 years up to 2005. In children born before 1990, the infant mortality rate had been 48 per 1,000. From 1990–94, a point at which things were improving, the infant mortality rate dropped to 31 per 1,000. But in the fifteen years since the HIV epidemic began, infant mortality had been swinging up again, trebling in the previous five years to 99 per 1,000 births. In KwaZulu Natal infant mortality increased from 28 per 1,000 live births in 1990–94 to 92 per 1,000 in 2000–04.[7] In a multicentre cohort study published in 2005, infants who were not breastfed had a 10-fold higher risk of dying from any cause and a three-fold higher risk of being hospitalised compared with predominantly breastfed babies.[8] Babies of HIV-positive mothers included in an intensive 'Formula-Plus' programme which ran in Haiti from mid-2001 to December 2003 had a 21% higher mortality rate despite receiving good medical care and frequent follow-up. 70% of those deaths occurred within the first six months of life.[9]

A 2004 report from Linkages (funded by USAID), in which modelling was done using risks of MTCT transmission versus risks of infant mortality in Africa, also concluded that not breastfeeding for the first four months of life presented much greater risks of mortality than breastfeeding by HIV-positive mothers.[1]

Michael Latham and Pauline Kisanga wrote in 2001[10] that in 1998 an estimated 590,000 infants worldwide acquired HIV from their mothers; 90% of these infants were in Africa. In many African countries, the HIV and AIDS pandemic was a major tragedy of unprecedented proportions, but even responsible health agencies had tended to exaggerate the role of breastfeeding in transmission. Research had shown that exclusive breastfeeding for four months, and possibly longer, greatly reduced the transmission of HIV from mother to child through breastfeeding. It was possible that an infant exclusively breastfed would have a healthy intact gut, which would likely reduce transmission of HIV well beyond six months if breastfeeding continued. In contrast the young infant fed infant formula or other animal milk products had a 'damaged' intestinal mucosa, more prone to infection with the virus.

Latham and Kisanga had found in their four-country assessment that there was a grossly exaggerated belief in transmission rates, even by senior and well-trained staff in government and UN agencies. But it was generally agreed, based on several reviews of the literature, that in a country or community where 30% of pregnant women were found to be sero-positive for HIV then only three of the 100 infants born to mothers attending an antenatal clinic would be HIV infected through breastfeeding. If only 10% of mothers were HIV-positive only one of 100 infants born would be infected through breastfeeding. On the other hand, if breastfeeding was undermined, or reduced in the whole population, because of fear of HIV transmission through breastfeeding, it meant that 97 out of 100 babies could suffer adversely, for the sake of the three who might be infected through breastfeeding, as outlined in the following diagram.

Ante-Natal Clinic	Sero-positive for HIV	Sero-positive for HIV
100 pregnant women	If: 30%	If: 10%
Then		
33.3% MTCT	10 infants	3.3 infants
33.3% through breastfeeding	3.3 infants	1.1 infants

Accepted Model of MTCT

This is sometimes stated as 1/3, of 1/3 of 1/3. If 1/3 are sero-positive, and 1/3 have MTCT, but only 1/3 of transmission is due to breastfeeding, you end up with only about three infants out of 100 infected with HIV through breastfeeding. Latham and Kisanga wrote that if fear of this problem was to lead to a spillover effect, reducing breastfeeding in a country or community, the negative effects would far outweigh the benefit.

What Latham and Kisanga had written in 2001 was almost prophetic. No provision had been made to monitor and evaluate infant health outcomes according to feeding method. This meant, in effect, that the PMTCT programme was subsequently scaled up and rolled out without any knowledge of whether the intervention employed – persuading mothers to formula-feed their babies – was going to be effective in reducing the number of babies who acquired HIV, or whether HIV-free survival of formula-fed babies would, as we suspected, be compromised.

Even in 2002, as the PMTCT sites in Botswana and other African countries were being rolled out, Anna Coutsoudis had also asked some uncomfortable questions which, in retrospect, seemed visionary:[12] 'In areas of high HIV prevalence, how appropriate is the move to promote replacement feeding by HIV-infected women by distributing free commercial formula milk? At the end of 1999 UNAIDS estimated that of the 36 million adults and children living with HIV/AIDS globally, 24.5 million live in sub-Saharan Africa. The global burden of HIV disease clearly lies in sub-Saharan Africa, home to some of the world's poorest countries, where the major cause of infant deaths is malnutrition and infectious diseases. At the same time UNICEF estimates that 1.5 million non-HIV related deaths per year can be prevented globally through breastfeeding. Does the risk of breastfeeding transmission warrant the risk of undermining the life-saving cultural practice of breastfeeding in resource-poor countries?'

It was not until after the full extent of the 2006 Botswana tragedy was revealed that results from other African PMTCT sites started to be formally published. It was almost as if before Botswana there had been editorial censorship of unfavourable results which didn't endorse replacement feeding by all HIV-positive mothers. Botswana served to shock the AIDS community into lifting the media blackout.

HIV-free survival in the research

The competing risks in the HIV and infant feeding debate were:

1. The risk of death due to HIV acquired through breastfeeding.
2. The risk of death due to common childhood illnesses, against which breastfeeding

was protective.

3. The additional risk of malnutrition, which exacerbated the risk of mortality when young children suffered infections such as pneumonia, diarrhoea or measles.

Thus the goal of any PMTCT programme was to keep children free of HIV infection and to reduce mortality risks. In the light of the need to measure the balance between these two risks, the international community now encouraged the use of a single index, HIV-free survival, which gave as the net result the number of children who were not infected *and* who had survived.[13] Sera Young, Caroline Chantry and Kiersten Israel-Ballard, who had begun research on inactivating the HIV virus in breastmilk, and continued to examine other aspects of HIV and infant feeding, noted that infants given replacement foods after a period of breastfeeding also suffered increased serious infections, including diarrhoea and pneumonia, faltering growth and death. They coined the term HIV-free 'thrival' as the main goal of PMTCT strategies, meaning that the HIV-exposed infant should not only survive, but also thrive.[14] Louise Kuhn subsequently wrote in 2012, 'only an HIV-uninfected child death is considered sufficiently severe to be counted as equivalent to an HIV infection. Thereby, the spectrum of other benefits of breastfeeding for maternal and child health is discounted.'[15]

The Botswana legacy

Following the reports of the floods in Botswana in early 2006, much more information was made available testifying to the risks of not breastfeeding. Researchers reported on morbidity and mortality due to formula-feeding in presentations made to the 31,000 delegates attending the August 2006 World AIDS Conference in Toronto:

- A prospective cohort study of over 1,400 children from rural and urban South Africa reported a cumulative six-month mortality estimate of 10% among exclusively breastfed infants vs 15% among formula-fed infants (eight out of 101 infants, all of whom died in the first three months of life). The risk of postnatal transmission by six months of age in exclusively breastfed infants who were negative at 4–8 weeks of age was 4.04%.[16]
- A small Ugandan study of babies followed up for 11–15 months found that a shorter duration of either exclusive breastfeeding or of total breastfeeding were both significantly associated with higher infant mortality.[17]
- A small study from south-western Nigeria, where babies were followed up for six months, showed that HIV-exposed formula-fed infants had higher morbidity and mortality due to diarrhoea, acute respiratory infection and sepsis than those whose mothers had chosen to exclusively breastfeed.[18]

The following year, at the February 2007 Conference on Retroviruses and Opportunistic Infections,[19] the question of safe infant feeding was one of the most talked-about topics, with some experts stating that women in most resource-constrained settings should no longer be advised to avoid breastfeeding or to wean early.

A 2010 review article by Louise Kuhn and Grace Aldrovandi looked at outcomes of stopping breastfeeding in order to reduce postnatal transmission of HIV, with a focus on the question of HIV-free survival.[20] They described how mothers in the PMTCT projects received the best possible help and support with replacement feeding, and extra safeguards likely to give the best results. Yet even so, babies who were not breastfed at all, or were weaned early, didn't fare as well as expected. All of the studies listed below included close monitoring and follow-up, and education or counselling which the investigators expected would make early weaning safe. Outcomes were worse with replacement feeding than with continued breastfeeding, except for the Nairobi study which has received negative reviews elsewhere. All but two were only reported after the 2006 Botswana tragedy suddenly made it clear how unsafe it was to suspend breastfeeding.

Researched studies showing the differences in health outcomes between replacement feeding and breastfeeding

The Nairobi Group, 2000

Only the famous Nairobi study was able to demonstrate a net benefit for HIV-free survival of artificial feeding.[21] Although only reported in 2000, the HIV-positive mothers were recruited into the study many years earlier, from 1992 onwards. The results from this study formed the basis for the policy to encourage HIV-positive mothers to choose replacement feeding for their babies, and formed the rationale for many studies that followed.

Pune, India, 2003

There was a significantly elevated risk of hospitalisation for HIV exposed babies who were formula-fed.[22]

Botswana, 2007, 2010

After the 2006 Botswana floods turned into a public health emergency it was found that formula-fed babies had a 25-fold risk of death due to diarrhoea compared to babies who were breastfed.[23,24]

PEPI, Malawi, 2006

Babies were enrolled between April 2004 and September 2009 in Blantyre, Malawi. The rates of morbidity were consistently higher among non-breastfed infants at various time intervals compared with breastfed infants. Cumulative mortality at 15 months was 3.5% for breastfed vs 6.4% for formula-fed infants. Cessation of breastfeeding was associated with acute morbidity events and cumulative mortality.[25,26]

Mashi trial, Botswana, 2006

Mortality was doubled at seven months for HIV-exposed, uninfected infants randomised to formula-feeding at birth – 9.3% for formula-fed vs 4.9% for breastfed babies.[13]

KIBS study, Kisumu, Kenya, 2007

Weaning at six months vs ad lib breastfeeding led to significantly higher rates of diarrhoea hospitalisations and growth faltering after weaning. Interventions to improve water safety were not effective in reducing morbidity.[27]

South Africa, 2007

Three criteria were found to be associated with improved HIV-free survival of babies whose mothers chose to formula-feed: piped water; electricity, gas or paraffin for fuel. Formula-feeding when these three criteria were not fulfilled led to the highest risk of HIV transmission or death. Within operational settings, the WHO/UNICEF guidelines were not being implemented effectively, leading to inappropriate infant-feeding choices and consequent lower infant HIV-free survival. There was no net benefit of formula-feeding for the babies of poor mothers.[28]

Côte d'Ivoire, 2007

Babies of 557 mothers who self-selected feeding choice had no increase in mortality or morbidity with either exclusive breastfeeding with early weaning at four months vs formula-feeding. There was, therefore, no net benefit to formula-feeding.[29]

Kampala, Uganda, 2007, 2010

Babies breastfed followed by early weaning at around four months had higher rates of diarrhoea and higher mortality due to other causes around the time of weaning compared to babies breastfed until around nine months. This study was interrupted by its Data Safety and Monitoring Boards due to increased morbidity after weaning.[30,31]

BAN study, Lilongwe, Malawi, 2007

In this study exclusive breastfeeding for six months was followed by rapid weaning. Babies were provided with a peanut-based food supplement similar to Plumpy'Nut at six months.[32] There was an increase in diarrhoea in exclusively breastfed infants weaned at six months.[33]

PEPI and NVAZ trials, Blantyre, Malawi, 2007 and 2010

A comparative trial in Malawi revealed that among breastfed and non-breastfed HIV-exposed infants and young children from birth–24 months early weaning was associated with increased risk of severe gastroenteritis and related mortality. Babies weaned later had significantly lower rates of diarrhoea and death compared to babies whose mothers were encouraged to wean at six months. Continued breastfeeding provided almost three-fold protection. This study was also interrupted by its Data Safety and Monitoring Board for increased illness after weaning.[34,35]

Rakai, Uganda, 2008, 2010

Infant mortality was increased more than six-fold among babies whose mothers chose to wean before six months rather than continuing breastfeeding beyond six months.[36,37] Babies who continued breastfeeding enjoyed higher rates of growth and protection from diarrhoeal disease and death and these benefits persisted into the second year of life to around 18 months.

Amata study, Rwanda, 2009

In this study, breastfeeding mothers received HAART. Only one child in the breastfeeding group became infected from 3–7 months, corresponding to a nine-month cumulative risk of postnatal infection of 0.5%. However cumulative mortality was almost twice as high (5.7%) for formula-fed compared to breastfed babies (3.3%). There was no net benefit of formula-feeding.[38]

Eldoret, Kenya, 2010

A retrospective study measured the combined endpoint of infant HIV status and mortality at three and 18 months at 18 HIV clinics in western Kenya where 2,477 babies were enrolled from February 2002 to July 2007. Documentation of feeding choice was poor, but of those who were documented, the results strongly suggested a benefit of antiretroviral prophylaxis in reducing infant death and HIV infection, but did not show a benefit at 18 months from the use of formula.[39]

Kesho Bora study group, Burkina Faso, Kenya, South Africa, 2012

Between 2005 and 2008, the Kesho Bora randomised controlled trial (RCT) funded by WHO enrolled HIV-infected pregnant women who were counselled to choose between exclusive breastfeeding for up to six months or replacement feeding from birth, as per WHO guidelines. At six months, weaned or never breastfed children were at a seven-fold higher risk of dying compared to children who were still breastfed, despite interventions to reduce risks associated with replacement feeding.[40]

ZEBS, Zambia, 2008–10

The ZEBS Study in Zambia[41–45] produced particularly tantalising results showing that there was no net benefit to early weaning. Some of the mothers did not comply with recommendations and the researchers then analysed the effects of early weaning and of non-compliance. Women were randomised to either stop breastfeeding at four months or to continue breastfeeding for their own preferred duration. Babies had better outcomes when their mothers received ART, and worse outcomes if they were weaned early. Health outcomes of infants whose mothers were assigned to breastfeeding followed by early weaning were tracked, but – since early weaning was not well accepted in the community – researchers also tracked the outcomes for babies whose mothers didn't adhere to the feeding groups that they were assigned to. Infants born to women who adhered to early weaning had worse outcomes than those whose mothers ignored their random assignment and continued breastfeeding. There was no net benefit to early weaning. Early weaning in fact led to a 2–4-fold increase in uninfected child mortality. Infants of mothers who refused to adhere to assignment to the extended breastfeeding group, and instead weaned early, also had worse outcomes.In the primary intent-to-treat analysis there was no benefit of early weaning at four months for HIV-free survival compared to the standard practice of continued breastfeeding. The magnitude of benefit (i.e. the amount of HIV prevented) was almost the same as the magnitude of the harm (i.e. the numbers of deaths caused in the population overall). The researchers extrapolated from these results that the magnitude of mortality caused by artificial feeding would be larger than the magnitude of HIV transmission prevented. So for women who were not yet at an advanced enough disease stage to require antiretroviral therapy for their own health (as per accepted protocols in place at the time), stopping breastfeeding at four months led to a three-fold increase in the combined outcome of HIV infection or death occurring between four and 24 months.

The dilemma

Louise Kuhn and Grace Aldrovandi succinctly summarised these unexpected results and the dilemma faced by those working with HIV-positive mothers and babies:[20]

> *'The increased risks of mortality among HIV-exposed uninfected infants due to artificial feeding might be justifiable if a net benefit in terms of HIV-free survival could be accomplished. However, other than in the original study in Nairobi, Kenya[21] in which no antiretroviral prophylaxis or treatment was available, this is not what has been found. In the clinical trial in Botswana there was no net benefit of artificial feeding on HIV-free survival. The reduced risk of HIV transmission as a result of formula feeding was outweighed by the increased risk of mortality among uninfected children.[13] Nor was there a net benefit for HIV-free survival of artificial feeding from birth vs. short breastfeeding in a study in Côte d'Ivoire.[29] At best, artificial feeding results in no improvements in health status. When implemented under real-world conditions, HIV-free survival has generally been worse, as shown in programs from South Africa and Uganda.[28,36] For example, in an evaluation of the South African national program, women's infant feeding choices bore little relation to their living circumstances. For women who lived in two of the poorer urban and rural sites, both HIV infection and death was increased among women who opted for formula feeding.'[28]*

In 2007, Jerry Coovadia and Anna Coutsoudis, commenting on recent developments, wrote:[46]

> *'The discourse on formula feeding or breastfeeding by HIV-positive mothers in developing countries has been mired in confusion or locked in robust disagreement. Recent data from ongoing and completed studies in Africa have suggested that the effects of avoidance of breastfeeding or cessation even at 6 months by HIV-positive mothers can be disastrous. This finding repeats what has been and remains the bedrock of public health policy for infants and children well before the HIV epidemic, and recognized through centuries of human experience... randomized controlled trials have shown that neither 'no breastfeeding' nor a short period of breastfeeding, holds any overall advantage over continued breastfeeding, as the decrease in HIV transmission is countered by an increase in infectious disease mortality.*
>
> *...The foregoing are exactly the consequences of formula feeding in poor populations that were recorded repeatedly in the last century, and which have been known for hundreds of years.[47–49] Many contemporary studies have taken care to adjust for confounding variables and to account for reverse causality.[50,51] The most consistent effect*

> *of the benefit of breastfeeding has been in terms of protecting against diarrhoea. Feachem and Koblinsky[52] reviewed 35 studies on diarrhoeal incidence from 14 countries and found consistent and clear evidence of the protective effect of breastfeeding. A further review of the literature by Victora[53] showed that in addition to breastfeeding reducing the incidence of diarrhoea, breastfeeding reduces the severity of diarrhoeal episodes, and case-fatality rates. Importantly, Victora's review highlighted the point that recently weaned infants may be more vulnerable. The child survival benefits of breastfeeding in developing countries have recently been reinforced by reliable data.[5,8]*
>
> *New studies among HIV-infected women in poor populations have demonstrated the impact on child health when formula milks replace breastfeeding, either from birth or during infancy. Diarrhoeal diseases are frequent, hospitalizations become necessary, growth and development falter, overt malnutrition supervenes, and mortality rates increase; socio-economic costs may also be incurred. Measures to make breastfeeding by HIV-infected women safe are urgently required. These findings confirm the historical experience in the pre-HIV era and require a response similar to that period, when international mobilization led to codification of policies for the protection, promotion and support of breastfeeding.'*

A final caution came from Kuhn and Aldrovandi, who reiterated that some of the strategies proposed to prevent HIV transmission, such as abstinence from breastfeeding or early weaning, also carry a cost in terms of lives of uninfected infants. The disadvantage of this approach is that it counts an HIV infection as equivalent to a death, a pessimistic approach and one that is out of date now that paediatric HIV infection can be successfully treated. It also stacks the deck in favour of interventions that prevent HIV transmission, but neglects the range of other non-fatal, but potentially serious, adverse outcomes associated with limiting breastfeeding.[20]

CHAPTER 22

ART and breastfeeding

The development of multi-drug combination therapy for the treatment of HIV is one of the great success stories of modern medicine. Over a period of approximately 10 years, antiretroviral treatment (ART) was developed and refined to the point that the risk of death following infection with HIV was reduced by almost 80%. Today, ART has transformed HIV from a catastrophic, fatal disease into a manageable, chronic illness.[1]

Without treatment, HIV-infected adults would die from AIDS in just over a decade. Over 90% of paediatric HIV occurred as a result of what we have come to call, for convenience, mother-to-child transmission (MTCT) – when the virus is passed to the baby of an infected mother, during pregnancy, birth or breastfeeding. One-third of infected babies died within a year, and half died by their second birthday.[2]

Without any intervention, the rate of MTCT of HIV ranged from at least 15% in industrialised countries to as much as 45% in developing countries.[3,4] The highest rates were found in African babies[5–11] and the difference in risk has always been put down to the fact that African women breastfeed.

The first antiretroviral drugs

The first drug to treat HIV was approved in 1987. In the next three decades many researchers conducted many studies on many therapies to reduce MTCT of HIV. These studies had an impressive array of acronyms: HIVNET 012, PACTG 076, PEPI, NAVI, ANRS, DITRAME, KIBS, Kesho Bora, BAN, SIMBA, Amata, MITRA and MITRA-Plus, SWEN, DREAM, ZEBS, ZVITAMBO, MASHI and Mma Bana studies, and no doubt many more. Different drugs, with various doses and durations of treatment, e.g. long-long, short-short, long-short, and any combination in between, were tried. At various times there was provision of sequential, alternating, delayed, prolonged, suspended, salvaged, single-dose, combined or multiple-drug treatment and most recently long-acting injectibles. To prevent and treat paediatric HIV there has been either infant prophylaxis or maternal therapy during pregnancy, during labour and birth, during breastfeeding, during all or only one of these. There has also been prophylaxis for the mother, for the baby, or both.

The quest by the AIDS community for prevention, treatment or cure has become a global industry. In 2006 I attended the eye-opening 2006 International AIDS Conference in Toronto as one of 31,000 delegates.[12,13] The abstract catalogue, the size of a telephone directory 8cm thick, was too heavy for my tote bag. Adding the acronym 'HIV' to any conceivable topic seemed to have been sufficient to attract research funding, and guarantee a place on the programme.

The US Department of Health and Human Services *Guidelines for the Use of Antiretroviral Agents in Adults and Adolescents Living with HIV* have been updated over 30 times.[14] Effective drug treatment, in the form of highly active antiretroviral therapy (HAART) is finally available, but it has been a long time coming. The cost in human life has been massive, with >75 million infections and >33 million deaths. There are 40 individual and combination medications approved for the treatment of HIV and one approved for the prevention of HIV infection,[15,16] and this means that today an HIV-infected individual on effective ART can live a normal life-span.[17,18] In 2019 a Canadian news outlet reported that an HIV-positive man had celebrated his 100th birthday.[19]

Viral load

Antiretroviral treatment works by suppressing the number of detectable viral copies in the blood, otherwise called the viral load. The goal is to reach an undetectable level, but different tests show different sensitivity, and when reading research articles it's wise to see what is meant by this term. Transmission of the virus between individuals – horizontally between sexual partners, or vertically from mother to child – is related to viral load. The percentage risk of passing on the virus according to the number of viral copies contained in one millilitre of a person's blood was quantified in a 1999 paper.[20] The longer an untreated individual has had HIV, the more the virus is able to replicate. As the immune system becomes progressively more compromised, the closer an infected individual moves towards developing active AIDS. Importantly, the higher the viral load the more infectious that person becomes to others.

Percentage risk of transmission	viral load, copies/mL
0	<1,000
16.6	1,000–10,000
21.3	10,001–50,000
30.9	50,001–100,000
40.6	>100,000
63.3	>100,000 no ART

Source: Garcia et al, 1999

Above average viral loads are associated with an increased risk of viral shedding in blood, plasma, genital secretions and breastmilk, leading to a higher risk of a mother infecting her baby by all routes.[21–24] A 1999 study from Thailand[21] found that mothers who transmitted HIV to their babies had four-fold higher viral levels at delivery compared to mothers whose babies were not infected. No transmission occurred at <2000 copies/ml. As viral RNA increased the odds ratio for transmission also increased linearly from 4.5 to 24.8. Two-thirds of transmission was due to viral load >10,000 copies/ml.

HIV transmission is also inversely related to an individual's CD4 count, which is a measure of how well the immune system functions; the higher a person's CD4 count, the healthier the individual. Until fairly recently, clinicians relied on the CD4 count to determine an individual's stage of disease; the lower the CD4 cell count, the higher the viral load. Treatment with ART was often rationed to individuals with a low CD4 count, and prescribed for short times, which led to viral rebound after the drug was discontinued – a bit like the resistance that has developed from similar treatment mishaps with antibiotics.

Treatment is not only good for the affected individual. While it reduces the viral load (nowadays to undetectable) as well as elevating a person's CD4 count, to halt progression of the disease and prolong life, it also reduces an HIV-positive individual's infectivity – the ability to pass on the virus to others. Thus it was found that provision of adequate antiretroviral therapy (ART) for HIV-infected mothers not only dramatically reduced the likelihood of her infecting her baby by any route, including through breastfeeding, but it also improved a mother's own health and prolonged her life, enabling her to care for her children as they grew up.

Early research on antiretroviral therapy

The first antiretroviral drug was zidovudine, initially developed as a cancer drug in the 1960s.[25] The drug was designed to interfere with the ability of a cancer cell's DNA to replicate, but when tested in mice it proved ineffective and was put aside. During the late 1980s and early 1990s, animal models of retroviral infection had demonstrated that zidovudine might prevent or alter the course of maternally transmitted HIV infection.[26,27] Heralded as a breakthrough, and pushed through in record time, zidovudine was approved by the US Food and Drug Administration on 19 March 1987 as an antiretroviral medication to treat HIV.

Zidovudine was initially tested in a randomised controlled trial on nearly 300 people diagnosed with AIDS. Half the participants received a placebo, but after only 16 weeks, Burroughs Wellcome stopped the trial on ethical grounds; the treatment group had only one death, but even in that short period the placebo group had 19. Activists and public health officials raised concerns about the prohibitive price tag of $8,000 per year, making the drug effectively unavailable to those who needed it. However, by 1990 zidovudine was beginning to be used to treat AIDS and AIDS Related Complex during pregnancy.[28] It was known to cross the placenta, but it was safe when used for short periods.[29,30]

PACTG 076 protocol, USA and France

Between April 1991 and the end of 1993, Edward Connor and colleagues recruited nearly 500 pregnant women from 14–34 weeks' gestation into a randomised, double-blind, placebo-controlled trial in the USA and France, subsequently known as the

PACTG 076 protocol, to test the efficacy of zidovudine in reducing MTCT.[31] The women had CD4 counts >200 cells/mm^3, with mildly symptomatic HIV disease, and no prior treatment with antiretroviral drugs. During late pregnancy they received oral zidovudine (100mg five times daily) for a median of 11 weeks (range, 0–26), then intravenously during labour (2mg per kilogram of body weight over a one-hour period, then 1mg per kilogram per hour until delivery). The babies also received zidovudine prophylaxis (2mg per kilogram orally every six hours for six weeks). The researchers chose a drug regimen that combined antepartum, intrapartum and neonatal therapy because the timing of maternal-infant transmission was uncertain. The dosing schedule reduced circulating levels of HIV and had minimal toxicity. Thirteen infants in the zidovudine group and 40 in the placebo group were infected, reducing the risk of maternal-infant HIV transmission by approximately two-thirds (8.3% vs 25.5%). The treatment was so successful that, based on the interim findings, the safety monitoring board terminated the trial and offered the drugs to women in the placebo group who had not yet delivered, and to their infants up to six weeks of age. From 1994, the regimen was then recommended as standard care in the United States.[32]

Connor and colleagues speculated that maternal zidovudine treatment may have reduced the viral load and diminished viral exposure of the foetus *in utero*, or at delivery, or both. However, some infants became infected despite treatment. The researchers thought that this may have happened due to transmission before treatment, inefficient suppression of maternal viral replication by zidovudine, or that mothers had not complied with the treatment regimen.

More information was gleaned during a follow-up study, showing the number of infants infected at 18 months of age, and the relationship between maternal viral load, the risk of HIV transmission and the efficacy of zidovudine treatment.[33] In both treated and untreated groups, transmission occurred at a wide range of maternal plasma HIV RNA levels. However, in the placebo group, a large viral burden either at entry or at delivery was associated with an increased risk of transmission: there was a 40% higher risk in the highest quartile of the RNA level. To prevent HIV transmission, the researchers recommended initiating maternal treatment with zidovudine regardless of the plasma level of HIV RNA or the CD4 count. Following this research, between 1994 and 1999 the number of babies born with HIV in developed countries dropped 78%.[34]

Thailand

It was thought that a drug regimen similar to the ACTG 076 regimen wouldn't be feasible in most developing countries, due to both complexity and cost. Annual national health budgets were often less than $10 per day and the cost of the drugs alone for the ACTG 076 regimen was at least eighty times that amount, whereas a 'short course' of zidovudine confined to the last four weeks of pregnancy and during labour would cost only $50.[35]

In Neil Shaffer's study conducted in Thailand from 1992 to 1994 the risk of MTCT of HIV for formula-fed babies was 24.2%.[21,36] In the March 1999 edition of the *Lancet*, he published the results of further research conducted from 1996 to 1997 as a collaboration between the US CDC, the Ministry of Public Health of Thailand and

Mahidol University. Using a simpler and less expensive regimen than the PACTG 076 for US and French mothers, pregnant Thai women who would not be breastfeeding were randomly assigned placebo or zidovudine twice daily from 36 weeks' gestation and during labour. The protocol was clearly 'logistically simpler', with a later start in pregnancy, shorter duration, less frequent dosing, orally rather than intravenously, and no infant treatment. Mothers in the treatment arm received three doses of zidovudine over the 25 days.[36] About 80% of the treatment effect was explained by lowered maternal viral concentrations at delivery. Transmitting mothers had a 4.3-fold higher viral load. No transmission occurred at <2000 copies/ml, most occurred at >10,000 copies/ml. This short course of antiretroviral therapy, in the absence of breastfeeding, was able to halve the risk of transmission from ~19% to 9%. It was concluded that it could thus prevent many HIV infections during late pregnancy and labour in the less-developed countries unable to implement the full PACTG 076 regimen. The hope was that, if implemented, thousands of perinatal HIV infections could be prevented in Thailand, where an estimated 20,000 HIV-infected women delivered infants each year.

Little concern appears to have been raised about the fact that although zidovudine had already been proven to be so effective in reducing perinatal transmission of the virus in the previous PACTG 076 trial that it was terminated early so that those in the placebo arm could receive treatment, the Thai research again included mothers who were only given a placebo.

Ivory Coast and Burkina Faso

Meanwhile, alongside the Thailand trial François Dabis and colleagues, in collaboration with the French Ministry of Co-operation, conducted randomised double-blind placebo-controlled trials in public clinics in Abidjan, Côte d'Ivoire, and Bobo-Dioulasso, Burkina Faso. Eligible women were recruited into the trial between September 1995, and February 1998, when enrolment to the placebo group was again stopped. All women were aged 18 or older, and had confirmed HIV infection at 36–38 weeks' gestation, i.e. only during the last 2–4 weeks of pregnancy. They were randomly assigned 300mg zidovudine twice daily until labour, 600mg at the beginning of labour, and 300mg twice daily for seven days postpartum, or matching placebo. Analyses were by intention to treat. The probability of HIV infection in the infant at six months was 18.0% in the zidovudine group and 27.5% in the placebo group, giving a 38% reduction in transmission despite breastfeeding.[37]

A further follow-up study was done in Abidjan, Côte d'Ivoire from April 1996 to February 1998. Wiktor and colleagues assessed the safety and efficacy of the shortened zidovudine regimen. Pregnant HIV-positive women attending a public antenatal clinic were enrolled at 36 weeks' gestation and randomly assigned placebo or zidovudine (300mg tablets), one tablet twice daily during pregnancy, one tablet at onset of labour, and one tablet every three hours until delivery. The median duration of the prenatal drug regimen was 27 days. All babies were breastfed. Among babies with known infection status at age three months, 16.5% in the zidovudine group and 26.1% in the placebo group were infected. The estimated risk of HIV transmission in the zidovudine and placebo groups were 12.2% and 21.7% at four weeks, and 15.7% and 24.9% at three months respectively.[38] Again, no concern was expressed about the use of placebo for HIV-positive women in these African settings, when the ability of zidovudine to almost halve transmission rates was already known.

The mechanism by which zidovudine blocked vertical transmission was still obscure. Given alone, the drug did not seem to lower viral concentrations to any great degree, so that although women with lower viral loads were less likely to pass the virus to their babies, it did not help by only reducing viral levels. It was believed that the drug might work primarily by blocking infection during delivery, when the infant's eyes, nose, mouth and gastrointestinal tract were exposed to virus in the secretions of the mother's reproductive tract.[39] At the same time there was also some concern that antenatal ART, which was discontinued after delivery, might actually increase viral load by causing a rebound effect during breastfeeding, reducing its overall efficacy in breastfeeding populations.[40–42] More research was needed.

How breastfeeding was seen to be a barrier to elimination of paediatric HIV

In the early phase of the ART research to prevent MTCT, estimates still blamed 'late postnatal transmission' (i.e. through breastfeeding) for as much as 42% of overall transmission.[43] In developing countries, shorter, simpler peripartum interventions had been shown to be effective in reducing transmission risk, but their application in populations where breastfeeding was commonly practised posed 'considerable challenges' according to François Dabis, who had conducted the ANRS studies in Côte d'Ivoire and Burkina Faso.[44] In an accompanying editorial in the *Lancet* on the Thai and West African trials, Lynne Mofensen noted that most transmission took place between eight and 45 days postpartum.[45] She wrote that the efficacy of zidovudine was clearly lower among breastfed than among non-breastfed babies and that there was a 'substantial risk' of transmission of HIV through breastmilk. According to the AIDS community it seemed futile to provide ART to save babies from MTCT during pregnancy and birth only to have them infected afterwards through breastfeeding, and the longer the duration of breastfeeding, the greater the cumulative risk.

The Italian Register for HIV in Children reported in 2002 that children who were breastfed were 10 times more likely to become infected than those who were bottle-fed.[46] The MTCT rate was 21.7% in 1985–95, but had risen to 53% from 1996–99. Not breastfeeding and receipt of ART were protective. Transmission risk was reduced by 76% by an incomplete zidovudine regimen, by 88% with a complete regimen and by 93% when the mother received combination ART. In the 1996–99 period the transmission rate was reduced to 2.4% when caesarean section, no breastfeeding and ART were combined.

Short-course ARV interventions to reduce postnatal transmission

Between November 1997 and April 1999, Laura Guay, who had previously worked in Zaire, conducted the landmark HIVNET 012 study at Mulago Hospital in Kampala, Uganda.[47] This was a randomised, double-blind, three-arm placebo-controlled Phase II clinical trial to determine the efficacy of two short-course ART drug regimens (oral zidovudine or oral nevirapine) against a placebo. Intended for PMTCT in resource-poor settings,[48] 626 mother-infant pairs were enrolled. Mothers were randomly assigned to receive either:

- nevirapine 200mg orally at onset of labour and 2mg/kg to their babies within 72 hours of birth, or
- zidovudine 600mg orally to the mother at onset of labour and 300mg every three hours until delivery, and 4mg/kg orally twice daily to their babies for seven days after birth.

Soon after it began, results of another study were released which led to the placebo arm being dropped. Almost 100% of the babies were still breastfeeding at 14–16 weeks. They were tested for HIV infection at birth, 6–8 and 14–16 weeks by HIV RNA PCR. The estimated rates of transmission in the zidovudine and nevirapine groups respectively were: 10.4% vs 8.2% at birth, 21.3% vs 11.9% by age 6–8 weeks, and 25.1% vs 13.1% by age 14–16 weeks. The researchers concluded that the nevirapine regimen, which lowered the risk of transmission by nearly 50% while breastfeeding was maintained, was a simple and inexpensive way to decrease MTCT of HIV in less-developed countries.

Single-dose nevirapine (sdNVP) subsequently became the mainstay of ARV prophylaxis in most developing countries, with one dose given to the mother at the onset of labour and one dose given to the infant within 72 hours after birth.[47] This single-dose nevirapine (sdNVP) regimen reduced MTCT by 50% in breastfeeding populations at four months of age, compared with a short course of zidovudine monotherapy, and was subsequently recommended by WHO as an interim PMTCT therapy until more effective and comprehensive interventions were available.[49]

The South African SAINT study provided further evidence that sdNVP and short-course zidovudine/lamivudine prophylaxis regimens were safe, effective, and could be easily provided at the onset of labour, even to women who were not attending antenatal clinics, proving that there were really few barriers to prevention of MTCT in resource-limited countries.[50]

As researchers cast around for measures which would be both effective and inexpensive, some of the treatment regimens became very complicated. Reporting in the 2000 *New England Journal of Medicine*, Lallemant and colleagues described an extremely elaborate study they had devised in Thailand.[51] Employing four different regimens of zidovudine, described as long-long, short-short, long-short, and short-long, 1,437 women received various durations of zidovudine treatment during pregnancy and labour. To avoid postnatal transmission, all the infants were formula-fed. Babies were tested at one, 45, 120 and 180 days. At the first interim analysis, the rates of transmission were 4.1% for the long-long regimen and 10.5 % for the short-short regimen. At this point the short-short regimen was stopped. But the researchers did establish that shorter treatment led to significantly higher *in utero* transmission (5.1% vs 1.6%).

Altogether, between 1999 and 2003 five trials in breastfeeding populations demonstrated the safety and efficacy of different short-course antiretroviral regimens.[52] However, over 800,000 babies had been newly infected during 2002 alone. While pharmaceutical companies had provided ART at reduced or no cost to resource-limited countries, it was 'mother-child health infrastructure' which seemed to be the sticking point – in other words, breastfeeding was still seen as a significant problem in 'countries where safe replacement feeding was not possible'.

Moving towards HAART

Although the use of simple, single-dose nevirapine-based PMTCT regimens was able to avert >30,000 infections in infants per year,[53] there was concern about nevirapine resistance in women and babies exposed to single-dose regimens.[54,55] In 2004 researchers had found that a nevirapine regimen in Kenya resulted in a transmission rate at 14 weeks of 18%, similar to the rate of 21% before the intervention, underlining the need for alternative strategies.[56] If initiated within six months of PMTCT therapy it seemed that previous exposure to single-dose nevirapine could impede nevirapine-based HAART's ability to suppress HIV.[57] Data from Botswana had found that initiation of nevirapine-based HAART soon after single-dose nevirapine could have a serious effect on suppression of the virus.[58] Despite WHO's edorsement, the issue of resistance to nevirapine continued to raise ethical and scientific concerns.[59–61]

Short-course zidovudine and single-dose nevirapine showed long-term relative efficacy among breastfeeding mothers until 18-24 months, but this was reduced somewhat due to postnatal transmission.[62–64] With the use of two or three-drug combinations during late pregnancy, during and after birth, MTCT could be reduced to 4–5% in breastfeeding mothers, or 2–3% with no breastfeeding.[65–67] These combined regimens came to be known as Highly Active Antiretroviral Therapy, or HAART. Combination antiretroviral therapy (cART) had been in use in the US as the standard of care since 1997 and AIDS-related deaths had been cut by 47% as a result.[68]

Maternal treatment or infant prophylaxis

Two randomised clinical trials from 2008 demonstrated that providing daily nevirapine to the breastfeeding infant also offered protection against HIV infection.[69,70] Once nevirapine was withdrawn, however, transmission risk returned unless the mother was receiving HAART. On the other hand, the HPTN 046 trial found that reduced rates of transmission at 6–9 months could be achieved with increased duration of prophylaxis for breastfeeding infants; 6.9% to six weeks,[70] 5.2% to 14 weeks,[69] and only 1.1% to 28 weeks,[71] so nevirapine for breastfed infants was recommended as an alternative prophylactic strategy for women with moderate to high CD4 cell counts who, as policymakers put it, 'did not require long-term HAART for their own health'.[72] A subsequent protocol was agreed whereby mothers could receive zidovudine prophylaxis from the second trimester of pregnancy until delivery, with daily oral nevirapine to the breastfed infant until all breastfeeding had ceased.[73] The HPTN 046 trial results, however, also confirmed that long-term infant nevirapine offered no additional benefit over maternal HAART. If women received HAART while breastfeeding, the monthly postnatal transmission risk was reduced by 80%. If the infant received extended nevirapine prophylaxis instead, the rate of transmission was reduced by 60%.[71]

Resource-rich countries

There had been a sharp difference in the success of treatments designed for developed countries vs developing countries. Within a year of publication of the PACTG 076 results, widespread implementation of the zidovudine prophylactic regimen, coupled with universal HIV counselling and testing, meant that HIV transmission to babies in the West decreased by two-thirds (from 25% to 8%). With the use of HAART and elective caesarean section, transmission rates were further decreased to <2%.[74] It was estimated that <400 infants per annum were born with HIV each year in the US.[75] Similar reports of success were achieved in Europe.[47] Where HIV-positive women had been treated with a combination of ARVs from early in pregnancy, longer treatment duration was found to be significantly more effective than shorter regimens in reducing viral load, reducing the risk of transmission during pregnancy and delivery to as low as 1–2%.[76] The combination of HAART, elective caesarean section, and postpartum formula-feeding virtually eliminated MTCT of HIV in the developed world.[50]

Maternal health and provision of antiretrovirals

The BHITS meta-analysis found that the risk of late postnatal transmission of HIV (i.e. through breastfeeding) was strongly associated with a lower CD4 cell count (<200 vs >500 cells/mm^3).[77] The authors suggested providing HAART to all HIV-infected pregnant women during the last weeks of their pregnancy and to breastfeeding mothers during the crucial first 4–6 months of lactation. From 2006 WHO also progressively recommended shifting away from single-dose nevirapine towards more effective alternatives.[78]

In earlier trials maternal treatment had only been provided to mothers who had low CD4 counts. Where a mother had a higher CD4 count, so-called ARV 'prophylaxis' was provided only during pregnancy, and was withdrawn once the baby was delivered, effectively leaving the mother to die. This practice was rationalised by saying that women with higher CD4 counts did not need antiretroviral treatment because they were not yet sick enough. In effect it meant that the mother was sacrificed after incubating a healthy baby.

Researchers working in the successful DREAM study in Mozambique, published in 2007, noted that it was difficult to have to tell a woman that she could avoid transmitting HIV to her child, but that nothing could be done for her own health. When they provided HAART to exclusively breastfeeding mothers regardless of their clinical, immunological or virologic status,[79] cumulative transmission to their babies between one and six months was reduced to only 2.2%.

Duration of maternal ART

Research published in 2010[80] found that the duration of HAART during pregnancy influenced the rate of *in utero* transmission. Transmission decreased with longer duration of therapy: the risk was 9.3% with less than four weeks of HAART, 5.5% with 4–16 weeks of HAART, and 3.5% with 16 to 32 weeks. If mothers received HAART for more than 32 weeks before the birth, there were no transmissions at all. Chibwesha and colleagues, in a study done in Zambia between 2007 and 2010, also found that the most important predictor of vertical HIV transmission in this cohort was time on HAART prior to delivery. Compared to women who had received HAART for at least 13 weeks prior to delivery, women on HAART for ≤ 4 weeks had a 5.2-fold increased odds of HIV transmission.[81] An exploratory analysis limited to women on HAART for fewer than 13 weeks demonstrated that for each additional week on HAART prior to delivery the odds of mother-to-child HIV transmission were reduced by 14%.

Surprisingly, programmes that proactively initiated treatment in sicker, pregnant women with low CD4 counts, who should therefore have been more infectious, consistently reported lower rates of postnatal transmission.[82–84] For breastfeeding mothers, it became clear that HAART used earlier in pregnancy was more effective than the same combination starting during labour and delivery. Viral load at enrolment and shorter duration of HAART significantly increased the risk of infant infection, whereas extended maternal or infant treatment or prophylaxis showed reduced postnatal HIV transmission through breastfeeding[85] even up to 12 months.[86]

Much improved results from the Kesho Bora[87] and other trials[88,89] underpinned WHO's 2010 decision to revise international guidelines for ARV to be used by pregnant and breastfeeding women.[90] Maternal triple ARV prophylaxis starting from the second trimester of pregnancy until all exposure to breastmilk ended was recommended. The unifying principle of the new guidelines was that effective maternal or infant antiretroviral-based prophylaxis to prevent MTCT was required in all instances.[72] Maternal HAART had since been shown to reduce postnatal HIV transmission four-fold compared to simpler regimens, e.g. single-dose nevirapine, even in times of severe socio-economic crisis.[91]

Cost

HAART not only improved the HIV-positive mother's health, but the DREAM study[79] had also found that the cost of ARVs for mothers was the same as the cost of formula for infants who were not breastfed. Intuitively it would seem more ethical as well as more cost-effective to provide HAART to the breastfeeding HIV-positive mother, to improve her health and prolong her life, than to use scarce funds for the purchase of formula to prevent MTCT through breastfeeding, placing the formula-fed infant at increased risk of other infections.

By 2009, significant reductions in the price of first-line antiretroviral medicines meant that low-income countries could provide a year's worth of ART at a median cost of US $137 per person. Over 50% of pregnant women living with HIV had access to antiretroviral medicines to prevent transmission of HIV to their infants. AIDS-related deaths dropped by 19% globally over the period 2004 to 2009.[92] The number of HIV infections among children also fell significantly – from 500,000 in 2001 to 370,000 in 2009 – as a result of expanded PMTCT programmes. In 2010 WHO also agreed that any infant-feeding strategy that included free provision of infant formula to HIV-infected mothers, even for a limited period of six months, would cost 2–6 times as much as life-long ARV treatment for mothers.[73]

The success of antiretroviral therapy to prevent MTCT during breastfeeding

Later studies showed that antiretroviral drugs given to the mother[69,70,79,88,89,93–95] or the infant[88,96–98] for up to six months after delivery could dramatically reduce MTCT during breastfeeding. And so the success of these studies at last provided the evidence for WHO to change its recommendation for continued breastfeeding with either maternal or infant prophylaxis.

In October 2009, as the lactation community held its collective breath, a further WHO Technical Consultation on HIV and infant feeding heard new information about the protective effects of HAART against HIV transmission through breastfeeding. This new body of research was described as 'transformational'.[99] Finally, as a result, WHO changed their guidance to recommend antiretroviral therapy for all pregnant women with CD4 counts less than 350 cells/ml and endorsed a return to breastfeeding:

> *'Evidence has been reported that antiretroviral (ARV) interventions to either the HIV-infected mother or HIV-exposed infant can significantly reduce the risk of postnatal transmission of HIV through breastfeeding. This has major implications for how women living with HIV might choose to feed their infants, and how health workers should counsel mothers when making these choices. The potential of ARVs to reduce HIV transmission throughout the period of breastfeeding also highlights the need for guidance on how child health services should communicate information about ARVs to prevent transmission through breastfeeding, and the implications for feeding of HIV exposed infants through the first two years of life.'*

In 2010 WHO and UNICEF formalised the 2009 Rapid advice.[73] Antiretroviral therapy regimens shown to be successful in significantly reducing the risk of HIV transmission through breastfeeding were described as 'a major breakthrough that should contribute to improved child survival'. In conjunction with the known benefits of breastfeeding to reduce mortality from other causes, this finding justified an approach that strongly recommended a single option as the standard of care.

Underpinning the new 2010 guidance was the research demonstrating that when mothers received effective ART, the level of virus in their blood (their viral load) could be suppressed to undetectable levels. This meant that the risk of transmission of HIV during a vaginal birth could be reduced to <1%. Furthermore, with maternal ART and six months exclusive breastfeeding, the risk of postpartum transmission of the virus could also be reduced to virtually zero. This will be further explored in Chapter 23.

The new recommendation finally brought HIV and infant feeding guidance in line with global breastfeeding recommendations outside the context of HIV. After six months exclusive breastfeeding, WHO recommended that breastfeeding should continue with the addition of household weaning foods for up to 12 months and in 2016 the recommendation for 12 months breastfeeding was extended to 24.[100]

From 2010 national authorities in each country could now decide which infant feeding practice, i.e. breastfeeding with an antiretroviral intervention to reduce transmission, or avoidance of all breastfeeding, would be primarily promoted and supported by maternal and child health services. This was a major shift in approach. While previously health workers were expected to focus on individual rights by individually counselling all HIV-infected mothers about various infant feeding options, and it was then for the mothers to decide between them, each country would now make the best recommendation based on public health considerations. The sting in the tail was the ambiguity about which recommendation was actually intended for developed countries: would they continue to promote formula-feeding by HIV-positive mothers? Or did the recommendation mean that if HIV-positive mothers were receiving ART they could breastfeed? This last question remains unanswered.

Meanwhile, further 2012 WHO guidelines for antiretroviral therapy for pregnant women and prevention of HIV infection in their infants[101] clarified several other ambiguities, including that reliance on CD4 counts would be dropped in favour of noting viral load. With proper ARV treatment, an HIV-positive mother's viral load becomes undetectable, not only protecting her own health and survival, but also reducing to virtually zero the risk of her baby acquiring HIV through her breastmilk.

In 2015 WHO removed the limitation on eligibility for treatment with full ART, and announced that all mothers who tested HIV-positive should receive effective ART from the time of diagnosis, whenever that occurred, regardless of CD4 T-lymphocyte count, and such treatment should continue for life.[102]

Rather than limiting ART for women to the time that they would incubate and give birth to just one HIV-free baby, they would now be able to live long enough to raise all their children, to enjoy a normal lifespan and even become grandmothers. Safer and more efficacious ARV drugs were becoming available and more affordable. WHO issued consolidated guidelines on the use of ART to include all age groups and populations and allowing a continuum of HIV care to be harmonised based on a public health approach.[103]

The battle to provide effective treatment for HIV had been a long time coming. WHO published the first guidelines on the use of antiretroviral therapy (ART) for HIV infection among adults and adolescents in 2002, and on the use of ARV drugs to prevent mother-to-child HIV transmission in 2004. The 2006 Updates introduced the concept of a public health approach, with simplified and harmonised ART regimens. In 2013, for the first time, WHO revised and combined these and other ARV-related documents into consolidated guidelines that addressed the use of ART for HIV treatment and prevention on a continuum across all age groups and populations. These were updated following an extensive review of evidence and consultations in mid-2015, and replaced by the 2016 consolidated guidelines on the use of antiretroviral drugs:

Previous antiretroviral protocols had been classified into therapeutic and preventive regimens:

- **Treatment:** In the past, mothers usually received ART for their own health based on their CD4 levels. They were eligible for treatment if their CD4 cell count fell below a certain number of viral copies per cubic millimetre of blood (usually <200mm^3 in the earliest studies and <350mm^3 or <500mm^3 in later studies).
- **Prophylaxis:** early treatment regimens provided pregnant or breastfeeding mothers with ARV prophylaxis to prevent vertical transmission to their babies which was

withdrawn after delivery of the baby, or when breastfeeding ended.

- **Current recommendations: HIV-positive** women should receive HAART; a combination or three or more drugs that attack the virus in several ways. ART should be initiated in all pregnant and breastfeeding women living with HIV regardless of WHO clinical stage and at any CD4 cell count and continued lifelong.[102]

Today there are over 30 different drugs which can be used. Neither ART nor HAART is a cure, but key to controlling both transmission and disease progression has been the necessity to reduce the infected individual's viral load to 'undetectable' (less than 50 viral copies/mm^3). Guidance on ART has been constantly updated as new research results have been released. Improving women's health so that they can continue to be vital and productive members of society, as well as care for their children, is of crucial importance but, in the rush to prevent another generation from being infected, remained unacknowledged for some time. Now it's known that if treatment is discontinued the virus becomes active again. This was not always the case, and much experimentation had to occur before the current recommendation was made that treatment needs to be taken for life, with meticulous adherence to treatment regimens to keep the virus at bay.

Thanks to the development of current antiretroviral regimens, the HIV-positive mother planning a pregnancy and giving birth today has an almost 100% chance of having a healthy baby, of being able to safely breastfeed, and of being able to raise her child in good health – a profound change from the dark days of 1985.

CHAPTER 23

EBF + ART, a winning combination

While I was spending time working at the WABA Secretariat in Penang in 2005, I came across an abstract of a paper published in 2003 by Dr Roger Shapiro from Harvard University. He described a pilot study conducted in Botswana, in preparation for further research on the use of antiretroviral drugs to prevent MTCT of HIV.[1]

Dr Shapiro and his colleagues wanted to know if HIV-positive mothers receiving ART would be adherent to a randomised feeding method – either breastfeeding or formula-feeding. The study yielded mixed results. At postnatal visits, nurses were tasked with expressing the breasts of new mothers who were allocated to formula-feeding to see if they were still lactating. Expression of drops or streams of breastmilk would be a marker for continued breastfeeding. It was found that 53% of the mothers were still producing breastmilk, and everyone suspected that they were closet-breastfeeding.

As a lactation consultant, what interested me were the methods the researchers used, which showed that their knowledge of breastmilk production and postpartum breast involution could do with some updating. This seemed to me to be another classic example of how better cooperation between the AIDS community and the lactation community might be useful in research on HIV and breastfeeding.

I immediately emailed Roger Shapiro to see if he could let me have a full-text copy of his article, which he kindly sent by return. When I thanked him I also gave a little information about how long it can take to suppress lactation after birth, and speculated that the mothers in his study might just be experiencing normal breast involution which can take 45 days, and I'd known even longer. He graciously replied to my comments and we had a little conversation back and forth about the difficulty in persuading African mothers to either exclusively breastfeed, or to exclusively formula-feed, because of the influence of older female relatives and cultural traditions. I said a little wistfully that what we really needed was research combining the protective effects of maternal ART *and* really, really exclusive breastfeeding (e.g. based on the low rates of MTCT with exclusive breastfeeding which had been achieved by the Coutsoudis and Iliff studies).[2,3] He wrote back that they were hoping that their HAART regimens would be effective in protection of transmission of HIV regardless of feeding method. And so we left it.

Roger Shapiro was to spend over two decades in Botswana, performing clinical trials and nationwide surveillance to improve health outcomes for HIV-infected pregnant women and their children.[4] He went on to oversee research programmes and clinical trials at 18 sites and acted as a research mentor bridging Boston and Botswana. His research has been used to direct health policy in Botswana and internationally, and through this work he has served as a scientific advisor to the World Health Organization for the development of guidelines for PMTCT, paediatric ART and infant feeding. This is an impressive set of accomplishments. But I believe that his greatest achievement has been conducting research which saved the day for breastfeeding in the face of HIV. His findings underpinned a global policy turnaround that enabled breastfeeding to be promoted once again in spite of HIV, and this resulted in the saving of millions of lives.

Between July 2006 and May 2008, Roger Shapiro and colleagues worked on the Mma Bana study (meaning 'mother of the baby' in Setswana). The results were published in the *New England Journal of Medicine* in 2010.[5] Mothers were provided with HAART during pregnancy and after birth, and they exclusively breastfed their babies for six months. Only two of 709 babies, a tiny 0.28%, became infected. Importantly, the reasons for those two failures were not random – they didn't just happen – they could clearly be identified:

- One of the mothers had medication adherence issues.
- The second mother had a baseline viral load of 171,000 copies/ml at recruitment at ~28 weeks of pregnancy. She was adherent to her medication, but her baby was born prematurely at 32 weeks' gestation and so she received antenatal ART for <4 weeks before commencement of breastfeeding, when she had a detectable HIV plasma RNA of 257 copies/ml.[6]
- Kahlert and colleagues, in examining this study, say in a 2018 article, 'Both mothers of the HIV-infected children started cART (combination antiretroviral therapy) with abacavir, zidovudine (AZT) and lamivudine only a short time before delivery (25 and 97 days)…'[7]

As previous research had hinted, and the Shapiro study now confirmed, it was *viral load* which determined transmission. HIV-positive mothers needed to have received HAART for long enough to show an undetectable level on a test. The results of this research, showing such a tiny percentage of transmission, were beyond our wildest dreams. This was the answer!

Virologic suppession at delivery is crucial

The researchers also found a stepwise effect in the efficacy of HAART to reduce viral load. It seemed to depend on a mother's baseline levels at the beginning of treatment, as well as on how long she received HAART during pregnancy. Risk factors for a lack of suppression of viral levels to less than 200 copies per millilitre at delivery included a higher baseline HIV RNA level and later gestational age at enrolment.

Baseline HIV RNA levels	Virologic suppression	
copies per millilitre	**NRTI group**	**protease inhibitor group**
≤1000	100%	96%
1001 to 10,000	99%	95%
10,001 to 100,000	95%	91%
≥100,000	90%	86%
Gestation in weeks	**NRTI group**	**protease inhibitor group**
26–27	99%	96%
28–30	95%	96%
31–34	91%	78%

Source: Shapiro R, New England Journal of Medicine *2010*

ART and exclusive breastfeeding

Soon, many similar studies became available from Tanzania, Mozambique, Rwanda, Uganda and Zambia, all providing maternal HAART during pregnancy and breastfeeding, and all helping mothers to exclusively breastfeed. All showed a reduction in the risk of transmission of HIV through breastfeeding to 1% or less – from the DREAM program in Mozambique, which began in 2007, to the Thomas research from Zambia, published in 2011. The research now seemed clear: providing the mother with treatment for her own health would reduce the quantity of virus in her blood and in her milk. When HAART was combined with exclusive breastfeeding to protect the infant gut from damage due to inflammation, the risk of postnatal MTCT of HIV became virtually zero. The results are shown in the table on pages 310–311 and are quite remarkable. These findings have crucial implications for the prevention of transmission of HIV through breastfeeding.

ART with continued breastfeeding to 12 months (following EBF to six months)

In late 2011, Dr Michael Silverman, Assistant Professor of Internal Medicine and Infectious Diseases at the University of Toronto, made a presentation at the 51st Interscience Conference on Antimicrobial Agents and Chemotherapy (ICAAC) in Chicago, Illinois.[8,9] He described results of research conducted in Lusaka, Zambia, where HIV-positive mothers had received a drug called Kaletra during late pregnancy and during 12 months' breastfeeding. The results were excellent.

Unsurprisingly, Dr Silverman had first-hand experience of the importance of protecting breastfeeding. He had worked on HIV/AIDS programs in Zimbabwe from 1999 to approximately 2008 at a time when the country had the fastest-shrinking economy in the world, an inflation rate of 7,000%, and eventually no infant formula.[10] As a lactation consultant who was involved in advocacy to preserve breastfeeding in the face of HIV, I appreciated this personal perspective. When I'd been working in Harare in 2002 events conspired to result in a situation where there was simply no infant formula for sale in the shops and pharmacies and this crisis lasted for months. Nor was it possible to buy fresh cows' milk, since the dairy farms, seized during the farm invasions of 2000, had gone out of production. At my antenatal breastfeeding preparation classes I'd abandoned discussion of infant feeding choice and resorted to begging my pregnant students to breastfeed: since the situation was so dire, babies who were not breastfed could starve. Then I focussed on how to bring in enough milk to breastfeed exclusively for a full six months. Motive and method. Faced with such a dilemma, 100% of the mothers at my antenatal classes complied and their babies thrived.

At the Chicago conference Dr Silverman described his 2008-09 research in Lusaka.[8] Nearly 300 pregnant HIV-positive women were recruited to receive HAART from 14–30 weeks' gestation and during breastfeeding for the first year of life. Babies were exclusively breastfed for the first six months and then continued breastfeeding with complementary foods until 12 months. This study was the first to record outcomes for babies in the 6–12 months period who had:

a. been exclusively breastfed for the first six months
b. continued breastfeeding with complementary foods from 6-12 months
c. mothers treated with full HAART for the whole period of breastfeeding

Three babies had become infected through breastfeeding (3/186 or 1.6%), all during the 6–12 month period. Dr Silverman explained the reasons for the transmissions during breastfeeding:

- One mother had a religious experience of cure at seven months and stopped taking her medications, but continued breastfeeding
- Another mother began drinking alcohol heavily and stopped taking her medication
- The third mother claimed good adherence but had a high viral load.

Like the infants in the Mma Bana study in Botswana, the Zambian babies also benefited from exclusive breastfeeding and maternal ART (EBF + ART). Of importance, there were *no* transmissions at all through breastfeeding when mothers had a very low viral load. WHO recommendations in place at the time were to exclusively breastfeed for six months and then rapidly wean. The Mma Bana research had clearly demonstrated that maternal HAART could dramatically reduce HIV transmission during exclusive breastfeeding. Now the Zambian study effectively laid to rest the lingering fear that if babies weren't weaned before they started solid foods during the second half of the first year this would place them at risk for HIV-transmission due to 'mixed feeding'. The lactation community had always suspected that mixed breastfeeding *after* six months would be far less risky. An exclusively breastfed infant reached this milestone with an intact, healthy intestinal mucosa and patterns of disease outside the context of HIV followed a pattern of very reduced infections. So this would be expected for HIV too. This was the first study to show that this might indeed be the case.

Postnatal HIV transmission rates <1% at 1–6 months where mother or baby received HAART and babies were exclusively breastfed (EBF + ART) (babies testing HIV+ in the first month were deemed to have been infected perinatally)

Reference	Duration of exclusive breastfeeding	Antiretroviral treatment and/or prophylaxis	Postnatal trans-mission	Determined by first infant HIV+ test result between...
Palombi et al 2007[a]	6 months	Maternal HAART from 25 weeks' gestation until weaning: infant sdNVP after birth	0.8% (2/251)	1–6 months
Kilewo et al 2008[b]	18 weeks	Maternal ZDV & 3TC from ~34 weeks' gestation to 1 week postpartum;Infant: ZDV & 3TC from 0-1 week, then 3TC alone during breastfeeding	1% (4/398)	6 weeks– 6 months
Kilewo et al 2009[c]	For a maximum of 6 months	Maternal HAART from 34 weeks' gestation to 6 months postpartum:Infant ZDV & 3TC to 1 week of age	0.9% (4/441)	6 weeks– 6 months
Marazzi et al 2010[d]	6 months: mothers advised to start weaning by 6 months ending within 2 months, but ? some breastfeeding 6–12 months	Maternal HAART ≥90days before delivery Infant sdNVP after birth	0.6% (2/313)	1–6 months
Peltier et al 2009[e]	6 months: mothers advised to wean at 6 months	Maternal HAART from 28 weeks' gestation to 7months postpartum:Infant sdNVP after birth + ZDV for 1 week	0.44% (1/227)	6 weeks– 9 months
Shapiro et al 2010[f]	Exclusive breastfeeding for 93% of infants to weaning: 71% breastfed >5months <1% breastfed >6months	Randomised and varied HAART regimens for mothers from 18-34 weeks' gestation until weaning: all mothers also received supplemental AZT during labour: Infant sdNVP after delivery plus 1 month AZT	0.28% (2/709)	1–6 months
Homsy et al 2010[g]	Exclusive breastfeeding for 92% for 4 months, weaned at 5 months	Maternal FDC, median duration 5.2-20.3 months preceding delivery and during breastfeeding: Infant sdNVP post birth or sdNVP + ZDV 1 week	0% (0/109)	6 weeks' of age– 6 weeks post weaning
Thomas et al 2011[h]	6 months	Maternal HAART from 34 weeks' gestation to 6 months postpartum: infant sdNVP at birth	0.8% (4/487)	6 weeks– 6 months

HIV transmission rates at > 12-18 months where mother continued HAART and baby continued breastfeeding with complementary foods

Reference	Duration of exclusive breastfeeding	Antiretroviral treatment and/or prophylaxis	Postnatal transmission	Determined by first infant HIV+ test result between…
Ngoma et al & Silverman 2011 [Ia] Ngoma et al 2015 [Ib]	Exclusive breastfeeding for 6 months + continued breast-feeding with complementary foods to 12 months Exclusive breastfeeding for 6 months + continued breastfeeding with complementary foods to 18 months	Maternal HAART from 14-30 weeks' gestation, continued during labour until cessation of breastfeeding. Infants received oral ZDV for 5 days postpartum	1.5% (3/201) 1.1% (2/186)	12 months 18 months
Gartland et al 2013 [II]	Exclusive breastfeeding for 6 months + continued breastfeeding with complementary foods to 12 months	Maternal HAART 28 weeks' gestation to cessation of breastfeeding; infant sdNVP + 7 days ZDV	1% (1/104)	12 months
Luoga et al 2018 [III]	Exclusive breastfeeding for 6 months + continued breastfeeding with complementary foods to 12 months	Maternal HAART, median duration 23 months; infant daily nevirapine 4-6 weeks.	0% (0/184) when maternal viral load was 100-1000 copies/ml	12 months

References

ART+ EBF to 6 months

a. Palombi L, Marazzi MC, Voetberg A et al. Treatment acceleration program and the experience of the DREAM program in prevention of mother-to-child transmission of HIV. *AIDS* 2007; 21(Suppl 4):S65–71.
b. Kilewo C, Karlsson K, Massawe A et al. Prevention of mother-to-child transmission of HIV-1 through breast-feeding by treating infants prophylactically with lamivudine in Dar es Salaam, Tanzania: the Mitra Study. *Journal of Acquired Immune Deficiency Syndromes* 2008;48(3):315–23.
c. Kilewo C, Karlsson K, Ngarina M et al (2009). Prevention of mother to child transmission of HIV-1 through breastfeeding by treating mothers with triple antiretroviral therapy in Dar es Salaam, Tanzania: the Mitra Plus study. *Journal of Acquired Immune Deficiency Syndromes* 52(3): 406–16.
d. Marazzi MC, Nielsen-Saines K, Buonomo E, Scarcella P, Germano P, Majid NA, Zimba I, Ceffa S, Palombi L. Increased Infant Human Immunodeficiency Virus-Type One Free Survival at One Year of Age in Sub-Saharan Africa With Maternal Use of Highly Active Antiretroviral Therapy During Breast-Feeding. *Pediatr Infect Dis J* 2009;28: 483–487 https://pubmed.ncbi.nlm.nih.gov/19483516/ (accessed 8 August 2020)
e. Peltier CA, Ndayisaba GF, Lepage P et al (2009). Breastfeeding with maternal antiretroviral therapy or formula feeding to prevent HIV postnatal mother-to child transmission in Rwanda. *AIDS* 23(18):2415–23.
f. Shapiro RL, Hughes MD, Ogwu A et al. Antiretroviral regimens in pregnancy and breast-feeding in Botswana. *New England Journal of Medicine* 2010;362(24):2282–94
g. Homsy J, Moore D, Barasa A et al (2010). Breastfeeding, mother-to-child HIV transmission, and mortality among infants born to HIV-infected women on highly active antiretroviral therapy in rural Uganda. *Journal of Acquired Immune Deficiency Syndromes* 53(1):28–35.
h. Thomas TK, Masaba R, Borkowf CB et al (2011). Triple-antiretroviral prophylaxis to prevent mother-to-child HIV transmission through breastfeeding -the Kisumu Breastfeeding Study, Kenya: a clinical trial. *PLoS Medicine* 8(3):e1001015. http://1.usa.gov/1wCtovS [Accessed 23 October 2014.

ART + continued breastfeeding with complementary foods to 12 months or beyond

Ia. Ngoma M, Raha A, Elong A, Pilon R, Mwansa J, Mutale W, Yee K, Chisele S, Wu S, Chandawe M, Mumba S and Silverman MS Interim Results of HIV Transmission Rates Using a Lopinavir/ritonavir based regimen and the New WHO Breast Feeding Guidelines for PMTCT of HIV International Congress of Antimicrobial Agents and Chemotherapy (ICAAC). 51st Interscience Conference on Antimicrobial Agents and Chemotherapy (ICAAC): Session 164, Abstract H1-1153. Presented September 19, 2011. Chicago Il, Sep19,2011. H1-1153 (presented by M Silverman).

Ib. Follow-up published paper to presentation in Chicago presented by M Silverman) Ngoma MS et al. Efficacy of WHO recommendation for continued breastfeeding and maternal cART for prevention of perinatal and postnatal HIV transmission in Zambia *Journal of the International AIDS Society* 2015, 18:19352 http://www.jiasociety.org/index.php/jias/article/view/19352 | http://dx.doi.org/10.7448/IAS.18.1.19352

II. Gartland MG et al, Field effectiveness of combination antiretroviral prophylaxis for the prevention of mother-to-child HIV transmission in rural Zambia, *AIDS* 2013 May 15; 27(8): doi:10.1097/QAD.0b013e32835e3937, https://www.ncbi.nlm.nih.gov/pmc/articles/PMC3836017/pdf/nihms521144.pdf/ accessed 5 August 2020

III. Luoga E et al, No HIV Transmission From Virally Suppressed Mothers During Breastfeeding in Rural Tanzania J Acquir Immune Defic Syndr 2018 Sep 1;79(1):e17-e20. doi: 10.1097/QAI.0000000000001758. https://pubmed.ncbi.nlm.nih.gov/29781882/ (accessed 6 Aug 2020)

I read about Dr Silverman's presentation in the 29 September 2011 issue of *Medscape* and I wrote to him the very next day to say how thrilled breastfeeding advocates would be with his results. He wrote back a few days later, letting me have a copy of his presentation, and giving more information.

> *'There have been a few updates since the abstract was submitted. I attach a copy of the talk that I gave. There have now been 3 transmissions, during breast feeding and all occurred in women with detectable viral loads, and during the time of complementary feeding. We are continuing to follow up these women (we hope to have all of the final results soon). One further transmission has just been documented (a few days ago, and so after this presentation) in a woman who stopped her meds at 2 weeks postpartum and then breastfed for a year (she decided that she did not believe that she was infected and so refused follow up). She unfortunately died of AIDS and her family brought the child in after over a year of breast feeding, and the child was positive. So overall our data suggests that breastfeeding with an undetectable viral load is safe in Africa and does support the new WHO guidelines for developing countries.'*

The Silverman research was finally peer-reviewed and published in the *Journal of the International AIDS Society* in 2015, showing Mary Ngoma as first author.[11] There were a few differences in the final paper, but the overall findings had not changed. HIV-positive mothers were started on zidovudine/3TC and lopinavir/ritonavir tablets at 14–30 weeks gestation and continued indefinitely thereafter. Women were encouraged to exclusively breastfeed for six months, complementary feed for the next six months and then cease breastfeeding at 12–13 months. Standard breastfeeding definitions obtained from UNICEF were used for the study:

> *Exclusive breastfeeding: Only breastmilk +medicines/vitamins.*
>
> *Mixed feeding: Breastmilk and non-human milk (including formula) and/or semi-solid/solid foods <6 months.*

Complementary feeding: Continued breastfeeding with the addition of solid or semi-solid foods >6 months.

Replacement feeding: No breastmilk at all, fed only non-human milk or semi-solids/solids.

All breastfeeding transmissions occurred >6 months of age. Not one of 215 babies who were negative at six weeks became positive before six months: i.e. no transmissions occurred in babies who were exclusively breastfeeding. Self-reported adherence to breastfeeding recommendations was requested at each visit. 92.8% of mothers exclusively breastfed until six months and 79% continued breastfeeding with complementary foods thereafter. Three of 201 babies became infected during the 6–12 month period. Of note, all mothers who transmitted the virus >6 months had a plasma viral load >1,000 due to poor adherence to their medication, as evidenced by missed dispensary visits, and their levels were higher than mothers who did not transmit the virus. The Ngoma-Silverman study was the only one at the time which recorded breastfeeding definitions carefully enough for us to see that transmission rates were extremely low in the 6–12 month period in babies who were still breastfed.

A further trial by Gartland and colleagues evaluated the effectiveness of HAART for 284 HIV-positive women from 28 weeks of pregnancy and their infants at nine clinics in rural Zambia between April 2009 and January 2011.[12] Four sites provided maternal ART until cessation of breastfeeding and mothers were encouraged to exclusively breastfeed for six months and then provide complementary feeds with continued breastfeeding until 24 months. At 12 months only one infant was infected; that baby had tested HIV-positive at two weeks, which would indicate that infection had occurred *in utero*. Thus no infections were recorded which could be attributed to breastfeeding. Regrettably, although exclusive breastfeeding was encouraged, there is no detail provided about how many mothers actually did so.

Between 1 January 2013 and 31 May 2016, Luoga and colleagues in Ifakara, southern Tanzania, recruited mothers who were on ART before delivery and whose babies had a negative HIV DNA PCR at 4–12 weeks, (ruling out the possibility of HIV transmission occurring *in utero* or at birth).[13] By the time their babies were born, mothers had received ART for an average of 23 months (range 4–52 months) and had a viral load of <1000 copies/ml. The babies were exclusively breastfed for six months and continued breastfeeding with complementary food for a median duration of 52 weeks (range 41–54 weeks). The final HIV serostatus, determined at a median age of 14 months, was known for 186 infants. There was no transmission of the virus through breastfeeding in mothers who adhered to their medications and whose viral load was suppressed. However, among 186 babies remaining at the end of the study (those not lost to follow-up or death) two babies (2/186, or 1%) tested HIV-positive.

- One of the babies had been born to a mother whose viral load five weeks after delivery was high (144,111 copies/ml).
- The other mother had an undetectable viral load at six weeks after birth, but shortly afterwards interrupted ART while continuing to breastfeed.

Effective ART means an undetectable viral load

From these studies the potential of ART to reduce the risk of transmission through breastfeeding is clear. Examination of the circumstances of babies who became infected showed that either their mothers had had treatment for too short a time, or they had stopped taking their medications altogether, as evidenced by high viral loads.

Since 2015, the World Health Organization has recommended lifelong ART for all HIV-positive women regardless of their CD4 counts and clinical stage of disease.[14] The main determinant of MTCT risk is maternal plasma HIV RNA viral load.[15] Perinatal HIV transmission has been reduced to virtually zero in European mothers who start ART before conception and maintain suppression of plasma viral load.[16] Achievement of an undetectable viral load through effective antiretroviral treatment allows HIV clinicians to feel confident of an extremely low risk of MTCT perinatal transmission in spite of vaginal vs caesarean delivery (the time of greatest risk of the baby becoming infected). In the United Kingdom the risk of MTCT before and during birth has been reduced to 0.1% when antenatal mothers have a viral load <50 copies/ml with an effective maternal HAART regimen.[17]

In literature which attempts to discourage HIV-positive women from breastfeeding, the crucial importance of effective ART for a long enough period to reduce a mother's viral load to undetectable, combined with the mother's determination to strictly adhere to her medications, are still not being accorded the acknowledgement that they deserve. Organisations with huge influence, such as the American Academy of Pediatrics[18] and the British HIV Association,[19] express concern that even when mothers receive full ART, there is still a risk of HIV transmission through breastfeeding.

Dr Ted Greiner and I wrote a short response to address these concerns in the 5 March 2013 issue of *Pediatrics*,[20] outlining the salient points in the Mma Bana study reported in the *New England Journal of Medicine* in 2010[5] and saying that the necessary safeguard of maternal ART adherence for a sufficient length of time to facilitate an undetectable viral load was not in place for the 2/709 (0.28%) of mothers who transmitted HIV postnatally to their babies. In particular, we cited the 2011 paper published by Chibwesha and colleagues,[21] which showed that the full effectiveness of ART in preventing vertical transmission is only achieved by meticulous maternal adherence to antiretroviral regimens for at least 13 weeks prior to delivery. Women on ART for <4 weeks had 5.2-fold increased odds of transmission.

Kesho Bora

Conscientious physicians working with HIV-positive mothers often cite the Kesho Bora study which received very wide publicity when it came out.[22] This research, published in 2011, covering five sites in Burkina Faso, Kenya and South Africa, had been funded by WHO.[23] Even as this study is widely cited as an example of how maternal ART during breastfeeding can reduce the risk of postpartum transmission, it is also held up as evidence that the risk of MTCT of HIV through breastfeeding is still unacceptably high in spite of maternal ART. With the benefit of hindsight, and the ability to compare what happened in Kesho Bora with other research, we can see how this misconception arises.

In Swahili (the lingua franca where I grew up in Kenya), Kesho Bora means 'tomorrow will be better', though this is more romantically translated by the researchers to mean 'a brighter future'. The Kesho Bora research ran from June 2005–August 2008 with the goal of assessing the efficacy of two PMTCT drug regimens, triple ART vs zidovudine/nevirapine, from 28–36 weeks' gestation until 6.5 months postpartum in >800 HIV-positive pregnant women. For the HAART vs zidovudine/nevirapine groups, 3.3% vs 5.0% of babies were infected at six weeks, and 5.4% vs 9.5% were infected at 12 months. Thus transmission which could be attributable to breastfeeding was 2.1% vs 4.5%. The Kesho Bora authors themselves pointed to similarities in the cumulative risk of transmission between their randomised study and the Peltier, Kilewo 2008, Marazzi and Thomas observational studies set out in the table above.[24–27] However, the risks of breastfeeding-associated transmission of HIV shown in these comparison studies were 0.5%, 0.6%, 1.0% and 0.9% respectively, suggesting a 2–4-fold increased risk for the Kesho Bora babies.

Closer scrutiny reveals what accounted for the differences. Only 70% of women in the Kesho Bora study had undetectable viral loads at delivery, and serial viral loads were not followed postpartum.[28] Less than half (only 45%) of the ever-breastfed Kesho Bora babies were breastfed *exclusively* up to the last available clinic visit before three months. Only 77% of mothers breastfed at all for 8–25 weeks.[29] Breastfeeding rates at four months of age varied between study sites, being 78% for Bobo-Dioulasso, 53% for rural KwaZulu Natal, 41% for Durban, 33% for Nairobi and 32% for Mombasa respectively.[30] While levels of sanitation and socio-economic status can partly explain this difference, national health policies also probably influenced counsellors. Standard advice in Nairobi was to stop breastfeeding at three months. In both Kenyan sites the child's HIV status was given to the mother at three months, providing mothers of uninfected children the opportunity to stop breastfeeding. In both South African sites, where proportionally higher numbers of women exclusively breastfed up to six months, information about the child's status was given 5.5 months after birth.

At first glance it seems counter-intuitive that the WHO-funded Kesho Bora study, which received a great deal of publicity in the press, did not pay more attention to WHO's own recommendations that HIV-positive mothers should exclusively breastfeed. However, the mothers were actually counselled according to WHO 'infant feeding recommendations' then in place and as published in 2003–04.[31] This guidance suggested that although exclusive breastfeeding during the first few months of life *might* be associated with a lower risk of HIV transmission than mixed feeding, research was still in progress to clarify the issue.

When I was challenged on the high risk of MTCT through breastfeeding apparently shown in the Kesho Bora study, by one of the clinicians who had been instrumental in updating the British HIV Association/Children's HIV Association guidance on HIV and breastfeeding, I replied, 'I don't know if WHO found that promotion and assistance with exclusive breastfeeding was too difficult, or if there were just too few mothers who did it for long enough to give a meaningful result... who knows? I know, of course, that getting mothers not to feed little bits of food and other liquids before six months is quite challenging, but it's certainly possible – and worthwhile, right?'[32] In any event, concluding that breastfeeding (even with ART) is risky based on the results of the Kesho

Bora study is to apportion blame unnecessarily. Most of the Kesho Bora babies were mixed fed and it is mixed feeding which poses the greatest risk of postnatally acquired HIV.

Opinion in the global north is perhaps overly pessimistic about the likelihood of success in reducing postnatal transmission while preserving breastfeeding. But rather than condemning breastfeeding out of hand, it's possible to pinpoint the reasons for the tiny percentage of apparent failures of ART to protect against transmission of the virus during breastfeeding. Adherence to ART has usually been compromised, viral load is consequently high, there has been mixed feeding, and transmission is more likely in those circumstances. Conversely, when HIV-positive mothers can be clearly informed about how ART + EBF works, about the life-saving possibilities of meticulous adherence to their antiretroviral medications, and about the importance of practising really exclusive breastfeeding, they don't have to forego breastfeeding.

CHAPTER 24

International HIV and infant feeding policy comes full circle

When the first PMTCT pilot projects began in the late 1990s and were scaled up in the new millennium, ART was available to very few HIV-positive mothers. This meant that for the majority the only intervention on offer was counselling to avoid breastfeeding, and free formula for the babies. There was almost no evidence to suggest that breastmilk substitutes, otherwise known as 'replacement feeding', would be acceptable, feasible, affordable, sustainable or safe. In fact research on formula-feeding in resource-poor settings in the 1980s had shown that it was *not* safe. Nevertheless, the original PMTCT programmes had directed almost all their prevention effort into offering HIV testing followed by carefully crafted counselling to undermine breastfeeding. Amid growing fears within the breastfeeding community that formula-feeding in resource-poor settings would lead to unacceptably high infant mortality,[1] global policy appeared firmly wedded to successful promotion of replacement feeding. Subsequent operational research suggests that untold numbers of babies died, not of postnatal HIV-transmission through breastfeeding, but due to the untried, untested – and largely unrecorded – withholding of their mothers' milk.

Had there been rigorous monitoring and evaluation of the pilot programmes, it is likely that promotion of replacement feeding would have ended before the full PMTCT initiative was scaled up and rolled out to thousands of sites worldwide. Failing that, the Botswana tragedy of 2005–06 should have sounded the final death-knell for promotion of artificial feeding to HIV-positive mothers in developing countries. There had been very high mortality rates of babies whose mothers had been persuaded to formula-feed. Investigators from the CDC concluded that breastfeeding was critical to infant survival in the developing world, even in the context of HIV.[2] Findings from the Zambia Exclusive Breastfeeding Study (ZEBS) provided further compelling evidence about the risks of early weaning on overall infant survival.[3] The ZEBS study, which began in 2001 and ended in 2004, confirmed that exclusive breastfeeding transmitted fewer infections than mixed feeding. It also established that early weaning was not effective in increasing the number of children who remained alive and HIV-free by two years of age.

Nevertheless, early in 2006 WHO published two revised training courses for health workers, which continued to follow the policy of promoting formula-feeding for the babies of HIV-positive mothers wherever possible:

1. **The January 2006 revised Baby Friendly Hospital Initiative Course.**[4] This replaced the 1992 Baby Friendly Hospital Initiative documents. It also included additional modules on HIV and infant feeding to be used if the maternity facility had a prevalence of more than 20% HIV-positive clients, and/or had a PMTCT programme. The 2006 BFHI criteria of 75% of mothers who should be breastfeeding on hospital discharge in order to obtain BFHI certification was less than the original 80% target set out in 1992–93. This total was further undermined by the possibility that assessments could exclude HIV-infected mothers *and* mothers who wished to maintain confidentiality about their HIV status and, on the face of it, would simply choose not to breastfeed.
2. **The 2006 WHO Integrated Infant and Young Child Feeding Counselling Course.**[5] This training combined the 1993 Breastfeeding Counselling and the 2000 HIV and Infant Feeding courses and subsequent updates up to 2005. Approximately 30% of the content was devoted to HIV and infant feeding, i.e. teaching about formula-feeding. Participants were reassured that after completing the course they would be able to counsel and support mothers to carry out WHO/UNICEF recommended feeding practices for their infants and young children from birth up to 24 months of age, and to counsel and support HIV-infected mothers to choose and carry out an appropriate feeding method for the first two years of life.

Unfortunately, these updates repeated the now outdated recommendations for replacement feeding in the context of HIV formulated several years earlier at the 2000 WHO HIV and Infant Feeding Technical Consultation and set out in subsequent documents released between 2000 and 2005. Though dated 2006, these important new teaching tools did not incorporate the major change agreed later in the year at the October 2006 WHO Technical Consultation on HIV and infant feeding, described below.

2006 WHO Technical Consultation

From 25–27 October 2006 WHO held another Technical Consultation on HIV and infant feeding in Geneva, the first to be convened in six years.[6] In the months leading up to the consultation, there had been intense activity behind the scenes by groups and individuals who were advocating for breastfeeding in the face of HIV, and who attempted, without success, to be represented at the meeting. Felicity Savage, now chairperson of the WABA Steering Committee, who had agreed to represent WABA in Geneva, in fact did not do so; she was also a consultant to WHO and perhaps there was a conflict of interest since it would be difficult to speak for preserving breastfeeding *and* for promoting replacement feeding – the position then taken by WHO. The International Lactation Consultant Association (ILCA), La Leche League International (LLLI) both members of WABA, and AnotherLook, which had several members also well-known to and involved with WABA, and all of whom were engaged in trying to protect, promote and support breastfeeding, made repeated requests to attend, but WHO replied with various excuses about why they couldn't do so. Thus the breastfeeding movement had no adequate representation at this important event. At the same time, the recent Botswana tragedy seemed to make protection of breastfeeding even more important than the AIDS community seemed to want everyone to believe. In the event, research which addressed HIV-free survival was successfully presented at the meeting and became impossible to ignore. Among the researchers themselves a growing lobby was pushing for greater support for exclusive breastfeeding. As it happened, the 2006 Technical Consultation ended without issuing an official statement on the outcome of its deliberations and in the following weeks there was considerable haggling over the text as successive drafts were negotiated between WHO and meeting participants.

Final 2006 HIV and Infant Feeding Policy

However, early in 2007 WHO published a series of documents emanating from the meeting; a Report of the Technical Consultation,[7] an Update based on the Consultation, [8]and a Review of Available Evidence.[9] The new guidance did contain one encouraging change reflecting a new caution about replacement feeding. Since 1997, UNAIDS/WHO/UNICEF policy had asserted that *when* replacement was safe then breastfeeding should be avoided. The big mistake had been the casual assumption of safety. The research released since Botswana, and now presented at the meeting, clearly blew this assumption out of the water. So now, finally, a revised recommendation introduced an important caveat, to suggest that *unless* formula-feeding was safe breastfeeding should continue to be recommended. To the breastfeeding movement, even though the new guidance still maintained a certain ambiguity, the new wording felt like a major concession:

- *Exclusive breastfeeding is recommended for HIV-infected mothers for the first six months of life **unless** replacement feeding is acceptable, feasible, affordable, sustainable and safe for them and their infants before that time.*
- ***When** replacement feeding is acceptable, feasible, affordable, sustainable and safe, avoidance of all breastfeeding by HIV-infected mothers is recommended.*
- *At six months, **if** replacement feeding is still not acceptable, feasible, affordable, sustainable and safe, **continuation** of breastfeeding with additional complementary foods is recommended, while the mother and baby continue to be regularly assessed. **All breastfeeding should stop** once a nutritionally adequate and safe diet without breast milk can be provided.*

2007 UNGASS

In 2007 WHO published guidance on global scale-up for the prevention of mother-to-child transmission of HIV[10] to report on a Declaration of Commitment of the UN General Assembly Special Session on HIV/AIDS. Depressingly, one of the UNGASS aims clearly endorsed the need for breastmilk substitutes:

Reduce the proportion of infants infected with HIV ...by ensuring that 80 per cent of pregnant women accessing antenatal care have information, counselling and other prevention services available to them, increasing the availability of and by providing access to HIV-infected women and babies to effective treatment ...including voluntary and confidential counselling and testing, ...and where appropriate, ***breast milk substitutes...***

Further teaching materials for formula-feeding

In 2007, WHO also published a trilogy of booklets giving detailed instructions about how to safely prepare infant formula in care settings,[11] and how to prepare formula for cup-feeding[12] or bottle-feeding[13] in the home. These publications were obviously designed to be used in both industrialised and resource-poor settings, e.g. where mothers might or might not have access to sterilisers, kettles or refrigerators.

In 2008 WHO published an updated HIV and Infant Feeding Counselling Tools Orientation Guide for Trainers,[14] which devoted a large number of pages to counselling HIV-positive mothers about choosing to formula-feed, and exploring the practical aspects needed to make and carry out such a decision.

In 2009 WHO published a Model Chapter on Infant and Young Child Feeding for medical students and allied health professionals,[15] which included information on HIV and infant feeding. Importantly, although published in 2009, its information is drawn from the 2007 WHO/UNICEF/UNFPA/UNAIDS HIV and infant feeding Update.[8] It failed to reflect the important change in HIV and infant feeding policy released later in November/December 2009 – i.e. later in the same year. In spite of the fact that it is clearly out of date, it remains on the WHO website to be used as a resource for medical students.

Evidence of morbidity and mortality due to formula-feeding

Meanwhile momentum was gathering for a change in the global policy promoting formula-feeding in the context of HIV. While provision of free formula to many HIV-positive mothers in resource-poor settings during the late 1990s had made replacement feeding affordable, and its acceptability and feasibility received quite generous coverage in the medical literature, an increasing number of questions about the safety and sustainability of replacement feeding began to be asked following publication of the Creek findings in Botswana, and the torrent of similar reports that soon followed. These papers confirmed that replacement feeding was risky for HIV-exposed babies in resource-poor settings compared to breastfeeding and conferred no child survival advantage.

At the February 2007 Conference on Retroviruses and Opportunistic Infections, HIV and infant feeding received a lot of attention.[16] Experts considered that women in most resource-constrained settings should no longer be advised to avoid breastfeeding or to wean early. New data from four countries was presented:

- In Uganda 11% of uninfected, non-breastfed infants had serious gastroenteritis and infant deaths rose sharply within 3 months after breastfeeding cessation.[17]
- In Malawi, gastroenteritis among recently weaned six-month old uninfected infants increased and mortality rose 22% compared to an earlier trial at the same site where

breastfeeding had lasted for two years.[18]

- In Kenya, early cessation of breastfeeding at six months for infants of mothers who had received HAART increased the risk of diarrhoea, hospitalisation and death compared to rates for babies who had been breastfed beyond 12 months.[19]
- In Zambia, stopping breastfeeding at four months resulted in less-than-anticipated reduction of HIV transmission, substantial mortality risk for infected babies, and did not improve HIV-free survival among uninfected infants at 24 months. The recommendation was that PMTCT programmes should strongly encourage breastfeeding for HIV-infected infants into the second year of life.[20]

In 2008 a paper from Uganda sounded a further note of warning about the risks of formula-feeding in rural Africa. Kagaayi and colleagues compared mortality and HIV-free survival of breastfed and formula-fed infants born to HIV-positive mothers receiving ART in a programme in Rakai District, Uganda,[21] where only 25% of women practised exclusive breastfeeding by one month postpartum. The cumulative 12-month probability of infant mortality for formula-fed infants was six times that of breastfed infants (18% vs 3%). The researchers concluded that formula-feeding should be discouraged in similar African settings.

Low risk of MTCT when HIV-positive mothers receive antiretroviral therapy

Simultaneously, several papers were published outlining very reduced rates of MTCT by any route (pregnancy, birth or breastfeeding) when mothers received appropriate ARVs for their own health, resulting in viral suppression. Between 2007 and 2009 at least 10 papers showed that rates of postnatal transmission ranging from 0.3%– 4% could be achieved when HIV-positive mothers practised both exclusive breastfeeding *and* received appropriate early prenatal, perinatal and postnatal treatment with antiretroviral medications:

2007	Kuhn	Zambia	3.92%[22]
2007	Coovadia	South Africa	4.04%[23]
2007	Palombi	Mozambique	0.8%[24]
2008	Thomas	Kenya	1.1%[25]
2008	Kilewo	Tanzania	1.2%[26]
2009	Kilewo	Tanzania	1%[27]
2009	Marazzi	Mozambique	0.6%[28]
2009	Chasela	Malawi	3%, 1.8%[29]
2009	Peltier	Rwanda	0.5%[30]
2009	Shapiro	Botswana	0.3%[31]

Change becomes inevitable: the 2009 revision of WHO Policy

In late 2008, barely two years after the 2006 meeting, WHO convened a further Technical Consultation. By this time, an estimated 33.4 million people were living with HIV, and AIDS was the leading cause of death among women of reproductive age.

There was now sufficient programmatic experience and published research to show the potential of ART to reduce HIV transmission during breastfeeding. A summary of the evidence, which included the papers noted above, was completed in October 2009[32] and new draft recommendations were circulated in preparation for a meeting of the full Guideline Development Group. They covered paediatric HIV-free survival, the risks of breastfeeding or replacement feeding, early cessation of breastfeeding, maternal access to ART, and support systems for mothers and the general population.

On 30 November 2009, on the eve of World AIDS Day, WHO simultaneously issued two complementary Rapid Advice documents; one on the use of ART for treating HIV-positive mothers to prevent transmission to their infants, and the other on HIV and infant feeding. These documents were directed towards policymakers, academics, health workers, national technical groups and international and regional partners providing HIV care and treatment services. The focus of the newly updated policy differed from previous global policy in two major respects:

1. It acknowledged the reality of a dual-standard in the recommendations deemed necessary for resource-rich and resource-poor areas.
2. It identified a paradigm shift in the human rights basis of the policy. There was a clear move away from the previous emphasis on individual human rights (maternal infant feeding choice) to one of public health (children's HIV-free survival at 18–24 months).

At last WHO acknowledged that exclusive breastfeeding in the first six months of an infant's life was associated with very much reduced risk of HIV transmission compared with mixed feeding with other milks or foods. Research was also presented showing that maternal ART could reduce the maternal viral load to undetectable, which was the key to reducing infectivity. Putting these two strategies together was pivotal, and WHO described this research as 'transformational'.

WHO 2009 Rapid Advice: use of antiretroviral drugs for treating pregnant women and preventing HIV infection in infants[33]

The first document on ARVs recommended two key approaches:

1. *Lifelong ART for HIV-positive women in need of treatment.*
2. *Prophylaxis, or the short-term provision of ARVs, to prevent HIV transmission from mother to child.*

This provided the basis for:

1. *Earlier ART for a larger group of HIV-positive pregnant women to benefit both the health of the mother and prevent HIV transmission to her child during pregnancy.*
2. *Longer provision of ARV prophylaxis for HIV-positive pregnant women with relatively strong immune systems who do not need ART for their own health.*
3. *Provision of ARVs to the mother or child to reduce the risk of HIV transmission during*

the breastfeeding period. ***For the first time, there is enough evidence for WHO to recommend ARVs while breastfeeding.***

This development would have very important implications for preserving breastfeeding in the face of HIV. Specific recommendations continued:

> *... Among breastfeeding infants, there is evidence that daily NVP for 6 weeks is efficacious in reducing HIV transmission or death.*
>
> *... The maternal component of this ARV prophylaxis strategy is the same as the one recommended in the 2006 guidelines,although the revised recommendation is to start earlier during pregnancy ... For breastfeeding infants, the panel placed a high value on an intervention that would allow safer breastfeeding practices in settings where breastfeeding is the norm... The panel also felt that these ARV guidelines should not recommend a target duration for breastfeeding; WHO will provide separate guidelines on HIV and infant feeding, in the context of ARVs.*
>
> *... The provision of maternal triple ARV prophylaxis during pregnancy in women who are not eligible for ART results in very low intrauterine and peripartum transmission rates... For breastfeeding infants, available data suggest that maternal triple ARV prophylaxis started in pregnancy and continued during breastfeeding is efficacious in reducing HIV transmission and infant death. The panel placed a high value on providing an intervention that would allow safer breastfeeding practices for as long as the child is exposed to breast milk.*

Researchers working on the DREAM study in Mozambique, which recruited pregnant HIV-positive mothers into their study between August 2005 and July 2006, had been among the first to identify that in developing country settings withdrawal of maternal ART once the baby was delivered was morally questionable. Continued maternal ART with exclusive breastfeeding resulted in postnatal transmission rates of only 0.6% from 1–6 months and greatly enhanced paediatric HIV-free survival.[34] In describing the rationale of the breastfeeding arm of their study the DREAM researchers had written that when proposals to protect the unborn child are accompanied by an immediate offer of treatment to the mother, outcomes improve significantly.

The new guidance recognised that in the same way that ART given during pregnancy could reduce viral load to undetectable levels and reduce MTCT at birth to <1%, whether through caesarean section or vaginal delivery,[35] so too, an undetectable viral load now showed an extremely low risk of transmission during the breastfeeding period. Continuing maternal medication after birth would be the standard of care in the industrialised world because it protected the mother's own health, allowing her to live longer.

The 2009 Rapid Advice responded to the need for continued treatment for all HIV-positive mothers after their children were born, rather than abandoning them to die once they had given birth to uninfected babies. From now on, HIV-positive mothers would be able to live a normal lifespan, enabling them to care for their new babies as well as their older children, and seeing an end to the growing number of AIDS orphans.

WHO 2009 Rapid advice on infant feeding in the context of HIV [36]

The new recommendations from the 2009 change of infant feeding policy also made a thorough and welcome exploration of the human rights rationale which had underpinned recommendations ever since 1997. This had affirmed the individual human right of an HIV-positive mother to choose her own infant feeding method. In a breastfeeding culture this had translated to the introduction of a novel choice *not* to breastfeed. The new guidelines now set out the need for HIV-positive mothers to receive counselling and *recommendations* based on evidence-based principles likely to safeguard public health, leading to the best chance for child survival, and the reasoning was clear:

- *National or sub-national health authorities should decide whether health services will principally counsel and support mothers known to be HIV-infected to* ***either****:*
    - *breastfeed and receive ARV interventions,*

    or

    - *avoid all breastfeeding*
- *The group …also considered the experiences of countries in implementing the current recommendations on HIV and Infant Feeding and the difficulty to provide high quality counselling to assist HIV-infected mothers to make appropriate infant feeding choices. The group noted that in highly resourced countries in which infant and child mortality rates were low, largely due to low rates of serious infectious diseases and malnutrition, HIV-infected mothers are strongly and appropriately* ***recommended*** *to avoid all breastfeeding. In some of these countries, infants have been removed from mothers who have wanted to breastfeed despite being HIV infected and even being on ARV treatment. In these settings, the pursuit of breastfeeding in the presence of safe and effective alternatives may be considered to constitute abuse or neglect.*
- *The advent of interventions that very significantly reduce the risk of HIV transmission through breastfeeding is a major breakthrough that should contribute to improved child survival. In considering the implications for principles and recommendations, the group extensively discussed why and how a focus on individual rights is important for public health activities.*

    ….The group considered that the effectiveness of ARVs to reduce HIV transmission is ***transformational*** *and in conjunction with the known benefits of breastfeeding to reduce mortality from other causes, justifies an approach that strongly recommends a single option as the standard of care in which information about options should be made available but services would principally support one approach. The group considered in general, '****What does the "reasonable patient" want to hear?' If there is a medical consensus in favour of a particular option, the reasonable patient would prefer a recommendation.***

    The group considered that mothers known to be HIV-infected would want to be offered ***interventions that can be strongly recommended*** *and are based on high quality evidence. The group considered that these did not represent a conflict with the individual patient's interests, either the infant's or the mother's.*
- *Pregnant women and mothers known to be HIV-infected should be informed of the infant feeding strategy* ***recommended by the national or sub-national authority***

to improve HIV-free survival of HIV-exposed infants and the health of HIV-infected mothers, and informed that there are alternatives that mothers might wish to adopt.

This principle is included to affirm that individual rights should not be forfeited in the course of public health approaches.

Skilled counselling and support in appropriate infant feeding practices and ARV interventions to promote HIV-free survival of infants should be available to all pregnant women and mothers;

The group considered that recommending a single option within a national health framework does not remove the need for skilled counselling and support to be available to pregnant women and mothers.

The ability of mothers to successfully achieve a desired feeding practice is significantly influenced by the support provided through formal health services and other community-based groups.

- *Breastfeeding, and especially early breastfeeding, is one of the most critical factors for improving child survival. Breastfeeding also confers many benefits other than reducing the risk of child mortality. HIV has created great confusion among health workers about the relative merits of breastfeeding for the mother who is known to be HIV-infected. Tragically this has also resulted in mothers who are known to be HIV uninfected or whose HIV status is unknown, adopting feeding practices that are not necessary for their circumstances with detrimental effect for their infants.*

  The group also noted how infant feeding, even in settings where HIV is not highly prevalent, ***has been complicated by messaging from the food industry and other groups with the result that mothers, who have every reason to breastfeed, choose not to do so based on unfounded fears****. In these settings, application of the International Code of Marketing of Breastmilk Substitutes has particular importance.*

The change from infant feeding choice to recommendation

This was a major change. The 1997 HIV and infant feeding policy had been achieved by suggesting that the risk of HIV transmission through breastfeeding was high and consequently mothers had the right to choose to formula-feed as a way to avoid that risk. It had been sold on the platform of human rights. I had been so troubled by this characterisation that I'd written a paper on it which had been published by the Lactation Resource Centre, part of the Australian Breastfeeding Association.[37]

Ruth Nduati, the researcher from Nairobi, had said during a 1998 WHO meeting that ethical promotion of infant feeding choice is only permissible in 'a balanced state of ignorance',[38] and we knew too much about the differences in health outcomes between breastfeeding and formula-feeding to be able to ethically endorse this position. Upholding the right of a mother to bodily integrity and not to breastfeed is a very Western concept, but it is seen as aberrant in most African societies where babies and breastfeeding are highly valued and there is great social stigma attached to not breastfeeding.[39] Grace John Stewart and Ruth Nduati wrote later, 'For the care provider and policy-maker the challenge has been how to distill and communicate the evidence base and recommendations accurately to allow an informed autonomous choice that optimizes beneficence and non-maleficence for mother and child. Rapid changes in messaging results in a mismatch between caregivers, mothers, and policy-makers—where on the ground the messages of yesterday have finally taken hold at the same time as changed messages are developed that need to be delivered.'

HIV is the only condition for which breastfeeding recommendations differ according to resources, leading to ethical questions surrounding parental autonomy in decision-making and the role of healthcare providers in the clinical counselling of HIV-positive women in high-income countries.[40,41] Brewster, writing about ethics, maintains, 'Since individual preferences are always affected by the way choices are framed by policymakers, it is impossible to avoid influencing a patient's choices.'[42] One of my colleagues in the AnotherLook advocacy group, formed by Marian Tompson in 2000 to take 'another look' at protection, promotion and breastfeeding in the context of HIV, gave the opinion:

> *'In the context of HIV, "informed choice" was fake. The HIV community needed a success story by the late 90s and was frustrated that PMTCT in the poor countries (the only place where vertical transmission was occurring in large numbers) was off limits because of the 1992 policy. The breastfeeding people in both UNICEF and WHO reported that suddenly, "for political reasons" the policy had to change. The... human rights oriented "informed choice" argument was used in the absence of any scientific data supporting the policy change to put down all who dared criticize it.*
>
> *Indeed, there was no interest in saving the lives of babies as long as they were prevented from getting HIV. Thus the purpose of the 11 pilot trials expected to reach 30,000 babies, as announced by WHO, UNICEF and UNAIDS in March 1998, was not to see if free formula resulted in an increase in HIV-free survival, but simply to test the logistical issues involved in getting the formula out there. UNICEF was bitterly criticized in a Wall Street Journal front page article for turning down the "charitable" formula being so kind heartedly offered by those endearing formula companies.*
>
> *Evidence for that "informed choice" as a human right in the HIV and infant feeding context was fake:*
>
> *1. It was not universal. Women in rich countries never enjoyed it. While some staff in UNAIDS once got riled up about this informally, not a peep of formal complaint about this ever issued from the mouths of any UN agency.*
>
> *2. It turned out only to be a temporary "right". It was reversed in the 2010 guidance when overwhelming evidence showed that its implementation was killing more babies than it saved.'*

Promotion of the 'rightness' of infant feeding choice is a marketing strategy used to good effect by industry. Bottle-feeding is socially acceptable and easily affordable in countries with low breastfeeding rates. The global north fervently defends the very seductive argument that mothers have the right to choose to formula-feed, even as all of us have a duty to act in the best interests of the child. To point out that the mother's right and the baby's rights are incompatible in this context is deeply unpopular. Yet back in 1997, having the HIV-positive mother make the choice about how her baby should be fed absolved health workers and governments from responsibility if the mother made a poor choice and the baby sickened or died. At the same time, there are very, very few acceptable medical reasons for *not* breastfeeding as identified by WHO,[43] and women themselves do not benefit when their babies don't survive and thrive.

The differences between infant formula and human milk are not trivial, but in the global north formula-feeding is seen as the normal way to feed babies. In the UK only one in 100 babies are exclusively breastfed to six months (the global recommendation) and only one in 200 continue to a year. Information about infant-feeding choice posted by the British Pregnancy Advisory Service on its website is typical of the kind of attitudes towards bottle-feeding that new mothers in Britain are exposed to.[44]

> *'Women are told that they are supposed to breastfeed exclusively for their baby's first six months, yet they find that they can't, or don't want to, do this... For policymakers, the huge gap between the target and the reality – that 99% of women don't meet that target – is problematic. While many health professionals do want to promote breastfeeding, they do not want new mothers to feel bad about themselves. To set a target that most people will not reach does not make for a credible policy; and in practice, as some midwives have warned, it can create defensiveness and other tensions between mothers and health professionals. The health benefits of breastfeeding tend to be presented as overwhelming, and imply that formula feeding will cause health problems. But the evidence shows a far less drastic difference between breastfed and formula-fed babies... Research into the social reasons why women breastfeed or formula feed indicate that the relative health benefits of breastfeeding are not the only issues at stake. The pain, discomfort and inconvenience that some mothers experience while breastfeeding, and their desire to share feeding with their partners, all provide an incentive to switch to, or supplement with, formula feeding in the first few months.'*

Lactation consultants in rich countries are tasked with endorsing the individual mother's unquestionable right to make her own infant-feeding decisions based on what she knows will work best for her. We are terribly careful not to provoke maternal guilt. We talk about maternal autonomy, bodily integrity and beneficence. And we extol these concepts at international meetings and export them to developing countries. But it's only in very privileged societies, with access to fuel, clean water, doctors, antibiotics and good hospitals, that mothers can forfeit breastfeeding and still have their babies survive. Even so, somehow a mother's right to choose *not* to breastfeed has been co-opted by feminist discourse into a universal right which seems often to supercede the baby's best interests. The differences between choice and capacity often become blurred in discussions about why mothers in developed countries 'need' formula; they cannot breastfeed because they receive little help, the system failed them, there are poor hospital practices, drugs during labour, poor maternity rights and so on. We use these reasons as justification for our low breastfeeding rates even as we fail to provide adequate training on breastfeeding and lactation management to our healthcare providers so that mothers can be practically assisted to breastfeed. This allows industry to promote its products to 'mothers who cannot or choose not to breastfeed'. But those of us who have received the training know that there is a vast difference between a mother who cannot breastfeed due to an inherent medical condition, and a mother who has so little social support that she feels she needs to sacrifice breastfeeding, or indeed a mother who chooses not to because she just doesn't want to. Ultimately almost all women *can* breastfeed, and the number who simply do not lactate in the normal way is less than one in 1,000.[45]

Thus infant feeding choice was so easy to sell to the international community in 1997. However, by 2009, the research showing the risk of formula-feeding was so compelling that international agencies had to acknowledge that breastfed babies survived in greater numbers and *recommendation* was substituted for choice. Molly Chisenga, a researcher from Zambia, put it well when she said, 'Women were influenced by health workers but, for several reasons, found it difficult to follow their advice. The recently revised international HIV and infant feeding recommendations may make the counselling process simpler for health workers and makes following their advice easier for HIV-infected women.'[46]

The accompanying recommendations in the WHO 2009 Rapid Advice were stated to reflect the most current evidence from research – for the global majority exclusive breastfeeding and antiretroviral therapy or prophylaxis (EBF+ART) would most likely give infants born to HIV+ mothers the greatest chance of HIV-free survival.

1. *Mothers known to be HIV-infected should be provided with lifelong antiretroviral therapy or antiretroviral prophylaxis interventions to reduce HIV transmission through breastfeeding according to WHO recommendations...*
2. *Mothers known to be HIV-infected (and whose infants are HIV uninfected or of unknown HIV status) should exclusively breastfeed their infants for the first 6 months of life, introducing appropriate complementary foods thereafter, and continue breastfeeding for the first 12 months of life. Breastfeeding should then only stop once a nutritionally adequate and safe diet without breast milk can be provided.*
3. *Mothers known to be HIV-infected who decide to stop breastfeeding at any time should stop gradually within one month. Mothers or infants who have been receiving ARV prophylaxis should continue prophylaxis for one week after breastfeeding is fully stopped. Stopping breastfeeding abruptly is not advisable.*
4. *When mothers known to be HIV-infected decide to stop breastfeeding at any time, infants should be provided with safe and adequate replacement feeds to enable normal growth and development...*
5. *Mothers known to be HIV-infected should only give commercial infant formula milk as a replacement feed to their HIV uninfected infants or infants who are of unknown HIV status, when specific conditions are met: (referred to as AFASS – affordable, feasible, acceptable, sustainable and safe in the 2006 WHO recommendations on HIV and Infant Feeding)*
   a. *safe water and sanitation are assured at the household level and in the community,* ***and,***
   b. *the mother, or other caregiver can reliably provide sufficient infant formula milk to support normal growth and development of the infant,* ***and,***
   c. *the mother or caregiver can prepare it cleanly and frequently enough so that it is*

safe and carries a low risk of diarrhoea and malnutrition, ***and,***

d. *the mother or caregiver can, in the first six months, exclusively give infant formula milk,* ***and,***
e. *the family is supportive of this practice,* ***and,***
f. *the mother or caregiver can access health care that offers comprehensive child health services.*

6. *Mothers known to be HIV-infected may consider expressing and heat-treating breast milk as an interim feeding strategy:*
   - *In special circumstances such as when the infant is born with low birth weight or is otherwise ill in the neonatal period and unable to breastfeed;* ***or***
   - *When the mother is unwell and temporarily unable to breastfeed or has a temporary breast health problem such as mastitis;* ***or***
   - *To assist mothers to stop breastfeeding;* ***or***
   - *If antiretroviral drugs are temporarily not available*
7. *If infants and young children are known to be HIV-infected, mothers are strongly encouraged to exclusively breastfeed for the first 6 months of life and continue breastfeeding as per the recommendations for the general population, that is up to two years or beyond.*

The clear recognition that breastfeeding, particularly when practised exclusively in the first months of life, rather than formula-feeding, would lead to greater numbers of HIV-exposed babies surviving past two years, was warmly welcomed as reflecting current evidence. This was what the recent research had shown again and again, and at last international policy would reflect these findings.

Expressed breastmilk

Breastfeeding advocates were disappointed however, about the information given on expressed breastmilk as a replacement feed for HIV-exposed babies. The following explanation had been added in the Rapid Advice:

> *...the group noted the paucity of programmatic data that demonstrates* [heat-treated expressed breastmilk's] *acceptability and sustainability at scale as an infant feeding strategy to improve HIV free survival. While reports are beginning to emerge describing its use in neonatal units or as a short-term approach in specific communities, the group was not confident to recommend this approach for all HIV-infected mothers who wish to breastfeed. More data is needed from a range of settings to understand what is needed from health systems to effectively support mothers in this approach. Evidence is needed to demonstrate that mothers can sustain adhering to the methodology over prolonged periods of time. Given the efficacy of antiretroviral drugs to prevent HIV transmission through breastfeeding, the role of heat-treatment of expressed breast milk as a truly feasible HIV prevention, child survival strategy is yet to be clarified. Until then, the group positioned the approach as an 'interim' strategy to assist mothers over specific periods of time rather than for the full duration of breastfeeding. The group endorsed the need for continued research in this area of HIV prevention and child survival.*

Confining the use of heat-treated breastmilk as an interim measure for use in special circumstances instead of endorsing its use as one more safe option for HIV-exposed babies in everyday situations, appeared to show unnecessary bias. As we saw in Chapter 11, there was adequate research to show that heat-treated expressed breastmilk was a safe, feasible and sustainable feeding method which could be completely controlled by the mother, was nutritionally and immunologically superior to infant formula, providing the baby with most of the components of breastmilk, and inactivated infectious HIV.[47–65] The claim that there was a paucity of programmatic evidence and knowledge of the degree of support which HIV-positive mothers might require to ensure success with exclusive breastmilk-feeding could only be made because of lack of support in the past for this feeding method and failure to investigate, document and acknowledge its success. The equipment and skills required to safely pasteurise breastmilk in the home are no more difficult to acquire or carry out than those needed to safely prepare infant formula. Consequently, heat-treated expressed breastmilk may be a safe feeding method for HIV-exposed babies in both developed and developing countries and should have been offered as another feeding option in all settings. Although it was disappointing and frustrating that this kind of research and experience had been so consistently dismissed by the UN agencies, the information about expressed breastmilk was more positive in the finalised 2010 WHO Guidelines (see paragraph 6 below).

WHO 2010 Guidelines on Infant Feeding in the context of HIV

In July 2010, following feedback on the 2009 Rapid Advice documents, WHO released the 2010 Guidelines on HIV and Infant Feeding, Principles relating how mothers were to be assisted, and Recommendations for Infant Feeding in the context of HIV and a Summary of Evidence.[66] The recommendations were as follows:

> ***1. Ensuring mothers receive the care they need***
> *Mothers known to be HIV-infected should be provided with lifelong antiretroviral therapy or antiretroviral prophylaxis interventions to reduce HIV transmission through breastfeeding according to WHO recommendations.*
> ***In settings where national authorities have decided that the maternal and child health services will principally promote and support breastfeeding and antiretroviral interventions as the strategy that will most likely give infants born to mothers known to be HIV-infected the greatest chance of HIV-free survival:***
>
> ***2. Which breastfeeding practices and for how long***
> *Mothers known to be HIV-infected (and whose infants are HIV uninfected or of unknown HIV status) should exclusively breastfeed their infants for the first 6 months of life, introducing appropriate complementary foods thereafter, and continue breastfeeding for the first 12 months of life. Breastfeeding should then only stop once a nutritionally adequate and safe diet without breast milk can be provided.*
>
> ***3. When mothers decide to stop breastfeeding***
> *Mothers known to be HIV-infected who decide to stop breastfeeding at any time should*

stop gradually within one month. Mothers or infants who have been receiving ARV prophylaxis should continue prophylaxis for one week after breastfeeding is fully stopped. Stopping breastfeeding abruptly is not advisable.

4. What to feed infants when mothers stop breastfeeding

When mothers known to be HIV-infected decide to stop breastfeeding at any time, infants should be provided with safe and adequate replacement feeds to enable normal growth and development. Alternatives to breastfeeding include:

• For infants less than six months of age:

– Commercial infant formula milk as long as home conditions outlined in Recommendation #5 below are fulfilled,

– Expressed, heat-treated breast milk (see Recommendation #6 below),

Home-modified animal milk is not recommended as a replacement food in the first six months of life.

• For children over six months of age:

– Commercial infant formula milk as long as home conditions outlined in Recommendation #5 are fulfilled,

– Animal milk (boiled for infants under 12 months), as part of a diet providing adequate micronutrient intake. Meals, including milk-only feeds, other foods and combination of milk feeds and other foods, should be provided four or five times per day. All children need complementary foods from six months of age.

5. Conditions needed to safely formula feed

Mothers known to be HIV-infected should only give commercial infant formula milk as a replacement feed to their HIV-uninfected infants or infants who are of unknown HIV status, when specific conditions are met:

a. safe water and sanitation are assured at the household level and in the community, ***and,***

b. the mother, or other caregiver can reliably provide sufficient infant formula milk to support normal growth and development of the infant; ***and,***

c. the mother or caregiver can prepare it cleanly and frequently enough so that it is safe and carries a low risk of diarrhoea and malnutrition; ***and***

d. the mother or caregiver can, in the first six months, exclusively give infant formula milk; ***and***

e. the family is supportive of this practice; ***and***

f. the mother or caregiver can access health care that offers comprehensive child health services.

These descriptions are intended to give simpler and more explicit meaning to the concepts represented by AFASS (acceptable, feasible, affordable, sustainable and safe).

6. Heat-treated, expressed breast milk

Mothers known to be HIV-infected may consider expressing and heat-treating breast milk as an interim feeding strategy:

• In special circumstances such as when the infant is born with low birth weight or is

otherwise ill in the neonatal period and unable to breastfeed; or
- *When the mother is unwell and temporarily unable to breastfeed or has a temporary breast health problem such as mastitis; or*
- *To assist mothers to stop breastfeeding; or*
- *If antiretroviral drugs are temporarily not available.*

7. When the infant is HIV-infected
If infants and young children are known to be HIV-infected, mothers are strongly encouraged to exclusively breastfeed for the first six months of life and continue breastfeeding as per the recommendations for the general population, that is up to two years or beyond.

In November 2010 UNICEF published a Community Infant and Young Child Feeding Counselling Package.[67] The Facilitator's Guide contained a 10-page section on training health workers on HIV and infant feeding which had been field-tested in Zambia in August 2010, and reviewed by WHO headquarters. One of the external reviewers was Felicity Savage of WABA.

Research finally showed that treatment was the best prevention for vertical transmission of HIV and resulted in reductions in both maternal and infant mortality. Sound public health principles were best served when mothers received ARV medication to protect their own health beyond the time of delivery and when they continued breastfeeding their babies. These transformational findings also finally permitted the option of breastfeeding in an industrialised country when that choice would also clearly benefit the HIV-positive mother and her baby.

It remained only for the most recent guidelines to be well disseminated, and for retraining of health workers to be undertaken and completed. Without full implementation on a global scale similar to that undertaken by the UN agencies in 2000, an unknown policy alone would not save lives. Refinements to the policy have been issued in the years since 2010, but essentially these guidelines remain current. The WHO website at the end of 2021[68] carries the following summary:

Mother-to-child transmission of HIV is the primary mode of HIV infection in infants. Transmission can occur during pregnancy, birth, or through breastfeeding. Decisions on whether or not HIV-infected mothers should breastfeed their infants are generally based on comparing the risk of infants acquiring HIV through breastfeeding, with the increased risk of death from malnutrition, diarrhoea and pneumonia if the infants are not exclusively breastfed.

Accumulating evidence has shown that giving antiretroviral medicines to the mother or the infant can significantly reduce the risk of HIV transmission through breastfeeding. National health authorities can refer to this evidence when formulating a strategy on infant feeding.

CHAPTER 25

If undetectable equals untransmissable, what about breastfeeding?

The story of the research showing the unqualified effectiveness of ART to suppress the quantity of virus in the blood of an HIV-infected man or woman, and subsequently to prevent him or her from passing on the infection horizontally, makes for remarkable reading.[1]

Vertical transmission (MTCT during pregnancy and birth)

Clinical evidence of the importance of viral load in the risk of transmission of HIV was highlighted in a report presented by Dr Karen Beckerman at the International AIDS Society conference in Geneva in July 1998. She described a small cohort of HIV-positive women in San Francisco who had received triple antiretroviral therapy during pregnancy. Previously, rates of transmission were 30% with no therapy and 10% with zidovudine monotherapy. Six mothers had already delivered and 10 mothers still pregnant had achieved an undetectable viral load with triple combination therapy, reducing transmission to a rate approaching zero.[2] Results showing that an undetectable viral load stopped a much higher rate of transmission warranted inclusion in the US DHHS guidelines to begin early ART.[3]

Effective ART reduces horizontal HIV infectivity to zero

The Rakai project

Two years later, in 2000, researchers from the Rakai project in Uganda reported a correlation between HIV in blood plasma and HIV transmission probability in sero-discordant couples (where one partner was HIV-positive and the other was not).[4] In a prospective cohort study of 415 couples, who were not receiving ART and who were followed up for a median of 22 months, the risk of HIV transmission increased with higher viral load. Each log increment in the viral load (the number of virus multiplied by a factor of ten) was associated with a 2.5-fold increased risk of infection. Conversely, and most importantly, there were *no* transmissions among 51 couples where the infected partner had a viral load below 1,500 copies/ml. Thus the risk of transmission of HIV with less than 1,500 copies of HIV RNA is negligible.

In a 2005 Spanish study of almost 400 sero-discordant couples before ART, or receiving early or late ART, no partner was infected when the infected partner had been treated with HAART.[5]

The Swiss study

In 2008, Pietro Vernazza and colleagues published the first high-profile evidence review that concluded that ART stopped transmission.[6] This paper was published in response to laws in Switzerland that criminalised an HIV-positive person if they had sex with an HIV-negative partner, even if condoms were used, or if a couple wanted to conceive with full consent. Reviewing more than 25 studies Vernazza and colleagues concluded that no transmissions occurred with ART. The estimated risk was less than 1 in 100,000 (0.001%) – and therefore effectively zero.

HPTN 052

In 2011, treatment with HAART so dramatically reduced the risk of HIV transmission for the uninfected partner of heterosexual couples in the HPTN-052 study[7] that it was stopped early so that all participants could be treated. HPTN-052 had recruited more than 1,700 couples, 97% of them heterosexual, from Malawi, Zimbabwe, South Africa, Botswana, Kenya, Thailand, India, Brazil and the US. The HIV-positive partners were randomised to either start ART immediately or to wait until their CD4 count dropped to 350 cells/mm (the then threshold in WHO guidelines for starting treatment). It soon became clear that HIV transmissions were almost exclusively occurring in the group waiting for ART and so the study was stopped early so that all HIV-positive participants could receive immediate treatment. Longer follow-up of HPTN continued for at least another four years and confirmed the strength of these early results.[8]

The PARTNER study

In 2009, a group of European researchers launched the prospective observational PARTNER study, enrolling sero-discordant couples at 75 sites in 14 countries where the HIV-positive partner was on ART, and where the couples were already not always using condoms (often for many years).[9–11] Early evidence of a strong link between the HIV viral load of an HIV-positive partner and the risk of transmission to an HIV-negative partner came from observational studies in sero-discordant heterosexual couples. Evidence from a randomised study of risk of HIV transmission in the context of virally suppressive antiretroviral therapy (ART) in heterosexual couples had been provided by the HPTN 052 trial, which reported a 96% reduction in linked transmissions in couples assigned to early (immediate) ART compared with couples assigned to delayed therapy. Researchers followed up both heterosexual and gay sero-discordant couples. One-third of the almost 900 couples were gay men and the study included detailed questionnaires on sexual activity to estimate risk based on actual exposure. In a planned early analysis, presented at the 2014 CROI conference in Boston, the study reported zero transmission of HIV between partners in over 44,000 sexual encounters without condoms, where viral load was undetectable (defined as <200 copies/ml). The PARTNER results also disproved previous concerns about viral load blips or other STIs – no transmissions were seen in the 91 couples where the positive partner reported an STI (approximately one-third of gay couples had open relationships). The final results, presented and published in July 2016, reported zero transmissions after 58,000 encounters without condoms.

The Opposites Attract study

The Opposites Attract study[12] was an observational prospective longitudinal cohort study of HIV transmission between male homosexual sero-discordant partners where the infected partner was receiving ART, running from 2012 to 2015 and conducted in clinics throughout Australia, Brazil and Thailand.[13] The HIV-positive partner's viral load was tested and the HIV-negative partner was tested for HIV antibodies at every clinic visit. The final results from 358 couples were reported at the 2017 International AIDS Society Conference in Paris.[14] There were zero transmissions after almost 17,000 acts of condom-less anal intercourse in homosexual male HIV-sero-discordant couples. These results provided strong support for the hypothesis that undetectable viral load prevents HIV transmission in homosexual men.

The PARTNER2 study

In order to provide an equal balance of evidence in transmission risk compared to that obtained for heterosexual couples, the PARTNER2 study continued to collect results in gay couples where the HIV-positive partner was taking virally suppressive ART to achieve a plasma HIV-RNA viral load of <200 copies/ml.[15] The PARTNER2 extension ran to the end of April 2018 and recruited and followed up gay couples only. At study visits, data collection included sexual behaviour questionnaires, HIV testing for the HIV-negative partner and viral load testing for the HIV-positive partner. Couples reported condom-less anal sex a total of 76,088 times. If a seroconversion occurred in the uninfected partner, anonymised phylogenetic analysis was done to identify linked transmissions. Thirty-seven per cent of 777 HIV-negative men reported condom-less sex with other partners. Fifteen new HIV infections occurred during follow-up, but none were phylogenetically linked within-couple transmissions, resulting in an HIV transmission rate of zero. These results provided a similar level of evidence that viral suppression in gay men resulted in no transmissions, similar to results previously generated for heterosexual couples. This meant that the risk of HIV transmission in gay couples through condom-less sex when HIV viral load is suppressed is also effectively zero. The findings supported the message of the U=U (undetectable equals untransmittable) campaign, and the benefits of early testing and treatment for HIV. Delegates attending the International AIDS conference in Amsterdam in July 2018 were electrified by the further information from the eight-year-long PARTNER trial. Publication of the results, notwithstanding their importance, had taken two years, possibly due to concerns that the results would undermine previous HIV prevention campaigns based on the need for consistent use of condoms.[15] A parallel can be drawn with the difficulty in making any headway with widely disseminating the zero risk of MTCT with exclusive breastfeeding and ART (EBF + ART) by HIV-positive mothers, since there is so much pre-existing support for formula-feeding, coupled with fears that relaxation of formula-feeding recommendations will spawn renewed enthusiasm for breastfeeding.

The huge financial investment in the AIDS industry had eventually borne results. Researchers looking at mutations, prevention strategies and myriad drug regimens had discovered a truly effective treatment which could simultaneously stop HIV in its tracks, allow people living with HIV to enjoy a normal lifespan without progression to AIDS, and prevent onward transmission to uninfected partners. By 2020, there had been no confirmed cases of HIV transmission from a person with an undetectable viral load in any studies. While the official cut-off point for an undetectable viral load as defined by the WHO ranged from <50 copies/ml in high-income countries to <1,000 copies/ml in low to middle-income countries, an *undetectable viral load is usually defined as under <200 copies/ml, which is also the measurement for viral suppression.*

Previous criminalisation of HIV

There had always been serious stigma attached to HIV infection. Criminal charges could be brought against an infected individual who deliberately or inadvertently infected an uninfected person if they did not disclose their HIV status. Since 2001, thirteen people were successfully prosecuted in the United Kingdom for giving their sexual partners HIV.[16] The laws used to prosecute criminal HIV transmission developed from existing assault laws: 'recklessly inflicting grievous bodily harm' in England and Wales and 'reckless injury' in Scotland. To secure a guilty verdict the prosecution had to prove that the person with HIV did, in fact, infect their partner, was aware of their HIV status and the risk of transmission, and did not obtain explicit consent to sex with an individual they knew had HIV. Hundreds of HIV-positive people have been imprisoned for many years for non-disclosure and often in the absence of actual transmission.[1,17]

The Swiss statement

In January 2008 a revolutionary statement on infectivity was issued by four of Switzerland's foremost HIV researchers, including Prof Pietro Vernazza. The statement said, 'After review of the medical literature and extensive discussion,' the Swiss Federal Commission for HIV/AIDS resolves that, 'An HIV-infected person on antiretroviral therapy with completely suppressed viraemia ("effective ART") is not sexually infectious, i.e. cannot transmit HIV through sexual contact.'[6,18–20] The statement, which had been published in the *Bulletin of Swiss Medicine* (*Bulletin des Médecins Suisses*) was initially intended to support heterosexual couples to conceive children naturally without facing legal charges when one member of the couple was HIV-positive and the other was HIV-negative (defined as sero-discordant), but the implications were far wider for doctors, for HIV-positive people, for HIV prevention and the legal system.

The Swiss statement set out several pre-conditions:

- *The HIV-positive person needed to be good at taking their meds and routinely seeing their doctor; and*
- *Their viral load needed to be undetectable for at least six months, and*

- *They had no other sexually transmitted infections (STIs).*

The statement became regarded as a landmark in the development of giving treatment to suppress viral load as an HIV prevention strategy known as Treatment as Prevention. Later its effectiveness came to be known as undetectable equals untransmittable (U=U).

Consensus statement

In July 2016 the Prevention Access Campaign issued the following consensus statement, endorsed by over 1,000 organisations from 102 countries.[21] (See box.) The Executive Director of CATIE, the Canadian AIDS Treatment Information Exchange, described developments leading up to release of the statement as 'the most significant development in the HIV world since the advent of effective combination therapy 20 years ago – people living with HIV with sustained undetectable viral loads can confidently declare to their sexual partners "I'm not infectious!" The "fabulousness" of this news cannot be overstated. With or without a condom, if you're undetectable you won't pass along HIV! This is an absolute game-changer and those who live with HIV can proudly share this information. At the same time, service providers working in HIV must get up to speed fast and share this far and wide with their communities. Let's get the word out!'

Zero or negligible: the burden of proof

Addressing concerns about use of the word 'negligible' vs 'zero' in statements about U=U, a member of the steering committee for the PARTNER studies made these points in a talk given to the Positive People's Forum held in Glasgow on 1 July 2017:[1]

> *...the semantic difference between zero risk and negligible risk, even when this theoretical risk is increasingly tiny (as with the Swiss statement), prevented some people saying that the risk was effectively zero. The most significant change... driven by the U=U campaign, has been for leading HIV scientists to now assert that a negligible theoretical risk is effectively zero... This reverses the scientific challenge from proving safety to proving risk. Purely theoretical risks are no longer a good enough level of evidence to sustain stigma and discrimination and certainly not criminalisation. Instead, there is no evidence to show that HIV transmission occurs when viral load is undetectable. People who want to assert the theory that HIV transmission might be possible, now have to provide some level of proof.*
>
> *A comprehensive body of evidence now supports the U=U statement... no cases of HIV transmission have been reported, over nine years since the Swiss statement set this challenge. This includes data for gay men, for couples that have anal sex, over periods when low-level viral blips are likely and even when STIs are present. In reality, even if the actual risk is zero, it is not healthy to think about anything in life as being risk-free. Even if at some point in the future an unlucky and rare case of transmission is reported with undetectable viral load, the U=U campaign is still right for closing the gap between zero and the real-life meaning of negligible in real terms.*

CONSENSUS STATEMENT, UNDETECTABLE = UNTRANSMISSABLE, 21 July 2016

Risk of sexual transmission of HIV from a person living with HIV who has an undetectable viral load

Messaging Primer & Consensus Statement

https://www.preventionaccess.org/consensus

There is now evidence-based confirmation that the risk of HIV transmission from a person living with HIV who is on Antiretroviral Therapy (ART) and has achieved an undetectable viral load in their blood for at least 6 months is negligible to non-existent. (Negligible is defined as: so small or unimportant as to be not worth considering; insignificant.) While HIV is not always transmitted even with a detectable viral load, when the partner with HIV has an undetectable viral load this both protects their own health and prevents new HIV infections.

However, the majority of people living with HIV, medical providers and those potentially at risk of acquiring HIV are not aware of the extent to which successful treatment prevents HIV transmission. Much of the messaging about HIV transmission risk is based on outdated research and is influenced by agency or funding restraints and politics which perpetuate sex-negativity, HIV-related stigma and discrimination.

The consensus statement below, addressing HIV transmission risk from PLHIV who havean undetectable viral load, is endorsed by principal investigators from each of the leading studies that examined this issue. It is important that PLHIV, their intimate partners and their healthcare providers have accurate information about risks of sexual transmission of HIV from those successfully on ART.

The following statement has also been endorsed by over 1,000 organisations from 102 countries.

People living with HIV on ART with an undetectable viral load in their blood have a negligible risk of sexual transmission of HIV. Depending on the drugs employed it may take as long as six months for the viral load to become undetectable. Continued and reliable HIV suppression requires selection of appropriate agents and excellent adherence to treatment. HIV viral suppression should be monitored to assure both personal health and public health benefits.

Endorsements, Updated 14 September, 2020 include:

"I just want to pay tribute to the U=U campaign, it has been astonishing. I think the time for excuses are over. I think it is very, very clear that the risk is zero. I very much think we have to promote this... if you are on suppressive ART you are sexually noninfectious and the time for excuses is over." Dr. Alison Rodger, lead author of

PARTNER2 at the International AIDS Conference - AIDS 2018 presentation (July, 2018)

"The science really does verify and validate U=U." Anthony S. Fauci, M.D., Director, NIAID, NIH, Speech at the United States Conference on AIDS (September, 2017)

"...studies have proven that when an individual living with HIV is on antiretroviral therapy and the virus is durably suppressed, the risk that he or she will sexually transmit the virus is negligible." Anthony S. Fauci, M.D., Director, National Institute of Allergy and Infectious Diseases; Carl W. Dieffenbach, Ph.D., Director, Division of AIDS, NIAID. NIH Statement on World AIDS Day 2016 (December, 2016)

"Among serodifferent heterosexual and MSM couples in which the HIV-positive partner was using suppressive ART and who reported condomless sex...there were no documented cases of within-couple HIV transmission" among 58,000 condomless sex acts. Reporting on PARTNER study, Dr Alison Rodger et al, Journal of the American Medical Association (July, 2016)

"Does this work over a long period of time for people who are anxious to be suppressed? The answer is absolutely yes, we now have 10,000 person years (of follow-up) with zero transmissions from people who are suppressed." Dr. Myron Cohen, Medpage, New England Journal of Medicine, (July, 2016)

"EATG calls for much better public information to be made available in Europe and globally about the prevention benefits of antiretroviral therapy (ART), and in particular (about) the fact that HIV-positive people with undetectable viral loads are not infectious. Widespread ignorance of this fact helps perpetuate stigma against and criminalisation of people living with HIV and it should be the subject of a funded public awareness campaign, possibly to run in conjunction with a PrEP awareness campaign." European AIDS Treatment Group (October, 2015)

"If people are taking their pills reliably and they're taking them for some period of time, the probability of transmission in this study is actually zero." Dr Myron Cohen, Chief, Division of Infectious Diseases, UNC School of Medicine, North Carolina, USA; Principal Investigator, HPTN 052 Interview with HIVPlus Mag (August, 2015)

"As the UK's leading voice for HIV health professionals, our backing for U=U is unequivocal. There should be no doubt about the clear and simple message that a person with sustained, undetectable levels of HIV virus in their blood cannot transmit HIV to their sexual partners...."This fact is a testament to the preventive impact of effective HIV treatment and highlights the need to maximise access to treatment in order to minimise and ultimately eradicate HIV transmission. Spreading the U=U message is also an important way to help reduce the stigma experienced by people living with HIV, whose sexual partners may fear infection unnecessarily." (BHIVA Chair, Prof Chloe Orkin, 17 July 2017)

Except for breastfeeding...

Notwithstanding the repeated assertions, backed up by the meticulous research in all scenarios, that U=U is true for every type of HIV transmission, whether horizontal, or vertical during pregnancy and birth, the assertion continues to be made that mother's milk poses a risk of HIV transmission to the breastfed baby even when mothers receive ART.

It is accepted today that there is no route of transmission which cannot be prevented by adequate antiretroviral therapy to infected individuals, e.g. during oral sex, vaginal sex and anal sex; between straight couples, gay couples or discordant couples (where one is infected, but the other is not), and between mother and baby in utero or during birth – every which way, in fact, except through breastfeeding.

AIDSMAP, a prominent AIDS support organisation in the UK, gave this advice December 2019:[22] 'If you have been on treatment for a while and it is working well, the risk during breastfeeding is low. It does however depend on your viral load, your own state of health, your baby's health and how long you breastfeed the child. *Breastfeeding is only recommended where formula feeding is not considered safe*, for example in low income countries.'

Those discouraging breastfeeding for HIV-exposed babies cite the existence of a viral reservoir of infected cells, maternal breast infections, failure of maternal ART, and inability of mothers to adhere to their drug regimens as reasons why breastfeeding should not be supported. These reasons, together with the belief in the safety and normality of formula-feeding for babies in the global north, serve to discourage breastfeeding by all but the most determined HIV-positive mothers.

No research from developed countries

The truth is that there has been no reported research or retrospective operational research on breastfeeding with HIV specifically from high-income countries where HIV-positive pregnant and lactating women are likely to be receiving the most up-to-date antiretroviral therapy (HAART or cART), as well as the monitoring of their own viral load and testing of their infants. This omission permits commentators on HIV and infant feeding to go unchallenged when they express misgivings about the safety of breastfeeding by HIV-positive mothers in the global north. They cite research from developing countries showing that ART has failed to completely protect against postpartum MTCT, such as the Mma Bana results from Botswana,[23] in which two infants had a positive HIV result during breastfeeding despite maternal ART. However, as set out in Chapter 23 these transmissions were due to inadequate treatment; one mother had received ART for only four weeks because she gave birth prematurely, and the other was shown to have a high viral load.

Another cited example is the meta-analysis published in 2017 to inform the WHO infant feeding guidelines. Six studies in low-income settings in which mothers started ART before or during their most recent pregnancy[24,25] gave an estimated postnatal transmission risk (excluding perinatal transmissions) of >1% up to six months of age. Two of the studies reported postnatal transmission up to 12 months of age, and the pooled estimate was close to 3%. However, there were considerable differences in the time of ART initiation during pregnancy and, unsurprisingly, a higher risk when mothers started ART later rather than earlier. There were also differences in the recommended duration of breastfeeding, the age at which infection in the infant was assessed, details on infant feeding modality and the definition of postnatal transmission. The quality of evidence for the risk of MTCT through breastfeeding from 6–12 months was low.

The PROMISE study

More recently, the Promoting Maternal Infant Survival Everywhere (PROMISE) trial has been cited again and again as evidence that breastfeeding is not completely safe, even when mothers receive HAART and where transmission was also shown to be <1%.[26] This was a dizzyingly complicated research project which recruited 5,400 HIV-positive pregnant women from 70 research sites in 15 countries across several continents. The PROMISE trial enrolled asymptomatic HIV-infected pregnant and postpartum women not eligible for ART according to local guidelines in place at the time (before the recommendation for universal access to HAART regardless of CD4 count). Women were randomly assigned proven antiretroviral strategies to assess relative efficacy for perinatal prevention plus maternal/infant safety and maternal health. One of the main difficulties involved persuading well women to accept and then adhere to ART.[27] Women not already receiving ART were strongly recommended to immediately initiate treatment to optimise their own health, but one-third of participants did not initiate ART after the initial counselling session, wanting more time to consider. Six sessions were required to attain 95% uptake. Women were assigned to different drug regimens and followed for HIV disease progression, vertical transmission and safety, as follows:

- In settings where maternal ART and replacement feeding was standard, eligible women were randomised within six weeks of delivery to continue – or stop – ART, and remain in follow-up for intense monitoring of HIV disease progression and adverse events in a protocol named 1077HS (for HAART standard).
- In settings where maternal ART was not standard for the prevention of vertical transmission, separate protocols were conducted in formula-feeding and breastfeeding groups respectively.
- Pregnant women who would breastfeed were randomised at 6-14 days *after birth* to triple ART – or prophylaxis – with zidovudine throughout pregnancy and delivery in the Antepartum Component – plus single dose nevirapine at delivery followed by a two-week 'tail' of tenofovir/emtricitabine.
- Women who did not access antenatal services could join around the time of delivery.
- Eligible mothers were randomised after delivery in the Postpartum Component to receive – or not receive – maternal ART, while some babies were randomised to receive ARV prophylaxis.
- Once the period of risk for vertical transmission was over – at delivery for non-breastfeeding mothers, or after weaning, or after 18 months of study intervention (whichever came first) for breastfeeding mothers, women receiving ART were randomised in the Maternal Health Component to continue – or stop – ART.
- Enrolled women who were not eligible for subsequent randomisations were followed in an observational cohort through study completion.

In this incredibly complicated study, the reported postnatal HIV transmission risk was 0.3% at six months and 0.7% at 12 months, with no difference between the arms where either breastfeeding mothers received HAART, or babies received ARV prophylaxis.

The significance of the PROMISE study is that apparently two breastfed babies were infected by mothers whose viral load was <40 copies/ml. It is difficult to ascertain the testing regimens for either mother to establish whether maternal adherence to ART was consistent with tested viral load.

The authors of the Swiss study express caution about the PROMISE methodology: 'Although these results confirm the low risk when cART is implemented, analysis of the HIV RNA for the whole breastfeeding period is currently not yet available to prove or disprove HIV MTCT whilst on fully suppressive cART. So far, we only have information from the first week postpartum, when 41% of women on cART had undetectable HIV plasma viral load.'[28]

The viral reservoir and breastfeeding

It has been suggested that ART during pregnancy and after delivery suppresses cell-free but not cell-associated HIV loads in breastmilk,[29] so that a residual CD4+ T-cell-associated reservoir of HIV is persistently present in the milk. It's thought that these latently infected CD4+ T-cells can transcribe HIV DNA and generate viral particles that are potentially 17 times more effective than their plasma counterparts in producing HIV antigens.

Old research is sometimes brought to bear to illustrate and talk up the risk of HIV transmission during breastfeeding. In a curious paper in which research conducted between 2001 and 2006 was not submitted for publication for eight years, Danaviah and colleagues begin, 'Exposure of the infant's gut to cell-associated and cell-free HIV-1 trafficking in breast milk remains a primary cause of mother-to-child transmission (MTCT)...'. They then go to postulate that DNA archived viruses stem from latently infected quiescent T-cells within breast tissue; MTCT can be expected to continue, albeit at low levels throughout lactation, *should interventions not effectively target these cells.*[30] The level of maturation of the infant's gut, mixed feeding and consequent inflammation of both mother's breast tissue and the baby's gut were all said to have an impact on the risk of transmission and the nature of the transmitted virus, which is not disputed. However, Danaviah and colleagues make the alarming observation that the infant's intestinal mucosa has an outsized surface area of approximately 200m^2 and constitutes a vast portal of entry to both cell-free and cell-associated HIV. Of particular note, mothers included in the small study where all babies had become infected through breastfeeding had only received single-dose nevirapine as prophylaxis.

In 2012, Philippe van de Perre and colleagues had given their opinion that recent studies of possible HIV reservoirs in breastmilk shed new light on features that influence HIV transmission through breastfeeding. The particular characteristics of breastmilk CD4+ T-cells that distinguish them from circulating blood lymphocytes (a high frequency of cell activation and expression of memory and mucosal homing markers) facilitate the establishment of HIV replication. Even during efficient ART, a residual stable CD4+ T-cell-associated reservoir of HIV was persistently present in breastmilk, a likely source of infection; only prophylactic treatment in infants – ideally with a long-acting drug, administered for the entire duration of breastfeeding – was likely to protect HIV-exposed babies against all forms of HIV transmission from breastmilk, including cell-to-cell viral transfer.[31]

When Shapiro and colleagues conducting the MASHI study looked at this in 2005 to compare HIV RNA and HIV DNA in women with low CD4 counts or active AIDS,[32] they found that among women who commenced HAART either shortly before or after delivery, no transmissions occurred through breastfeeding over seven months of follow-up. Within two months, almost all women in the HAART group had suppressed HIV RNA viral loads to <400 copies/ml compared with two-thirds who did not receive treatment. There was no correlation between HIV DNA load in breastmilk and baseline plasma HIV RNA load overall. Most of the mothers had only received HAART for 86–112 days (median 98 days), whereas subsequent research shows that the longer the duration of maternal treatment, the lower the risk of HIV transmission to their babies. Shapiro and colleagues reported:

> *'We did not detect a significant effect of HAART on breast-milk HIV DNA load. Similar findings were noted in previous studies of cell-associated genital secretions, where proviral DNA remained detectable in the cervicovaginal fluid of up to one-half of women receiving HAART, and in the semen of men receiving HAART. HAART may reduce the HIV DNA load in breast milk over time, as long-lived HIV-infected macrophages in breast milk are eventually replaced. This delay in cell-associated viral reduction, compared with cell-free virus reduction, has been demonstrated in peripheral blood and lymph-node mononuclear cells. The duration of treatment in our cohort is probably typical for women who start HAART during late pregnancy, so a potential risk for cell-associated HIV-1 transmission despite the use of HAART may remain in such patients. The magnitude of cell-associated breast-milk HIV-1 transmission is unknown. The risk posed by high loads of cell-free HIV-1 RNA in breast milk is better documented, as is the association between cell-free virus and transmission in studies during the peripartum period and in animal models.'*

Other cell types in breastmilk such as macrophages, CD4+ progenitor T-cells, and dendritic cells, could also be involved in transmission.[31] Hence, the Nairobi group in 2008 believed that even in the face of ART, latent reservoirs in breastmilk could still replicate and plasma viral suppression did not equate to breastmilk viral suppression.[33] Moselholm and colleagues in 2019 say it is unknown if this holds true for women on long-term ART or whether any newer drugs influence these latent T-cells.[29] As ART is being implemented globally for all women living with HIV there is an increasing need to better define the viral reservoir in women receiving ARV drugs, to clarify the potential of these cells to produce infectious virus and to define a viral threshold in breastmilk for increased transmission risk.[34]

First evidence of latency

When, where, and how HIV latency is established is still the object of intensive investigations. In the absence of ART, activated CD4+ T-cells represent the main target for HIV and die rapidly upon infection. Only a minute fraction of these cells survive and enter the pool of persistent and long-lived latently infected cells.[35] The capacity of HIV to lie dormant within specific types of cells and at extremely low frequencies suggests that it can establish latency under rare circumstances.

The first evidence for this was demonstrated in 1995, before the implementation of combination ART: Chun et al isolated resting CD4+ T-cells from the blood of individuals with active HIV infection and observed that a small fraction of these cells harboured integrated HIV genomes and could produce viral particles upon stimulation *ex vivo*.[36] In 1997, the implementation of effective ART revealed the clinical importance of this pool of latently infected cells: three studies reported the presence of a small number of persistently infected cells harbouring replication-competent HIV in individuals on suppressive ART. Although these cells were extremely rare (around one in one million resting CD4+ T-cells), the reservoir was long-lived, with an estimated half-life of 44 months,[37,38] indicating that ART alone would not eradicate the pool of latently infected cells in a lifetime.

The latent reservoir of HIV was demonstrated in 2003 using an assay in which resting cells from patients were activated to reverse latency. Viruses released from individual latently infected cells were expanded in culture. This viral outgrowth assay was used to demonstrate the remarkable stability of the latent reservoir. At a half-life of 44 months and at this rate of decay, it would take >70 years for a pool of just 10^6 cells to decay completely.

Twenty years after discovery of latent virus, the precise nature of the HIV reservoir remains unclear. A recently published article describing the multi-faceted nature of HIV latency by Caroline Dufour and colleagues[35] offers additional explanation. Viral reservoirs have been defined as 'cell types or anatomical sites where replication-competent forms of the virus persist with more stable kinetic properties than in the main pool of actively replicating virus'.[39,40]

During untreated HIV infection, the majority of infected cells are short-lived: HIV viraemia is sustained by a dynamic process involving continuous rounds of new infection. Initiation of ART leads to a dramatic reduction in the levels of viral replication and in the frequency of infected cells. Residual viraemia persists and can originate from low levels of ongoing replication or, more likely, from the continuous production of viral particles from stable reservoirs. The majority of infected cells in HIV-positive individuals receiving ART do not produce viral particles and are defined as latently infected cells. Any infected cell with a half-life of more than two days, which corresponds to the average half-life of productively infected cells,[41,42] may represent a reservoir for HIV.

Using ultrasensitive methods to quantify and characterise traces of persisting virus in HIV-positive individuals who receive fully effective ART, two types of viral reservoirs that could both contribute to HIV persistence have been identified:

- Firstly, suboptimal diffusion of ART in lymphoid tissues allows the virus to replicate at low levels, suggesting that ART is not fully efficient. HIV-specific CD8+ T-cells may not be able to access anatomical sites in which ongoing replication occurs, for example in the germinal centre of second lymphoid organs or in immune-privileged organs such as testes.

- Secondly a small pool of latently infected cells that persists for decades in people living with HIV receiving ART.[43–45] Latently infected cells can be defined as cells harbouring integrated and intact proviruses *that do not actively produce infectious virions, but have the capacity to do so upon stimulation.*

Memory CD4+ T-cells represent the major cellular reservoir for HIV. While it was originally thought that the pool of latently infected cells was largely composed of cells harbouring transcriptionally silent genomes, recent evidence indicates that several factors make these cells nonproductive.

Attempts to eliminate the viral reservoir: the search for a cure

Effective ART has transformed HIV from a lethal disease which progresses to AIDS and death to a chronic but manageable disease, like diabetes. Nevertheless, researchers are still aiming for a complete cure. More than 20 years since the development of ART, it has still not been possible to eradicate HIV completely. HIV persists in cellular and anatomical reservoirs that show minimal decay during ART. The viral reservoir has thus been extensively studied in order to bring about the complete elimination of HIV – rather than merely managing the disease through continuous antiretroviral therapy. The persistence of HIV in a small pool of long-lived latently infected resting CD4+ T-cells is a major barrier to viral eradication – a goal which has long frustrated HIV researchers.

Finding ways to eliminate the latent reservoir for HIV has become a major research focus. The persistence of a latent form of the virus in a small population of resting memory CD4+ T-cells prevented a cure. But viral genes are not expressed at significant levels unless the T-cell has been activated.[46] There has been a dramatic increase in optimism that HIV infection may be curable if the problem of the latent reservoir can be overcome. One critical issue going forward is how to measure this, since there is currently no clinical assay for the latent reservoir. Because of the low frequency of latently infected cells, large sample volumes are required, typically 180ml of blood. Most HIV proviruses are defective and PCR assays do not distinguish defective from replication-competent proviruses.

It's likely that all infected individuals will require interventions directly targeting the reservoir to achieve a cure. One way to bring HIV out of its hiding place and into the open where it can be treated is to identify and expose virus hidden away in lymphoid and other tissues. Attempts to eradicate HIV have adopted a shock-and-kill strategy combining the reactivation of latent proviruses ('shock') and the elimination of the resulting productively infected cells ('kill'), with the hypothesis that viral clearance of virus-expressing cells by the immune system will reduce the size of the latent reservoir.[35] HIV-infected individuals receive 'treatment holidays' from antiretroviral drugs to stimulate latent virus to start proliferating again so that it can be 'seen' and subsequently eliminated.

We need to remember that when ART is stopped so that virus can replicate it is a very diferent strategy, the opposite in fact, to urging absolute adherence to drug regimens in

HIV-positive pregnant and lactating mothers in order to maintain an undetectable viral load which protects against MTCT. But somehow the idea that the viral reservoir can be deliberately activated by suspension of ART has enabled many in the AIDS community to point out that ART alone cannot eradicate HIV in infected individuals. Instead they insist that persistence of viral reservoirs in the peripheral blood and lymphoid tissues of the breastfeeding mother renders her continually infectious. Like all good arguments, there is a ring of truth to it, but we can ask whether it tells the whole story.

Cell-free vs cell-associated virus in breastmilk

A 2014 paper from the Nairobi group[34] identified one question remaining to be elucidated: the molecular mechanism of virus transmission in MTCT – i.e. whether the most infectious form is free virus or an infected cell. Cell-free (RNA) and cell-associated (DNA) virus had both been detected in maternal blood (plasma), breastmilk and genital secretions, and virus levels in these fluids had all been correlated with MTCT. A number of epidemiologic studies of breastfeeding and intrapartum transmission had suggested that cell-associated virus might be relatively more important.

The Nairobi group had previously looked at this question.[33] Although they found that cell-free and, to a lesser extent, cell-associated HIV RNA levels in breastmilk were reduced with HAART, there was no significant reduction in the reservoir of infected cells. They thought that this could contribute to breastmilk HIV transmission. Notably, however, at the time that their research was conducted it had yet to be discovered that HAART needed to be taken for at least 13 weeks in order to fully reduce viral load to undetectable and thus be protective against MTCT. Milligan and Overbaugh concluded 'It has been difficult to isolate infectious HIV from breast milk, perhaps because levels are low, and past efforts in our lab were unsuccessful; however, there have been at least two reports of HIV being cultured from breastmilk'.[34,47,48] These studies isolated the virus from cellular and cell-free fractions of breastmilk, suggesting that infectious virus may exist in either form. HIV RNA levels are typically 100 times lower in breastmilk than in blood.[49] HIV DNA has also been detected in breastmilk CD4+ T-cells and macrophages.[31]

RNA vs DNA

A science overview on the AVERT website[50] explains that, being a retrovirus, HIV stores its genetic information using RNA instead of DNA. Once the proviral DNA enters the cell nucleus, it binds to the host DNA and then the HIV DNA strand is inserted into the host cell DNA. HIV integrase inhibitors have been developed to block the transfer of the HIV DNA strand into the host cell DNA. HIV then remains dormant within the cellular DNA. This stage is called latency and the cell is described as 'latently infected'. It is these long-lived cells of the immune system that form a 'reservoir' of HIV infection in the body. They are difficult to detect, even when using the most sensitive tests, unless the CD4 cell becomes 'activated' by encountering an infectious agent.

More than 20 years after the discovery of the viral reservoir, its precise nature remains unclear. Dufour and colleagues write, 'Production of viral proteins by latently infected cells appears to be rare.'[35] This suggests that several blocks may contribute to the inability of persistently infected cells to produce infectious viral particles. HIV-infected cells are found in multiple tissues after years of ART. Dufour describes how, in addition to blood, persistently infected cells are found in the lymph nodes, gut, central nervous system, lungs, bone marrow and genital tract. Postmortem studies revealed the presence of HIV DNA in all 28 tissues analysed. Since gut-associated lymphoid tissue (GALT) and lymph nodes are particularly enriched in persistently infected cells during ART, lymphoid tissues may represent a favourable environment for the establishment of viral latency.

Antiretroviral drugs and the viral reservoir

Two types of antiretroviral drug have been developed to stop the action of reverse transcriptase and the creation of proviral DNA:[50]

1. Nucleoside and nucleotide reverse transcriptase inhibitors (NRTIs and NtRTIs) block HIV production, terminating the chain.
2. Non-nucleoside reverse transcriptase inhibitors (NNRTIs), a particular type of ART, block HIV production by binding directly to the reverse transcriptase enzyme.

A 2015 extensive and careful follow-up study of latent reservoir decay found that despite including patients who had been receiving new classes of antiretroviral drugs, such as integrase inhibitors, the decay rate of the latent reservoir is almost exactly the same as that reported in 2003, with the half-life measured being 43 months.[51] The fact that the decay rate measured in the 2015 study was no different from that measured more than a decade previously confirms that the stability of the latent reservoir is not determined by treatment regimens. As long as the regimen produced a complete or near-complete arrest of new infection events, the decay of the reservoir was determined by the biology of the resting memory T-cells that harbour persistent HIV. Nonnucleoside reverse-transcriptase inhibitors and protease inhibitors possess a remarkable potential to inhibit viral replication. At clinical concentrations, the best protease inhibitors can actually produce a 10 billion–fold inhibition of a single round of HIV replication. Thus, even the early combination therapy regimens may have produced complete or near-complete inhibition of new infection events in drug-adherent patients.

What is known today?

A relatively large fraction and possibly the majority of latently infected cells do not produce viral particles. Accordingly, production of viral proteins by latently infected cells appears to be rare[52,53] and several impediments may contribute to the inability of persistently infected cells to produce infectious viral particles.

Experts have determined that plasma HIV viraemia can be suppressed and maintained below the limits of detection for prolonged periods of time in the vast majority of HIV-infected individuals who receive effective ART.[54] Multiple studies have failed to identify strong evidence for ongoing viral replication in individuals receiving new-generation antiviral drugs.[35,55–58] Thus, the clinical outcome for those who have access to these drugs is dramatically improved.

Current treatment recommendations are sophisticated and effective: WHO guidelines recommend initial treatment with two nucleoside reverse transcriptase inhibitor (NRTI) + one integrase inhibitor as the first-line treatment of HIV among adults, including pregnant women.[59] An increasing proportion of pregnant and lactating women have already been receiving HAART for many years.

In high-income countries today there is high coverage of antenatal HIV screening. Current guidance recommends maternal HAART from diagnosis and to be continued for life. This means that almost all pregnant HIV-positive mothers fulfil what Kahlert called a 'best scenario',[28] beginning with early diagnosis and prompt treatment with HAART from the first trimester, reducing their viral load so effectively that they qualify to safely give birth to their babies vaginally. The time of greatest risk of MTCT of HIV is around the 24 hours of birth, yet due to the effectiveness of this regimen, obstetricians no longer recommend routine caesarean section. Thus the recommendation for a vaginal delivery can be used as a marker for a viral load sufficiently undetectable to also allow for safe breastfeeding.

People who start ART and reach an undetectable viral load within nine months have a low chance of experiencing a viral load greater than 200 copies/ml, the criteria considered to be a viral rebound.[60] The rebound risk decreases steadily over the next seven years.[61] A considerable body of research suggests that having a viral load <200 means that there is an extremely low risk of transmission; the risk may in fact be zero. Self-awareness of recent adherence patterns may help reduce any doubt surrounding an individual's viral load between tests. Results from the ongoing multicentre UK CHIC study, published in the *Lancet* in 2017, included data on 16,101 HIV-positive participants. Individuals who began treatment with three or more ARVs achieved full viral suppression (a viral load <50 copies/ml) within nine months of starting treatment. According to the new study's lead author, Andrew N. Phillips, an epidemiologist and biostatistician at University College London, the research highlighted a 'small but real risk that people taking ARVs who have incomplete adherence but have not actually interrupted treatment may develop a viral load >200 at some point between tests. But I suspect, but don't know, that most of the rebounds observed in our study occurred in people who did not have consistent high adherence in the recent period before the rebound.' In other words, individuals taking ARVs arguably have considerable control over preventing viral rebound by sticking to their daily drug regimen.

Replication-competent proviruses are present in only one in one million CD4+ T cells in the blood,[43,44] whereas HIV DNA quantification typically measures frequencies that are two to three orders of magnitude higher. This difference is due to a large proportion of HIV genomes presenting various defects preventing them from replicating. In the blood, defective proviruses represent 95%–98% of the viral genomes, and these defects accumulate rapidly in the course of infection. Only a few studies have investigated the presence of intact or replication-competent genomes. Therefore, the exact contribution of these anatomical reservoirs to the pool of persistently infected cells remains largely unknown.[35]

Multiple studies highlight the cellular mechanisms that contribute to the non-productive state of HIV-infected cells during ART. The majority of persistently infected cells do not produce viral particles during ART. These latently infected cells are maintained through both cell survival signals, preventing HIV-infected cells from death, and cell division signals, promoting the expansion of HIV-infected clones. Several studies over the past 10 years have clearly demonstrated that clonal expansions occur in the persistent HIV reservoir. These infected clones wax and wane during ART.

Adherence

According to long-time HIV and infant feeding researcher, Mary Glenn Fowler, the largest remaining barrier to eliminating perinatal HIV transmission is overcoming poor adherence to lifelong ART regimens.[62] She asserts that this is a worldwide problem. Several studies have recorded that adherence to maternal ART during the postpartum period is worse than before birth. Naturally, decreased adherence has been associated with increases in breastmilk viraemia and increased risk of postpartum transmission. Prior to 2016, ART was reserved for HIV-infected pregnant women with signs of immunosuppression or clinical AIDS. HIV-positive women received antiretroviral prophylaxis during pregnancy, and they or their infants received prophylaxis during lactation, but drugs were withdrawn later. As many as one-quarter of women were lost to follow-up after their babies' first birthday as they transferred from maternity services to general ART clinics. Among women on life-long ART, one recent study showed that a significant minority of women taking ART pre-conception enter antenatal care with detectable viraemia.[63] After initial viral suppression with ART during pregnancy, a number of studies showed decreased rates of viral suppression at 12 and 24 months postpartum, putting the breastfeeding infant at risk of postnatal infection.

Reports of women who either seem to be reluctant to begin ART during pregnancy, or who maintain poor adherence to ART during breastfeeding, thus risking transmission of MTCT of HIV to their babies, are at odds with what I hear from pregnant or breastfeeding HIV-positive mothers themselves. It would seem to be a no-brainer: whether they live in South Africa, Kenya, England or Germany, every single one is single-mindedly committed to being meticulously adherent to her medications, firstly so that her baby will not become infected, but also due to each mother's recognition that she needs to maintain her own health during her years of mothering all her children until they are grown up and independent.

U=U for breastfeeding?

In a 2018 article Catriona Waitt, Philippe Van de Perre and colleagues ask if the campaign Undetectable=Untransmittable (U=U), established for the sexual transmission of HIV, can be applied to the transmission of HIV through breastfeeding.[64] European and American guidelines now say that mothers with HIV who wish to breastfeed should be supported, with increased clinical and virological monitoring. They propose a roadmap for collaborative research to provide the missing evidence required to enable mothers who wish to breastfeed. Does the success of U=U for sexual transmission make it applicable in breastfeeding?

Clinical guidelines from high-income countries all make a first recommendation against breastfeeding with HIV, even though recent updates from several countries now acknowledge that women who choose to breastfeed should be supported to do so.[65] At the same time, in low-income settings, WHO recommends breastfeeding for at least six months and continuing up to 12 or 24 months.[66] Waitt and colleagues perceptively identify the reasons for the difference in approach:

> *'The recommendations are based on the same sources of data, but the balance of benefit versus harm of breastfeeding differs. In low-income settings, the morbidity and mortality from infection in infants receiving formula milk outweighs the risks of HIV transmission through breastmilk, because of unclean water and lost protection from maternal antibodies in breastmilk.'*

Questioning the significance of cell-associated virus and the relationship between transmission in women with or without suppressed viral load, Waitt and colleagues ask, does this still hold true for women on long-term ART? If HAART can prevent transmission from HIV-positive men with sexually transmitted infections, can it not also prevent transmission from mother to baby during sub-clinical mastitis? Do any newer drugs influence cell-associated virus? What is the genuine rate of transmission? Very low rates are reported in the context of suppressive ART, and most transmissions can be explained through detectable virus or poor adherence. Waitt and colleagues urge as a research priority establishment of a registry of mother–infant pairs to capture any transmissions. Fortunately such a registry exists in England,[67] and by July 2019 it had recorded 90 HIV-positive mothers who had breastfed, 57 with results indicating no transmissions.[68] Haberl and colleagues' recent paper reports on a further 42 cases from Germany.[65] The task remaining is to publish these findings in a format which can be easily accessed and scrutinised by clinicians in first world countries.

A Swiss Statement for breastfeeding

Christian Kahlert, together with Pietro Vernazza, the Swiss researchers who worked on the original research underpinning the Swiss Statement, wrote an article in the *Swiss Medical Weekly* in 2018 defending breastfeeding in the presence of ART.[28] Combined antiretroviral treatment (cART) has reduced MTCT of HIV to virtually zero in industrialised countries, where strictly bottle-feeding is recommended for HIV-infected mothers, and to as low as 0.7% after 12 months in low-resource settings, where breastfeeding is strongly encouraged. Given the theoretically very low risk of transmission by breastfeeding with cART, and the advantages and benefits of breastfeeding, also in industrialised countries, the strong recommendation to HIV-infected mothers to refrain from breastfeeding in this setting may no longer be justified. cART is able to fully suppress HIV RNA in body compartments and fluids including blood, rectal tissue, genital secretions, lymph node tissue and breastmilk.[69] Thus HIV transmission is effectively reduced when cART is implemented, resulting in an undetectable plasma viral load.

The Swiss group defined an 'optimal scenario' with virtually zero risk of HIV MTCT when a pregnant woman:

1. is adherent in taking her cART,
2. receives regular clinical care, and
3. has a suppressed HIV plasma viral load of <50 RNA copies/ml throughout pregnancy and breastfeeding.

In a recent WHO-commissioned systematic review which summarised the literature on transmission of HIV through breastfeeding by mothers on cART, several cases of transmission were identified, but none fulfilled the optimal scenario criteria.[25] In a literature review to identify cases where HIV MTCT did occur, Kahlert and colleagues were not able to identify a single case of HIV transmission via breastfeeding while mothers complied with the 'optimal scenario'.

Comparing breastfeeding with other situations that carry a risk of HIV transmission suggests a very low risk of HIV MTCT via breastmilk. While cell-associated HIV could theoretically constitute an additional risk, breastmilk contains many inhibitors of viral replication which can inactivate a large proportion of cell-free virions present in breastmilk. For horizontal transmission, large studies have shown that the presence of HIV in secretions does not represent a risk for infection if HIV viral load is suppressed.[70,71]

It certainly looks as if U=U can be clinically applied to breastfeeding. Could it then be that the decision to exclude breastfeeding in spite of the evidence is down to politics?

'It is politics that determines whose truth is heard.'

Penny van Esterik, York University

CHAPTER 26

Breastfeeding by HIV-positive women in the global north

Shortly after the discovery that HIV could be transmitted through breastfeeding, the US Centers for Disease Control and Prevention (CDC) recommended that women at risk for infection with the AIDS virus should be advised of the possibility of transmission via breastmilk. Using the rationale that infant formula was safe, affordable and culturally acceptable, they suggested that women testing HIV-positive in the United States avoid breastfeeding.[1] These recommendations were echoed by most other industrialised countries: Sweden,[2] Canada,[3] Britain,[4] and Australia.[5]

In high-income countries most practitioners still prefer to interpret official guidance as meaning that HIV-positive mothers should be discouraged from breastfeeding, though that is not strictly the case. But the prevailing attitude appears to be that when formula-feeding is considered to be safe, why would a mother want to take a chance of passing HIV to her baby through breastfeeding?

Different guidance for developed vs developing countries

The about-turn in WHO recommendations, as set out in the WHO 2009 Rapid Advice on HIV and infant feeding, for a single policy approach for different countries (either breastfeeding with maternal/infant ARVs or no breastfeeding at all) was met with considerable confusion by breastfeeding counsellors and lactation specialists, wherever they worked. While the recommendation for a return to breastfeeding in resource-poor areas was welcome, was guidance for bottle-feeding in the global north being endorsed? Even if the mothers were on ART? It was very murky.

From the beginning it had often been assumed in the developed countries that HIV infection was confined to gay men and intravenous drug users. But infection among women had been growing. Across the countries of the global north; the USA, Canada, UK, Europe, Australia and New Zealand, the patterns of HIV infection in women are very similar.

The United Kingdom

By 1990 there had been 82 pregnancies reported among HIV-positive women in the UK, increasing to 1,394 by 2006. Injecting drug use as the reported risk factor declined from almost half in 1990–93 to a tiny 3% in 2004–06, while the proportion of women born in sub-Saharan Africa increased from half to three-quarters in the same period. Overall transmission of HIV to infants declined from nearly 20% in 1990–93 to only 1% in 2004–06 due to increasing provision of ART in pregnancy. By this time 90% of infected people had been born in sub-Saharan Africa (83% in Zimbabwe), and two-thirds were diagnosed within two years of arrival.[6] Thus a high proportion of HIV-positive women in England who acquired HIV through heterosexual contact were of African origin. An unknown number were illegal aliens or asylum seekers with uncertain immigration status. By 2008, 50% of HIV-positive individuals were infected heterosexually, 67% were black African, 20% were white, 63% were women, and 110 babies had been infected through MTCT. By the end of 2009, HIV prevalence was very low at between 0.1–0.5% of the population. The latest figures available show that the UK has a relatively small, concentrated HIV epidemic, with an estimated 101,600 people living with HIV in 2017.[7] Breastfeeding by HIV-positive mothers is strongly discouraged. A prominent AIDS support organisation gives this advice on its website: 'In the UK and other high-income countries, the safest way for a mother living with HIV to feed her baby is to bottle feed using formula milk.'[8]

Europe

By the end of 1984, there had been nearly 800 cases of AIDS reported in Europe, with western Europe being most badly affected. Modes of transmission vary greatly by country. HIV disproportionately affects men who have sex with men and migrants from sub-Saharan Africa. Of over 24,000 people who were diagnosed in 2008, 42% acquired their infection via heterosexual contact and 30% were female.[9] A recent European Collaborative Study found that 41% of HIV-positive women who had late diagnosis of HIV were black African,[10] but 90% of all pregnant HIV-positive women in Europe received ART and there were only 268 cases of MTCT for the whole region.[11]

A recent presentation at the International Workshop on HIV and Women in Boston, Massachusetts, in March 2020, and a follow-up paper, describes 42 HIV-positive mothers at 15 treatment centres in Germany who had breastfed their babies between May 2009 and July 2020.[12] Over time, an increasing number of mothers wanted to breastfed rising from one in 2009 to 13 in 2018. Duration of breastfeeding varied from a single breastfeed of colostrum to 104 weeks. All women except one elite controller (an individual whose immune system can control viral replication without drug therapy) received ART. Breastfeeding was clearly becoming more popular. The study authors called for guidelines to implement more detailed recommendations, and monitoring and follow-up of mothers and babies. A 2020 Belgian paper describes case histories of two HIV-positive mothers who breastfed with close supervision, also with good outcomes.[13] There is an urgent need for prospective national and European data collections to further improve HIV prevention of mother-to-child transmission (PMTCT) through breastfeeding.

USA

The first cases of what would later become known as AIDS were reported in the United States in June 1981.[14] By 1996, at the time of the Vancouver AIDS conference, women were increasingly becoming infected with HIV and, as in Africa, at an earlier age than men. HIV/AIDS was now disproportionately affecting women from ethnic minority backgrounds and was increasingly reflecting horizontal transmission.[15] Heterosexual transmission now accounts for 24% of new diagnoses, more cases than at the beginning of the epidemic. In 2016 HIV was the fifth leading cause of death for Black women aged 35–44. Over 250,000 women are living with HIV today and Black women account for nearly two-thirds of new HIV diagnoses in this group.[16]

In March 2009 Washington DC reported an HIV prevalence of at least 3% among people over 12 years of age, a rate similar to some parts of sub-Saharan Africa. Black women represented more than a quarter of HIV cases in the district of Columbia, and approximately 58% were infected heterosexually.[17] In Minnesota, of 60 births in 2009, about half were to HIV-positive African-born mothers, who were reported to present a particular challenge because breastfeeding was both a cultural norm and an economic necessity, and because African-born women feared revealing their HIV status if they didn't breastfeed.[18]

Canada

The Canadian Paediatric and Perinatal AIDS Research Group (CPARG) had been tracking cases of MTCT of HIV since 1990.[19] Before the advent of ART, 84% of HIV-positive mothers received their HIV diagnosis after they became pregnant, but in 2014 97% had received ARVs before giving birth. Canada reported that 10,000 women had HIV in 2006, 34% of all new positive tests were in women[20] and 65% of these were in women between the ages of 19 and 49.[21] Virtually all perinatal transmissions in the past few years have occurred in undiagnosed women, who have not received optimal prenatal care and/or ART. However, breastfeeding remained contraindicated, even among women receiving HAART with suppressed viral loads.[3] Some Canadian authorities also recommended that seronegative women who engaged in high-risk behaviour which could result in HIV infection during the postpartum period should also be advised about the potential dangers of breastfeeding during seroconversion.

Three studies from Canada's perinatal HIV surveillance programme, presented at the 8th International AIDS Conference on HIV Pathogenesis, Treatment and Prevention in Vancouver in 2015,[22] found that each year an average of 200 babies were born to HIV-positive women. Of almost 3,900 women, half were foreign-born, and of those, 71% emigrated from Africa, mainly from Ethiopia, Congo, Zimbabwe and Nigeria. Today, Canada has virtually eliminated MTCT of HIV primarily because of high rates of prenatal testing and ready access to ART. Women with HIV living in Canada are advised to avoid breastfeeding, regardless of plasma HIV viral load and use of cART.[23] In a 2018 interview on HIV and infant feeding, reported by CATIE, Canada's Dr Mona Loutfy, Professor, Women's College Hospital at the University of Toronto, described how they counsel HIV-positive mothers who wish to breastfeed:[24]

'We have to approach this discussion with an empathetic frame of mind. Being pregnant is stressful enough; adding discussions of infant feeding and HIV transmission adds yet another layer of stress. My patients come to me expecting me to have done my homework – to know the literature and understand what the evidence is telling us. I ensure that I have done that and do my best to convey this information. Support should be offered to women regardless of their choice. And with the very open discussions that we have, in over 95% of the cases, women choose to formula feed. Even if they experience sadness with not breastfeeding, they most often articulate this choice as supporting their baby's health.'

Australia

National policy was revised in 2006 to recommend antenatal HIV testing for all pregnant women. Screening had identified a four-fold increase in perinatal exposure from 1982–2006.[25] The increased incidence of HIV-infection occurred largely in women from countries with a high HIV prevalence, such as sub-Saharan Africa. MTCT was 45% among children whose mothers were not screened during pregnancy, and was 47% among women who used no interventions. As HIV rates fell dramatically among gay and bisexual men, new HIV diagnoses attributed to heterosexual sex rose 14% between 2016 and 2017. Heterosexual sex accounted for one in four new HIV diagnoses in 2017 (238 people: 145 men and 93 women). New HIV diagnoses in men that were attributed to heterosexual sex (rather than injecting drugs) rose 19% over the previous five years.[26] By the end of 2017, women comprised almost one in seven of all HIV diagnoses, with a median age of 30.[27] While there had been a decrease in homosexual infections from 2014, there had been a 19% increase in cases attributed to heterosexual sex during the same period. By the end of 2017, women comprised almost one in seven of all HIV diagnoses, with a median age of 30.[28] In 2019 new HIV diagnoses among heterosexual men overtook those for men who have sex with men for the first time. By 2020 it was estimated that there were 3000 women living with HIV in Australia, 10% of the HIV-infected population. An estimated 400-500 of women were undiagnosed.[29] One-third of HIV-positive women were born outside Australia. There are few specific guidelines for breastfeeding in the context of HIV, and the guidance simply says, 'At present, breastfeeding is contra-indicated when a mother is known to be HIV positive (specialist advice is needed for each individual case.'[30] An Australian colleague advised me that they used British guidance from BHIVA in 2019 for an HIV-positive mother who wanted to breastfeed.

New Zealand

Perinatal HIV levels remain very low with no infected babies born in New Zealand since 2007 and only one infection in a child born overseas in 2018. Diagnoses among heterosexual people infected overseas increased sharply from 2002 to 2006[31] due to a large increase in migrants and refugees from countries with high HIV prevalence, when screening was not compulsory. Africans remained the only ethnicity over-represented until 2015 but from 2018 Asians comprise 30% of new diagnoses. New Zealand also refers to the BHIVA guidance, including specifically quoting wording used advising against referral to child protection services.

Coercion of HIV-positive mothers to formula-feed

George Kent, author of *HIV/AIDS, Infant Feeding, and Human Rights*,[32] appeared as a witness in the 1998 case of Kathleen Tyson,[33] an HIV-positive mother living in the US who was prevented from breastfeeding her baby. His account serves to illustrate how HIV-positive mothers who have indicated an intention to breastfeed have been coerced into complying with national recommendations prohibiting breastfeeding:

> *'...some women who have been diagnosed as being infected with HIV have been pressured into using breastmilk substitutes such as infant formula to feed their infants. Is that warranted? In some cases this pressure has gone well beyond gentle urging by concerned health workers, and has taken the form of strong coercion by government agents. For example, in Los Angeles, a woman diagnosed as HIV-positive was confronted by social workers from the Child and Family Services agency because she was breastfeeding her child. They told her to go with them and have herself and her baby tested, or they would take the baby. On the way to the testing site the officials stopped to buy infant formula, and demanded that the woman stop breastfeeding immediately.*
>
> *On September 17, 1998, Kathleen Tyson of Eugene, Oregon, then six months pregnant, was told that her blood tests indicated that she was HIV-positive. Her son, Felix, was born on December 7, 1998. He appeared to be healthy in every way. Less than 24 hours after his birth, Ms. Tyson was pressed by a paediatrician to treat Felix with AZT, an antiretroviral drug, and to not breastfeed him.*
>
> *Having studied the issue along with her husband, she declined to accept that advice. Within hours, a petitioner from Juvenile Court came to her hospital room, and issued a summons for her to appear in court two days later. She and her husband were initially charged with "intent to harm" the baby, but the petition, dated December 10, 1998, said that the child "has been subjected to threat of harm." When the Tysons appeared in court, they were ordered to begin administering AZT to Felix every six hours for six weeks, and to stop breastfeeding completely. The court took legal custody of the infant, but allowed the Tysons to retain physical custody so long as they obeyed the court's orders. A hearing was held in Eugene from April 16 to April 20, 1999. The judge ruled against the Tysons. Thus, the State retained legal custody of Felix. The Tysons retained physical custody on the condition that, as ordered, Felix would not be breastfed.*
>
> *I have a special interest in the Tyson case because I was asked to serve as an expert witness on its human rights aspects. However, after I was sworn in, the judge said that human rights considerations were irrelevant, and asked me to step down. (Kent, 1999a; 1999b). In another case, in Camden, England, a woman who had been diagnosed as HIV positive was ordered by the courts to have her infant tested for HIV. She and her partner refused, and they fled the country with the child, partly out of fear that if the child were to be tested and found to be HIV-negative, the mother might be ordered to stop breastfeeding (BBC News, 1999). They were fearful partly because they were aware of the outcome in the Tyson case in Oregon.*
>
> *There have been other cases in which women diagnosed as HIV-positive have been forced to have their infants tested for HIV or to accept particular drug treatments.'*

Another case in the USA which attracted negative press for breastfeeding in 2005 was that of Eliza Jane Scovill, who died aged three and a half after having been breastfed by her HIV-positive mother, Christine Maggiore, who had refused antiretroviral therapy. The parents were AIDS denialists and refused to have their daughter tested, but a post-mortem found that the little girl had suffered from the opportunistic infection *Pneumocystis jirovecii*. Expert opinion determined that she had died of AIDS-related causes.[34] Her mother also died a short time later.

A 2014 article[35] found that Canadian HIV-positive women may be subject to a high degree of unwelcome surveillance, and experience disappointment in not being permitted to breastfeed. There are unique concerns for mothers living with HIV who are recommended to avoid breastfeeding yet live in a social context of 'breast is best'. Author Saara Greene recorded narrative interviews with HIV-positive mothers from across Ontario who described a range of feelings; balancing feelings of loss and self-blame with the view of responsibility, 'good mothering', and social and cultural norms across geographical contexts. Ted Greiner and I wrote a letter in response to the Greene article pointing out that the safety of formula-feeding may be exaggerated and referencing the current UK and USA (AAP) guidance[36] described later in this chapter, which concedes that when an HIV-positive mother adherent to ART, with an undetectable viral load, wishes to breastfeed, then she should be supported to do so.

Child protection and safeguarding in the UK

In the UK, breastfeeding by HIV-positive mothers has often been framed as a potential safeguarding issue and the tone has been quite menacing. In the past, no consideration was given to the real possibility that a baby may be born already infected. Child protection advice issued by authorities in the English Midlands in 2010[37] warned that breastfeeding led to a high risk of transmission, with child protection implications, and hinted that testing of the baby can identify HIV infection in the mother:

> *HIV is never in itself a child protection issue. However …the interests of the child must be the paramount consideration for all professionals involved with the family, regardless of their specific role …recent research into the role that ante-natal treatment and breastfeeding play in transmission raises new practice issues about promoting the health and welfare of infants… Parents may fear that child protection procedures will be used to coerce them into making decisions about testing and treatment about which they are unhappy… There is clear evidence that the risk of transmission can be greatly reduced by interventions such as anti-retroviral drug treatment, elective caesarean section and* ***the avoidance of breastfeeding****.*
>
> *Once women are aware of their HIV infection, most choose to accept interventions that will reduce the risk of vertical transmission and protect their babies. Most women will agree a plan with medical and midwifery staff for the management of the pregnancy and birth* ***and will agree not to breastfeed*** *…Children's social care should be consulted where parents appear to be refusing intervention to reduce the risk of vertical transmission… The referral should be actioned as soon as concerns become evident due to the fact that appropriate interventions are time-limited… a pregnant woman may*

> *decline some or all of the interventions offered,* ***or may indicate that she intends to breastfeed****. Under UK law, unborn children do not have any legal status, and pregnant women cannot be compelled to have an HIV test, to accept medication or to undergo a caesarean delivery. However… children's social care should become involved where there is concern that an unborn child may be at future risk of significant harm. Such involvement can include convening a pre-birth child protection conference, placing the unborn child on the Child Protection Register and agreeing a plan to protect the baby as soon as she/he is born. Following the birth, the baby has rights of her/his own, including a right to 'the highest attainable standard of health and to facilities for the treatment of illness' (UN Convention on the Rights of the Child: Article 24). Consideration may need to be given to whether the baby is suffering, or is likely to suffer, significant harm (Children Act 1989: Section 47) and whether action is needed to safeguard the baby. In practice, concerns will arise at this stage where parents are …****breastfeeding where safe alternatives are available…*** *The conclusion of the assessment may be that the baby is at increased risk of being infected with HIV as a result of actions or inactions by the parents. A decision will need to be made whether this constitutes a risk of significant harm, and therefore whether child protection procedures and legal intervention are indicated… Professionals should maintain collaborative working and refer to existing procedures in order to ensure that the diagnosis of HIV within a family does not prejudice the assessment or outcomes of any child protection/welfare concern.*

Interestingly, the authorities have no capacity to intervene before the birth, but afterwards it would be possible for them to turn up at the mother's bedside to protect the baby from suffering what might be construed as significant harm through breastfeeding. And ironically, there has never been any recognition that formula-feeding is, in its own right, intrinsically harmful, costing the British NHS approximately £40 million per annum on their own calculations for 2009–10 to treat infections which would be avoided by breastfeeding.[38]

Marielle Gross and colleagues also articulate some of the problems in the US:[39]

> *HIV-exposed US infants disproportionately experience health risks that could be mitigated by breastfeeding. In 2013, mortality for black infants was more than double that of white infants, chiefly attributed to greater burdens of prematurity and SIDS. Since preconception cART is associated with prematurity and low birthweight, the HIV-exposed infants least likely to contract HIV are most likely to be harmed by not breastfeeding. Socioeconomically disenfranchised infants would especially benefit from decreased diabetes, obesity, and asthma, plus a higher IQ with corresponding adult educational attainment and income. While donor breastmilk may partially alleviate consequences of current policy, most HIV-exposed infants do not have access to banked milk, and breastfeeding itself is more beneficial, feasible, and cost-effective. Discouraging women living with HIV from breastfeeding may inadvertently contribute to poor health outcomes among vulnerable infants and women, systematically reinforcing racial inequity by deepening disparities in health and wealth.*

Parents remain afraid that they could be accused by child protection authorities of harming their child by breastfeeding. One of my clients told me she 'knew her baby was safe until the cord was cut'. I found it chilling that she felt so threatened. HIV-positive mothers and those attempting to support HIV-positive mothers in various first world countries who have reached out to me over the years for information about the possibility of breastfeeding in the context of HIV are always afraid of coercion. The consequences of mother-baby separation can be catastrophic. Part of my care plan may include retaining the services of a lawyer, before birth, to provide legal representation within the hospital setting if necessary, to ensure that the baby will not be removed from the mother. A mother facing such a threat has to be very brave to persevere, yet so strong is her wish to breastfeed that she will often be prepared make these plans.

In 2008, I received a request for information from an Australian lactation consultant for such a mother. I sent my colleague a bundle of papers and research articles and we had some correspondence which ended when she reported sadly that the mother had had to agree to abandon her plans to breastfeed. Her doctors had said it was too risky, and were threatening her with loss of custody of her baby. Two years later, an article published in the *Journal of Paediatrics and Child Health*, the official journal of the Australasian Paediatric Association, described a very similar case.[40] My colleague confirmed that it was the same one. The Australian paediatricians described their care of a clinically well, pregnant HIV-infected woman wishing either to breastfeed or provide her child with pasteurised expressed breast milk. The mother was receiving ART, had an undetectable viral load, and a CD4 cell count of more than 500 cells/ml. Citing research showing that one litre of ingested breast milk equates to one act of unprotected sex and the Coovadia 2007 study (discussed in Chapter 8) in which lapses in exclusive breastfeeding had led to a disappointingly high risk of breastfeeding-associated transmission, the paediatricians had recommended formula-feeding, claiming a duty of care to protect the infant. They also thought that heat treatment of breastmilk couldn't be recommended due to its inconvenience and the risk of mixed feeding. The evidence for this claim was not cited. As HIV is inactivated by heat treatment, their caution seemed unwarranted. To prevent either breastfeeding or breastmilk-feeding, the case was ultimately referred antenatally to child protection services.

The Australian case had been reported in July 2010 and my colleagues Ted Greiner and Kiersten Israel-Ballard and I decided to put together a response, which was eventually published in the journal *AIDS* in September the following year[41] (further discussed in Chapter 29). The Australian article was a poorly evidenced opinion that failed to justify threatening a mother with loss of custody of her child. It had been sadly obvious to the IBCLC and to me that the doctors' threats had caused her to abandon her plans to breastfeed, but my article with Ted and Kiersten was too late to save this situation.

Christina's story, which follows in the next chapter, is another example of the pressure that is still applied, although she found a way around it. Others are not so lucky.

HIV-positive mothers who want to breastfeed

An increasing number of HIV-positive women now living in the global north do want to breastfeed and some of them are desperate for more help to do so. Pregnancy and the birth of a new child are especially vulnerable times in a woman's life and navigating this journey with an HIV diagnosis can be extremely challenging. Formula-feeding comes at high social and personal cost, and there are significant structural, cultural and personal barriers to formula-feeding for women living with HIV in the UK, three-quarters of whom are of African origin.[42]

British HIV-positive mothers who are prevented from breastfeeding experience severe distress and stigma. In 2012 Jacquie Ayugi de Masi, an employee of NAM, a charity based in the United Kingdom that works to change lives by sharing information about HIV and AIDS, described eloquently the distress they experience:[43]

> *'Stigma and discrimination is still huge within African communities, leading to late HIV diagnosis, leading to poor health. Breast feeding symbolises motherhood but also an achievement (fertility) for both partners. African women living with HIV in London are advised not to breast feed. They find it extremely difficult to justify to their husbands/ partners and the wider African community. During my visit to an African community organisation, sitting in during their HIV-positive support group session, one service user, Ms A, stated "Whenever family members, relatives and friends come to visit us, my husband tells me to prepare the food and when the visitors arrive, I should greet them, show them the baby, then go to the bedroom, because he doesn't want our visitors asking questions why I am not breast feeding, he doesn't want people to start talking and spreading rumours, it will only bring him shame.'*

Ayugi de Masi also describes the words of another mother, who said:

> *'I am from Nigeria, and in Nigeria everybody knows everybody and word travels faster than lightning. Everybody knows nowadays in Africa and UK that if an African woman does not breast feed her baby then she must be HIV-positive. For this reason I would rather let my baby cry until I get into a secure and private place, like a toilet, and feed my baby'.*

Another service user relates:

> *'I was OK when going for my antenatal classes with my midwife but when my support was shifted to the health visitors, they immediately asked me why I wasn't breast feeding, and I told them I was HIV-positive, since that time I feel they treat me differently, like they were afraid of touching my baby, constantly coming to visit me at home, one even advised me, 'now that you are aware of your HIV status you should try and not have other children'. I was hurt, ashamed and felt dirty.'*

These are heartbreaking descriptions. I have had African women breaking down and sobbing on the phone when they describe how important breastfeeding is to them. They say that if they are not allowed to breastfeed they will not feel 'like a real woman' or a 'proper mother'. Although most HIV-positive mothers in the UK are of African origin, not all of them are. My clients come from all backgrounds. Caucasian mothers can be equally devastated by the loss of breastfeeding that an HIV diagnosis may bring.

Early in 2020 Michele Griswold and Jesica Pagano-Therrien published a paper in the

Journal of Human Lactation looking at the social and emotional experiences of infant feeding for women living with HIV in high-income countries and the ethical implications surrounding clinical recommendations to avoid breastfeeding.[44] Conducting a literature search of 900 papers, they found that only six, from just two countries, Canada and the UK, met the inclusion criteria. HIV-positive women living in high-income countries have been poorly served. The findings are slightly summarised below:

> *Participants expressed the importance of breastfeeding as part of their maternal identity or self-worth with breastfeeding being inseparable from their role as a mother. Specifically, 'good' mothers breastfeed, and 'bad' mothers do not. Health-related messaging like 'breast is best' contributed to internal feelings of guilt for not being able to provide what they perceived to be the best nutrition and bonding experience for their infants. Mothers expressed powerful emotional responses to receiving a diagnosis of HIV and the inability to breastfeed their children with emotions ranging from guilt and disappointment to 'devastation'. Experiences reported include rape, trauma, and violence leading to a sense of hopelessness, self-neglect and, for some, suicidal ideation. Simultaneously, a sense of strength and resilience was realized through connections to others with similar experiences, and through feeling that their children gave them reason to live. Many of the women had emigrated to high income countries from African countries with unique implications for infant feeding counseling. In contrast to 'acculturalization,' whereby over time cultural practices are voluntarily relinquished, 'deculturalization' can be understood in the context of infant feeding as surrendering the 'mental and physical abilities to continue the practices'. Deculturalization was noted across studies, and was manifested in deep emotional responses to the loss of breastfeeding. Women expressed the cultural importance of breastfeeding and associated feeling 'unnatural' and 'not womanly' with avoidance of breastfeeding.*
>
> *...Women living with HIV often reported feeling pressured to breastfeed by family yet pressured to avoid breastfeeding by healthcare providers. Internal conflicting feelings were reported about the painful choice between disclosure of HIV status to family members versus the emotional energy spent on devising lies to explain why they were not breastfeeding. And 'some women went to great lengths to conceal the fact that they were feeding their baby formula'. Relocation and familial disclosure further marginalized and isolated these women, and for a few, the pressure may have resulted in them partially breastfeeding their infants.*
>
> *Political landscapes may also be of considerable concern. Criminalization laws pertain to the willful transmission of HIV and at least 60 countries have enacted related laws to cover this. Because women bear the reproductive burden of birth and breastfeeding, current criminalization laws as they pertain to HIV disproportionately affect women. HIV+ women who leave their home countries where exclusive breastfeeding is recommended and arrive in countries where the avoidance of breastfeeding is strongly recommended, face the additional burden of possible criminalization simply because they may not know about the laws. Alternatively, criminalization laws provide further examples of extreme surveillance that may isolate HIV+ women from seeking infant feeding counseling.*

Griswold and Paggano-Therrien conclude that women in high-income countries living with HIV deserve the highest standard of lactation care and counselling available. Healthcare professionals are ethically obliged to provide it.

Until late 2009, HIV and infant feeding policy in the UK was covered by two sets of recommendations formulated in 2004[45] and 2008[46] containing a somewhat ambiguous mix of outdated research combined with human rights rationales favouring support for the mother's infant-feeding decision on the one hand, and somewhat coercive language on the other.

Asylum seekers

In October 2009 I was asked by the Children's Commissioner to make an assessment of infant feeding at Yarl's Wood Detention Centre in Bedford, England, where failed asylum-seeking mothers were held with their babies pending deportation back to their countries of origin (e.g. Uganda, Malawi, Cameroon). For refugee women, support for formula-feeding combined with scanty assistance to breastfeed often tips the scales in favour of risky decision-making in terms of the baby's health and future food security. My findings were included in a report on the detention and arrest of children awaiting deportation.[47]

There were many African mothers and babies at Yarl's Wood. Medical staff knew that many of the detainees had HIV. I found that infant formula and feeding equipment was provided for free, and all mothers of young babies had inappropriately fed their babies formula even if they had arrived at the detention centre breastfeeding. Two-thirds had weaned prematurely. Staff in the detention centre made no attempt to guide mothers in the correct preparation of formula, saying how mothers fed their babies was their own choice. Mothers would often add an extra scoop of powder to the bottle to make the mix stronger for hungry babies. I enquired of the staff what arrangements for feeding the babies were made in preparation for their enforced removal back to their home countries? I learned that mothers are given bottles with only enough formula to feed their babies on the flight home. In effect, they would descend the steps of the aircraft in Lilongwe or Kinshasa or Harare with hungry babies and empty bottles. Formula is often expensive in developing countries and sometimes it is unobtainable. Safe preparation of formula requires clean piped water and sterilising facilities. Returning refugees are likely to have access to few resources. At Yarl's Wood, no thought had been given to the possibility that failed migrant women might not have access to these luxury items in their home countries, yet they had been encouraged to abandon breastfeeding while living in England. My recommendations included suggestions to remedy this hazardous situation. Mothers, whether HIV-positive or not, need their healthcare providers to tailor specific anticipatory care that will take their individual circumstances into consideration for the whole time that their babies will need milk feeds (estimated by WHO to be two years).

BHIVA consultation to update guidance

In early 2009, I was invited to submit a report outlining the concerns about current British HIV and infant feeding policy to Lord Eric Avebury, a Member of the House of Lords who worked on a Parliamentary Select Committee looking at HIV/AIDS. I compiled a very comprehensive report running to over 15 pages. It was sent on to the

Secretary of State for Health, who passed it to the Minister for Health. They wanted more information, and I wrote another 16 pages. Eventually I received confirmation that the report and correspondence would be forwarded to a joint committee of the British HIV Association and representatives of the Expert Advisory Group on AIDS 'to help inform their deliberations'. BHIVA and the EAGA were hosting a joint consultation on HIV and infant feeding in the next few months. They received a substantial number of responses, expressing diverse and often conflicting views, but it seemed that Lord Avebury's interest in the plight of HIV-positive mothers in the UK had really helped. At the next conference of the British HIV Association in April 2010, paediatrician Dr Gareth Tudor-Williams of the Children's HIV Association made a presentation on 'Changing UK Practice: influence from resource-poor settings including new infant feeding guidance'[48] in which he mentioned that he had heard from the House of Lords on the matter. In November 2010 the revised joint British HIV Association/Children's HIV Association (BHIVA/CHIVA) Position Statement on Infant Feeding in the UK was released[49] and in March 2011 the document was formally published in *HIV Medicine*.[50]

In a careful and well-worded combination of conventional advice with acknowledgement of the dilemmas faced by the majority of HIV-positive mothers living in the UK (the largest majority of whom were African women from normally breastfeeding cultures), the new BHIVA/CHIVA position paper succeeded in formulating guidelines which were largely appropriate to the target population they were designed to protect. In particular, and using extremely clever wording, they included *both* the single-policy recommendations contained in the new WHO recommendations (a recommendation for replacement feeding, *and* support for breastfeeding), as well as the recommendation that if women chose the latter course, they were not to be reported to child protection services. The plight of asylum-seekers was acknowledged too.

- *BHIVA/CHIVA continue to recommend that, in the UK, mothers known to be HIV-infected, regardless of maternal viral load and antiretroviral therapy, refrain from breast feeding from birth.*
- *In the case of women with HIV infection whose immigration status is uncertain or who are applying for asylum, who have refrained from breast feeding and whose babies are being fed with infant formula milk, it should be recognized that removal of the infant from the UK to a setting where continued formula feeding is not feasible, affordable, sustainable and safe would represent a direct threat to the health and life of the child.*
- *New data emerging from observational cohort studies and randomized controlled studies in Africa, in settings where refraining from breast feeding is less safe than in the UK, show low rates (0–3%) of HIV transmission during breast feeding in mothers on HAART. BHIVA/CHIVA acknowledge that, in the UK, the risk of mother-to-child transmission through exclusive breast feeding from a woman who is on HAART and has a consistently undetectable HIV viral load is likely to be low but emphasize that this risk has not yet been quantified. Therefore, complete avoidance of breast feeding is still the best and safest option in the UK to prevent mother-to-child transmission of HIV.*
- *BHIVA/CHIVA recognize that occasionally a woman who is on effective HAART and has a repeated undetectable HIV viral load by the time of delivery may choose, having*

carefully considered the aforementioned advice, to exclusively breastfeed. Under these circumstances, child protection proceedings, which have until now been appropriate, must be carefully considered in the light of the above and emerging data. While not recommending this approach, ***BHIVA/CHIVA accept that the mother should be supported to exclusively breastfeed*** *as safely, and for as short a period, as possible.*

- *In the very rare instances where a mother in the UK who is on effective HAART with a repeatedly undetectable viral load chooses to breastfeed, BHIVA/CHIVA do not regard this as grounds for automatic referral to child protection teams.*
- *Maternal HAART should be carefully monitored and continued until 1 week after all breast feeding has ceased. Breast feeding, except during the weaning period, should be exclusive and all breast feeding, including that during the weaning period, should have been completed by the end of 6 months. The 6-month period should not be interpreted as the normal or expected duration of breast feeding in this setting but as the absolute maximum, as exclusive breast feeding is not recommended beyond this period under any circumstances. The factors leading to the maternal decision to exclusively breastfeed should be regularly reviewed and switching to replacement feeding is advocated as early as possible, whether this be after 1 day, 1 week or 5 months. It is acknowledged that this strategy will result in a period of mixed feeding and that there are no data to describe the risk related to this during fully suppressive maternal HAART. The Writing Group, however, considered this to be preferable to continuing exclusive breast feeding to 6 months followed by weaning over a period of several weeks, recognizing that less than 1% of mothers in the UK are exclusively breast feeding at 6 months.*
- *Prolonged infant prophylaxis during the breast-feeding period, as opposed to maternal HAART, is not recommended. Whilst serious adverse events were not reported in infants given nevirapine for up to 6 months there are currently insufficient safety data to advocate this approach given the particular safety concerns regarding the use of nevirapine in adults uninfected with HIV. The use of nevirapine for longer than the 2–4 weeks currently recommended for post-exposure prophylaxis is not advised.*
- *Intensive support and monitoring of the mother and infant are recommended during any breast-feeding period. To ensure continued antiretroviral effectiveness, we recommend monthly maternal viral load testing. To identify any drug toxicity or HIV transmission in the infant, monthly assessment is advised. The timing of follow-up testing for the infant to exclude HIV infection must be adjusted according to the time of last possible exposure. Education to identify factors that might increase the risk of transmission, despite HAART (e.g. mastitis or cracked nipples), should be given and the resources to enable switching to safe alternatives should be in place.*

This approach simultaneously protects babies, mothers and healthcare providers. If breastfeeding does take place, the recommendation for exclusive breastfeeding during the first six months, due to the acknowledged risks of mixed feeding, is clear and unambiguous. The suggestion for monthly checks of the viral load of the breastfeeding mother and the HIV status of the breastfed affords the opportunity to fill the gap in research on MTCT in breastfed populations in the industrialised world. Such data have, of necessity, been exclusively provided by resource-poor countries for the simple reason that, until that time, breastfeeding by HIV-positive mothers in the richer countries had been effectively prohibited. In a welcome move, it recommended that HIV-exposed formula-fed babies of mothers with failed immigration applications should not be deported to resource-poor settings due to the risks to their future health, survival and food security.

These were the first recommendations formulated by any industrialised country to adequately provide physicians and healthcare workers with sufficient flexibility, within clearly defined parameters, to protect and support breastfeeding by HIV-positive mothers when that feeding method would be appropriate to their particular individual circumstances. This Position Statement could act as an example and useful precedent for other medium and resource-rich countries to emulate in the future and in fact that has happened. They have served as a template to countries in the global north (e.g. Australia and New Zealand) pending development of their own country-specific guidance, and importantly they formed an example for the USA to follow.

US HIV and infant feeding recommendations

In 2008 the American Academy of Pediatrics Policy statement on testing and prophylaxis for PMTCT in the US Committee on Pediatric AIDS[51] had given the recommendation that an HIV-positive mother should be 'counselled not to breastfeed the infant.'

The National Institutes of Health, in an updated guideline dated 24 May 2010,[52] also recommended that 'where safe infant feeding alternatives are available and free for women in need, HIV-infected women should not breastfeed their infants. Postnatally, mothers should be advised that although antiretroviral therapy is likely to reduce free virus in the plasma, the presence of cell-associated virus (intracellular HIV DNA) remains unaffected and may therefore continue to pose a transmission risk.'

However, in late January 2013, there was a major breakthrough. Using wording very similar to that employed by BHIVA, the American Academy of Pediatrics similarly revised its recommendations to support breastfeeding by HIV-positive mothers.[53] They also used a very similar rationale to the British guidance, in effect reversing the previous ban on breastfeeding by HIV-positive women. Like BHIVA, the AAP's guidance makes a clear first recommendation for formula-feeding, but then permits and encourages clinicians to support HIV-positive mothers in specific ways if they want to breastfeed. The text reads:

> *Physicians caring for infants born to women infected with HIV are likely to be involved in providing guidance to HIV-infected mothers on appropriate infant feeding practices. It is critical that physicians are aware of the HIV transmission risk from human milk and the current recommendations for feeding HIV-exposed infants in the United States. Because the only intervention to completely prevent HIV transmission via human milk is not to breastfeed, in the United States, where clean water and affordable replacement feeding are available, the American Academy of Pediatrics recommends that HIV-infected mothers not breastfeed their infants, regardless of maternal viral load and antiretroviral therapy.*
>
> *Recent studies in Africa have revealed that 6 months of antiretroviral prophylaxis, either daily infant nevirapine or a triple-drug antiretroviral regimen administered to the*

mother, significantly reduced postnatal transmission risk to 1% to 5%. On the basis of these data, the World Health Organization (WHO) published revised feeding guidelines for infants born to HIV-infected mothers living in resource-limited settings where infectious disease and malnutrition are major causes of infant mortality and replacement feeding is not feasible. In such settings, the WHO recommends exclusive breastfeeding for the first 6 months of life, followed by complementary foods and breastfeeding through 12 months of age, accompanied by postnatal infant or maternal antiretroviral prophylaxis to reduce HIV transmission during breastfeeding.

However, neither infant nor maternal postpartum antiretroviral prophylaxis completely eliminates the risk of HIV transmission via human milk. In the United States, with current interventions, mother-to-child HIV transmission during pregnancy and labor is very low at under 1%. Breastfeeding transmission rates with antiretroviral prophylaxis administered to either the infant or the mother, although low, are still 1% to 5%, and transmission can occur despite undetectable maternal plasma RNA concentrations. Maternal prophylaxis with triple-drug regimens may be less effective if first started during the postpartum period or late in pregnancy, because it takes several weeks to months before full viral suppression in human milk is achieved. Antiretroviral drugs taken by the mother have differential penetration into human milk, with some drugs achieving concentrations much higher or lower than maternal plasma concentrations.

An HIV-infected woman receiving effective antiretroviral therapy with repeatedly undetectable HIV viral loads in rare circumstances may choose to breastfeed despite intensive counseling. This rare circumstance (an HIV-infected mother on effective treatment and fully suppressed who chooses to breastfeed) generally does not constitute grounds for an automatic referral to Child Protective Services agencies. Although this approach is not recommended, a pediatric HIV expert should be consulted on how to minimize transmission risk, including exclusive breastfeeding. Communication with the mother's HIV specialist is important to ensure careful monitoring of maternal viral load, adherence to maternal therapy, and prompt administration of antimicrobial agents in instances of clinical mastitis. Infant HIV infection status should be monitored by nucleic acid (plasma HIV RNA or DNA) amplification testing throughout lactation and at 4 to 6 weeks and 3 and 6 months after weaning. Breastfeeding by an infected mother with detectable viral load or receiving no antiretroviral therapy despite intensive counseling represents a difficult ethical problem that requires consultation with a team of experts to engage the mother in a culturally effective manner that seeks to address both her health as well as her child's.

The optimal strategy for management of breastfeeding women with suspected acute HIV infection is unknown. In such circumstances, the mother should undergo appropriate evaluation (i.e., plasma HIV RNA test as well as an HIV antibody test, because the antibody test result may be negative in acute infection), and breastfeeding should be stopped until HIV infection is confirmed or ruled out. Mothers should be assisted to pump and store expressed milk until a confirmatory test result is available and supported with skin-to-skin care to maintain milk supply; if HIV infection is ruled out, breastfeeding can resume. If the mother is found to be HIV infected, the infant should undergo age-appropriate HIV diagnostic testing evaluation, with follow-up testing at 4 to 6 weeks and 3 and 6 months after breastfeeding cessation if the initial test result is negative.

Professor Ted Greiner, my friend from AnotherLook, and I were delighted by the AAP Statement, but we felt that there were one or two uncertainties which could be clarified. We put together a letter to *Pediatrics*, which was published almost immediately:[54]

> *In December 1998, a mother recently diagnosed as HIV-positive lost legal custody of her newborn to the State of Oregon because she wanted to breastfeed. She was charged with Intent to Harm and, in order to retain physical custody, the mother had to agree not to breastfeed, nor to feed her baby any stored breastmilk.*
>
> *Recent publication of the American Academy of Pediatrics' (AAP) policy document on HIV and infant feeding may prevent such an eventuality from happening again, at least under certain conditions. While the guidance contains a clear recommendation, echoing national policy since 1985, that HIV-infected mothers should formula-feed, it also provides for some flexibility; an HIV-infected mother living in the United States, on effective treatment and with full viral suppression, may still wish to breastfeed, and this does not constitute automatic grounds for referral to child protective agencies.*
>
> *Instead, a pediatric HIV expert should be consulted about how to minimize transmission risk, including through exclusive breastfeeding, careful monitoring of maternal viral load, adherence to maternal ART, prompt treatment of any clinical mastitis, and infant HIV-testing throughout lactation and at 4-6 weeks and 3-6 months after cessation of breastfeeding.*
>
> *This wording reflects recent research outlined in current global HIV and infant feeding and antiretroviral (ART) recommendations. It has important implications for healthcare providers, who are to make a clear infant feeding recommendation to HIV-infected mothers, but ultimately support the mothers' choices.*
>
> *We would point out that while the AAP statement cites a paper by Shapiro et al. as evidence that postnatal transmission can occur even with full ART and undetectable viral load, these safeguards were not in place for the 2/709 mothers who transmitted postnatally in that study. One mother had medication adherence issues. The other had a baseline viral load of 171,000 copies/mL at recruitment at ~28 weeks of pregnancy, received antenatal HAART for <4 weeks before delivery at 32 weeks' gestation, and had a detectable HIV-1 plasma RNA of 257 copies/mL at commencement of breastfeeding.*
>
> *Confirmatory results from a more recent pilot program involving 194 Zambian HIV-positive women and their infants also showed that the only postnatal transmissions during not only 6 months exclusive breastfeeding but also 6 months of continued breastfeeding, occurred in women who were non-adherent to their medications.*
>
> *The effectiveness of full ART in preventing vertical transmission is achieved by maternal adherence to antiretroviral regimens for at least 13 weeks prior to delivery. Women on HAART for <4 weeks may have a 5.2-fold increased odds of HIV transmission.*
>
> *The AAP decision to accommodate the option of breastfeeding in the context of HIV will enable careful monitoring and documentation of outcomes in resource-rich settings. Since nearly all research on postnatal transmission of HIV to date has, of necessity, come from developing countries, such data are currently lacking. The new policy constitutes a far-reaching and enlightened revision for which the AAP can be congratulated.*

The AAP Statement was reaffirmed in August 2016.[55]

The CDC took a somewhat different position, issuing guidance on 21 March 2018 as follows:

> *Taking HIV medicine as prescribed can make a person's viral load very low – even so low that a test can't detect it (called an undetectable viral load). We don't know if a woman with an undetectable viral load can transmit HIV to her baby through breastfeeding. Being undetectable very likely reduces the risk, but we don't know by how much. In the United States, where safe alternatives to breastmilk are available, a woman living with HIV should avoid breastfeeding, even when viral load is undetectable.*[56]

Clinicians will see the conflict between the guidance given by these two important organisations.

European guidance

The latest European AIDS Clinical Society update was issued in October 2020[57] and contains a small section on pages 19–21 on pregnancy and breastfeeding. The format follows the British and US example of recommending against breastfeeding and then providing guidance for when it does take place. The European guidance goes a little further, however, in suggesting a lactation suppressant (cabergoline) on weaning and to prevent 'covert breastfeeding':

> *Breastfeeding*
>
> • *The topic of feeding intentions should be discussed with a pregnant woman as early as possible in pregnancy, together with providing education and support to the mother*
>
> • ***We advise against breastfeeding**, as in high-income settings the optimal way to prevent mother-to-child transmission is to feed infants born to mothers living with HIV with formula milk*
>
> *- To reduce the potential physical and emotional discomfort associated with breast engorgement, together with the risk of covert breastfeeding, women living with HIV should be given cabergoline to suppress lactation after delivery*
>
> ***• In situations where a woman chooses to breastfeed, we recommend input from an interdisciplinary team including adult HIV specialist, paediatrician and obstetrician/gynecologist***
>
> *- We recommend monthly follow-up during the whole breastfeeding period with increased clinical and virological monitoring of both the mother and the infant. Measurement of drug concentrations in the milk could be done to inform clinical practice*
>
> *- **Maternal HIV-VL >50 copies/mL should result in a stop of breastfeeding, providing cabergoline and support from interdisciplinary team and a nursing specialist***
>
> *- Immediate consulting by the interdisciplinary team should be provided in case of signs and symptoms of mastitis, infant mouth or gut infections*
>
> *- Currently there is no evidence supporting PrEP recommendation for the infants who*

are breastfed
- After stopping the breastfeeding, the child should undergo routine diagnostics as recommended in HIV-exposed children

Reviews and updates in the UK

Since 2011, the British guidance on HIV and infant feeding has been reviewed and updated several times. The clever phrasing enables clinicians to provide a recommendation which absolves them from any risk of any possibility of postpartum transmission through breastfeeding, but at the same time it also opens the door to providing a way that they can help mothers who have their heart set on breastfeeding by supporting maternal choice.

The Safer Triangle booklet

Regrettably, countering the excellent recognition of the importance of breastfeeding contained in their 2019 updated guidance, BHIVA also issued a new practical breastfeeding guidance booklet. It urges mothers to follow 'The Safer Triangle', defined as: 'No Virus + Happy Tums + Healthy Breasts for Mums'. This kind of cutesy language is reported to have been collected from health workers, and may be used by British midwives, but it is not the way African women would speak.[58] Nor would it really be appropriate in other countries who have co-opted our guidance. The highly negative tone, with repeated suggestions of weaning to formula for every small problem, while offering no preventive care or strategies to resolve breastfeeding difficulties, makes this booklet out of touch with the lived reality of most breastfeeding HIV-positive mothers. The take-home message is that if undertaken at all, all sorts of things can go wrong, requiring formula supplementation which in turn raises a risk of mixed feeding so that breastfeeding needs to be abandoned as soon as possible. The information seems to be at odds with the spirit and intention of the BHIVA guidance itself. It also reveals another missed opportunity for collaboration between the lactation community and the AIDS community, which could have led to development of more user-friendly, up-to-date and evidence-based materials for the mothers who need them.

Old prejudices persist. Although the BHIVA and AAP guidance permits breastfeeding by HIV-positive mothers, there are other organisations and individuals who choose to interpret these very nuanced guidelines differently, preferring to focus only on the initial recommendations for formula-feeding in the early paragraphs of both documents.

Generally speaking, there has been a remarkably consistent distrust of breastfeeding in the face of HIV, notwithstanding the transformational finding that vertical transmission can be virtually eliminated with exclusive breastfeeding and maternal ART.[59–61] Clearly, different positions are taken by different groups of experts. We are effectively caught in a Catch-22 situation. Practitioners in the industrialised countries are distrustful of research from developing countries until it can be replicated in Europe or North America. But because breastfeeding by HIV-positive mothers has been so successfully discouraged in Europe and North America since 1985, all research has, of necessity, been conducted in the global south. We have reached an impasse.

National surveillance: a well-kept secret

But perhaps there is some preliminary data, after all? At the 2018 conference of the British HIV Association, a Clinical Nurse Specialist called Paula Seery, who worked in the infectious disease service of a well-known London hospital, made the startling revelation that since 2012 no fewer than 40 babies had been breastfed by HIV-positive mothers in the UK and there had been *no transmissions.*[62] Furthermore, they had all been officially registered with the UK National Surveillance of HIV in Pregnancy and Childhood (NSHPC) service, a comprehensive, population-based surveillance register, in place since 1990, that collected demographic and clinical data on all pregnant women living with HIV, their children, and all HIV-infected children in the United Kingdom and Ireland.[63] In 2020, the NSHPC was placed under the umbrella of the Integrated Screening Outcomes Surveillance Service (ISOSS). ISOSS carries out this work on behalf of the NHS Infectious Diseases in Pregnancy Screening Programme: Data on supported breastfeeding (in accordance with BHIVA guidelines) has been collected since 2012, with enhanced surveillance since August 2018. The website says that 'Patient data is collected without consent by ISOSS with PHE Regulation 3 approval.' Maternity and paediatric respondents are contacted for information including all monthly infant test results for the duration of breastfeeding. Details are recorded by phone about a mother's reasons for wanting to breastfeed, who she has shared her HIV status with, her drug therapy, how long she breastfeeds, whether breastfeeding is exclusive, and infant HIV status.

At the International AIDS Conference in Mexico in July 2019 Dr Helen Peters, from UCL Great Ormond Street Institute of Child Health, gave a presentation about British HIV-positive mothers who had been supported to breastfeed for various periods of time, ranging from 1 day to 2 years. These cases had been recorded by the National Surveillance of HIV in Pregnancy & Childhood (NSHPC).[64] Mothers of 90 babies had been supported to breastfeed for various periods of time ranging from one day to two years (median duration seven weeks) and 'results show no vertical transmission among supported breastfeeding cases so far'. In September 2021, Dr Peters gave a powerpoint presentation expanding on this data at the Children's HIV Association conference about British HIV-positive mothers, 83% of whom had been born abroad, who had breastfed their babies between 2012 and 2019.[65] Breastfeeding duration varied from 1 day to 2 years or is ongoing amongst over 130 reports of planned and/or supported breastfeeding among women on fully suppressive therapy since 2012. In January 2021, I heard from the ISOSS Co-ordinator that it wasn't possible to draw any conclusions about breastfeeding-associated transmission from this data because 'only 57 of these infants had infection status confirmed and a number of infants were lost to follow-up so their infection status remains unknown. Of these 130 cases, interviews have been carried out for 95. Infection status has not yet been confirmed in many cases and monitoring is ongoing.'[66]

The existence of a register, recording so many babies who have not been infected through breastfeeding, is very encouraging. However, it's disappointing that this data, so badly needed, remains unavailable and under-reported. It would be so helpful if clinicians were able to discuss local relevant information and experience of the risk and benefits to patients who want to talk about whether they can safely breastfeed their own babies. The data can inform future HIV and infant feeding guidance. Informed choice means that mothers, and their support teams, need access to these statistics.

Withholding support

Disappointingly, one more constraint has been added to the challenges already faced by HIV-positive mothers living in the UK: the risks associated with undergoing blood tests during the escalating Coronavirus pandemic. Monthly testing of maternal viral load and infant HIV status, designed to monitor and safeguard the health of mother and baby, were already described by some as an 'additional testing burden', but now this is apparently a reason to prohibit breastfeeding. On 25 March 2020, two days after the first national lockdown had been announced, BHIVA issued a Statement[67] which read:

> *Monitoring by HIV physicians may be reduced based on clinician assessment of HIV treatment and its efficacy but with a minimum of one initial contact/bloods (virtual or in person), one second trimester contact (virtual or in person) and one final visit in person at 36/40 for bloods and confirmation of the birth plan. Should further support be required antenatally and/or postnatally, virtual follow-up by phone is encouraged.* ***Breastfeeding should be discouraged as it requires monthly maternal and infant viral load follow-up for the duration of the breastfeeding period and for 2 months post-cessation of breastfeeding.***

Was this response justified? Once again breastfeeding was seen as dispensable. Supporting it was too dangerous. Nevertheless, sometimes ignorance is bliss: a client unaware of this guidance was able to pre-book blood tests for herself and her baby, and has not experienced any difficulty in obtaining monitoring of her viral load and the baby's HIV status throughout the last year in spite of Covid restrictions. Fortunately, now that the lockdown has been lifted, BHIVA has removed this recommendation from its website.

HIV-positive women's breastfeeding ambitions

When, thanks to the efficacy of current antiretroviral therapy, the risk of mother-to-child transmission of HIV *in utero*, during birth or during breastfeeding can be reduced to virtually nil, it should no longer be necessary for HIV-positive women to forgo their reproductive aspirations. Not only is it safe for them to embark upon a pregnancy and deliver their children vaginally, but research continues to document improved health outcomes for breastfed vs non-breastfed babies, even in the context of HIV and even in the global north. And if the new Coronavirus pandemic has taught us anything, it is that our survival may depend on a robust immune response – likely to be maximised by having been breastfed as an infant.[68]

CHAPTER 27

Mothers' stories

Data presented at local and overseas conferences have described the current experiences of British HIV-positive women who want to breastfeed.[1] Common reasons included bonding with the infant, health benefits for the child, pressure from family or friends, concerns about disclosure of HIV status, and worries about the cost of formula. Three-fifths of the HIV-positive mothers who had not breastfed reported that they had been questioned by friends, families or members of their community and two-thirds said they had lied about their reasons for not breastfeeding.

Since 2010, WHO guidance on HIV and infant feeding has incorporated up-to-date findings on the effectiveness of maternal HAART to prevent postpartum transmission. The supporting background documents are detailed and thorough, with a focus on HIV-free child survival rather than merely a reduction in mother-to-child transmission of HIV by breastfeeding avoidance.[2]

However, many British practitioners believe that the WHO guidelines are not generally applicable to the UK setting. HIV-positive mothers living in resource-rich settings are mistakenly led to believe that there is no evidence base to support safe breastfeeding. The assumption is that because they have access to clean water and safe infant feeding alternatives then formula-feeding is safer. This belief is unfounded. It may in part stem from the cultural norm of bottle-feeding in much of the global north, and in part from misleading reporting of research results.[3] But in fact, there is substantial evidence of increased morbidity associated with formula-feeding even in developed countries.[4]

The best care gives the best opportunity to have a good outcome

If extremely low rates of postpartum transmission can today be achieved in resource-poor settings, how much more likely is breastfeeding to be safe in the resource-rich countries? A mother with HIV living in the global north has access to as much preventive care as she can possibly need to protect her baby from MTCT.[5] Today's mother is screened for HIV in the first trimester of pregnancy so that if an HIV infection is identified, she receives ART immediately. This is long enough (>13 weeks)[6] to achieve an undetectable viral load (<50 copies/mm^3), pivotal to eliminating maternal infectivity, by the time the baby is born.[7] So long as she is diligent about adhering to her ART, the risk of her baby becoming infected *in utero* or during birth is tiny. Even though the evidence is clear that labour and birth carries the greatest risk of MTCT, clinicians in the UK are so confident in the ability of ART to reduce viral load in the birth canal to undetectable levels that they now promote vaginal delivery.[8] Logically then, if a mother's HIV infection is sufficiently controlled to have a vaginal birth, then it is also low enough to enable breastfeeding.

Since 2015, nine out of 10 pregnancies in British women have been diagnosed before conception and three-quarters of mothers are receiving ART by the time they conceive.[9] Antenatal HIV screening, and obstetric care and management during pregnancy, have all contributed to a decline in the rate of vertical transmission from 2% in 2000–01 to 0.3% in 2012–14. In 2018, the last year that figures for infections in newborns were available, no babies were infected. By July 2019, the National Surveillance of HIV in Pregnancy and Childhood programme reported that in 90 HIV-exposed babies who had been breastfed for as little as one day to as long as two years, and 'after breastfeeding had stopped... results show no vertical transmissions among supported breastfeeding cases so far...'[10]

Mothers who realised their dreams

The following mothers' stories are shared with the permission of three gallant and persistent mothers who contacted me for information about breastfeeding with HIV. I feel privileged to have accompanied them on their journeys as they worked around and overcame the different challenges they faced. Their determination to follow their dreams to breastfeed their babies made them a joy to work with. Names and places have been changed to protect the identities of the mothers, their babies and their healthcare providers.

Anna's story

Anna had been diagnosed with HIV a couple of years before she became a mother for the first time. Her first baby, born eight years earlier, had been bottle-fed. By the time she became pregnant with her second baby, Anna was unaware that new research on breastfeeding with HIV had emerged. She had her heart set on a water birth so she had contacted a national organisation of doulas for help and advice. Anna's doula also suggested that if she would like to breastfeed, this might be possible despite the barriers put in place during her first pregnancy. She referred Anna to me for more detailed information.

Anna contacted me when she was about six months pregnant. Anna writes:

'[my doula] signposted me to various weblinks, which proved invaluable. I continued with my research into HIV, and started to read the many articles and links from Pamela. I then compiled all the latest information, research and evidence from her, which I needed to discuss with my midwifery team, obstetrician, paediatrician and specialist

GUM consultant. I also finalised a birth plan which detailed clearly my wishes and plans for this birth, which I shared with my medical team.'

Anna's obstetrician and midwife expressed concern. They hadn't worked with a mother with HIV who wanted to breastfeed before. Since formula-feeding was considered to be safe, wouldn't breastfeeding pose an avoidable risk of HIV transmission to the baby?

Help with positioning and latching the baby to the breast after birth would be provided by Anna's doula, while I supplied written information on how she could manage her own lactation as her milk came in, and during the crucial early weeks of breastfeeding. She shared this with her obstetric team, midwives, nurse specialists and health visitors as she quickly became an active partner in her own healthcare.

Anna then had a two-hour consultation with her GUM specialist consultant, to cover areas of concern surrounding breastfeeding with HIV. They went through each topic, one by one, in great detail. Fortuitously, the GUM consultant was himself the father of four babies who had been exclusively breastfed. While careful, he was more open and more knowledgeable than the very cautious members of the obstetric team. While he was reluctant to provide broad guidance which might contradict existing policy, he did agree to facilitate breastfeeding for Anna personally. He was extremely thorough, and looked closely at Anna's patient history, all clinical aspects, including routine test results, allergic reactions, toxicity, resistance to drugs, compliance, responsibility, attendance at the clinic and existing knowledge and expectations. He also discussed with Anna drug regimens and implications of transfer of maternal antiretroviral drugs into breastmilk. They discussed the possibility of maternal drug adjustment as the baby matured and grew, and risks and benefits of several courses of action. They covered the baby's own post-birth prophylaxis, how the baby's health would be monitored and the tests that could be done. The GUM specialist was especially concerned about breast or nipple problems, and the risk of transmission of HIV through mastitis. Perhaps the baby could receive additional post-exposure prophylaxis should there be concerns about elevated viral levels in breastmilk. Anna stated her plan to wean to formula if symptoms of mastitis became obvious. Planned duration of breastfeeding was also discussed in detail. Great care was taken to cover every small yet important detail.

The GUM specialist also took the time to seek appropriate professional advice from another specialist consultant in London and arranged to meet with Anna's paediatrician the following week to discuss her case further, so that they could look at all options and make a decision on what the best course of action would be.

The GUM consultant followed these meetings by writing a very clear and detailed care plan outlining the kinds of breastfeeding situations that might be encountered and what advance arrangements were to be put in place and written into Anna's medical notes. In the case of any breast or nipple infections, arrangements were also made to have her milk tested at a lab in London. The baby would receive four weeks of ARV prophylaxis after birth. Maternal viral load had been undetectable during pregnancy, and would be tested as soon as possible after birth and repeated monthly. Special arrangements were made with the laboratory so that viral load results could be received within 2–3 days (rather than the normal three weeks) so that, if Anna had a blip in her viral load, or if there was any other concern about elevated viral levels, she could quickly switch the baby to replacement feeding.

Anna gradually became aware that she and her team were pioneers. Many of the concerns expressed by her healthcare providers were because no mother with HIV living in her area had indicated a wish to breastfeed before, so they were all breaking new ground. The hospital would need to write protocols to cover all the eventualities she had discussed with her GUM specialist, her paediatrician and members of the obstetric team. She wrote:

> *'I am delighted that after taking all of these things into account that they will stand by me as one of the first HIV+ mothers to choose breast feeding in [my area]. I feel so proud and empowered to have stood up for my right to choose how I feed my baby, championing the superiority of breast milk over any formula and facing into the challenges along the way. Honestly, if this can even open the door for just one other mum in the future or even just open the minds of HCPs, it will all have been worth it. I hope breast feeding my baby will be safe and the right choice in the end, I am not under-estimating the risk or concerns of those around me. However the research, no matter how recent, is there. Other mothers have successfully breast fed their children and with all this risk management in place, there is no reason why my baby and I can't be a success story for the books too.'*

Since the possibility of breast or nipple problems was the factor causing the most worry, I provided Anna with a lot more information about preventive self-care, and suggested that she consider hiring a breast pump to promptly resolve any milk stasis or engorgement in the early days after the birth when milk production really got going. We had extensive correspondence about what to expect, including what was normal, what would be of concern, and how she could promptly institute strategies to head off plugged ducts or mastitis at the first symptoms. I also sent a lot of information on the transfer of antiretroviral drugs into breastmilk and information on the likely effects on the baby.

Anna's baby boy was born at term, with her doula in attendance, via the perfect water birth she had dreamed of. The baby breastfed really well in the first few days, losing only 6.5% of his birthweight, well within normal range, and then gained a whopping 65g (>2oz) per day exclusively on mother's milk. Breastfeeding went so well that by the time he weaned at nine months he was at the 98th percentile on the weight chart. The only concern was that he developed the beginnings of eczema, so Anna went on a dairy elimination diet and his symptoms resolved. He was exclusively breastfed for six full months and then very gradually weaned from the breast. Night-time weaning was a little challenging, but Anna managed this creatively by gently changing over to formula milk by bottle after six months and substituting a dummy for comfort-sucking. She made sure to prevent breast engorgement as she weaned and was glad to be warned about the possibility of weaning grief, which can be normal at the end of breastfeeding.

The baby's HIV screening consistently came back negative. Anna noted, 'In addition his antibodies declined since birth, despite breastfeeding and by 9 months they were nil. This has made me so happy as even with the extended period of mixed feeding from 6–9 months, it has made no impact on the baby's HIV risk.'

Anna wrote of her own HIV management:

'During my time breastfeeding I was attending the clinic for monthly viral load checks, all of which were undetectable, even under the latest lab technology which screens down to 20 copies of the virus per ml of blood, which is really very tiny amounts. It was very reassuring to know that my bloods are so stable and consistent.'

Finally, Anna's breastfeeding experience had been so successful that her paediatrician requested a first-hand account.

'Dr [...] has asked me to put together a case study on my perspective and experience as a parent throughout our journey, as a learning tool for junior doctors. I am thrilled to do this as it was always part of my motivation to educate others and open their minds to new possibilities, so I am very happy to do this for the next generation of doctors in this field!'

Finally, Anna's doula wrote up her case history, outlining the success of her ambition to breastfeed her baby and containing the following useful summary, which was published by the national organisation of doulas:[11]

This piece, by Doula UK member Anne Glover, was first published in The Doula *magazine.*

What made a difference:

1. Mum has been HIV+ for more than 10 years with no risk factors, and is meticulous with her medication. She has never missed a single appointment, and has been on the same combination ART (anti-retroviral therapy) for years now, achieving a consistently undetectable VL (viral load) long before and during pregnancy.
2. Lab agreed to turn round any of mum's VL tests within 3 days instead of 3 weeks to support the level of monitoring requested by her medical team – without this support the GUM specialist probably would not have agreed to oversee breastfeeding at all.
3. Having the most up to date research and evidence on HIV+ and breastfeeding to enable a full discussion with the medical team early on in the pregnancy.
4. Addressing breastfeeding issues, potential problems and preventive measures, and being equipped with knowledge on mastitis, sore/bleeding nipples, home pasteurisation. Awareness of local support, e.g. hospital grade pump, breastfeeding counsellor, health visitors.
5. GUM specialist can overrule other HCPs. Luckily this mum's GUM specialist had 4 EBF babies of his own although he could not support breastfeeding as a matter of course. The interpretation of the BHIVA guidance led him to conclude that formula feeding remains the first choice feeding option

for HIV+ women in [area] under his care, for clinical and ethical reasons. However he wrote a letter of instruction to all the medical teams involved after taking time to seek appropriate professional advice from another specialist consultant in London. He explained that he had to take a very detailed look at patient history covering all clinical aspects, including routine test results, allergic reactions, toxicity, resistance to drugs, compliance, responsibility, attendance to clinic and existing knowledge and expectation of HIV+ and breastfeeding. GUM specialist and Paediatrician met to discuss all options and made a decision on the best course of action.

Result!

- Obstetrician wrote in the maternity notes that mum wished to have a water birth and breastfeed, including that she had researched feeding in depth.
- Paediatrician wrote in her maternity notes that mum wishes to breastfeed and he supports her decision (massive step plus a humungous success for mum).
- GUM specialist took time to seek professional advice from another specialist consultant in London.
- Health visitor reassured mum that they would be looking out for her and would support her and help with technique to ensure optimal latch.
- Midwifery team assessed the birthing pool and deemed it safe for water birth without concern of cross infection.
- [Area] revolutionary and ground breaking for HIV + mothers. One of the first HIV+ mums to choose breastfeeding in [area].
- It has forced the [area] Hospital in [city] to produce their own guidance on HIV+ and breastfeeding for the first time.

Recommendations:

- Consider your options
- Do the research and know what you are talking about
- Share your knowledge, provide the evidence
- Discuss your options very fully with your medical team well in advance
- Make your wishes known
- Obtain the support of your medical team
- Risk management

Briony's story

Briony wanted to find out whether it was possible to breastfeed with HIV even before she became pregnant. She had heard, through a friend, about a presentation I had given on HIV and breastfeeding at a local mother-support organisation annual conference. A nurse by profession, Briony had been diagnosed with HIV eight years previously, was in a happy relationship with a lovely man and they were hoping to conceive a child. She wanted to learn more, because – as she eloquently described – 'Feeling that I can't breastfeed has always been one of the things that has upset me the most about having the disease.'

We were able to discuss her hopes and ambitions for feeding this very planned baby and within less than two months, Briony let me know that she was pregnant, with the baby due just before Christmas. Briony had always had a high CD4 count, and she had commenced antiretroviral 'treatment as prevention' in preparation for conception. Her viral load was undetectable and her CD4 count remained high. In the following weeks I sent her a whole list of articles outlining the most up-to-date research, together with web links and information sheets about the importance of exclusive breastfeeding, how to 'manage' lactation and maximise breastmilk production, and strategies for breast self-care.

Briony set about letting her healthcare team know of her ambition to breastfeed and a short time later she wrote,

> *'My doctor has been really supportive, and so has the specialist midwife, they both have experience with people doing it'. Briony had a long appointment with her doctor 'and spent most of the time talking about breastfeeding. I think she quite enjoys our discussions and needs them, in the sense that she needs to be able to document that we are informed and sentient, in our decision making and also that the decisions are joint and not in any way one sided. I have just sent her all of the informative bits from your emails, as she is very interested and supportive. From what I understand there is a monthly meeting about all of the HIV+ve women within the [area] Trust once a month. This is attended by GUM HIV doctors, the specialist obstetricians and specialist midwives but I'm not sure whether there is a paediatric input. They are all very interested to hear about our decision making process, some individuals being more supportive than others. From what I can gather there are more women choosing to breast feed but still not many, and only in areas where there is perhaps more prevalence and therefore experience and more people to have the opportunity of open minds.'*

Briony was now leaning even more towards a decision to breastfeed and we had long phone calls to talk about anticipatory care: initiating breastfeeding after birth, how to know the baby was 'getting enough', and the need for good postnatal care. She had arranged with a local breastfeeding counsellor to receive hands-on help with positioning and attaching the baby to the breast after the birth and she had found a breast pump. She would be meeting with her midwife soon, and had arranged to attend antenatal classes. I urged her to make a formal, written birth plan.

In the next week she met with all the midwives and wrote,

> *'The appointment with [...] had a great outcome but a shaky start. I turned up to find the specialist midwives there waiting. I felt like I had been ambushed and that they were there with bad news. However, they were there to discuss and document my wishes/plans for the birth and beyond. They have organised for me to meet with one of the birth centre midwives so that when I turn up they don't panic and start questioning the safety of the water birth etc... They were also positive and supportive about the breast feeding, and*

will keep me in for a few days until they are confident that I am confident with what I'm doing.'

The baby was born just before her due date. Briony had a lot of help from her midwives, checking the baby's latch, and her milk came in well as expected. She did have one sore nipple, and we discussed strategies to resolve that. She attended a breastfeeding clinic where the nurses confirmed they were happy with the way the baby was breastfeeding and the nipple healed well.

The baby had gained >50g per day from hospital discharge to 10 days of age, and continued to gain really exceptional amounts of weight on her mother's milk alone, but she remained very unsettled and colicky. We began to suspect she might be reacting to cows' milk proteins and possibly also soy in the mother's diet. Over the next few weeks Briony kept a careful food diary, and she began to realise that the baby became colicky and unhappy every time she ate out. I sought information about allergens in breastmilk and implications for the infant gut mucosa from my colleague Maureen Minchin in Australia,[12] author of *Milk Matters: Infant Feeding and Immune Disorder*. Maureen's opinion was reassuring.

Because of Briony's lifestyle and own need to eat regularly due to the medications she was taking, it became increasingly difficult to avoid foods which upset the baby. Briony herself began to experience health problems, developing chest pain, with suspected pleurisy or pulmonary embolism, when the baby was four weeks old, and she was later found to have a pelvic infection.

And so at six weeks, Briony made the difficult decision to wean the baby off the breast. During the changeover from breastfeeding to bottle-feeding with a hypoallergenic formula, and so as to avoid the possibility of mixed feeding such a young baby, Briony fed the baby home-pasteurised breastmilk for several days. She was careful to suppress lactation gradually and gently by expressing her breasts to comfort until she slowly stopped producing milk and she suffered no breast problems.

Although Briony felt sad about weaning, she felt she had made the right decision in her individual circumstances. She was pleased that by taking so much time and trouble to investigate and plan, she had fulfilled a long-held ambition. The baby had had a great start in life and Briony had ensured initial mother-baby bonding, which had been one of her main motivations. The baby's post-birth HIV test and all testing in the following weeks and months came back negative. This was a great outcome.

A second pregnancy

Six months later Briony was pregnant again, this time with twins. She decided she would like to breastfeed these babies too, even though she was aware of the challenges. During the pregnancy Briony started to plan for the possibility that the babies might be born early, and/or might need some supplementation in the first few days, so she explored the possibility of accessing donor breastmilk and we discussed the many implications of this. We also covered in depth the need to maximise breastmilk production in the early postpartum in order to ensure adequate breastmilk for two babies for a full six months.

With the endorsement of her midwives, Briony had also explored the possibility of expressing colostrum during late pregnancy. Her aim was to have a stash of breastmilk/colostrum ready to feed her babies during the first couple of days before her milk came in. I provided links and more info gleaned from the lactation literature. She had also arranged with two friends who would be willing to donate their breastmilk for her babies as necessary. However, there was some concern about this:

> *'At a multi-disciplinary team meeting of there has apparently been discussion about me using another woman's breast milk if I need to and its safety with respect to HIV. They are concerned that the other milk would contain different antibodies/allergens etc and could possibly cause gut irritation and therefore increase the risk [of transmission of HIV] to the babies'.*

We thus explored the use of pasteurised banked milk, and whether the hospital would agree to arrange this in advance (as they had for another HIV-positive mother I'd worked with previously). We also discussed how much milk would be needed during the first few days, how to compute the quantity based on the babies' weights, World Health Organization guidance on the use of breastmilk in the context of HIV and generally how to plan for a possible caesarean section birth, since one twin was in the breech position. I contacted Professor Coutsoudis in South Africa for her expert opinion on the safety of mixed feeding with mother's milk and either raw donor or pasteurised breastmilk and received a reassuring reply by return which I passed on to Briony for her multidisciplinary team.

Briony's twin girls were born at nearly 36 weeks, by emergency caesarean section, each baby weighing well over 2kg. Briony suffered several unexpected and significant birth injuries, which made moving around very difficult and required pain relief and treatment with antibiotics. Her iron levels also dropped, leading to the potential for delayed milk production. Both babies were sleepy at first, a characteristic of pre-term babies, and the larger twin lost a significant amount of weight and was slower to begin breastfeeding. While the babies were learning to breastfeed, they were fed banked donor milk via nasogastric tube, before graduating to cup-feeding. As well as breastfeeding direct, Briony also stimulated her own milk production with pumping and altogether this was hard work and it was quite a difficult time. At just over a week old, the babies perked up and started breastfeeding with more competence. However, just as things were starting to go well there followed a period of several days when there were many concerns coming all together. Briony developed an MRSA infection in her wound, causing a lot of pain and requiring that mother and babies were all isolated together and treated with antibiotics. Briony had to go back to theatre twice: for debridement of her wound, and to have it re-stitched. Twin two had some bleeding after needing to have her nasogastric tube replaced several times, raising the risk of injury and exposure to the virus in breastmilk. The possibility of extending twin two's zidovudine prophylaxis beyond four weeks was raised, as infant prophylaxis for six weeks is the standard of care in developing countries. Then it was found that both babies had lost considerable weight as the changeover was made to more breastfeeding and less supplemental banked milk. However, once the babies started taking more of mother's own milk directly at the breast, they started to regain the lost weight.

Finally mother and babies were discharged home. Briony found being at home much easier, but the frequent breastfeeding needed by newborn twins is very hard work, and there was also an older toddler to care for. Briony wanted to increase her breastmilk supply so as to build up a stash of expressed milk and needed information about the use of domperidone as a galactogogue. We talked about what to do if the babies seemed unsettled, but in fact breastfeeding continued to go very well, the babies thrived, and galactogogues were definitely not needed. The babies were exclusively breastfed for six months, with one baby weaning slightly later than the other. Briony was easily able to suppress lactation after stopping breastfeeding with no breast problems.

Looking back, Briony wrote:

> *'I fed them both up to 6 months, slightly longer with [twin 1] They had 48 hours of my frozen milk before beginning formula and they starting weaning a few days later. I didn't rush it! I was very sad to stop but at least felt that I really had gone as far as I could. All the support I received was incredible. Maybe because they were all prepared for it after [first baby] but it was certainly very positive. I was surprised at times about the support I had surrounding some of the decisions we made. It turned out that most people were actually behind our decision. All three of my children have strong healthy immune systems supported by breastfeeding... They are 5, 5 and 6 now, and have never been sick. The bond it gave me and my children, the healthy start in life it gave them, the benefits of breastfeeding – I don't think I did the wrong thing.'*

Christina's story

Christina wrote to me from Europe in early 2017, wanting to explore the possibility of breastfeeding her second baby, due in six weeks. She had discovered that she was infected with HIV 14 years previously. She hadn't needed antiretroviral treatment for many years, but had now been on triple antiretroviral therapy for seven years in order to protect her HIV-negative partner. Her CD4 count was around 800–1,000 cells/mm^3 and she had an undetectable viral load. Her first baby, now aged 15 months, had been born more than 10 weeks prematurely, and had been bottle-fed. She was very happy with her doctor, who had supported her decision to conceive naturally because she had good viral control, but the doctor had less knowledge about breastfeeding with HIV. Christina was concerned not to put her baby at risk, and wanted more information. Breastfeeding was taboo in her country and she didn't know anyone who had done it. She had found me after reading the WABA HIV Kit.[13]

I confirmed that the very best way of taking her ambition forward would be to enlist the support of her doctors, the baby's paediatrician and her HIV clinicians. The most up-to-date information was that there was a very low risk of transmission of the virus (0–<1%) when the mother:

1. Has an undetectable viral load at birth
2. Is receiving full antiretroviral therapy for the whole time that she breastfeeds
3. Is absolutely adherent to her antiretroviral therapy during at least 13 weeks of pregnancy, and for the full time that she will be breastfeeding

Also that the baby:

1. Will receive antiretroviral prophylaxis for the first 4–6 weeks after birth
2. Will be exclusively breastfed (receive absolutely no other foods/formula or liquids, not even water) for the first six months of life.

I sent several articles and web links. In view of the short time left before the baby was due, I offered to try and find a local IBCLC for help with the first few days of breastfeeding. It would be very important that Christina knew how to position and attach her baby to the breast so that breastfeeding was effective and comfortable. It was also necessary to resolve any over-production of breastmilk in the first few days as her milk came in.

Christina wanted to talk about her main concerns:

- Discussing breastfeeding with her doctor because of the stigma of this feeding method in her country
- ART drugs passing to the baby through breastmilk and the implications of this
- Duration of ARV prophylaxis for the baby
- The possibility of pasteurising her breastmilk

I sent more articles covering these concerns, and confirmed that in the UK we were finding that breastfeeding with HIV was still very unusual. The doctors initially had concerns about liability issues, but it seemed that when they read the research and talked to their colleagues, they became very supportive. They often monitored the mother's health, and her viral load, very carefully, and conducted frequent HIV tests on the baby. I suggested that she share with her medical advisors the current recommendations of the British HIV Association and the American Academy of Pediatrics. In particular several years ago there had also been possible child protection concerns so that, in order to protect my clients from any possibility of coercion, I used to suggest that they might like to engage the services of a lawyer/attorney in advance. The new guidance made this no longer necessary. I also sent info sheets on exclusive breastfeeding with HIV, why it was important, how to achieve it, and how to suppress lactation should that be necessary. In addition, recent research meant that WHO had changed their guidance for mothers who were receiving ART to suggest that it was safer to continue breastfeeding beyond six months and up to 24 months.

Christina and her partner went through the materials, discussed the issues, and she shared these resources with her HIV clinician, letting her know that she would like to breastfeed. She received a reply by return which she had translated for me:

> *'We agree, the risk is tiny and probably zero in cases [such as yours] where the plasma viral load is undetectable. But even in this case I do not think that you will find a doctor in [area] who gives you a formal 'agreement' for breastfeeding, insofar as it is possible in [area] to have safe artificial feeding. Now, given the data of the literature and under strict conditions of surveillance, you can personally and without our 'agreement' make this choice of this type of breastfeeding... This is something that has happened a long time ago*

> *on transmission in the context of sero-different couples and unprotected sexual relations where many couples had made this choice without the endorsement of their doctor! Talk to gynecologist to get her opinion.'*

This reiterated the common response, that because formula-feeding was deemed safe in the global north, breastfeeding was seen to be an unnecessary risk for the baby.

Christina also sent the materials to her gynaecologist who, after long discussions, granted her request, explaining that in her situation breastfeeding would be acceptable, but the situation was complicated. The fear was that other women might learn about her plan and want to breastfeed too and for them it would not be recommended. Her gynaecologist recommended finding a paediatrician who would agree to provide care for a breastfed child. This was not easy and the paediatrician, who was obliged to agree to do the follow-up, was not in favour of breastfeeding the baby.

Three weeks later, Christina phoned to say that her 37 week, 2.3kg baby girl had been born at 5.30am that morning. The baby was born healthy and was breathing on her own, and she had held her, but as well as being early, this was not the birth Christina had planned. After her waters had broken, the hospital staff had more or less coerced her, due to her HIV status, into having a caesarean section, saying it would not be safe to have a vaginal birth due to too long a period of ruptured membranes. Christina was very surprised by this advice because her first child had been born vaginally, and the circumstances surrounding the beginning of labour were similar. She and her husband had refused at first, but the staff had been very insistent and in the end the parents felt they had to agree.

By the time Christina phoned, the staff had already taken the baby to the hospital nursery, and fed her formula. They were adamant that this was necessary because the baby was premature and as a result her blood sugar levels were at the lowest limit of safety. They told Christina that she couldn't breastfeed now since this would mean that the baby was being mixed fed, which was too dangerous because of the risk of HIV transmission to the baby. Due to the caesarean section, mother and baby would be in the hospital for four days.

This meant that Christina's careful plans to breastfeed had been sabotaged. But she was undeterred. She had refused medication to dry up her milk and now planned to express her own milk for her baby, to pasteurise it to inactivate any virus, and then change over from breastmilk-feeding to direct breastfeeding as soon as she possibly could. In other words, these developments had not changed her wish to breastfeed. We talked about how she could achieve this end:

1. It would be possible to hand express colostrum today and tomorrow
2. From about day three postpartum she could obtain a breast pump, and pump her breasts. It would be very important to express milk as often as it took to avoid over-fullness. Even if the staff didn't support provision of pasteurised milk for the baby, it would be wise to maintain good breast care to avoid mastitis, and the hospital staff should be obliged to assist with this.
3. I attempted to talk Christina through how to hand express, which was complicated

because of the language difficulties. I arranged to send links to videos of manual expression and suggested she ask for midwife help with this too.

4. Christina seemed confident that she could express breastmilk for the baby quite easily for a couple of weeks. I anticipated she might have to wait until she went home in order to actually feed the pasteurised breastmilk to the baby. In the meantime I arranged to contact a colleague who had special expertise for her opinion[12] about how long it might take the baby's gut to heal from the effects of early formula-feeding once she was no longer exposed to it; i.e. how long would Christina need to feed the baby pasteurised expressed breastmilk for before she could safely make the switch to breastfeeding direct?
5. Christina would request a hospital visit from local IBCLCs so that she could receive practical help with manual expression of breastmilk, provision of a pump, and later assistance to position/attach baby to the breast.
6. I just listened as Christina told me about her huge disappointment over the caesarean section birth, her worry that she had missed the irreplaceable opportunity to breastfeed her baby in the first hour after her birth, and the attempt to frustrate her wish to breastfeed at all. These were no small things, and I was privately outraged and heartbroken for her. I urged her to be calm about them for now, since her baby was healthy and strong, and she was already planning for damage control in providing her milk, and because they were disappointments she would be better able to work through later when she was recovered from her surgery, back in her own home and feeling stronger.

Maureen Minchin and I had some correspondence about infant intestinal flora, disappearance of bifido and lacto species associated with formula-feeding, and the implications of whether the mother herself had been breastfed, but the bald fact was that there was actually no research. I also did a little digging around for information on stool testing to assess newborn bowel integrity, which had been particularly directed towards the risk of necrotising enterocolitis for formula-fed premature babies. Maureen thought that feeding pasteurised breastmilk for at least three weeks would be necessary if the baby was receiving a mixture of pasteurised and fresh donor milk. Meanwhile, in the hospital, Christina was hand expressing and had accessed a pump and she was asking about milk storage and the logistics of pasteurising different quantities of collected breastmilk.

Mother and baby were discharged home on day four after the birth, and Christina immediately started feeding her home-pasteurised (flash-heated) breastmilk to the baby. Her milk was coming in well and she was finding the process easy. We discussed the quantities that the baby would need based on her weight and age in days, and the need to pump possibly more milk than the baby was taking for now, and freezing the rest.

A week later, Christina wrote, '[Baby] only drinks my pasteurized breast milk and this is a great joy for me. I did not think that one day my child would drink my milk!' The baby was gaining weight really well, and her parents were astonished at how much milk she was taking. Christina was now pumping 850–900ml in each 24 hours, 160ml at a time every three hours in the day, with a longer 4–5 hour interval at night. She was looking forward to teaching her baby to breastfeed. Meanwhile she was holding her baby skin-to-skin against her breast during bottle-feeding, and her let-down reflex was triggered by just watching the baby sucking the bottle. It was all so hopeful. The midwife who was now visiting Christina at home was becoming very interested in breastfeeding with HIV and asked to read the papers that Christina had collected on the subject. She would be available to help with latching when the time came.

As breastfeeding-direct day came closer, I provided anticipatory care and urged patience as the baby learned to breastfeed, but this preparation was completely unnecessary. Christina was ecstatic, 'I write to tell you that it worked very very well with breastfeeding. She took the breast as if she always did it, and didn't need the bottle. That is a big relief for us!' We talked about how to avoid sore nipples and Christina found that the tenderness she felt during the first few breastfeeds resolved easily. We also discussed how breastfed babies may need more frequent feeding because they may take less milk each time than bottle-fed babies. The changeover from bottle-feeding to breastfeeding went very well. Christina continued to pump if the breasts became overfull, and the baby's father sometimes fed expressed breastmilk while she pumped so the work was shared. Mother, father, big brother and baby were enjoying their time together.

As Christina feared, the baby's one-month check-up at the hospital did not go so well. She phoned to say she was worried that the baby was given sugar-water to reduce the pain of the blood test – did this constitute a lapse in exclusive breastfeeding? I confirmed that this would most likely be within the definition of prescribed medications, but I suggested next time she might take some expressed breastmilk for the purpose, or breastfeed immediately after the procedure instead. Christina had also been upset by the attitude of the paediatrician towards her decision to breastfeed. The paediatrician cited a colleague's opinion about the findings of the Kesho Bora study,[14] which showed a high transmission rate of 5.4% MTCT of HIV in spite of maternal ART. I wrote to Christina pointing out that the Kesho Bora mothers had followed protocols from 2005, 12 years earlier, which had promoted formula-feeding and premature weaning. So in fact very few of the Kesho Bora mothers had exclusively breastfed and most had weaned before three months. Consequently the comparatively high rate of MTCT in that study was misleading. The pediatrician had suggested extending the baby's ARV prophylaxis, originally planned for one month, for the entire period that Christina was breastfeeding. I sent Christina links to the most recent WHO global guidance on breastfeeding and the use of antiretroviral drugs, for her to share with the baby's paediatrician.[15–17] We also discussed the possibility of reverting to feeding pasteurised breastmilk if she was worried, but she said that she was really enjoying breastfeeding now, it was giving her a lot of pleasure, the baby was thriving, gaining 46g/day, and that rather than change her feeding method she would prefer to change her paediatrician! For while she felt confident that she was not putting her daughter at risk of contamination, the lack of support from the medical profession weighed heavily on her.

When the baby was six weeks old, Christina reported that she experienced a few days of more frequent breastfeeding, which may have been a growth spurt, or a few 'frequency days'. We reviewed lactation management and how to increase or decrease her breastmilk supply as needed, according to the baby's demand. She was reassured to know that fluctuations in the baby's appetite were normal and she took this small challenge in her stride. When the baby developed oral thrush Christina needed information about when to be worried about this, i.e. if there was any bleeding from the baby's mouth or the mother's nipples, but this was not the case. The paediatrician prescribed antifungal medication and it cleared very quickly. I began to hear from Christina less frequently as she was becoming more and more confident in her ability to meet her baby's needs through breastfeeding.

The family were planning an overseas holiday and Christina was thinking about weaning after they returned. We discussed local and international recommendations for when breastfeeding should stop. She would not be returning to work until the baby's first birthday and was eager to continue breastfeeding past six months if possible. The WHO 2016 Global guidance[16] now supported continued breastfeeding with the addition of weaning foods for up to two years.

This was also confirmed with a retired paediatrician with whom she had been in contact from the beginning and who wrote to her:

> *'I think you can diversify your baby's diet while continuing to breastfeed. Sudden stops at 6 months were advised in the absence of treatment of the mother, which is no longer the case at present. For me there is no risk or the risk is virtually zero in your case where under treatment you are undetectable for a long time. Do as you please.'*

This made Christina very happy as she maintained her plans to continue breastfeeding past six months.

Quarterly follow-up appointments with her daughter's regular pediatrician were always very difficult for Christina, but she always honoured them. The next I heard from her was just as the baby was turning one, and they were still breastfeeding. She wrote that it had been very difficult to introduce solid food. Her little one was fussy, she didn't like vegetables, though she would take a little fruit. She was now taking a little formula, but was still breastfeeding a lot, especially at night. And she enjoyed it a lot.

I heard from Christina again when the baby was 15 months. She wanted to talk about weaning completely as she had understood that the benefit of breastfeeding had greatly diminished and that there was no longer any advantage in continuing. The baby had quadrupled her birthweight and now that she was attending nursery she had begun eating fish, meat and eggs. She used to breastfeed in the morning when she dropped her daughter off at the nursery, in the afternoon when she picked her up, and in the evening, but no longer at night. Her blood test results, carried out every six months, were good.

The paediatrician who was monitoring her baby recommended that she stagger her medication to reduce as much as possible the amount of the drug that would be ingested by her daughter. For once she was able to reassure Christina and she decided to continue, as breastfeeding was still important for both of them. However, Christina's doctor suggested that she change her ARV treatment. This caused Christina great concern about the toxicity of the new treatment for her daughter, but her doctor did not agree. Not wanting to contradict her doctor, she preferred to ask another doctor to prescribe her usual treatment and to change her treatment only after weaning.

Christina wanted to make final weaning from the breast as easy as possible for her little girl since breastfeeding was still important to her. I sent her information and strategies for substituting other physical comfort and contact, as well as other activities and foods to take the place of breastfeeding, the benefits of weaning gradually, and an info sheet on how to suppress lactation.

In the end Christina breastfed her little girl for the full two years and later she shared with me how special the experience was to her:

> *'I had agreed with [...] to breastfeed her until she was 2 years old. Towards the end we had managed to have a rhythm of 2 breastfeeds per day and finally weaning went pretty well, maybe because we had talked about it quite a bit together. I have such a beautiful memory of this experience with my daughter! She's in very good health, the tests always good.'*

CHAPTER 28

Helping an HIV-positive mother who wants to breastfeed

Can an HIV-positive mother breastfeed? Those working with breastfeeding mothers are likely to encounter this question sooner or later. Initially, it may seem like a difficult question to answer. The information is nothing if not conflicting, and it is scattered all over the place. IBCLCs are very conscious that they could be stepping outside their mandate. But ultimately, it's important to remember that – as with every other breastfeeding situation – our job is to ascertain a mother's goals, and provide her with information. Thereafter it's up to her to make the decision about how to feed her baby, with the help of her healthcare providers.

Kahlert and colleagues, who have raised the issue of U=U (undetectable=untransmissable) guidance for breastfeeding mothers as well as for other groups affected by HIV,[1] suggest:

> *'The decision for or against breastfeeding must follow the process of shared decision making with any woman wishing to breastfeed. This process requires that the HIV-infected mother receives comprehensive and unbiased information that empowers her to understand the risks and benefits of each decision. The healthcare provider's role in this process is to supply all the required information for the decision-making process in an unbiased manner, and to understand and respect the woman's preference and autonomy. Ideally, after exchanging this information and discussing all potential risks and benefits, a decision is made that can be shared by all the involved partners. This decision process should take place before delivery.'*

1. Breastfeeding goals

The first task is to ascertain how your client would really like to feed her baby, and learn what she knows about breastfeeding with HIV. Is this her first baby? Will this be her first breastfeeding experience? If this will be a second or subsequent baby, was she supported to breastfeed the previous baby and if so, how did it go? How long does she envisage breastfeeding for? What medical advice has she received about her pregnancy? Does she have the support of the baby's father? Who knows that she has HIV? Will her friends and family help her with care and support in the early weeks and months (as hopefully they would for any new mother?) Taking a full history and listening to the mother's hopes and concerns can be illuminating. Learning as much as possible beforehand will help you build a full picture of what your client wants and help you explore with her what will be possible, and what will not, and help you to tailor a realistic care plan for her.

2. Safety checks

What medications is the mother receiving, and when did she start antiretroviral treatment (recommended for at least 13 weeks before the birth)? Does she understand the vital role of meticulous adherence to her medications in order to maintain an undetectable viral load – the key to PMTCT by all routes? What is her current viral load? Does she understand the importance of regular monitoring of her own viral load and the need for frequent testing for the baby – usually monthly? What medical advice has she received about her pregnancy? Will she be having a vaginal delivery? Is she planning an elective caesarean section?

3. Share resources

One of the first things I do is to send my new client, on my letterhead, a list of articles and web links on HIV and breastfeeding (see box). If she has difficulty accessing them, I send the articles as attachments. The resources fall broadly into three categories:

1. Summary articles about HIV and breastfeeding (see box) which will contain references that can also be accessed if necessary.
2. National and international HIV and breastfeeding recommendations.
3. Breastfeeding and lactation management sheets I have developed over the years on initiating and maintaining breastfeeding, the importance of exclusive breastfeeding and how to achieve it, breast care including how to avoid and resolve postpartum engorgement, and resolve sore nipples, blocked ducts and mastitis, how to increase or decrease breastmilk production, home pasteurisation of breastmilk, and lactation suppression for use during elective or recommended weaning.

I suggest that the mother reads the resources on the list and comes back to me with questions or comments so that we can fully discuss any points that seem unclear. I encourage her to share whatever I send with her doctors. It's important that everyone is on the same page and that all healthcare providers are happy to support the mother in her ambition to breastfeed. I always offer to be available to answer questions from any member of the mother's healthcare team.

4. Mother to discuss her wish to breastfeed with her healthcare team

I strongly suggest that the mother then discuss her wishes and plans, and share information from the resource list, with:

- her HIV clinicians
- her obstetrician
- her paediatrician
- the midwives, and hospital/maternity staff who will be delivering the baby at home or in the hospital

Ideally, these discussions will take place well in advance of the baby's due date. We all have the same goal – the best health of the mother and her baby – and it's very helpful if all concerns are discussed and resolved before the birth. It's crucial too that everyone providing any care to the mother or the baby is working together as a multidisciplinary team, and that neither they nor the mother have to deal with any surprises or uncertainty about the mother's wish to breastfeed the baby from birth and throughout the first few days and weeks. It may be helpful if the mother can obtain written guidance/permission about breastfeeding from her HIV consultant (usually the healthcare provider who correlates the different aspects of care of mother and baby) and if all other members of the team have copies in advance. Written birth and breastfeeding plans in the records of the right members of the healthcare team will be helpful in reducing the chance of misunderstandings later.

Mothers typically say that they make a prenatal appointment with their consultant and that it may take a good couple of hours to go through all the questions and concerns. The HIV consultant may then smooth the way with the other members of the healthcare team, and may also put in place orders for HIV tests for the baby, and viral load tests for the mother, so that the health of both mother and baby can be monitored very carefully, and so that everyone can be reassured and prompt action can be taken should there be any unexpected results. Planning appointments for all these tests, well in advance, can be very worthwhile.

5. Need for legal representation?

Things should not go wrong if the mother already has the help and support of her healthcare team as set out above, but misunderstandings due to staff turnover can arise; e.g. the new midwife, the stand-in health visitor, or someone else who has not been involved in the mother's planning right from the beginning. In the past I have sometimes felt the need to suggest to my clients that they might like to explore in advance of the birth whether they are likely to need protection from those who may think they have a duty to apply safeguarding standards to 'protect' the baby from breastfeeding by an HIV-positive mother. In view of the ambiguous nature of some of the HIV and infant feeding guidelines, or misinterpretation of the guidance, and in view of some of the case histories that have been reported, mothers might consider retaining a solicitor for legal advice and representation before the birth. The legal advisor must be happy to make an urgent hospital visit if necessary. I have sometimes found a legal advisor for the mother myself. Hopefully their services will not be required, but I feel better being prepared.

6. Be ready to supply additional information

It's helpful if the IBCLC or counsellor can be ready to supply the healthcare team with any other documentation or references should they be requested. As her due date nears it's also helpful for the mother to receive specific information about how to manage breastfeeding and breastmilk production in the first days and weeks of breastfeeding. I make sure that I send or resend information sheets on why exclusive breastfeeding is so important, how to achieve exclusive breastfeeding (lactation management techniques like preventing engorgement) and how to suppress lactation should this be necessary.

7. Specific help with positioning and attachment, initiating and maintaining breastfeeding

The mother may need videos or other teaching aids showing how to attach the baby to the breast. I usually ask her if she would like a referral to an experienced IBCLC near her who can make a home visit to provide practical assistance with latching the baby to the breast if necessary, though hopefully hospital staff will have already covered this. It's important that anyone who provides assistance is skilled in latching babies, and that they will not suggest tongue-tie surgery or any procedure which would cause bleeding or damage to the baby's oral anatomy. The lactation consultant should also be familiar with helping mothers exclusively breastfeed since any supplementation at all would compromise breastfeeding: i.e. the baby needs to either be exclusively breastfed, *or* exclusively formula-fed. If formula is really necessary then using home-pasteurised breastmilk in place of breastfeeding direct will avoid any risk of mixed feeding. This might need to be continued for three weeks after formula supplementation has ended (see Christina's story).

8. Be available for ongoing help and follow-up

I expect to provide ongoing assistance and answers to questions for as long as the mother will be breastfeeding, whether that is days, weeks, six months or even a couple of years. A mother with HIV will have exactly the same questions and concerns as any other mother, but with the added underlying consideration that any breastfeeding before six months must be exclusive. While nipple problems and breast pathologies need to be prevented and avoided for all mothers, there is an extra urgency if a mother has HIV; if they do occur, they need to be minimised and treated very promptly. There is always the possibility that the mother might need to feed her own pasteurised breastmilk if there is nipple damage or a breast infection.

I leave the mother with my contact details so that she can contact me any time of the day or night in the first few days as she works to establish breastfeeding. I urge her to call me for a small concern immediately, rather than leaving it until it turns into a bigger problem. This can be invaluable when something unexpected happens so that she can receive help and the opportunity to brainstorm about a way around the difficulty. I expect to be available to answer large and small questions from the time the mother contacts me until the baby is weaned from the breast. In almost all respects this is the care that we would provide to any mother-baby pair. For a mother with HIV everything is that tiny bit more complicated. I expect to share with my client anything relevant to her situation from the latest papers on HIV and breastfeeding. From the mother I like to be kept up to date with the baby's weight gain to assess that exclusive breastfeeding is going well, and to suggest interventions if there are questions. I also like to have viral load and HIV test results for her and her baby, so that I can note them on her records together with any medical advice she receives, and her clinicians' opinions about her continued breastfeeding. For an HIV-positive mother there may be special considerations around confidentiality; some mothers may not wish their GPs or even family members to know their HIV status.

9. Weaning

A mother with HIV is likely to wean her baby from the breast earlier than normal. She may also need to wean her baby before she would really wish, but her first concern will be to keep her baby safe and free from the virus. Hopefully she will make the decision about the best time to wean with her HIV clinician and healthcare providers. My protocol on cessation of breastfeeding is based on expressing or pumping to comfort as often as necessary, leaving the breasts just a little over-full, until no more breastmilk is being produced. It usually takes about two weeks. It is especially necessary that an HIV-positive mother does not put herself at risk for mastitis, and that she is able to access prompt medical care, as well as help with good lactation management if she experiences any symptoms. She may also appreciate information about weaning grief and extra support as she goes through this process. I like a last infant HIV test result for my own peace of mind and to be able to celebrate this special mother's very significant accomplishment.

10. Helping a mother meet her goals

It's not an easy thing to negotiate the roadblocks to breastfeeding with HIV, and the mother who is determined to do it and succeeds will be justly proud all her life of what she has accomplished. For the lactation consultant, working in such a situation can be a very intense experience. Few scenarios can be more professionally challenging than being invited to assist an HIV-positive mother to succeed in breastfeeding her baby – something that has often been a long-held ambition – when so many obstacles are put in her way. When she succeeds, few situations are more rewarding.

Additional Reading:

- Morrison P, Back to the Future on HIV and Breastfeeding; the findings that transformed policy. Powerpoint from GOLD 2013 online conference, available at www.hivbreastfeeding.org
- Morrison P, Practice Update: HIV and breastfeeding, Essentially MIDIRS, August 2014;5(7):38-9, available at page 38, http://www.midirs.org/em-aug2014-worldbreastfeedingweek/
- Morrison P and Faulkner Z, HIV and breastfeeding: the unfolding evidence, Essentially MIDIRS, Dec/Jan 2015;5(11):7-13, https://www.midirs.org/wp-content/uploads/2014/12/272-MID-EM-December-2014-p7-12.pdf
- Morrison P, Should HIV+ mothers breastfeed? Women's Health Today blog, January 2018 https://womenshealthtoday.blog/2018/01/25/should-hiv-mothers-breastfeed/
- Morrison P, What HIV-positive women want to know about breastfeeding, World AIDS Day 2013 issue of Fresh Start, Trinidad & Tobago, 1 December 2013, available at http://issuu.com/freshstartbybeststart/docs/fresh_start_supplement_final (see pages 8-12)

- Morrison P, Israel-Ballard K, Greiner T, Informed choice in infant feeding decisions can be supported for HIV-infected women even in industrialized countries, AIDS 2011, 25:18071811 e-pub ahead of print AIDS, 1 August 2011, final version 24 September 2011, PMID: 21811145 http://www.ncbi.nlm.nih.gov/pubmed/21811145
- Morrison P. Breastfeeding for HIV-Positive Mothers, Breastfeeding Today, Nov 2014, republished on La Leche League International Website Nov 2018 https://www.llli.org/breastfeeding-for-hiv-positive-mothers/
- WABA 2018 Updated HIV and WABA 2018 Updated HIV and breastfeeding Kit, six modules, available at www.hivbreastfeeding.org (NB Unfortunately the AAP guidance mentioned in (1) above has been omitted from this set of documents; this decision was taken by the reviewers and without the knowledge of the authors of the papers.)
- Young SL, Mbuya MNN, Chantry CJ, Geubbels EP, Israel-Ballard K, Cohan D, Vosti SA and Latham MC,Current Knowledge and Future Research on Infant Feeding in the Context of HIV: Basic, Clinical, Behavioral, and Programmatic, Adv. Nutr 2011;2: 225–243, doi:10.3945/an.110.000224 available at http://www.ncbi.nlm.nih.gov/pmc/articles/PMC3090166/ (accessed 26 Oct 2019)
- Morrison P, Update on HIV and breastfeeding, Leader Today LLLI, link, 4 Apr 2019 https://www.llli.org/update-on-hiv-and-breastfeeding-public/?fbclid=IwAR2aJPJE8cYK4fFLFy5anEOokFQSM9nQppMHzVaYwVpQILs_v1uRdwv3vvw (accessed 5 April 2019)
- Doula UK, Case study on HIV and breastfeeding in N. Ireland (my case) https://doula.org.uk/hiv-breastfeeding-case-study/
- Gross M et al, Breastfeeding HIV, Evidence for new policy, J Law, Med & Ethics 2019 https://journals.sagepub.com/doi/abs/10.1177/1073110519840495 (accessed 29 Aug 2019)
- Well Project, Breastfeeding and HIV in the Era of U=U; Research Policy and Lived Experiences, US Conference on AIDS, Sept 6, 2019 https://www.thewellproject.org/news-press/breastfeeding-and-hiv-era-uu-highlights-growing-discussion (accessed 15 November 2020)

National & International recommendations:

- WHO 2010, Guidelines on HIV and infant feeding. Principles and recommendations for infant feeding in the context of HIV and a summary of evidence, ISBN 978 92 4 159953 5 available at http://whqlibdoc.who.int/publications/2010/9789241599535_eng.pdf
- WHO-UNICEF 2016, Guideline: Updates on HIV and Infant Feeding, http://apps.who.int/iris/bitstream/10665/246260/1/9789241549707-eng.pdf
- WHO 2016, Consolidated guidelines on the use of antiretroviral drugs for treating and preventing HIV infection: recommendations for a public health approach – 2nd ed. ISBN 978 92 4 154968 4 available at http://www.who.int/hiv/pub/arv/arv-2016/en/
- Morrison P, History of HIV & Infant Feeding policy development in UK for World Breastfeeding Trends Initiative, 18 March 2016. (attachment) and WBTi Blog, Part II on HIV and breastfeeding, 4 Jan 2019
- American Academy of Pediatrics Infant Feeding and Transmission of HIV in the US http://pediatrics.aappublications.org/content/131/2/391
- British HIV Association guidelines for the management of HIV in pregnancy and postpartum 2018 (2019 interim update) https://www.bhiva.org/file/5bfd30be95deb/BHIVA-guidelines-for-the-management-of-HIV-in-pregnancy.pdf (accessed 18 January 2020) Section 9.4 Infant feeding, page 88 onwards
- BHIVA HIV and breastfeeding your baby https://www.bhiva.org/file/5bfd3080d2027/BF-Leaflet-1.pdf NB Breastfeeding management information in Leaflet 1 is poor, suggest seek additional input from an IBCLC.
- BHIVA General info on infant feeding https://www.bhiva.org/file/5bfd308d5e189/BF-Leaflet-2.pdf
- LCGB website HIV and breastfeeding page (concise recommendations) https://www.lcgb.org/resources/hiv-breastfeeding/

CHAPTER 29

Advocacy, politics, spillover and lessons learned

HIV has always been a political hot potato. The early response to the HIV epidemic in the industrialised world was one of 'denial, blame and punishment'[1] and in many ways, much of the early stigma surrounding HIV infection has persisted.

Of the early pandemic, WHO describes how:

> *'Leading political figures carefully avoided even mentioning the word AIDS, while those infected were subjected to an appalling series of discriminatory and stigmatizing actions by many people, including members of the health care profession and the judiciary who were charged with protecting the human and civil rights of everyone. HIV-infected children were barred from schools, while HIV-infected adults were dismissed from their jobs, thrown out of their apartments, excluded from serving in the military, segregated within prisons and prevented from immigrating or even visiting many countries. Some were even targets of serious physical violence.... The disinterest and inaction displayed by governments and entire societies bordered on criminal negligence.'*

As breastfeeding experts today work to counter old prejudices about the risks of breastfeeding in the context of a new disease, Covid-19,[2] they are often reminded of the lessons learned regarding breastfeeding in the context of HIV; there are several parallels.

The politics of HIV and breastfeeding

Once breastfeeding was known to be a vector of HIV transmission from mother to child, it effectively became an endangered practice. The breastfeeding movement has been lucky to have some extremely passionate and dedicated allies within its ranks, but the perceived risk of HIV transmission, and the exaggeration of that risk, has created ongoing problems. Milk banking worldwide was seriously affected, as was the Baby Friendly Hospital Initiative. The formula industry justified more aggressive marketing of its products because of HIV. Endorsement of formula-feeding as a safe feeding method and free distribution by UNICEF provided the seal of approval for mothers in developing countries and we live with the consequences today.

The struggle to preserve breastfeeding in the face of HIV has revealed unexpected instances of personal prejudice and institutional neglect, often by the very organisations and people who had previously championed breastfeeding – those who should have known how important breastfeeding was to child survival. As the world faces another pandemic due to Covid-19, there are lessons to be learned from the story of HIV and breastfeeding. Fearing the consequences of mismanagement of lactation and suspension of breastfeeding due to infection of mothers or babies with Coronavirus, which they at first worried might turn out to be just as serious as those posed by HIV, colleagues have shown a renewed interest in the successes achieved in policy and management of breastfeeding in the context of HIV. What we have learned about viruses, viral load and PCR testing and immunological properties of breastmilk while monitoring HIV has helped us to more readily understand and respond to Covid-19 and especially to question prohibitions against breastfeeding.

Advocacy by the breastfeeding community

We are fortunate today to be able to build on lessons from the past. After I had been contacted by my first HIV-positive client in 1995, I became aware of the alarming lack of guidance about breastfeeding with HIV. Apart from the 1985 US and European recommendations for formula-feeding, there was very little to go on. No professional association had weighed in to the debate. The research was patchy and hard to find. So, for my own use, I started searching the medical journals and collecting all the small snippets of information I could find. In response to a request for information from La Leche League South Africa in 1998, I sent them my file, and they invited me to speak at their annual conference in Johannesburg later that year. Virginia Thorley, another invited speaker from Australia, submitted my presentation to *Breastfeeding Review*, which published it,[3,4] and so began my role in advocating internationally to preserve breastfeeding in the face of HIV.

AnotherLook

Early in 2000 Marian Tompson, one of the original mothers who had founded La Leche League International in 1956, gathered together a group of people who were especially interested in breastfeeding and HIV. Marion had been quietly talking to researchers, and keeping records of health outcomes for American HIV-positive mothers who, notwithstanding the pressure to formula-feed, were actually breastfeeding their babies. In some cases, the attitude of policymakers and health authorities in North America and Europe bordered on persecution and some of these women had gone underground.

With the goal of revisiting some of the misinformation surrounding the subject, Marian named the new group AnotherLook. As the PMTCT pilot sites in developing countries were being scaled up, breastfeeding was becoming ever more marginalised and I was thrilled to be invited to join the new group. The AnotherLook membership comprised activists, researchers, doctors, La Leche League Leaders, IBCLCs, nutritionists, a political scientist, a virologist, a paediatrician, an HIV-positive mother and even one or two AIDS denialists. Our diversity was part of our strength, and we communicated via email because we were truly international, being scattered around the world in southern Africa, the Caribbean, the US, Canada, Asia and Europe. It was rare that we all agreed on everything, but under Marian's leadership we searched and researched, reviewed and discussed, collaborated and co-operated, debated, drafted and edited. We examined in minute detail any research which apparently showed that breastfeeding caused HIV in infants. We picked apart how researchers defined breastfeeding. We looked at their backgrounds and possible conflicts of interest. We scrutinised how and when HIV infection in infants was determined, and what distinguished infection through breastfeeding from infection during pregnancy, labour or birth, as a result of hospital or medical procedures, or even through pre-chewed food.

Working singly or in groups, we wrote many articles and submitted them to the major medical journals: the *Lancet*,[5] the *British Medical Journal*,[6] the *Bulletin of the World Health Organization*,[7] *Breastfeeding Abstracts*,[8] the *Journal of Human Lactation*,[9–12] *Health Care for Women International* (Canada)[13], *MIDIRS* (UK)[14,15] *AIDS*,[16] the *Journal of the American Medical Association*,[17] *Pediatrics*, the *Archives of Pediatric & Adolescent Medicine*,[18] *PloS Medicine*,[19] the *Journal of Acquired Immune Deficiency Syndrome*,[20] the *Australian Lactation Resource Centre Topics in Breastfeeding*,[21] the *Journal of Lactation Consultants of Great Britain*,[22] *AIDSTAR-One for USAID/PEPFAR*,[23] *Fresh Start* in Trinidad,[24] *Breastfeeding Today*,[25]and WBTi in Pakistan.[26]

We gave radio and television interviews in the USA, Canada, Zimbabwe and Trinidad and Tobago. Marian had meetings and interviews with some of the most respected HIV experts in the world. In her autobiography[27] she writes, 'During those first two years, I met with researchers at Georgetown University Medical, the National Institutes of Health, the FDA, congressional aides, and directors of government agencies. I met and talked with former president Jimmy Carter....' Marian also participated in roundtable discussions at the American Public Health Association Annual meeting, and gave presentations at Breastfeeding Coalition conferences hosted by the United States Breastfeeding Committee. She spoke at LLL-hosted health provider seminars in many different countries. AnotherLook members also presented at conferences and seminars for breastfeeding counsellors, lactation professionals, doctors and nursing staff in North America,[28–30] South Africa,[31] Australia,[32–36] Trinidad,[37] Canada,[38,39] Malaysia,[40] Spain,[41,42] England,[43–46] and at online webinars hosted from Australia,[47–49] Canada,[50] and Hong Kong.[51] Following the WHO's about-turn in 2010 to once again support breastfeeding by HIV-positive mothers, AnotherLook became less active, but members remain in touch, and still share concerns, resources and news, particularly in view of the new risks to breastfeeding promotion posed by Covid-19.

The WABA-UNICEF HIV Colloquium

In 2002 Ted Greiner, who had been a prominent member of the breastfeeding movement for several decades, co-ordinated a WABA-UNICEF HIV Colloquium in Arusha, Tanzania.[52] This was the first international meeting to bring together specialists from the breastfeeding movement and experts on HIV. Ted, with his former professor, Michael Latham, had begun setting the scene for this event, meeting and talking with UNICEF friends, several years before. His main hope was that bringing these two organisations together would improve collaboration, and that the AIDS community would be more willing in the future to include input from the breastfeeding community.[53] At the Colloquium he said:

> *'Policy formulation, research and program implementation related to HIV and infant feeding have so far failed adequately to involve persons and organisations with breastfeeding expertise. The NGOs have watched in frustration as policy, research and program activities have ignored good practice and lessons learned from the past. In the best case this has resulted in a lot of 'reinventing the wheel'. It is likely that it has also resulted in a good deal of unnecessary human suffering and perhaps death. This oversight needs to be redressed as soon as possible...[including] the interesting question of why the UN policy had to be changed in 1997. Obviously the arguments used, that a more equitable and human rights approach was needed, somehow only applied to [the developing world]. The NGOs have always been concerned about the role of industry in the background.'*

There were some excellent presentations by UNICEF and UNAIDS personnel such as Connie Osborne and David Clark, as well as by friends in the breastfeeding community, Peter Iliff of ZVITAMBO, Ellen Piwoz of LINKAGES and other activists and advocates. Discussions focused on assessment of risk of HIV transmission through breastfeeding versus the risk of not breastfeeding at all. The outcome of interest was overall infant health and survival, not just levels of HIV transmission. It would be many years before HIV-free survival was endorsed as the major goal of PMTCT initiatives, but the Arusha event in 2002 may have been where it was first raised.

Stephen Lewis, the UN Special Envoy for HIV/AIDS in Africa, who subsequently headed the UN agency for women, noted in his keynote address the tragic consequences of the epidemic on women:[54]

> *'There has never been in modern history, such a horror story, around a communicable disease, for women. It's as though Darwin had said natural selection doesn't address the survival of the fittest, it addresses the elimination of an entire gender. It seems to me that that's the backdrop for this conference – the extraordinary vulnerability and unbelievable decimation of women across the continent. I want to point out to you that the world has watched this unfold for the last several years and has barely raised a finger... When I was leaving UNICEF in 1999, ...we were talking about questions of infant feeding and replacement feeding. There were people in UNICEF – all males, every one of them – who argued determinedly that UNICEF should turn itself over to formula feeding – that UNICEF should understand that the evidence that was coming in about the transmission of the virus through breast milk meant that we had to abandon the commitment to breastfeeding that we had had for years. Formula feeding had to be embraced; that it would be the end of the organisation if we didn't tell women what to do – and that became the ultimate expression of the argument: women should not so much be counselled and given information, but they should be told explicitly what to do.'*

Stephen Lewis ended with some advice:

> *'It's terribly important, I think, that WABA, in a respectful but determined way, launches criticism, even of its friends. UNICEF should feel distinctly uncomfortable with WABA on occasions – sure WABA can partner with UNICEF, I partnered with UNICEF, they're nice people. But it doesn't mean that you can't take issue with them on occasion, as it doesn't mean you can't take issue with the UN generally... I do want to encourage you to feel that circumstance should not stop you from what you are doing. You are fighting for the survival of women and infants, recognising the excruciating dimension of HIV transmission, addressing it in a sophisticated, knowledgeable and sympathetic way...'*

In 2004 Ted coordinated another WABA workshop on HIV and breastfeeding in Zambia.[55] I was sad not to be able to attend this one. Participants brainstormed, mapped out areas of concern and made plans for development of future resources and advocacy. They also visited PMTCT programme sites to get first-hand information, and were able to confirm that the records being kept by UN employed nurses did not reflect what was really happening on the ground where in fact a substantial proportion of babies fed free formula, especially when started from birth, had died.

In May 2006, Dr Penny van Esterik coordinated a WABA/York University workshop in Toronto, entitled 'Gender, Child Survival and HIV/AIDS; From evidence to policy'.[56] WABA believed it was important to enhance cooperation between women's groups on the issue of HIV and breastfeeding. Penny, as a long-time expert in politics and breastfeeding, had also been involved in WABA activities for many years. She observed:

> *'Each shift in framework provided new ways to understand the disease. Blood and semen rather than breastmilk were of most interest. When attention focussed on semen as the carrier fluid, we learned a great deal from gay men's groups. When the circulating medium was blood, we learned from hemophiliac support groups. What gets revealed when we look at breastmilk as the carrier fluid? What new processes can be understood when we look at mothers who breastfeed in the context of HIV/AIDS and at breastfeeding support groups? How do the questions change? For example, why was replacement feeding supported as an intervention rather than exclusive breastfeeding, when it has long term survival benefits for infants? And how can groups working to support breastfeeding mothers further support the research and policy work of AIDS advocacy groups?'*

This was an intensely interesting and useful meeting for advocates of different groups to meet and find common ground.

I flew to Toronto again in August 2006, where Ted Greiner had coordinated a special PATH symposium on HIV and breastfeeding to be held during the course of the huge International AIDS Conference hosting 31,000 delegates from all around the world. I listened to Bill Gates and Bill Clinton, as well as Jerry Coovadia and many breastfeeding experts, as outlined in Chapter 21. The *New York Times* reported, 'in the only conference session dedicated to infant feeding and newborn nutrition, PATH senior nutritionist Ted Greiner and senior program officer Christina Kramer presented, with other experts, an examination of standing policies about HIV transmission and breastfeeding. PATH staff are leading the effort to act on new evidence that exclusive breastfeeding not only reduces HIV transmission, but also increases infant survival'.[57,58]

Not all plain sailing

While the breastfeeding movement had many successes, there were also setbacks. AnotherLook members worked for months on an examination of the Dunn meta-analysis which had quantified the risk of MTCT through breastfeeding at 14%.[59] The Dunn paper had been cited so often, yet 'breastfeeding' had been so poorly defined. Looking back, what happened to our paper typified the lack of transparency surrounding HIV and infant feeding that we repeatedly came up against. Since it was impossible to publish, we put it up on the AnotherLook website[60] with the legend:

> *'This paper has been submitted to Lancet (where the Dunn paper was originally published in 1992), the British Medical Journal in 2004 and the Journal of Human Lactation in 2005 and was rejected by all three. Lancet gave no reasons. BMJ sent the paper for review to a scientist with significant financial conflicts of interest with the formula industry. That reviewer implied that the Nduati studies from Kenya had largely supplanted Dunn, a contention we challenge here and in a letter published in JAMA. The JHL reviewer recommended against publication because the Dunn paper is so old. They noted that there is newer research, but only provided two citations for conference abstracts, not fully documented peer-reviewed papers, and one mathematical model, which is of course fully dependent on various assumptions, some of which we question.'*

My professional association, the International Lactation Consultant Association, had adopted wording in their first position paper on HIV and infant feeding, dated 2002, which appeared to have been lifted directly from the UNAIDS guidance promoting replacement feeding. My efforts to have this changed met with no success whatsoever. One prominent ILCA member frankly judged my criticism as 'not appropriate', and another promised that if I stopped complaining, she would use her influence to get the board to revisit it. It never happened.

Three years later, as part of a WABA-ILCA collaboration, I was invited to submit a paper on HIV and infant feeding to ILCA's professional publication, the *Journal of Human Lactation*. I worked on it for months. Somewhere after draft 11 I realised that as fast as I addressed one objection, a different reviewer would raise another. My wording was described as 'too judgemental'. In withdrawing my submission, I responded,

> *'During March and April I spent 5 weeks in Penang to work with WABA on HIV and infant feeding and while there I had the opportunity to access more information in the area of how the research on HIV and infant feeding is applied in the PMTCT sites, the difficulties experienced by counsellors, and the constraints of achieving safe and sustainable formula-feeding in resource-poor settings, etc. It is difficult to lay out the facts without sounding judgemental, even if the intention is to be objective, e.g. that less*

than 10% of HIV+ mothers receive antiretroviral therapy or any intervention other than HIV and infant feeding counselling, that the evidence base for safe replacement feeding in developing countries of high HIV prevalance simply does not exist, or that mortality rates for non-breastfed HIV-exposed babies are not in the public domain, that at some sites mothers run out of formula, that formula may take up 60% of PMTCT budgets...'

In 2006, I was able to provide input into a revised ILCA Position Paper, which has since become out of date, and by 2021 has not been replaced. In 2015 the ILCA Board invited me, with my colleague Penny Reimers, who had had many years' experience working on the front line with Professor Anna Coutsoudis in South Africa, to draft a new Position Paper on HIV and infant feeding. Penny and I put together a document which eventually ran to 22 drafts, setting out the current research and then incorporating all the concerns that the board and reviewers submitted over several months. Eventually, however, our work turned out to have been in vain. ILCA advised that they would simply not be publishing any more position papers, either ours on HIV or others on the use of donor milk, safe sleep and infant feeding in emergencies. These were all contentious issues on which ILCA members who work daily with breastfeeding mothers would have appreciated clear guidance, but it seemed that the board were worried about liability. They explained, 'While we all agree that ILCA should be leaders in understanding and disseminating knowledge about lactation, there is an understanding that it is not the place of ILCA to make medical recommendations that go beyond lactation knowledge, particularly recommendations that may differ from the recommendations of the medical authorities in some countries.' We agreed. We had been careful not to give medical advice, but to recommend that HIV-positive mothers share information received from their lactation consultants with their medical doctors. Ironically, the then president of ILCA recently wrote, 'The scarcity of research and counseling guidelines regarding infant feeding, coupled with an increasing awareness from [healthcare professionals] that [women living with HIV] in high income countries may want to breastfeed, is at best concerning and at worst a potential breach of ethical responsibility on the part of healthcare professionals.'[61]

Inexplicably, WABA too sometimes appeared to be reluctant to advocate for breastfeeding and HIV. After initial enthusiasm, there was sometimes unexpected withdrawal of support for various projects. People would spend months or even years putting together a plan only to find that it was abandoned at a critical point, or even that their appointment had been reversed, thus missing opportunities to collaborate and work with researchers and organisations that could have taken the breastfeeding and HIV agenda forward.

WABA had employed me as a consultant on HIV and infant feeding in 2005. My first task had been to compile up-to-date information, not only to inform a revision of the existing ILCA position paper, but also to produce a set of documents for a WABA HIV Kit. I worked from home in England and travelled to Penang several times a year to spend time at the secretariat, to update and brainstorm, and network with those attending the Global Partners' Forum. It was intensely interesting work. I loved everything about my job and really enjoyed working with the WABA folk in the office. After much research, taking many opinions and incorporating multiple recommendations from WABA allies around the world, the first version of the HIV Kit was ready for review in May 2007. And there it sat for the next year and a half. Eventually I learned that the Kit was to be rewritten by someone else. To be sure, my current version had questioned UNICEF and WHO policy promoting replacement feeding in developing countries, and I was told, 'We *must* agree with WHO.' Ironically, if the 2007 version had been published it would have shown that we had come up with the same recommendations as WHO (exclusive breastfeeding with ART) a full two years before the WHO 2009 Rapid Advice was issued. I suspected that this was the very problem; Felicity Savage, a prominent WABA member of the Steering Committee, was also a consultant to WHO, and perhaps WABA could not be seen to pip them at the post.

Success in the global north

In 2009 I was invited to make a submission to Lord Avebury, a member of the British Parliamentary Select Committee on HIV/AIDS and the House of Lords (see Chapter 26). My report was passed to the Secretary of State for Health, before going forward to a joint committee of the British HIV Association and the Expert Advisory Group on AIDS to inform and update national HIV and infant feeding advice. In 2010 the revised national policy was released giving details of how HIV+ mothers who wished to breastfeed their babies should be supported to do so.[62] In 2013 the American Academy of Pediatrics released an almost identical guidance paper.[63] Similar guidance from the authorities in Germany and Austria, and Switzerland, has been subsequently issued.[64] Finally, HIV-positive mothers in the global north could breastfeed without fear.

In 2011, I learned that the WABA HIV Kit was still not finished, and now the situation had completely changed since WHO now promoted exclusive breastfeeding with maternal ART. I offered to work on it again, and finally it was published in time for World AIDS Day in 2012. In 2017, I began work on a further update, this time helped by a Brazilian colleague, Regina da Silva. The Kit was given a final review by colleagues at the Academy of Breastfeeding Medicine, an American organisation for doctors with special expertise in lactation and breastfeeding. The final updated version was published in July 2018.[65] But there was still one last glitch. A few days later, Regina and I noticed that the American Academy of Pediatrics recommendations allowing for breastfeeding with HIV,[63] which we had carefully included, had simply quietly been deleted from the text. Upon enquiry, the WABA secretariat explained:

> *'As we went through the kit with ABM, the text in section 4 that you are referring to was taken out to avoid more confusion. Although the AAP policy statement (2013) is quite clear that '**Therefore, in the United States, where there is access to clean water and affordable replacement feeding, the AAP continues to recommend complete avoidance of breastfeeding as the best and safest infant feeding option for HIV-infected mothers, regardless of maternal viral load and antiretroviral therapy**', there appear to be discussions within the US on this topic. For now, we will leave it at that. The main focus is anyhow on the WHO/UNICEF guidance.'*

It's unclear why WABA would have gone along with an American doctors' organisation's wish to exclude support for breastfeeding with HIV when the American Academy of Pediatrics had already endorsed it. The attitude seemed to be that this was a topic that was behind us now and we needed to move on. In late 2018 another of the WABA consultants who had been asked to update a very useful and beautifully put together resource book let me know that she had been instructed in her rewrite to omit the whole section on HIV because it was 'no longer relevant'.[66] My colleague had refused, and the idea of the update had been dropped.

Different advice for developed and developing countries

When WHO reversed its position so that it would once again support breastfeeding in the context of HIV, the breastfeeding movement was overjoyed. There was only one aspect which worried us; there seemed to be a double standard between recommendations for breastfeeding with ART in the global south compared with recommendations for formula-feeding in the global north: 'National health authorities are encouraged by WHO to identify the most appropriate infant feeding practice (*either* breastfeeding with ARVs *or* the use of infant formula) for their communities. The selected practice should then be promoted as the *single standard of care*.'[67] Did this mean that the industrialised countries would still effectively prohibit breastfeeding by HIV-positive mothers? Or did we dare hope that HIV-positive mothers in England, the US or Europe would be permitted to 'breastfeed with ARVs'? It seemed that 'the use of infant formula as the single standard of care' was intended for countries where formula was seen to be safe. It was hard to ignore the double standard that breastfeeding was considered to be criminal when posing a higher risk but that advising, facilitating (via free formula) and even pressuring a mother into bottle-feeding, even when it clearly results in the child's death, was not associated with the slightest hint of professional malfeasance.[68]

Politics and pressure

The Rapid Advice also retained anomalies in the quantification of risk of HIV transmission through breastfeeding. A rather high risk estimate of 5% had been taken from the WHO-supported Kesho Bora studies. The Kesho Bora mothers had followed HIV and infant feeding protocols designed in 2005, breastfeeding exclusivity had been low, and duration had been short, with predictably disappointing results. Of concern, WHO had ignored research showing the very reduced risk of postpartum transmission with exclusive breastfeeding and antiretroviral therapy for either mother or baby. There had been at least 10 known study results released between 2003 and 2009 (when the Rapid Advice meetings were held) which had achieved better outcomes, with results ranging in descending order of risk from 3%[69] down through 1.8%[70] 1.2%,[71] two at 1.1%,[72,73] 1%,[74] 0.8%,[75] 0.6%,[76] 0.4%,[77] and 0.3%,[78] right down to 0%.[79] The Americans were aware of these good numbers; during 2009, I had completed work for USAID/PEPFAR/AIDSTAR-One, on a table identifying them.[80] The results were known by the time that WHO compiled the data for its Rapid Advice. By omitting them were they seeking to exaggerate the fear of HIV transmission through breastfeeding? This omission seemed reminiscent of when WHO excluded the 1999 Coutsoudis exclusive breastfeeding results[81,82] from the 2000 WHO policy documents.

The possibility of HIV-positive mothers providing heat-treated expressed breastmilk to their babies, in preference to formula, was also negatively described in the Rapid Advice, the assertion being that the research had not been done. It had. The extensive research by Kiersten Israel-Ballard and Caroline Chantry is thoroughly described in Chapter 11. I was an author of the first Chantry paper on heat treatment, published in 2000. I had also lobbied Helen Armstrong of UNICEF, sending her case histories documenting that breastmilk-feeding was possible. The negativity about heat-treated breastmilk seemed like another example of the way that information could be framed to fit a political narrative – in effect institutional prejudice being presented as evidence-based medical fact.

Selective application of the U=U principle

In treating health conditions there is always an acceptance of the risk-benefit ratio of various interventions. As discussed in Chapter 25, U=U is now accepted in almost every situation where HIV could be transmitted. If the infected partner has an undetectable viral load then the risk to the uninfected partner is considered to be negligible. This principle has recently even been extended to HIV-positive donors who wish to give blood to the Blood Transfusion Service.[83] Yet HIV-positive mothers who wish to breastfeed their babies still face stigma and exaggeration of the risk of transmission through breastmilk.

Promotion of formula-feeding

Over the years HIV and infant feeding policy has evolved dramatically. The late 1990s saw recommendations enacted allegedly on the basis of human rights, urging respect and support for mothers' (uninformed) infant feeding choices, in order to ensure that the feeding of breastmilk substitutes, or 'replacement feeding' as it was euphemistically called, would avoid postnatal transmission of HIV. Broadly speaking, endorsement of maternal choice to make formula-feeding possible was promoted in settings where breastfeeding was the norm, while prohibitions on breastfeeding were imposed in countries where most babies were formula-fed, thus favouring universal formula-feeding. That these guidelines had a political component cannot be ruled out; much of the breastfeeding advocacy literature acknowledges and describes unexpected commercial and economic influences driving infant feeding policy, and it is well-known that industry is permitted to provide input into national and international infant-feeding policy documents, in and out of the context of HIV. One breastfeeding advocate suggested that 'the early days of the AIDS crisis in the 1980s coincided with excess milk stores in the European Union, resulting from EU intervention policies to artificially raise the price of milk. The concept that the provision of infant formula might have a contribution in the fight against AIDS led to huge commercial efforts to enter African markets. Free samples were given and research was funded. Early research advised against breastfeeding thus providing European industries with an opportunity for an altruistic intervention which solved a European problem and extended European business.'[84]

Obstructive policies

The recent recommendation against breastfeeding with HIV, imposed two days after the national Covid-19 lockdown in March 2020, on the rationale that it would be too difficult or too unsafe for mothers and babies to attend hospitals or clinics for blood tests, is just one example of the manipulation of a national crisis to discourage breastfeeding. 'Insufficient data' sounds plausible and 'lost to follow-up' is a frequent refrain in studies everywhere looking at HIV transmission through breastfeeding. Recent reshuffling of government departments and reassignment of responsibility for who is tasked with collecting and sorting the data used for the Enhanced Surveillance Register on breastfeeding by HIV-positive mothers is another. Is political fall-out surrounding mishandling of the Covid-19 pandemic serving to obscure accountability for delivering this crucial information to both clinicians and mothers, preventing informed decision-making regarding breastfeeding with HIV?

Jargon

In the political minefield of HIV and breastfeeding, the use of jargon has often been used as a political tool to hide intent. Meaning is important and unclear terminology can be employed to either lull or alarm. Terms like 'replacement feeding' can soothe the general public into believing that this is simply an alternative type of feeding method being recommended for use by HIV-infected women. But these words can also act as a secret code understood perfectly by international agencies and charity donor organisations to mean infant formula, a commercially manufactured cows' milk-based substitute for mother's milk, which can profoundly and negatively affect the health and ultimately the survival of recipient babies and can swallow up large proportions of PMTCT budgets. Today the commonly used descriptions 'infant feeding' or 'infant and young child feeding' (IYCF) are defended as generic terms which include breastfeeding both babies and toddlers – and they also act as a smokescreen to hide what else we feed to infants and young children.

In the case of HIV, calls for confidentiality have often been used to maintain secrecy and sometimes even to mislead; for example the HIV-positive mother who is advised to tell her friends that she's bottle-feeding because she didn't have enough milk. Politically correct and misleading jargon has often been employed in the lactation field to maintain the personal or political agenda of the individuals, groups and organisations who use it. For many years, those promoting breastfeeding were discouraged from using the word 'breast' in case it offended anyone. More recently, the transgender movement in the global north, increasingly converging with Black activism, is demanding the use of 'inclusive' language – 'families' or 'lactating parents' in place of 'mothers', or 'chest-feeding' instead of 'breastfeeding'. Use of jargon in this context is especially confusing since it is African women in the global south who not only bear the heaviest burden of HIV, but who also place a high value on motherhood. They expect recognition of their role in conceiving, gestating, bearing and breastfeeding babies. In the HIV and infant-feeding literature, the very definition of 'breastfeeding' is already obscure; we need to insist on clarity in this context.

Spillover

'Spillover' is the term that describes the spread of artificial feeding among untested mothers who do not breastfeed, either from fear of HIV infection, or because bottle-feeding has been popularised. Provision of free formula in the PMTCT sites in developing countries normalised bottle-feeding even as it failed to record or publish mortality of non-breastfed babies.[85] Karen Moland and colleagues, writing in the *International Breastfeeding Journal* in 2010,[86] observed:

> *'It remains a legacy of the decade that the 2001 guidelines became extremely influential as they coincided with the large scale roll-out of the PMTCT programme, and were fundamental in the training of a generation of postnatal PMTCT counsellors. It is most probable that the ambiguous policy on breastfeeding launched in these guidelines will have long lasting repercussions for public health efforts on infant feeding in sub-Saharan Africa for years to come. It may take years for national programmes and health services to overcome the confusions created in the wake of the WHO's 2001 infant feeding recommendations.'*

These words were prophetic. Spillover from the policies and practices of the last 15 years will be hard to reverse. Spillover was first identified after the 2006 flooding in Botswana, when it was discovered that bottle-feeding rather than HIV infection caused most mortality.

South Africa probably has the highest spillover of formula-feeding in sub-Saharan Africa today. In the early 2000s, the PMTCT programme recommended replacement feeding for infants of women living with HIV, and provided free infant formula at public sector health facilities.[87] Owing to fears of HIV transmission, a decade-long suspension of support for breastfeeding in any public messaging began. Today's mothers would have been aware as they were growing up that government clinics were handing out free formula. They may have also incorrectly believed that formula-feeding was practised through choice, since – in order to avoid stigma and preserve confidentiality – HIV-positive mothers were counselled to lie about their reasons for not breastfeeding. In 2012, following the 2009–10 WHO about-turn in policy, the South African government ceased providing free infant formula and instead scaled up access to lifelong triple ART. However, it's not hard to see how spillover occurred and the implications are concerning. South Africa is the trend-setter for the rest of Africa, and what happens in the south eventually spreads north.

The very successful implementation of UN HIV and infant feeding recommendations has left a terrible legacy. Dr Chantell Witten, a prominent nutritionist in South Africa, conducted her doctoral studies on infant feeding in a typical low-income area burdened by high levels of unemployment, violence and crime, high rates of under-five mortality and stunting combined with poor living conditions, and low levels of social capital.[88] She found high rates of formula-feeding. Although mothers knew about the health benefits of breastfeeding for their infants, babies' crying, frequent breastfeeding and short sleep cycles would be interpreted and internalised as negative responses to their breastmilk. Stressed mothers were likely to turn to formula. Worldwide, formula-feeding is seen to liberate women from the demands of motherhood.[89] Yet formula is unaffordable for the majority of South African families: one-third live below the poverty line, and the cost can equate to the entire family income. Consequently, many mothers opt for mixed feeding and/or dilute the formula to make it stretch further. Keeping bottles clean is equally challenging since one-third of households don't have a safe source of drinking water in the home. Gastroenteritis (9%) and lower respiratory tract infections (17%) continue to be leading causes of under-five mortality. Nearly one-third of pediatric hospital mortality in 2015 was due to acute malnutrition. Breastfeeding would have been protective against nearly all these deaths, yet sales of infant formula in South Africa expanded four-fold from 2003 to 2018, reaching Rand 2 billion in 2018. Sales are projected to triple again by 2023.

Following patterns well known in the west, there is increasing social acceptance of the reasons mothers give for not breastfeeding. Spillover is perpetuated by human rights concepts imported from the global north and exploited by industry. In recent years the Nestlé Nutrition Institute has ramped up contact with health professionals, such as through nutrition symposia at universities in southern and eastern Africa,[90,91] in spite of the South African government's efforts, through the 2011 Tshwane Declaration, to provide renewed support for breastfeeding.[92] For a third-world country that practised almost universal breastfeeding two decades ago, positive attitudes towards formula-feeding have been easily and quickly assimilated. It will not be easy to put the genie back in the bottle.

Lessons learned

We've come a long way in the last 25 years. While the number of women with HIV who become pregnant every year has remained static since 1999 at 1.3 million, the number of new HIV infections in their babies has decreased by more than 60% from 450,000 to 160,000. The reduction in the number of babies infected by HIV is an unqualified success story. The only intervention for PMTCT in 2000 was counselling and provision of free formula; today ART and continued breastfeeding can save the lives of both the HIV-positive mother and her baby.

At the end of 2019 the world was hit by the Covid-19 pandemic. Breastfeeding advocates are already noting similarities in guidance about whether babies should be separated from Covid-19-infected mothers at birth, and indeed whether they should be breastfed. Before it could be properly researched, once again the initial reaction was that breastfeeding was risky.[93] To save lives, policymakers and medical personnel need to be mindful not to repeat the mistakes of the past.

The way forward

We haven't quite finished the work of advocacy for preserving breastfeeding in the face of HIV until mothers in the global north can receive the same kind of support for breastfeeding as those in the global south. If breastfeeding wasn't so important we could let it go, but it is, and we can't.

The struggle to defend and preserve breastfeeding through the threat posed by HIV has been daunting. Jean Humphrey, one of the researchers at the ZVITAMBO project in Harare, Zimbabwe, whose own research helped to confirmed the value of exclusive breastfeeding, revealed that, after all, the tragedy of the pandemic and the deaths of millions of babies may not have been in vain. Their legacy was to reveal on a huge *in vivo* scale the life-saving value of mother's milk, and the risks of *not* breastfeeding:[94]

> *'Ironically, the HIV epidemic may be the best thing that ever happened to breast-feeding. It is difficult to imagine an experiment that could provide more compelling momentum for breast-feeding promotion than the natural one the HIV epidemic has provided: an incurable disease that infects up to 30%–40% of antenatal women in some African countries and is transmitted to infants through breast-feeding leads UN agencies and governments to promote and even freely provide formula for exposed infants. Moreover, scores of these infants are already under surveillance by scientists measuring and documenting numerous indices of infant health. In short, the HIV epidemic and our efforts to ameliorate its effect on children provided an ethical opportunity to observe what happens when large number of infants living in conditions of poverty are not breast-fed. If these observations lead to stronger breast-feeding policy and programming that in turn reduce the 1.4 million child deaths occurring each year due to suboptimal breast-feeding, we will have created one of the epidemic's very few silver linings.'*

About the author

Pamela Morrison has been speaking and writing about breastfeeding and HIV since 1995. A former La Leche League Leader, in 1990 she became the first IBCLC in Zimbabwe, where she worked in private practice and served as a member of the Zimbabwe National Multi-sectoral Breastfeeding Committee, as a BFHI trainer and assessor, and assisted with development of national WHO Code legislation and HIV and breastfeeding policy. She was a consultant to the World Alliance for Breastfeeding Action, authoring the WABA publication, International Policy on HIV and Breastfeeding: a Comprehensive Resource.

Since 2005 she has lived and worked in private practice in the UK until her recent retirement. She continues to be active in advocating for mothers with HIV who wish to breastfeed their babies.

Acknowledgements

I'm grateful beyond words to the HIV-positive mothers and their babies who have contacted me through the years and shared with me their hopes and dreams, their challenges, fears, frustrations, and successes, as well as pictures of their beautiful healthy babies. I cannot thank you by name, but my admiration of your courage and gallantry knows no bounds.

I've been guided and helped on my quest to tell this story by the wonderful help and generosity of many special people. My grateful thanks are extended to all of you, and you know who you are, for sharing your thoughts, knowledge, expertise, experiences, papers, up-to-date research findings, reviews, published and yet-to-be published papers, and your own very valuable opinions.

Lastly I'm forever thankful to my husband Alan, and my sons Ian, Bryn and Shaun for the gift of mothering and breastfeeding. I loved it all so much that I turned it into a career.

Glossary

Abrupt weaning – immediate cessation of breastfeeding which may be forced on the infant by the mother or on the mother and infant by others.

AFASS – Acceptable, feasible, affordable, sustainable and safe – the conditions set out in the first years of WHO policies promoting the use of breastmilk substitutes for HIV-exposed babies.

AIDS – Acquired Immunodeficiency Syndrome: the active pathological condition that follows the earlier, non-symptomatic state of being HIV-positive.

Antiretroviral drugs (ARV) – the medicine used to treat HIV infection or prevent HIV transmission, including from mother to child or between sero-discordant couples; and to prevent people from acquiring HIV when they are exposed (post-exposure and pre-exposure prophylaxis).

Antiretroviral therapy (ART) – the use of a combination of two or three or more ARV drugs for treating HIV infection to reduce their viral load. ART involves lifelong treatment.

B cells –a type of lymphocyte of the immune system which make antibodies against antigens.

Breastmilk substitute – any food being marketed or otherwise represented as a partial or total replacement for breastmilk, whether or not suitable for that purpose.

CD4 cells (also known as T4 or helper T cells) – lymphocytes (a type of white blood cell), which are important in immune responses. These are the main target cells for HIV. Their numbers decrease during HIV infection, and their level is used as a marker of progression of the infection.

Cell-associated virus – HIV which lives inside the cell, measured as HIV DNA.

Cell-free virus – parts of the virus (virions) not associated with a cell, measured as HIV RNA.

Cessation of breastfeeding – completely stopping breastfeeding, which includes no more suckling at the breast.

Child – a child, usually aged 0–5 years.

Clade B HIV – the sub-group (clade) of the type of HIV (Group M) affecting men who have sex with men, and found in Europe and North America.

Clade C HIV – the sub-group (clade) of the most common type of HIV (Group M). It is the dominant form in southern Africa, eastern Africa, India, Nepal, and parts of China.

Cohort – group of subjects who have shared a particular event together during a particular time span, e.g. a research study.

Commercial infant formula – a product that meets the applicable Codex standard for being the sole source of nutrition for an infant.

Complementary food – any food, whether manufactured or locally prepared, used as a complement to breastmilk or to a breastmilk substitute, when additional nutrients are needed once an infant reaches six months of age.

Codex Alimentarius Standards – internationally recognised standards of food and food safety, developed by a Commission established by WHO and FAO.

Counselling – a type of talking therapy that allows a person to talk about their problems and feelings and be listened to with empathy in a confidential and dependable environment.

Cup feeding – feeding an infant or child using a cup.

DNA – a self-replicating material which is present in nearly all living organisms as the main constituent of chromosomes. It is the carrier of genetic information.

ELISA – an Enzyme Linked Immunosorbent Assay HIV test which identifies antibodies to HIV in an infected person's blood.

Epidemic – the occurrence of more cases of disease than expected in a given area or among a specific group of people over a particular period of time. In a generalised HIV epidemic**:** HIV is firmly established in the general population. HIV prevalence is consistently over 1% among pregnant women. Most generalised HIV epidemics are mixed in nature, where certain (key) subpopulations are disproportionately affected.

Ex vivo – outside the body

Exclusive breastfeeding – the infant receives only breastmilk without any other liquids or solids, not even water, except for oral rehydration solution or drops or syrups of vitamins, minerals or medicines. When expressed milk is given, the preferred term is exclusive breastmilk-feeding.

Failure-to-thrive (FTT) – a condition of malnutrition where a baby fails to gain sufficient weight for his age, most likely due to insufficient calorie intake, also described as **faltering growth** in the UK. Babies with FTT are more likely to fall prey to infections, and take longer to recover.

Formula-feeding – commercially manufactured infant milk that is formulated industrially in accordance with applicable Codex Alimentarius standards, usually based on cows' milk, but may also be made from goats' milk or soy proteins. **2nd on,**

Full breastfeeding – means exclusive *and* almost exclusive breastfeeding which means that no other liquid or solid from any other source enters the infant 's mouth, *or* that occasional tastes of other liquids, traditional foods, vitamins and/or medicines have been given.

GUM – genitourinary medicine, a clinic providing sexual and reproductive health services, often has overarching responsibility for the health care of an HIV+ woman and her baby in the UK.

HAART – Highly Active Antiretroviral Therapy – a combination of three or more different antiretroviral drugs given at the same time.

Healthcare worker – a person who is involved in the provision of health services to a user, including lay counsellors and community caregivers.

Heat-treating milk – heating or pasteurising milk on a stove or in a commercially manufactured pasteuriser to inactivate pathogens, e.g. bacteria and viruses.

HIV – the human immunodeficiency virus. There are two types of HIV: HIV-1 and HIV-2. The vast majority of people living with HIV infections globally have HIV-1. This text uses HIV to mean HIV-1.

HIV-exposed infant or child – an infant or child born to a mother living with HIV whose HIV status is unknown pending an HIV test.

HIV-free survival – describes the status of an infant or young child born to an HIV-infected mother who remains both HIV-uninfected (confirmed negative HIV status) and also has not died of other causes over a defined follow-up period, commonly reported at 18 months or 24 months of age. This concept has emerged as a consensus outcome to evaluate different prevention strategies.

HIVp24 antigen – a viral protein that makes up most of the viral core and which is present in the blood serum of newly infected individuals during the short period between infection and seroconversion, making p24 antigen assays useful in diagnosing primary HIV infection.

HIV-infected – people who are infected with HIV, whether or not they are aware of it, often written as HIV-positive or HIV+.

HIV-negative (HIV-) – refers to people who have had an HIV test and who know that they tested negative, or to young children who have tested negative.

HIV-positive (HIV+) – abbreviatiation commonly used to describe a person living with HIV who has had an HIV test and who knows that they tested positive, or to young children who have tested positive. Also written as HIV-infected.

HIV status unknown – people who either have not taken an HIV test or who have had a test but do not know the result. Sometimes written as HIV?

Human Immunodeficiency Virus (HIV) – a viral infection which destroys parts of the body's immune system, see HIV above.

In vitro – cultured in a laboratory

Intention to treat analysis – a method for analysing results in a prospective randomised study where all participants who are randomised are included in the statistical analysis and analysed according to the group they were originally assigned, regardless of what treatment (if any) they received.

International Board Certified Lactation Consultant (IBCLC) – a healthcare professional who specialises in the clinical management of breastfeeding and must recertify every five years either by exam or by continuing education. An IBCLC works in a wide variety of settings, to facilitate an optimal breastfeeding experience for mothers and babies. IBCLCs provide leadership, advocacy, professional development, and research in the lactation field. In 2021 there are approximately 33,500 IBCLCs practising in 125 countries around the world.

Lactogenic – a substance inducing the secretion of milk.

Low/high HIV prevalence – low HIV prevalence refers to settings with less than 5% prevalence in the population surveyed; high HIV prevalence refers to settings with 5% prevalence or more.

Infant – a baby less than 12 months of age.

Informed choice – receiving or acquiring sufficient information with which to reach a knowledgeable decision.

Mixed feeding – an infant younger than six months of age is given other liquids and/or foods together with breastmilk. This could be water, other types of milk or formula or any type of solid or ready-to-use therapeutic foods.

mm^3 – cubic millimetre, a unit of measurement to determine the amount of virus or the number of CD4 cells in the blood.

Mother-to-child transmission of HIV (MTCT) – also known as vertical transmission, parent-to-child transmission (PTCT), paediatric transmission or HIV-transmission to infants. MTCT is the term most often used for HIV transmission during pregnancy (prenatal), birth (perinatal) or breastfeeding (postnatal), because the immediate source of the child's HIV infection is the mother. Consensus on the use of one or other of these terms has not been reached. Some people advocate for use of terms which avoid the blame for infection seeming to be the responsibility of the mother alone, when she is likely to have been infected through unprotected sex with an infected partner, often the child's father.

NAT test – Nucleic acid testing technologies that are developed and validated for use at or near to be point of care that can be used for early infant HIV testing.

Neonate – an infant aged from birth to 28 days.

Non-consensual sex – sexual assault or rape.

Opportunistic infection – an infection that can infect people when their immune system is weakened, as with HIV infection, but not when they are healthy.

Option B+ – currently recommended, means immediate provision to HIV-infected women of antiretroviral drugs which are continued for life regardless of their CD4 count, to protect their own health and to prevent vertical transmission of the virus to their babies and their sexual partners.

Pandemic – an epidemic of infectious disease that has spread across a large region; for instance multiple continents, or even worldwide.

Parent to child transmission or PTCT – vertical transmission. This term is used to avoid the blame for infection seeming to be the responsibility of the mother alone, when she is likely to have been infected through unprotected sex with an infected partner, often the child's father. MTCT remains the most commonly used term, and may be more accurate, although consensus on the use of one or other of these terms has not been reached.

Paediatric HIV – HIV in children. This term is used in connection with the child's infection and illness, whatever the source and to recognise that not all children's infections come from the mother.

Partial breastfeeding – a baby is receiving some breastfeeds but is also being given other food or food-based fluids, such as formula milk or weaning foods.

PCR (Polymerase Chain Reaction) test – a type of test which can identify viral copies in the blood and other body fluids, including breastmilk.

Perinatal/perinatally – describes the period surrounding birth.

Perinatal transmission – defined as HIV transmission from mother to child during the very end of pregnancy, labour and delivery.

Person living with HIV – an individual who has tested HIV-positive on an HIV test.

Phylogeny – the study of evolutionary history and relationship between or among a group of species, to allow understanding how a species has evolved.

PMTCT – prevention of mother-to-child transmission, often used to describe preventive programmes.

Post-exposure prophylaxis (PEP) – the provision of ARVs to an individual who has potentially been exposed to HIV-infection in body fluids such as blood, bloodstained saliva, breastmilk, genital secretions, and cerebrospinal, amniotic, peritoneal, synovial, pericardial or pleural fluid. HIV PEP should be offered and initiated as early as possible in all individuals with an exposure that has the potential for HIV transmission, preferably within 72 hours.

Postnatal transmission – usually vertical transmission of HIV during the breastfeeding period, measured as occurring 4–6 weeks after birth until three months after weaning from the breast in a baby who is breastfed. Specifically, the infant must have had a negative HIV PCR test at birth and at 30 days of age, and then has either a positive PCR result or, if older than 18 months, shows a positive HIV antibody test result. Most postnatal transmission is through the breastmilk of a woman living with HIV, but this definition may also include accidental infection, such as through pre-masticated foods, an infected needle or through child sexual abuse.

Postnatal/postnatally – the period from birth to six weeks of age.

Pre-Exposure Prophylaxis (PrEP) – the use of ARV drugs before HIV exposure by people who are not infected with HIV in order to block the acquisition of HIV.

Premastication – pre-chewing food to break it down for an individual who cannot chew for themselves, e.g. by a mother or other caretaker for a baby during the weaning process.

Primary prevention – measures designed to prevent the onset of a given health care problem, e.g. health protection education and typically considered the most cost-effective form of healthcare.

Rapid test or RDT testing – HIV testing recommended for settings where laboratory services are weak or absent. The Rapid test allows a quick turnaround, does not require specialised equipment, and can be operated by trained non-laboratory personnel, including lay service providers.

Replacement feeding – the process of feeding a child who is not receiving any breastmilk with a diet that provides all the nutrients the child needs until the child is fully fed on family foods. During the first six months, this should be with a suitable breastmilk substitute. Often used as a euphemism for formula-feeding.

RNA – ribonucleic acid, one of the three major *biological* macromolecules that are essential for all known forms of life (along with DNA and proteins). A central tenet of molecular *biology* states that the flow of genetic information in a cell is from DNA through *RNA* to proteins: 'DNA makes *RNA* makes protein'.

Self-testing – a process in which a person collects a specimen, performs a test and interprets the test result by themselves in private.

Sero-discordant partner – a partner in a sexual relationship who is of a different HIV-status to the other, e.g. one partner is HIV-infected and the other is not.

Spillover – a term used to describe the spread of artificial feeding among mothers who either know that they are HIV-negative or do not know their HIV status – they do not breastfeed, or they breastfeed for a short time only, or they mix-feed, because of unfounded fears about HIV, or misinformation, an increased availability of breastmilk substitutes or the perception that artificial feeding is becoming the norm.

Stigma – a mark or sign of disgrace or discredit associated with HIV infection.

Sub-Saharan Africa – the area of the continent of Africa that lies south of the Sahara Desert.

Suppressed viral load – when a person living with HIV has a viral load (HIV RNA) which is reduced to an undetectable level on an HIV test.

Transactional sex – a relationship involving the giving of gifts or services in exchange for sex with the definite motivation to benefit materially from the sexual exchange. Often the participants frame themselves not in terms of prostitutes/clients, but rather as girlfriends/boyfriends, or sugar babies/sugar daddies and they are particularly common in sub-Saharan Africa, where they often involve relationships between older men and younger women or girls.

Undetectable viral load – when a person living with HIV under ART has their viral load reduced to a very low level, usually <40 copies/ml, depending on the test.

Vaginal lavage –vaginal disinfection with diluted chlorhexidine (0.2%) during labour and delivery.

Vertical transmission – transmission of HIV that occurs from a mother living with HIV to her infant. This may occur *in utero*, in the peripartum period or postnatally through breastfeeding. Also called mother-to-child transmission or MTCT.

Viral load – a measure of the number of viral particles present in an organism or environment, especially the number of HIV viruses in the bloodstream, usually written as the number per cubic millimetre (mm^3).

Viral suppression – a viral load below the threshold for detection using viral assays.

Weaning – has multiple meanings and thus should be avoided in technical communication. It may mean beginning the process of feeding the infant other food or drink apart from breastmilk. It can also refer to the process of reducing breastfeeding or

even complete cessation of breastfeeding.

Woman vs mother – these terms have been used interchangeably: woman when portraying her in a holistic manner and mother when specifically referring to her role as the mother of an infant or young child.

Young child – a toddler or child from 12–36 months of age.

References

Introduction: The untold story of breastfeeding and HIV

1. Riordan J, AIDS and Breastfeeding: The Ultimate Paradox. *J Hum Lact* 1993;9(1):3-4.
2. Innocenti Declaration on the Protection, Promotion and Support of Breastfeeding https://www.unicef.org/nutrition/index_24807.html (accessed 25 August 2020)
3. A separate ethnic group in their own right in Zimbabwe, see https://en.wikipedia.org/wiki/Coloureds
4. HIV-1 is the predominant type worldwide, and for simplicity, and in line with other discussions and writings on the topic, unless otherwise stated throughout most of this book will also be referred to simply as HIV.
5 Borrowed from: Africa, the forgotten continent, *Jordan Times*, 6 January 2003, a speech by Paul Wolfowitz, president of the World Bank, June 2005.
6. Timberg C and Halperin D. *Tinderbox: how the West sparked the AIDS epidemic and how the world can finally overcome it*, The Penguin Press 2012. ISB 978-1-59420-327-5, page 198.
7. Avert, Funding for HIV and AIDS, https://www.avert.org/professionals/hiv-around-world/global-response/funding (accessed 18 November 2020)
8. US DHHS, Guidance for Counseling and Managing Women Living with HIV in the United States Who Desire to Breastfeed, Dec 24, 2019, https://aidsinfo.nih.gov/guidelines/html/3/perinatal/513/counseling-and-management-of-women-living-with-hiv-who-breastfeed
9. Title adapted from Morrison P, A matter of life or death: the untold story of HIV, Breastfeeding and Child Survival, presented for the World Alliance for Breastfeeding Action (WABA), at the Asia-Pacific Institute for Broadcasting Development Conference on Global Media Strategies for HIV and AIDS. Hotel Nikko, Kuala Lumpur, 28 May 2007, http://www.waba.org.my/whatwedo/hiv/pdf/MediaConferenceHandouMay2007.pdf (accessed 8 January, 2011)

Chapter 1: What is HIV?

1. Cell biologies by the numbers, http://book.bionumbers.org/how-big-are-viruses/
2. Koonin EV, Wolf YI, Evolution of microbes and viruses: a paradigm shift in evolutionary biology? *Front Cell Infect Microbiol.* 2012;2:119. Epub 2012 Sept 13, http://www.ncbi.nlm.nih.gov/pubmed/22993722
3. Lawrence CM, Menon S, Eilers BJ, Bothner B, Khayat R, Douglas T, Young MJ. Structural and functional studies of archaeal viruses. *J Biol Chem.* 2009 May 8;284(19):12599-603. Epub 2009 Jan 21, available at http://www.ncbi.nlm.nih.gov/pubmed/19158076?dopt=Abstract
4. *New York Times*, Welcome to the Virosphere, 24 March 2020, https://www.nytimes.com/2020/03/24/science/viruses-coranavirus-biology.html .
5. Burdick A, Monster or Machine? A Profile of the Coronavirus at 6 Months, Our "hidden enemy," in plain sight. *New York Times*, Monster or Machine, 2 June 2020, https://www.nytimes.com/2020/06/02/health/coronavirus-profile-covid.html (accessed 3 June 2020)
6. Society for General Microbiology, see http://www.microbiologyonline.org.uk/about-microbiology/introducing-microbes/viruses
7. Information for this section taken from Wikipedia http://en.wikipedia.org/wiki/HIV (16 September 2012) and Avert, http://www.avert.org/hiv-virus.htm (22 Oct 2012)
8. Beccera JC, Bildstein LS, Gach JS. Recent insights into the HIV/AIDS Pandemic, *Microbiol Cell* 2016;3(9):451-475, http://microbialcell.com/researcharticles/recent-insights-into-the-hivaids-pandemic/ (accessed 12 Jan 2020)
9. Trinidad & Tobago National AIDS Coordinating Committee, Facts about HIV/AIDS http://www.health.gov.tt/downloads/DownloadItem.aspx?id=251
10. The Body website, http://www.thebody.com/content/30024/hiv-transmission.html?ic=4001 (accessed 7 Sept 2012)
11. Israel-Ballard K, HIV in breastmilk killed by flash-heating, new study finds, Demonstration of flash-heating breastmilk, UC Berkeley, 15 May 2007 http://www.berkeley.edu/news/media/releases/2007/05/21_breastmilk-video.shtml
12. UNAIDS blog, HIV transmission filmed live by French scientists, 28 May 2018 http://www.unaids.org/en/resources/presscentre/featurestories/2018/may/hiv-transmission-film
13. Rodger A et al. Risk of HIV transmission through condomless sex in MSM couples with suppressive ART: The PARTNER2 Study extended results in gay men. *AIDS* 2018, 23-27 July 2018, Amsterdam. Late breaker oral abstract WEAX0104LB. http://programme.aids2018.org/Abstract/Abstract/13470 https://tinyurl.com/y6tweapv
14. Alcorn K, Stem cell transplant has cured HIV infection in 'Berlin patient' say doctors. The search for a cure. AIDSMAP News, 13 December 2010, http://www.aidsmap.com/page/1577949/
15. Insert to story by Simeon Bennett, *Bloomberg*, AIDS Vaccine Sleuths Find New Clues as 30-year Hunt

Continues, 10 Sept 2012, http://www.bloomberg.com/news/2012-09-10/aids-vaccine-sleuths-find-new-clues-as-30-year-hunt-continues.html (accessed 13 Sept 2012)

16. TAC Electronic newsletter, 27 November 2008
17. Hutter G et al, Long-term control of HIV by CCR5 Delta 32/Delta 32 stem cell transplantation, *New England Journal of Medicine* 360(7) 692-8. https://www.nejm.org/doi/full/10.1056/nejmoa0802905
18. Heidi Ledford, Souped-up antibody fends off HIV, *Nature*, 8 July 2010 doi:10.1038/news.2010.341 http://www.nature.com/news/2010/100708/full/news.2010.341.html
19. Moore PL et al. Evolution of an HIV glycan-dependent broadly neutralizing antibody epitope through immune escape. *Nat Med.* 2012 Oct 21. doi: 10.1038/nm.2985. http://health-e.org.za/documents/65ed0a18ee383f46bfbaca3f6d0151ec.pdf
20. Thom A, Antibodies offer AIDS vaccine clue, Health-e, 24 October 2012, available at http://health-e.org.za/news/article.php?uid=20033834 (accessed 31 October 2012)
21. Poropatich K and Sullivan DR Jr. Human immunodeficiency virus type 1 long-term non-progressors: the viral, genetic and immunological basis for disease non-progression. *Journal of General Virology* (2011), 92, 247–268 DOI 10.1099/vir.0.027102-0, available at http://vir.sgmjournals.org/content/92/2/247.long
22. UNAIDS, HIV This Week, Issue: Issue #88 - January 29, 2011, http://hivthisweek.unaids.org/post/long-term-non-progressors
23. Rhodes DI, Ashton L, Solomon A, Carr A, Cooper D, Kaldor J and Deacon N for the Australian long-term nonprogressor study group. Characterization of Three *nef*-Defective Human Immunodeficiency Virus Type 1 Strains Associated with Long-Term Nonprogression. *Journal of Virology* 2000; 74(22:10581-10588 http://jvi.asm.org/content/74/22/10581.full.pdf+html
24. Gus Cairns, Elite controllers may self-vaccinate against active HIV infection, gene study suggests, *AIDSMAP News*, 28 August 2020 https://www.aidsmap.com/news/aug-2020/elite-controllers-may-self-vaccinate-against-active-hiv-infection-gene-study-suggests
25. Jiang C-Y et al. Distinct viral reservoirs in individuals with spontaneous control of HIV-1. *Nature*, early online publication, 26 August 2020. http://www.doi.org/10.1038/s41586-020-2651-8
26. Chomont N. HIV enters deep sleep in people who naturally control the virus. *Nature*, 26 August 2020. http://www.doi.org/10.1038/d41586-020-02438-7
27. Kaul R et al. Late seroconversion in HIV-resistant Nairobi prostitutes despite pre-existing HIV-specific CD8+ responses. *J Clin Invest.* 2001 Feb;107(3):341-9. http://www.jci.org/articles/view/10714
28. Piot P with Marshall R, *No time to lose; a life in pursuit of deadly viruses*, WW Norton & Company, New York, London 2012 (p 158) ISBN 978-0-393-06316-5

Chapter 2: The origins of HIV

1. Leppard K et al. *Introduction to Modern Virology*. Blackwell Publishing Limited, 2007 ISBN 1-4051-3645-6.
2. James Gorman, How do bats lives with so many viruses? *New York Times*, 28 January 2020 https://www.nytimes.com/2020/01/28/science/bats-coronavirus-Wuhan.html (accessed 29 January 2020)
3. Scientific Veterinary Committee Subgroup, Bovine Immunodeficiency Virus report, 24 June, 1996, available at http://ec.europa.eu/food/fs/sc/oldcomm4/out32_en.pdf (accessed 18 June 2012)
4. Bruce Ingersoll, AIDS Cousin Infects Cattle; No Danger Seen, *Wall Street Journal*, 31 May 1991. http://aidsinfobbs.org/articles/wallstj/91/136.txt
5. Cornell University, College of Veterinary Medicine, Feline Immunodeficiency Virus (FIV) Brochure, 2002 at http://www.vet.cornell.edu/fhc/brochures/fiv.html (accessed 18 September 2012)
6. Piot P with Marshall R, *No time to lose; a life in pursuit of deadly viruses*, WW Norton & Company, New York, London 2012, ISBN 978-0-393-06316-5
7. Peeters et al. Risk to human health from a plethora of simian immunodeficiency viruses in primate bushmeat. *Emerg Infect Dis* 2002;8(5):451-7. https://www.ncbi.nlm.nih.gov/pubmed/11996677 (accessed 4 October 2018)
8. Gao F et al Origin of HIV-1 in the chimpanzee Pan troglodytes troglodytes, *Nature* 1999;397(6718:436-441 https://www.ncbi.nlm.nih.gov/pubmed/9989410
9. Ho DD, Neumann AU, Perelson AS, Chen W, Leonard JM, Markowitz M. 1995. Rapid turnover of plasma virions and CD4 lymphocytes in HIV-1 infection. *Nature* 373:123–126. https://www.ncbi.nlm.nih.gov/pubmed/7816094 (accessed 5 October 2018)
10. Wei X, Ghosh SK, Taylor ME, Johnson VA, Emini EA, Deutsch P, Lifson JD, Bonhoeffer S, Nowak MA, Hahn BH, et al. 1995. Viral dynamics in human immunodeficiency virus type 1 infection. *Nature* 373: 117–122. https://www.ncbi.nlm.nih.gov/pubmed/7529365 (accessed 5 October 2018)
11. Li et al, Rates and dates of divergence between AIDS virus nucleotide sequences. *Mol Biol Evol* 1988 Jul;5(4):313-30. https://www.ncbi.nlm.nih.gov/pubmed/3405075 (accessed 4 October 2018)
12. Wikipedia, Subtypes of HIV, https://en.wikipedia.org/wiki/Subtypes_of_HIV (accessed 28 September 2018)
13. Sharp PM & Hahn BH (2011) 'Origins of HIV and the AIDS pandemic' *Cold Spring Harbour Perspectives in Medicine* 2011;1(1):a006841 (accessed 6 October 2018)
14. John Weber and Keith Alcorn, Conference Report Origins of HIV and the AIDS Epidemic *Medscape HIV/*

AIDS 6(4), 2000

15. Mauclere P et al. 1997. Serological and virological characterization of HIV-1 group O infection in Cameroon. *AIDS* 1997;11: 445–453. https://www.ncbi.nlm.nih.gov/pubmed/9084791 (accessed 1 October 2018)
16. Peeters et al Geographical distribution of HIV-1 group O viruses in Africa. *AIDS* 1997;11: 493–498. https://www.ncbi.nlm.nih.gov/pubmed/9084797 (accessed 1 October 2018)
17. Simon F et al Identification of a new human immunodeficiency virus type 1 distinct from group M and group O. *Nat Med* 1998;4:1032–1037. https://www.ncbi.nlm.nih.gov/pubmed/9734396 (accessed 1 Oct 2018)
18. Vallari A et al, Confirmation of putative HIV-1 group P in Cameroon. *J Virol* 2011:85: 1403–1407. https://www.ncbi.nlm.nih.gov/pubmed/21084486
19. Plantier C et al, A new human immunodeficiency virus derived from gorillas, *Nat Med* 2009 Aug;15(8):871-2. doi: 10.1038/nm.2016. Epub 2009 Aug 2. https://pubmed.ncbi.nlm.nih.gov/19648927/ (accessed 28 January 2021)
20. Hemelaar J, The origin and diversity of the HIV-1 pandemic. *Trends in Molecular Medicine* 2012;18(3):182-192 https://www.cell.com/trends/molecular-medicine/fulltext/S1471-4914(11)00210-3 (accessed 30 September 2018)
21. Worobey M et al, Island biogeography reveals the deep history of SIV. *Science* 2010;329(5998):1487 https://www.ncbi.nlm.nih.gov/pubmed/20847261 (accessed 4 October 2018)
22. Keele BF et al, Chimpanzee Reservoirs of Pandemic and non-pandemic HIV-1, *Science* 2006; 313(5786):523-526 http://science.sciencemag.org/content/313/5786/523 (accessed 4 Oct 2018)
23. Korber et al, Timing the ancestor of the HIV-1 pandemic strains. *Science* 2000;288(5472):1789-96 https://www.ncbi.nlm.nih.gov/pubmed/10846155
24. Lemey P et al, The molecular population genetics of HIV-1 group O. *Genetics* 2004;167(3):1059-68, https://www.ncbi.nlm.nih.gov/pubmed/15280223 (accessed 4 October 2018)
25. Worobey et al, Direct evcidence of extensive diversity of HIV-1 in Kinshasa by 1960, *Nature* 2008;(7213):661-4 https://www.ncbi.nlm.nih.gov/pubmed/18833279 (accessed 4 October 2018)
26. Lemey P, Pybus OG, Wang B, Saksena N, Salemi M and Vandamme A-M, Tracing the origin and history of the HIV-2 epidemic, *Proceedings of National Academy of Science U S A*. 2003 May 27; 100(11): 6588–6592, http://www.ncbi.nlm.nih.gov/pmc/articles/PMC164491/pdf/1006588.pdf (accessed 22 October 2012)
27. Hooper E, Sailors and star-bursts, and the arrival of HIV. *British Medical Journal* 1997;315:1689. https://www.bmj.com/content/315/7123/1689 (accessed 1 October 2018)
28. Faria et al, HIV epidemiology. The early spread and epidemic ignition of HIV-1 in human populations. *Science* 2014;346(6205):56-61. https://www.ncbi.nlm.nih.gov/pubmed/25278604
29. Science News Staff, Oldest surviving HIV virus tells all. 3 Febr 1998, reporting on David Ho's research, presented at the 5th Conference on Retroviruses and Opportnistic Infections in Chicago) http://www.sciencemag.org/news/1998/02/oldest-surviving-hiv-virus-tells-all (accessed 30 Sept 2018)
30. Ledford H, Tissue sample suggests HIV has been infecting humans for a century. *Nature* doi:10.1038/news.2008.1143 https://www.nature.com/news/2008/081001/full/news.2008.1143.html (accessed 6 October 2018)
31. *The Atlantic*, August 2019 https://www.theatlantic.com/science/archive/2019/08/hiv-genome-two-decades-before-its-discovery/596272/ (accessed 9 January 2020)
32. Wikipedia History of Kinshasa, https://en.wikipedia.org/wiki/History_of_Kinshasa (accessed 1 Oct 2018)
33. Pepin J, Expansion of HIV in colonial Leopoldville, 1950s, *Sex Transm Infect*. 2012 Jun;88(4):307-12. doi: 10.1136/sextrans-2011-050277. Epub 2012 Feb 11. https://www.ncbi.nlm.nih.gov/pubmed/22328643 (accessed 1 Oct 2018)
34. Schneider WH and Drucker E, Blood Transfusions in the Early Years of AIDS in Sub-Saharan Africa, *Am J Public Health* 2006;96:984–994. http://www.ncbi.nlm.nih.gov/pmc/articles/PMC1470624/pdf/0960984.pdf (accessed 6 October 2018)
35. Zimbabwe Ministry of Health Zimbabwe National HIV and AIDS Estimates. Harare: Zimbabwe Ministry of Health, 2003 as cited by, Takarinda K et al , Factors Associated with Ever Being HIV-Tested in Zimbabwe: An Extended Analysis of the Zimbabwe Demographic and Health Survey (2010–2011). PLoS ONE 2016;11(1): e0147828. https://doi.org/10.1371/journal.pone.0147828 (accessed 6 October 2018)
36. Keim B Early Spread of AIDS Traced to Congo's Expanding Transportation Network, *National Geographic*, https://news.nationalgeographic.com/news/2014/10/141002-hiv-virus-spread-africa-health/ (accessed 1 October 2018)
37. Hooper E, *The River; a journey back to the source of HIV and AIDS*, 1999 Penguin Books, England. ISBN 9780140283778
38. Wikipedia, United Nations Operation in the Congo, https://en.wikipedia.org/wiki/United_Nations_Operation_in_the_Congo (accessed 2 October 2018
39. Jackson Regine, The Failure of Categories: Haitians in the United Nations Organization in the Congo, 1960 – 1964. *The Journal of Haitian Studies*, 2014: 20 (1) DOI: 10.1353/jhs.2014.0001, https://www.researchgate.net/publication/267557516_The_Failure_of_Categories_Haitians_in_the_United_Nations_Organization_in_the_Congo_1960_-_1964 (accessed 1 Oct 2018).

40. Kuiken C et al, Genetic Analysis Reveals Epidemiologic Patterns in the Spread of Human Immunodeficiency Virus, *Am J Epidemiology* 2000; 152(9):814-822 https://academic.oup.com/aje/article/152/9/814/59564 (accessed 2 Oct 2018).
41. Worobey M, Gilbert M, Pitchenik A et al. Exodus and genesis: the emergence of HIV-1 group M subtype B. Oral abstract 149, 14th Conference on Retroviruses and Opportunistic Infections, 2007, Chicago, Illinois.
42. Collins S, Clade-B HIV-1 infection in Haiti predates global subtype-B virus, HIV i-Base, 4 Apr 2007 reporting on 14th CROI Conference 2007, http://i-base.info/htb/2650 accessed 30 Sept 2018
43. Gilbert MT, Rambaut A, Wlasiuk G, Spira TJ, Pitchenik AE, Worobey M. 2007. The emergence of HIV/AIDS in the Americas and beyond. *Proc Natl Acad Sci* 104:18566–18570 https://www.ncbi.nlm.nih.gov/pubmed/17978186
44. Kiwanuka N, Robb M, Laeyendecker O, Kigozi G,Wabwire-Mangen F, Makumbi FE, Nalugoda F, Kagaayi J, Eller M, Eller LA, et al. 2010. HIV-1 viral subtype differences in the rate of CD4þ T-cell decline among HIV seroincident antiretroviral naive persons in Rakai district, Uganda. *J Acquir Immune Defic Syndr* 54: 180–184. https://www.ncbi.nlm.nih.gov/pubmed/17978186 (accessed 5 October 2018)
45. Kalish et al. The Sequential Introduction of HIV-1 Subtype B and CRF01_AEin Singapore by Sexual Transmission: Accelerated V3 Region Evolution in a Subpopulation of Asian CRF01 Viruses. *Virology* 2002;304, 311–329 http://people.biology.ucsd.edu/satish/Science/MePapers/kalish.pdf (accessed 1 Oct 2018)
46. Pokrovskii VV, Eramova IIu, Deulina MO, Lipetikov VV, Iashkulov KB, Sliusareva LA, Chemizova NM, Savchenko SP. An intrahospital outbreak of HIV infection in Elista [Article in Russian] *Zh Mikrobiol Epidemiol Immunobiol.* 1990 Apr;(4):17-23.
47. Avert, HIV strains and types, https://www.avert.org/professionals/hiv-science/types-strains (accessed 28 Sept 2018)
48. US Centers for Disease Control and Prevention. 1981. Pneumocystis pneumonia—Los Angeles. MMWR 1981:30:1-3
49. Greene WC, A history of AIDS: Looking back to see ahead *Eur. J. Immunol.* 2007. 37: S94–102, https://onlinelibrary.wiley.com/doi/epdf/10.1002/eji.200737441 (accessed 2 October 2018) ,
50. Shilts R. *And the Band Played On. Politics, People and the AIDS Pandemic*, Souvenir Press 2011, ISBN 9780285640191.
51. US Centers for Disease Control, Current Trends Update on Acquired Immune Deficiency Syndrome (AIDS) --United States *MMWR* Sept 24 1982/31(37);507-508,513-514
52. Barré-Sinoussi F, Chermann JC, Rey F, Nugeyre MT, Chamaret S, Gruest J, Dauguet C, Axler-Blin C, Vézinet-Brun F, Rouzioux C, Rozenbaum W, Montagnier L. Isolation of a T-lymphotropic retrovirus from a patient at risk for acquired immune deficiency syndrome (AIDS). *Science.* 1983 May 20;220(4599):868-71. https://www.ncbi.nlm.nih.gov/pubmed/6189183 (accessed 30 September 2018)
53. Gallo R & Montagnier L, The Discovery of HIV as the Cause of AIDS. *N Engl J Med* 2003; 349:2283-2285 https://www.nejm.org/doi/full/10.1056/NEJMp038194 (accessed 30 September 2018)
54. Robbins KE, Lemey P, Pybus OG, Jaffe HW, Youngpairoj AS, Brown TM, Salemi M, Vandamme A-M and Kalish ML, U.S. Human Immunodeficiency Virus Type 1 Epidemic: Date of Origin, Population History, and Characterization of Early Strains. *J Virol.* June 2003:77(11);6359–6366. http://www.ncbi.nlm.nih.gov/pmc/articles/PMC155028/pdf/2541.pdf (accessed 22 October, 2012)
55. M. Worobey et al., "1970s and 'Patient 0' HIV-1 genomes illuminate early HIV/AIDS history in North America," *Nature* 2016;539(7627):98-101 https://www.ncbi.nlm.nih.gov/pubmed/27783600 (accessed 5 October 2018)
56. UNAIDS Global HIV & AIDS statistics — 2020 fact sheet https://www.unaids.org/en/resources/fact-sheet (accessed 19 November 2020)
57. UNAIDS data 2019 https://www.unaids.org/sites/default/files/media_asset/2019-UNAIDS-data_en.pdf (accessed 19 November 2020)

Chapter 3: The rise and rise of the HIV pandemic

1. Altman L, Rare cancer seen in 41 homosexuals, *New York Times* 3 July 1981, https://www.nytimes.com/1981/07/03/us/rare-cancer-seen-in-41-homosexuals.html accessed 12 October 2018 2. *MMWR Weekly*, Pneumocystis pneumonia, Los Angeles, June 5, 1981 / 30(21);1-3 https://www.cdc.gov/mmwr/preview/mmwrhtml/june_5.htm (accessed 12 October 2018)
3. Timberg C and Halperin D, *Tinderbox: How the West sparked the AIDS epidemic and how the world can finally overcome it*, The Penguin Press, New York, 2012, ISBN 978-1-59420-327-5
4. Merino HI et al, Screening for gonorrhea and syphilis in gay bathhouses in Denver and Los Angeles, *Public Health Rep* 1979;94(4):376-379. https://www.ncbi.nlm.nih.gov/pmc/articles/PMC1431782/?page=1 (accessed 18 October 2018)
5. Shilts R. *And the Band Played On. Politics, People and the AIDS Pandemic*, Souvenir Press 2011, ISBN 9780285640191.
6. UNAIDS, Global HIV & AIDS statistics — September 2018 fact sheet, http://www.unaids.org/en/resources/fact-sheet

7. Greene WC, A history of AIDS: Looking back to see ahead *Eur. J. Immunol.* 2007. 37: S94–102 https://www.ncbi.nlm.nih.gov/pubmed/17972351 (accessed 22 Jan 2020)
8. Gestoft J et al, Severe acquired immunodeficiency in European homosexual men, *Br Med J (Clin Res Ed)* 3 July 1982;285(6334):17-9, https://www.ncbi.nlm.nih.gov/pubmed/6805793 (accessed 18 Oct 2018)
9. Centers for Diseae Control and Prevention. Epidemiologic notes and reports imunodeficiency among female sexual partners of males with Acquired Immune Deficiency Syndrome (AIDS) – New York. *MMWR Weekly* 31(52);697-698 https://www.cdc.gov/mmwr/preview/mmwrhtml/oooo1221.htm
10. Man-Chiu Poon et al, Acquired Immunodeficiency Syndrome with Pneumocystis carinii Pneumonia and Mycobacterium avium-intracellulare Infection in a Previously Healthy Patient with Classic Hemophilia: Clinical, Immunologic, and Virologic Findings. *Ann Intern Med* 1983;98(3):287-290, http://annals.org/aim/article-abstract/696316/acquired-immunodeficiency-syndrome-pneumocystis-carinii-pneumonia-mycobacterium-avium-intracellulare-infection (accessed 18 Oct 2018)
11. *BBC News*, What is the contaminated blood scandal? By Nick Triggle, Health correspondent, 14 June 2019 https://www.bbc.co.uk/news/health-48596605 (accessed 22 Jan 2020)
12. Wikipedia, https://en.wikipedia.org/wiki/Elizabeth_Glaser (accessed 23 January 2020)
13. HIV.gov, https://www.hiv.gov/hiv-basics/overview/history/hiv-and-aids-timeline
14. Barré-Sinoussi F et al. Isolation of a T-lymphotrophic retrovirus from a patient at risk for acquired immune deficiency syndrome (AIDS). *Science* 1983;220(4599):868-871, https://www.ncbi.nim.nih.gov/pubmed/6189183 (accessed 19 September 2018)
15. *Hutch News*, 6 questions with the woman who discovered HIV, 28 August 2014 http://www.fredhutch.org/en/news/center-news/2014/08/6-questions-Nobel-scientist-Francoise-Barre-Sinoussi-discovered-HIV.html (accessed 13 April 2015)
16. Gallo R et al, Frequent detection and isolation of cytopathic retroviruses (HTLV-III) from patients with AIDS and at risk for AIDS. *Science* 4 May 1984;224(4648):500-3 https://www.ncbi.nlm.nih.gov/pubmed/6200936 (accessed 19 October 2018)
17. Marx JL et al, Strong new candidate for AIDS agent.*Science* 04 May 1984:224 (4648):475-477, http://science.sciencemag.org/content/224/4648/475 (accessed 19 October 2018)
18. Gallo R and Montagnier L, The Discovery of HIV as the Cause of AIDS, *N Eng J Med* 2003:349:2283-2285, https://www.ncbi.nlm.nih.gov/pubmed/14668451 (accessed 20 October 2018)
19. Case K, Nomenclature: Human Immunodeficiency Virus. *Annals of Internal Medicine* 1986;105(1):133, http://annals.org/aim/article-abstract/700592/nomenclature-human-immunodeficiency-virus (accessed 19 October 2018.
20. WHO 2006, HIV/AIDS in Europe Moving from death sentence to chronic disease management https://www.who.int/hiv/pub/idu/hiv_europe.pdf (accessed 11 Jan 2020)
21. Avert, HIV and AIDS in Eastern Europe and Central Asia, https://www.avert.org/professionals/hiv-around-world/eastern-europe-central-asia (accessed 11 January 2020)
22. Home of the WABA HIV Kit www.hivbreastfeeding.org
23. Beccera JC, Bildstein LS, Gach JS. Recent insights into the HIV/AIDS Pandemic, *Microbiol Cell* 2016;3(9):451-475, http://microbialcell.com/researcharticles/recent-insights-into-the-hivaids-pandemic/ (accessed 12 Jan 2020)
24. Human Dignity Trust, Map of countries that criminalize LGBT people, https://www.humandignitytrust.org/lgbt-the-law/map-of-criminalisation/ (accessed 28 Aigst 2020)
25. Yebra G et al, Analysis of the history and spread of HIV-1 in Uganda using phylodynamics. *J Gen Virol* 2015;96(Pt7);1890-1898, https://www.ncbi.nlm.nih.gov/pmc/articles/PMC4635457/ (accessed 20 October 2018).
26. Serwadda D et al, Slim disease: a new disease in Uganda and its association with HTLV-III infection. Lancet 1985;2(8460):849-852. https://www.ncbi.nlm.nih.gov/pubmed/2864575 (accessed 10 January 2020).
27. homas I, The History of AIDS in Africa, *Black History 365*, 25 Aug 2015 https://www.blackhistorymonth.org.uk/article/section/real-stories/the-history-of-aids-in-africa/
28. Fassin D and Schneider H, The politics of AIDS in South Africa: beyond the controversies. *British Medical Journal.* 2003;326(7387): 495–497. https://www.ncbi.nlm.nih.gov/pmc/articles/PMC1125376/ (accessed 10 January 2020)
29. *Harvard School of Public Health Magazine*, Spring 2009. The human cost of South Africa's misguided AIDS policies describing doctoral thesis by Pride Chigwedere, https://www.hsph.harvard.edu/news/magazine/spr09aids/ (accessed 10 January 2020).
30. Piot P and Quinn T, Response to the AIDSpandemic - a global health model, *N Engl J Med* 2013; 368:2210-2218, DOI: 10.1056/NEJMra1201533 https://www.nejm.org/doi/full/10.1056/NEJMra1201533 (accessed 11 Jan 2020)
31. Chipato T, McCann T, August 1997, Interventions to Reduce Mother to Child HIV transmission in Zimbabwe, Model project prepared for UNAIDS
32. Mahomed K, Kasule J, Makuyana D et al 1991, Seroprevalence of HIV infection amongst antenatal women in greaater Harare, Zimbabwe. *Central African Journal of Medicine* 37(19):322-325, https://www.ncbi.nlm.nih.gov/pubmed/1813126 (accessed 10 January 2020)
33. Mbizvo MT, Mashu, Chipato T et al 1996, Trends in HIV-1 and HIV-2 prevalence and risk factors in

pregnant women in Harare, Zimbabwe. *Central African Journal of Medicine 42(*1):14-21. https://www.ncbi.nlm.nih.gov/pubmed/8868380 (accessed 10 January 2020)
34. UNAIDS/WHO 1998, Report on the global HIV/AIDS report, http://data.unaids.org/pub/report/1998/19981125_global_epidemic_report_en.pdf (accessed 10 Janary 2020).
35. UNICEF The State of the World's Children 1995 https://www.unicef.org/sowc/archive/ENGLISH/The%20State%20of%20the%20World%27s%20Children%201995.pdf (accessed 10 January 2020)
36. John GC, Nduati RW, Mbori-Ngacha D, Overbaugh J, Welch M, Richardson BA, Ndinya-Achola J, Bwayo J, Krieger J, Onyango F, and Kreiss J 1997, Genital Sheddiing of Human Immunodeficiency Virus Type 1 DNA during Pregnancy: Association with Immunosuppression, Abnormal Cervical or Vaginal Discharge, and Severe Vitamin A Deficiency. *Journal of Infectious Diseases* 175:57-62. https://www.ncbi.nlm.nih.gov/pubmed/8985196 (accessed 10 January 2020)
37. Sandala L, Luri P, Sunkutu MR, Chani EM, Hudes ES, Hearst N, 1995. 'Dry sex' and HIV infection among women attendng a sexually transmitted diseases clinic in Lusaka, Zambia. *AIDS*. 9 Suppl 1:S61-8 https://www.ncbi.nlm.nih.gov/pubmed/8562002 (accessed 10 January 2020)
38. Beksinska M, Rees HV, Kleinschmidt I, McIntyre J. The practice and prevalence of dry sex among men and women in South Africa: a risk factor forsexually transmitted infections? *Sex Transm Inf* 1999;75:178–180
39. UNAIDS, AIDS Epidemic Update, December 2003 http://data.unaids.org/pub/report/2003/2003_epiupdate_en.pdf (accessed 20 October 2018)
40. Lewis S, final address at the XVI International Conference on AIDS, Toronto, 18 August, 2006
41. Susan S. Hunter. *Black death: AIDS in Africa*. 2003.Palgrave Macmillan: New York, New York, USA. ISBN: 1-4039-6244-8
42. Lewis S, Speech at United Nations, New York, 12:30 PM, Friday, March 17, 2006.
43. WHO Global Health Observatory Data, https://www.who.int/gho/hiv/en/ (accessed 26 August 2020)

Chapter 4: Routes of infection of babies, mothers, fathers and others

1. *MMWR Weekly*. Unexplained Immunodeficiency and Opportunistic Infections in Infants -- New York, New Jersey, California. 17 Dec 1982, https://www.cdc.gov/mmwr/preview/mmwrhtml/00001208.htm (accessed 18 Oct 2018)
2. Ziegler JB, Cooper DA, Johnson RO, Gold J. Postnatal transmission of AIDS-associated retrovirus from mother to infant. *Lancet*. 1985 Apr 20;i(8434):896-8. https://www.ncbi.nlm.nih.gov/pubmed/2858746 (accessed 21 Oct 2018)
3. Morrison P and Faulkner Z, HIV and breastfeeding: the unfolding evidence, *Essentially MIDIRS*, Dec/Jan 2015;5(11):7-13, https://www.midirs.org/wp-content/uploads/2014/12/272-MID-EM-December-2014-p7-12.pdf
4. Thiry L et al. Isolation of AIDS virus from cell-free breast milk of three healthy virus carriers. *Lancet*. 1985 Oct 19;2(8460):891-2. https://www.ncbi.nlm.nih.gov/pubmed/2864603 (accessed 21 Oct 2018)
5. Bucens M, Armstrong J, Stuckey M 1988, Virologic and electron microscopic evidence for postnatal HIV transmission via breastmilk. In: Fourth International Conference on AIDS, Stockholm. Frederick Md: University Publishing Group. Abstr #5099.
6. Goudsmit J, et al 1988, Virological and electron microscopic evidence for postnatal HIV transmission via breast milk. Presented at Fourth International Conference on AIDS, Stockholm, June 12-16, Abstract 5009.
7. Milligan C & Overbaugh J, The Role of Cell-Associated Virus in Mother-To-Child HIV Transmission, *J Infect Dis* Dec 2014;210 Suppl 3(Suppl 3):S631-40. https://pubmed.ncbi.nlm.nih.gov/25414417/ (accessed 4 July 2020)
8. Lehman DA, Farquhar C. Biological mechanisms of vertical human immunodeficiency virus (HIV-1) transmission. *Rev Med Virol* 2007; 17:381–403. 2, 31
9. Lewis SH, Reynolds-Kohler C, Fox HE, Nelson JA. HIV-1 in trophoblastic and villous Hofbauer cells, and haematological precursors in eight-week fetuses. *Lancet* 1990; 335:565–8.
10. Wofsy CB, Cohen JB, Hauer LB et al. Isolation of AIDS-associated retrovirus from genital secretions of women with antibodies to the virus. *Lancet* 1986;1:527-529.
11. Kreiss J, Willerford DM, Hensel M et al. Association between cervical inflammation and cervical shedding of human immunodeficiency virus DNA. *J Infect Dis* 1994;170:1597-601.
12. John GC, Nduati RW, Mbori-Ngacha D, Overbaugh J, Welch M, Richardson BA, Ndinya-Achola J, Bwayo J, Krieger J, Onyango F, and Kreiss J. Genital Sheddiing of Human Immunodeficiency Virus Type 1 DNA during Pregnancy: Association with Immunosuppression, Abnormal Cervical or Vaginal Discharge, and Severe Vitamin A Deficiency. *Journal of Infectious Diseases* 1997;175:57-62.
13. Zijenah L, Mbizvo MT, Kasule J, Nathoo K, Munjoma M, Mahomed K, Maldonado, Madzime S and Katsenstein D. Mortality in the first 2 years among infants born to HIV-infected women in Harare, Zimbabwe. *Journal of Infectious Diseases* 1998;178:109-13.
14. Hoffman RM, Black V, Technau K, van der Merwe KJ, Currier J, Coovadia A, Chersich M. Effects of Highly Active Antiretroviral Therapy Duration and Regimen on Risk for Mother-to-Child Transmission of HIV in Johannesburg, South Africa. *J Acquir Immune Defic Syndr.* 2010;54(1): 35–41. doi: 10.1097/

QAI.0b013e3181cf9979, http://www.ncbi.nlm.nih.gov/pmc/articles/PMC2880466/

15. UNAIDS. Technical update: mother-to-child transmission of HIV. 2000.
16. De Cock KM, Fowler MG, Mercier E, De Vincenzi I, Saba J, Hoff E, Alnwick DJ, Rogers M, Shaffer N, Prevention of mother-to-child HIV transmission in resource-poor countries; translation research into policy and practice. *JAMA* 2000;283:1175-1182
17. Kwiek JJ, Mwapasa V, Milner DAJ, et al. Maternal-fetal microtransfusions and HIV-1 mother-to-child transmission in Malawi. *PLOS Med* 2006; 3:e10.
18. Kwiek JJ, Arney LA, Harawa V, et al. Maternal-fetal DNA admixture is associated with intrapartum mother-to-child transmission of HIV-1 in Blantyre, Malawi. *J Infect Dis* 2008; 197:1378–81
19. The International Perinatal HIV Group. The mode of delivery and the risk of vertical transmission of human immunodeficiency virus type 1—a meta-analysis of 15 prospective cohort studies. *N Engl J Med.* 1999;340(13):977-87.
20. Mofenson LM, Lambert JS, Stiehm ER, Bethel J, Meyer WA 3rd, Whitehouse J, Moye J Jr, Reichelderfer P, Harris DR, Fowler MG, Mathieson BJ, Nemo GJ. Risk factors for perinatal transmission of human immunodeficiency virus type 1 in women treated with zidovudine. Pediatric AIDS Clinical Trials Group Study 185 Team. *N Engl J Med.* 1999;341(6):385-93.
21. Wilfert CM and McKinney RE. When Children Harbor HIV, Defeating AIDS: what will it take? *Scientific American Special Report* 1998
22. Mofensen LM 1994, Epidemiology and determinants of vertical HIV transmission. *Semin Pediatr Infec Dis* 5:253-65.
23. Grosskurth H, Mosha F, Todd J, Mwijarubi E, Klokke A, Senkoro K, Mayaud P, Changalucha J, Nicoll A, ka-Gina G et al. Impact of improved treatment of sexually transmitted diseases on HIV infection in rural Tanzania: randomized controlled trial. *Lancet* 1995;346: 530-536.
24. Moodley D et al. High HIV incidence during pregnancy: compelling reason for repeat HIV testing. *AIDS* 2009;23:1255-59.
25. Goedert JJ, Duliege AM,Amos CI, Felton S,Biggar RJ. High risk of HIV-1 infection for first-born twins. The International Registry of HIV-exposed Twins. *Lancet* 1991;338:1471–5.
26. Bulterys M, Chao A, Dushimimana A, KagerukaM, Nawrocki P, Saah AJ. HIV-exposed twins. *Lancet* 1992;339:628.
27. Duliege AM, Amos CI, Felton S, Biggar RJ, Goedert JJ. Birth order, delivery route, and concordance in the transmission of human immunodeficiency virus type 1 from mothers to twins. International Registry of HIV-Exposed Twins. *J Pediatr.* 1995;126(4):625-32. https://pubmed.ncbi.nlm.nih.gov/7699546/ (accessed 25 Mar 2021)
28. Scavalli CPS et al. Twin pregnancy as a risk for mother-to-child transmission of HIV-1: trends over 20 years. *AIDS* 2007;21: 993 – 1002.
29. Jackson JB, Musoke P, Fleming T, Guay LA, Bagenda D, Allen M, Nakabiito C, Sherman J, Bakaki P, Owor M, Ducar C, Deseyve M, Mwatha A, Emel L, Duefield C, Mirochnick M, Fowler MG, Mofenson L, Miotti P, Gigliotti M, Bray D, Mmiro F. Intrapartum and neonatal single-dose nevirapine compared with zidovudine for prevention of mother-to-child transmission of HIV-1 in Kampala, Uganda: 18-month follow-up of the HIVNET 012 randomised trial. *Lancet.* 2003 Sep 13;362(9387):859-68.
30. Jamieson DJ. Read JS, Kourtis AP, Cesarean delivery for HIV-infected women: recommendations and controversies. *American Journal of Obstetrics & Gynecology* S96-S100, Supplement to September 2007 issue doi: 10.1016/j.ajog.2007.02.034 https://www.ajog.org/article/S0002-9378(07)00270-0/abstract (accessed 31 January 2020).
31. American College of Obstetricians and Gynecologists. Scheduled cesarean delivery and the prevention of vertical transmission of HIV infection: ACOG committee opinion no.: 219: ommittee on Obstetric Practice. *Int J Gynaecol Obstet* 1999;66:305-6.
32. Read JS, Newell MK. Efficacy and safety of cesarean delivery for prevention of mother-to-child transmission of HIV-1. *Cochrane Database Syst Rev* 2005;4:CD005479.
33. Preble EA and Piwoz EG, *HIV and infant feeding: A chronology of research and policy advances and their implications for programs,* The Linkages Project and the Support for Analysis and Research in Africa (SARA) Project, the Academy for Educational Development, USAID Bureau for Africa. 1998 https://files.eric.ed.gov/fulltext/ED479277.pdf (accessed 2 Dec 2018)
34. Southern SO. Milk-borne transmission of HIV: characterization of productively infected cells in breast milk and interactions between milk and saliva. *J Hum Virol.* 1998;1:328-337. https://www.ncbi.nlm.nih.gov/pubmed/10195260 (accessed 21 Jan 2020)
35. Miotti PG, Taha TE, Kumwenda NI, Broadhead R, Mtimavalye LA, Van der Hoeven L, Chiphangwi JD, Liomba G, Biggar RJ. HIV transmission through breastfeeding: a study in Malawi. *JAMA.* 1999 Aug 25;282(8):744-9 https://www.ncbi.nlm.nih.gov/pubmed/10463709 (accessed 22 January 2020)
36. Van de Perre P, Simonon A, Msellati P et al 1991, Postnatal transmission of human immunodeficiency virus type 1 from mother to infant - a prospective cohort study in Kigali, Rwanda. *N Engl J Med* 325:593-598.
37. Humphrey JH, Marinda E, Mutasa K, Moulton LM, Iliff PJ, Ntozini R, Chidawanyika H, NathooKJ, Tavengwa N, Jenkins A, Piwoz EG, Van de Perre P, Ward BJ on behalf of the ZVITAMBO study group. Mother to child transmission of HIV among Zimbabwean women who seroconverted postnatally:

prospective cohort study. *BMJ* 2010;341:c6580 doi:10.1136/bmj.c6580, http://www.ncbi.nlm.nih.gov/pmc/articles/PMC3007097/ (accessed 18 April 2013)
38. Dunn DT, Newell ML, Ades AE, Peckham CS. Risk of human immunodeficiency virus type 1 transmission through breastfeeding, *Lancet* 1992 Sep 5;340(8819)585-588. https://www.ncbi.nlm.nih.gov/pubmed/1355163 (accessed 14 January 2020)
39. Morrison P, HIV and infant feeding: to breastfeed or not to breastfeed: the dilemma of competing risks. Part 1. *Breastfeed Rev.* 1999 Jul;7(2):5-13, https://www.ncbi.nlm.nih.gov/m/pubmed/10453705/
40. Morrison P, HIV and infant feeding: to breastfeed or not to breastfeed: the dilemma of competing risks. Part 2. *Breastfeed Rev.* 1999 Nov;7(3):11-20. https://www.ncbi.nlm.nih.gov/m/pubmed/10943427/
41. Kuhn L and Aldrovandi G, Chapter 20, Pendulum swings in HIV-1 and infant feeding policies; Now halfway back. In AP. Kourtis and M. Bulterys (eds.), Human Immunodefi ciency Virus type 1 (HIV-1) and Breastfeeding, *Advances in Experimental Medicine and Biology* 743, DOI 10.1007/978-1-4614-2251-8_20, © Springer Science+Business Media, LLC 2012.
42. Crowe D, Kent G, Morrison P & Greiner T, Commentary: revisiting the risk of HIV infection from breastfeeding, 2006, *AnotherLook* http://www.anotherlook.org/papers/g/english.pdf (accessed 4 December 2018)
43. Nduati R, John G, Mbori-Ngacha D, Richardson B, Overbaugh J, Mwatha A, Ndinya-Achola J, Bwayo J, Onyango FE, Hughes J, Kreiss J. Effect of breastfeeding and formula feeding on transmission of HIV-1: a randomized clinical trial. *JAMA.* 2000 Mar 1;283(9):1167-74 available at https://www.ncbi.nlm.nih.gov/pubmed/10703779 (accessed 28 October 2018).
44. De Cock KM, Fowler MG, Mercier E, De Vincenzi I, Saba J, Hoff E, Alnwick DJ, Rogers M, Shaffer N, Prevention of mother-to-child HIV transmission in resource-poor countries; translation research into policy and practice. *JAMA* 2000;283:1175-1182 available at https://www.ncbi.nlm.nih.gov/pubmed/10703780 (accessed 14 January 2020).
45. Coutsoudis A, Breast-feeding and HIV transmission, *Nutrition Research Reviews* 2001;14:191–206 https://pdfs.semanticscholar.org/a039/e451250fc41dc669637bbc056183b68f4174.pdf (accessed 16 November 2018)
46. Kuhn L, Aldrovandi G. Pendulum Swings in HIV-1 and Infant Feeding Policies: Now Halfway Back. *Adv Exp Med Biol.* 2012;743:273-87. http://www.ncbi.nlm.nih.gov/pubmed/22454357
47. WHO 2004, (prepared by Ellen Piwoz) What are the options? Using formative research to adapt global recommendations on HIV and infant feeding to the local context. https://apps.who.int/iris/bitstream/handle/10665/42882/9241591366.pdf (accessed 29 August 2020)
48. Leroy V, Karon JM, Alioum A et al. Postnatal transmission of HIV-1 after a maternal short-course zidovudine peripartum regimen in West Africa. *AIDS* 2003; 17: 1493–1501.
49. John GC, Nduati RW, Mbori-Ngacha DA et al. Correlates of mother-to-child human immunodeficiency virus type 1 (HIV-1) transmission: association with maternal plasma HIV-1 RNA load, genital HIV-1 DNA shedding, and breast infections. *J Infect Dis.* 2001; 183: 206–212.
50. Richardson BA, John-Stewart G, Hughes JP et al. Breast milk infectivity in human immunodeficiency virus type 1 mothers. *J Infect Dis.* 2003; 187: 736–740.
51. Semba RD, Kumwenda N, Hoover DR et al. Human immunodeficiency virus load in breast milk, mastitis, and mother-to-child transmission of human immunodeficiency virus type 1. *J Infect Dis.* 1999; 180: 93–98.
52. Read JS, Newell ML, Dabis F, Leroy V. Breastfeeding and late postnatal transmission of HIV-1: An individual patient data meta-analysis (Breastfeeding and HIV International Transmission Study). XIV International AIDS Conference, Barcelona, Spain. Abstract TuOrB1177, July 2002.
53. Embree JE, Njenga S, Datta P et al. Risk factors for postnatal mother-child transmission of HIV-1. *AIDS* 2000;14: 2535–2541.
54. Ekpini ER, Wiktor SZ, Satten GA et al. Late postnatal mother-to-child transmission of HIV-1 in Abidjan, Cote d'Ivoire. *Lancet* 1997;349: 1054–1059.
55. Coutsoudis A, Pillay K, Spooner E et al. Influence of infant-feeding patterns on early mother-to-child transmission of HIV-1 in Durban, South Africa: a prospective cohort study. South African Vitamin A Study Group. *Lancet* 1999; 354: 471–476.
56. Coutsoudis A, Pillay K, Kuhn L et al. Method of feeding and transmission of HIV-1 from mothers to children by 15 months of age: prospective cohort study from Durban, South Africa. *AIDS* 2001; 15: 379–387.
57. World Alliance for Breastfeeding Action, HIV Kit, adapted from Ellen Piwoz, Presentation on HIV and breastfeeding, WABA-UNICEF HIV Colloquium, Arusha, Tanzania, 2002
58. Piwoz EG and Ross JS, Use of population-specific infant mortality rates to inform policy decisions regarding HIV and infant feeding. *J Nutr* 2005;135:1113-1119
59. Iliff PJ, Piwoz EG, Tavengwa NV, Zunguza CD, Marinda ET, Nathoo KJ, Moulton LH, Ward BJ, the ZVITAMBO study group and Humphrey JH. Early exclusive breastfeeding reduces the risk of postnatal HIV-1 transmission and increases HIV-free survival. *AIDS* 2005;19:699–708 https://www.ncbi.nlm.nih.gov/pubmed/15821396 (accessed 10 December 2018)
60. Pokrovskii VV, Eramova IIu, Deulina MO, Lipetikov VV, Iashkulov KB, Sliusareva LA, Chemizova NM, Savchenko SP. An intrahospital outbreak of HIV infection in Elista [Article in Russian] *Zh Mikrobiol Epidemiol Immunobiol.* 1990 Apr;(4):17-23.

61. Mike Elkin, Libya's HIV-infected Babies, *Daily Beast*, March 2011, http://news.yahoo.com/s/dailybeast/20110311/ts_dailybeast/12849_libyashivinfectedbabies_1 (accessed 16 March 2011).
62. B Longo, G Liuzzi, V Tozzi, G Anzidei, M A Budabbus, O A Eljhawi, M I Mehabresh, A Antinori, E Girardi, U Visco-Comandini, Child-to-mother transmission of HIV by breastfeeding during the epidemic in Benghazi, Libya. IAC 2006 Toronto Conference Abstract.
63. Little KM, Kilmarx PH, Taylor AW, Rose CE, Rivadeneira EM and Nesheim SR, A Review of Evidence for Transmission of HIV From Children to Breastfeeding Women and Implications for Prevention *Pediatr Infect Dis J* 2012;31:938–942. http://www.ncbi.nlm.nih.gov/pubmed/22668802 (accessed 8 September 2019)
64. Thorley V. Sharing breastmilk: wet nursing, cross feeding, and milk donations. *Breastfeed Rev.* 2008;16:25–29. https://www.ncbi.nlm.nih.gov/pubmed/18546574 (accessed 25 Jan 2020)
65. Ramharter M, Chai SK, Adegnika AA, et al. Shared breastfeeding in central Africa. *AIDS*. 2004;18:1847–1849. https://pubmed.ncbi.nlm.nih.gov/15316347/
66. Shisana O, Connolly C, Rehle TM, et al. HIV risk exposure among South African children in public health facilities. *AIDS Care*. 2008;20:755–763. https://www.ncbi.nlm.nih.gov/pubmed/18728983 (Accessed 25 Jan 2020)
67. Sidley P. Wet nursing increases risk of HIV infection among babies. *BMJ*. 2005;330:862 https://www.ncbi.nlm.nih.gov/pmc/articles/PMC556184/ accessed 25 January 2020.
68. WHO 2003, HIV and infant feeding: guidelines for decision makers, https://apps.who.int/iris/bitstream/handle/10665/43864/9241591226.pdf (accessed 15 Jan 2020)
69. Azad F, Rifat MA, Manir MZ, Biva NA (2019) Breastfeeding support through wet nursing during nutritional emergency: A cross sectional study from Rohingya refugee camps in Bangladesh. *PLoS ONE* 14(10): e0222980. https:// doi.org/10.1371/journal.pone.0222980 https://journals.plos.org/plosone/article?id=10.1371/journal.pone.0222980 accessed 25 January 2020
70. WABA 2018 HIV Kit, See Module 7, Section 4, The importance of breastfeeding to infant and young child health and HIV-free survival, page 19 on www.hivbreastfeeding.org or https://waba.org.my/understanding-international-policy-on-hiv-and-breastfeeding-a-comprehensive-resource/ (accessed 25 January2020)
71. Sanders L, Backwash from nursing babies may trigger infection fighters. *Science News* 2015, https://www.sciencenews.org/blog/growth-curve/backwash-nursing-babies-may-trigger-infection-fighters (accessed link, 25 January 2020)
72. Ezeonwumelu I, Bártolo I, Martin F et al, Accidental Father-to-Son HIV-1 Transmission During the Seroconversion Period, *AIDS Research and Human Retroviruses* https://www.liebertpub.com/doi/pdfplus/10.1089/AID.2018.0060 (accessed 2 September 2018).
73. Rachel Rettner, Father Transmits HIV to Newborn Son in Rare Case: How Did It Happen? *Live Science* Sept 28, 2018. https://www.livescience.com/63710-father-transmits-hiv-to-son-rare-case.html
74. Will Dunham, HIV can be passed to babies in pre-chewed food, *Health News*, Reuters, Feb 6, 2008 http://www.reuters.com/article/healthNews/idUSN0631284520080206?sp=true
75. Gaur A et al.. Practice of Offering a Child Pre-masticated Food: An Unrecognized Possible Risk Factor for HIV Transmission. CROI 2008, conference abstract 613b. 15th Conference on Retroviruses and Opportunistic Infections, Boston , 3-6 February 2008.
76. Gaur A et al, Practice of feeding premasticated food to infants: a potential risk factor for HIV transmission, *Pediatrics* 2009; 124(2):658-66. doi: 10.1542/peds.2008-3614. Epub 2009 Jul 20. https://www.ncbi.nlm.nih.gov/pubmed/19620190
77. Ruth Hope, personal communication, August 2009
78. Habicht J-P, Zhang Y, Pelto GH, Premastication and HIV, *Pediatrics*, 3 August 2009 http://pediatrics.aappublications.org/cgi/eletters/124/2/658
79. Centers for Disease Control and Prevention (CDC). Premastication of food by caregivers of HIV-exposed children--nine U.S. sites, 2009-2010. *MMWR* 2011 Mar 11;60(9):273-5. http://www.ncbi.nlm.nih.gov/pubmed/21389930
80. Maritz ER, Kidd M, Cotton MF, Premasticating food for weaning African infants: a possible vehicle for transmission of HIV. *Pediatrics* 2011 Sep;128(3):e579-90. doi: 10.1542/peds.2010-3109. Epub 2011 Aug 28. https://www.ncbi.nlm.nih.gov/pubmed/21873699 (accessed 28 January 2020).
81. James Hall, Pre-chewing your baby's food can lead to HIV, 14 September 2011, *Swazi Observer*, http://www.observer.org.sz/index.php?news=29764
82. Labraña Y1, Alvarez AM, Villarroel J, Wu E. Premastication: a new way of transmitting HIV. First pediatric case reported in Chile [article in Spanish] *Rev Chilena Infectol.* 2013 Apr;30(2):221-2. doi: 10.4067/S0716-10182013000200014. http://www.ncbi.nlm.nih.gov/pubmed/23677162 (accessed 28 January 2020).
83. Dan Wiessner, HIV-Positive Saliva Not a 'Deadly Weapon' - NY Court, *Reuters Health Information*, 10 June 2012, http://www.medscape.com/viewarticle/765295?src=nl_topic
84. Balamane M, Winters MA, Dalai SC, Freeman AH, Traves MW, et al. (2010) Detection of HIV-1 in Saliva: Implications for Case-Identification, Clinical Monitoring and Surveillance for Drug Resistance. *Open Virol J* 4: 88–93. https://www.ncbi.nlm.nih.gov/pubmed/21673840 (accessed 28 January 2020).
85. Liuzzi G, Chirianni A, Clementi M, Bagnarelli P, Valenza A, et al. (1996) Analysis of HIV-1 load in

blood, semen and saliva: evidence for different viral compartments in a cross-sectional and longitudinal study. *AIDS* 10: F51–56 https://www.ncbi.nlm.nih.gov/pubmed/8970677 (accessed 28 January 2020)

86. Wahl A, Swanson MD, Nochi T, Olesen R, Denton PW, et al. (2012) Human Breast Milk and Antiretrovirals Dramatically Reduce Oral HIV-1 Transmission in BLT Humanized Mice. *PLoS Pathog* 8(6): e1002732. doi:10.1371/journal.ppat.1002732 https://journals.plos.org/plospathogens/article?id=10.1371/journal.ppat.1002732 (accessed 28 Jan 2020).

Chapter 5: HIV testing and monitoring the stage of disease

1. Rubinstein A, Sicklick M, Gupta A, et al. Acquired immunodeficiency with reversed T4/T8 ratios in infants born to promiscuous and drug-addicted mothers. *JAMA* 1983;249(17):2350–6
2. Preble EA and Piwoz EG, *HIV and infant feeding: A chronology of research and policy advances and their implications for programs,* The Linkages Project and the Support for Analysis and Research in Africa (SARA) Project, 1998, the Academy for Educational Development, USAID Bureau for Africa.
3. Krishen Samuel, How HIV works: what are the symptms of seroconversion? AIDSMAP, May 2019
4. HIV Test. Michigan Medicine, https://www.uofmhealth.org/health-library/hw4961 (accessed 8 February 2020)
5. AIDSMAP What is P 24 Antigen https://www.aidsmap.com/about-hiv/faq/what-p24-antigen (accessed 5 February 2020).
6. CATIE HIV testing technologies September 2019. https://www.catie.ca/en/fact-sheets/testing/hiv-testing-technologies (accessed 4 February 2020)
7. AIDSMAP What is the window period for HIV testing? June 2019 https://www.aidsmap.com/about-hiv/what-window-period-hiv-testing
8. Delaney KP et al, Time from HIV infection to earliest detection for 4 FDA approved point of care tests, Abstract No. 565, Conference on Retroviruses and Opportnistic Infections, Boston, Massachusetts, March 4-7. 2018.
9. WHO, In vitro diagnostics and viral load testing. https://www.who.int/diagnostics_laboratory/faq/viral_load/en/ (accessed 8 February 2020)
10. The International Perinatal HIV Group. The mode of delivery and the risk of vertical transmission of human immunodeficiency virus type 1—a meta-analysis of 15 prospective cohort studies. *N Engl J Med.* 1999 Apr 1;340(13):977-87. https://www.ncbi.nlm.nih.gov/pubmed/10099139 (accessed 9 February 2020)
11. Townsend CL, Cortina-Borja M, Peckham CS, de Ruiter A, Lyall H, Tookey PA. Low rates of mother-to-child transmission of HIV following effective pregnancy interventions in the United Kingdom and Ireland, 2000-2006. *AIDS.* 2008 May 11;22(8):973-81 https://www.ncbi.nlm.nih.gov/pubmed/18453857
12. Shapiro RL, Hughes MD, Ogwu A, Kitch D, Lockman S, et al. Antiretroviral Regimens in Pregnancy and Breast-Feeding in Botswana. *New England J Med* 2010;362:2282-94. http://content.nejm.org/cgi/rechprint/362/24/2282.pdf (accessed 17 June 2010)
13. British HIV Association guidelines for the management of HIV in pregnancy and postpartum 2018 (2019 interim update) Section 9.4 Infant feeding, page 88 https://www.bhiva.org/file/5bfd30be95deb/BHIVA-guidelines-for-the-management-of-HIV-in-pregnancy.pdf (accessed 18 January 2020).
14. American Academy of Pediatrics, Policy Statement, Committee on Pediatric AIDS, Infant Feeding and Transmission of Human Immunodeficiency Virus in the United States https://pediatrics.aappublications.org/content/131/2/391 (accessed 2 August 2018).
15. Paul Kidd, Phylogenetic analysis as expert evidence in HIV transmission prosecutions, *HIV Australia* 2016; 14(1) https://www.afao.org.au/article/phylogenetic-analysis-expert-evidence-hiv-transmission-prosecutions/ (accessed 27 August 2020)
16. S Collins, HIV-i-Base, reporting on the BHIVA 2017 conference, Arena and Convention Centre, Liverpool, 4-7 April 2017
17. Grabowski MK and Redd AD, Molecular tools for studying HIV transmission in sexual networks, *Curr Opin HIV AIDS* 2014;9(2):126-133. https://www.ncbi.nlm.nih.gov/pmc/articles/PMC4109889/ (accessed 8 February 2020)
18. Morrison P, HIV and infant feeding: to breastfeed or not to breastfeed: the dilemma of competing risks. Part 1. *Breastfeed Rev.* 1999 Jul;7(2):5-13, https://www.ncbi.nlm.nih.gov/m/pubmed/10453705/?i=6&from=/12179305/related
19. Creek TL, Sherman GG, Nkengasong J, Lu L, Finkbeiner, Fowler MG, RivadeneiraE , Shaffer N. Infant human immunodeficiency virus diagnosis in resourcelimited settings: issues, technologies, and country experiences. *Am J Obstet & Gynecol,* Supplement 2007;S64-S71
20. Rivera DM, Medscape Pediatric HIV Infection Workup, Updated: Jun 25, 2019 https://emedicine.medscape.com/article/965086-workup (accessed 5 February 2020).
21. Cadman H & Tobaiwa O 1996, The HIV test explained. *Zimbabwe Science News* 30(3):85-90.
22. Monforte AA, Novati R et al. Early diagnosis of HIV infection in infants. *AIDS* 1989;3:391-395
23. Ehrnst A, Lindgren S, Dictor M et al. HIV in pregnant women and their offspring: evidence for late transmission. *Lancet* 1991;338:203–7. https://www.ncbi.nlm.nih.gov/pubmed/1676777 (accessed 8 February 2020)
24. WHO 2003, HIV and infant feeding: guidelines for decision makers, https://apps.who.int/iris/bitstream/

handle/10665/43864/9241591226.pdf (accessed 15 Jan 2020)

25. Bryson YV, Luzuriaga K, Wara DW. Proposed definitions for in utero versus intrapartum transmission of HIV-1. *N Eng J Med* 1992;327:1246-1247, https://www.ncbi.nlm.nih.gov/pubmed/1406816
26. Morrison P and Faulkner Z, HIV and breastfeeding: the unfolding evidence, *Essentially MIDIRS*, Dec/Jan 2015;5(11):7-13, https://www.midirs.org/wp-content/uploads/2014/12/272-MID-EM-December-2014-p7-12.pdf
27. National Institutes for Health (USA) NIH, Panel on Treatment of HIV-infected Pregnant Women and Prevention of Perinatal Transmission. Recommendations for Use of Antiretroviral Drugs in Pregnant HIV-1-Infected Women for Maternal Health *and* Interventions to Reduce Perinatal HIV Transmission in the United States. Revisions to the April 29, 2009 version pp 7-9. Note that recommendations are updated on a regular basis and most recent information is available on the AIDSInfo website http://aidsinfo.nih.gov
28. National Institutes for Health, Recommendations for Use of Antiretroviral Drugs in Pregnant HIV-1-Infected Women for Maternal Health and Interventions to Reduce Perinatal HIV Transmission in the United States. Initial Postnatal Management of the HIV Exposed Neonate. 14 Sept 2011 update. http://aidsinfo.nih.gov/guidelines/html/3/perinatal-guidelines/188/initial-postnatal-management-of-the-hiv-exposed-neonate
29. Carter M, AIDSMAP News http://www.aidsmap.com/en/news/8CB638BC-AE0F-4698-9F67-B39B5C23C915.asp
30. Gulia J et al. HIV Seroreversion Time in HIV-1–Uninfected Children Born to HIV-1–Infected Mothers in Malawi. *J Acquir Immune Defic Syndr* 2007;46: 332–337.
31. Nastouli E et al. False-positive HIV antibody results with ultrasensitive serological assays in HIV uninfected infants born to mothers with HIV. *AIDS* 2007;21: 1222 – 1223.
32. Morrison P, HIV and infant feeding: to breastfeed or not to breastfeed: the dilemma of competing risks. Part 2. *Breastfeed Rev.* 1999 Nov;7(3):11- 20. https://www.ncbi.nlm.nih.gov/m/pubmed/10943427/?i=2&from=/10453705/related
33. Mok J 1993, Breastmilk and HIV-1 infection. *Lancet* 341:930-931.
34. Nduati RW, John GC, Richardson BA, Overbaugh J, Welch M, Ndinya-Achola J, Moses S, Holmes K, Onyango F and Kreiss JK 1995, Human immunodeficiency virus type 1-infected cells in breast milk: association with immunosuppression and vitamin A deficiency. *Journal of infectious Diseases* 172:1461-8.
35. Dunn DT, Newell ML, Ades AE, Peckham CS 1992, Risk of human immunodeficiency virus type 1 transmission through breastfeeding, *Lancet* 340(8819)585-588.
36. John GC, Nduati RW, Mbori-Ngacha D, Overbaugh J, Welch M, Richardson BA, Ndinya-Achola J, Bwayo J, Krieger J, Onyango F, and Kreiss J, Genital Sheddiing of Human Immunodeficiency Virus Type 1 DNA during Pregnancy: Association with Immunosuppression, Abnormal Cervical or Vaginal Discharge, and Severe Vitamin A Deficiency. *Journal of Infectious Diseases* 1997;175:57-62.
37. Kreiss J 1997, Breastfeeding and vertical transmission of HIV-1. *Acta Paediatr Suppl* 421:113-117.
38. Semba R, Miotti PG, Chiphangwi JS, Saah AJ, Cnner JK, Dallabetta GA, Hoover DR, Maternal vit A deficiency and mother-to-child transmission of HIV-1. *Lancet* 1994;343(8913):1593-7.
39. Ekpini ER, Wiktor SZ, Satten GA, Adjorlolo-Johnson GT, Sibailly TS, Ou CY, Karon JM, Brattegaard K, Whitaker JP, Gnaore E, De Cock KM, Greenberg AE 1997, Late postnatal mother-to-child transmission of HIV-1 in Abidjan, Cote d'Ivoire. *Lancet* 1997;349(9058):1054-1059.
40. Karlsson K, Massawe A, Urassa E, Kawo G, Msemo G, Kazimoto, Lyamuya E, Mbena E, Urassa W, Bredberg-Raden U, Mhalu F, Biberfeld G. Late postnatal transmission of human immunodeficiency virus type 1 infection from mothers to infants in Dar es Salaam Tanzania. *Pediatric Infectious Disease Journal* 1997;16(10):963-7.
41. Humphrey JH, and the ZVITAMBO Study Group. Mother to child transmission of HIV among Zimbabwean women who seroconverted postnatally: prospective cohort study. *BMJ* 2010;341:c6580 doi:10.1136/bmj.c6580, http://www.bmj.com/highwire/filestream/400641/field_highwire_article_pdf/0/bmj.c6580 (accessed 17 May 2013)
42. Ten Years of HAART: Foundation for the Future, *Medscape*, https://www.medscape.org/viewarticle/523119 (accessed 3 March 2020)
43. Latham MC, Kisanga P, Current status of proection support and promotion of breastfeeding in four African countries: actions to protect, support and promote breastfeeding in Botswana, Kenya, Namibia and Uganda, based on a rapid review 2 Oct – 3 Nov 2000, Prepared for UNICEF ESARO March 2001
44. WHO 2010 Recommendations on the diagnosis of HIV infection in infants and children. Geneva: World Health Organization. http://www.who.int/hiv/pub/paediatric/diagnosis/en
45. WHO 2014, Supplement to the 2013 consolidated guidelines on the use of antiretroviral drugs for treating and preventing HIV infection http://www.who.int/hiv/pub/guidelines/arv2013/arvs2013upplement_march2014/en
46. WHO 2015. Consolidated guidelines on HIV testing services. http://www.who.int/hiv/pub/guidelines/hiv-testing-services/en

Chapter 6: Breastfeeding: why it matters

1. Morrison P, How Often does breastfeeding really fail?, *Breastfeeding Today*, 19 February 2016, https://

www.llli.org/how-often-does-breastfeeding-really-fail/

2. Raju, TN (2011). Breastfeeding is a dynamic biological process—not simply a meal at the breast. *Breastfeeding Medicine*, 6(5), 257-259. https://www.ncbi.nlm.nih.gov/pmc/articles/PMC3199546/pdf/bfm.2011.0081.pdf (accessed 27 February 2020).
3. Ziegler JB et al. Postnatal transmission of AIDS-associated retrovirus from mother to infant. *Lancet*. 1985 Apr 20;i(8434):896-8. https://www.ncbi.nlm.nih.gov/pubmed/2858746 (accessed 21 Oct 2018).
4. Jelliffe DB and Jelliffe EFP, *Human Milk in the Modern World; Psychosocial, Nutritional and Economic Significance*, Second Edition, Oxford University Press, ISBN 0 19 442362 X, first published 1978, reprinted with corrections 1979.
5. Young SL, Mbuya MNN, Chantry CJ, Geubbels EP, Israel-Ballard K, Cohan D, Vosti SA and Latham MC, Current Knowledge and Future Research on Infant Feeding in the Context of HIV: Basic, Clinical, Behavioral, and Programmatic, *Adv. Nutr* 2011;2: 225–243, doi:10.3945/an.110.000224 http://www.ncbi.nlm.nih.gov/pmc/articles/PMC3090166/ (accessed 26 Oct 2019)
6. KidsHealth, Breastfeeding vs Formula Feeding http://web.archive.org/web/20160916145548/http://kidshealth.org/en/parents/breast-bottle-feeding.html (accessed 19 November 2018)
7. NHS Start4Life, Breastfeeding Bottle-feeding, https://www.nhs.uk/start4life/baby/breastfeeding/bottle-feeding/ (accessed 18 November 2018.)
8. Hastings, G., Angus, K., Eadie, D. et al. Selling second best: how infant formula marketing works. *Global Health* 16, 77 (2020). https://doi.org/10.1186/s12992-020-00597-w https://globalizationandhealth.biomedcentral.com/articles/10.1186/s12992-020-00597-w (accessed 3 September 2020)
9. WHO Health Topics Breastfeeding website http://www.who.int/topics/breastfeeding/en/ (accessed 16 November 2018
10. Minchin M, *Breastfeeding Matters: what we need to know about infant feeding*. Alma Publications, Australia, 1985.
11. Minchin M. *Infant Feeding and Immune Disorder*, Trilogy, 2015. ISBN-10: 0959318313, ISBN-13: 978-0959318319
12. Sankar MJ, Sinha B, Chowdhury R, Bhandari N, Taneja S, Martines J, et al. Optimal breastfeeding practices and infant and child mortality: a systematic review and meta-analysis. *Acta Paediatr* 2015; 104 (Suppl. 467):3–13.
13. Edmond et al Delayed breastfeeding initiation increases risk of neonatal mortality. *Pediatrics* 2006;117(3):e380-6. http://www.ncbi.nlm.nih.gov/pubmed/16510618
14. Jones G, Steketee R, Black R, Bhutta Z, Morris S. How many child deaths can we prevent this year? *Lancet*. 2003;362:65–71. https://www.ncbi.nlm.nih.gov/pubmed/12853204 (accessed 5 May 2020)
15. Keith Hansen, A Vice President for Human Development of the World Bank Group, *Lancet* https://www.thelancet.com/journals/lancet/article/PIIS0140-6736(16)00012-X/fulltext (accessed 25 March 2021)
16. Lawrence Ruth and Robert, *Breastfeeding: A guide for the medical profession, 8th edition*, Elsevier, ISBN: 9780323357760
17. World Health Organization, International Code of marketing of breast-milk substitutes, Geneva 1981 http://www.who.int/nutrition/publications/Guidelines_english.pdf
18. Jennifer Stanton, Obituary, Dr Cecily Williams, *The Independent* 16 July 1992. https://www.independent.co.uk/news/people/obituary-dr-cicely-williams-1533501.html
19. IOCU, https://archive.wphna.org/wp-content/uploads/2014/03/1939_Cicely_Williams_Milk_and_murder.pdf (accessed 3 September 2020)
20. Brown A. What do women lose if they are prevented from meeting their breastfeeding goals? *Clinical Lactation*, 2018;9(4):200-207. http://dx.doi.org/10.1891/2158-0792.9.4.200 (accessed 9 December 2018)
21. International Board of Lactation Consultant Examiners, History, https://iblce.org/about-iblce/history/ (accessed 28 February 2020).
22. International Lactation Consultant Association, What is an IBCLC, http://www.ilca.org/why-ibclc/ibclc (accessed 15 November 2018)
23. Breastfeeding Support, Latching and attachment, https://breastfeeding.support/category/latching-attaching/ (accessed 15 November 2018).
24. Mannel R, Martens PJ, Walker M, Core *Curriculum for Lactation Consultant Practice, International Lactation Consultant Practice,* 2014, Jones & Bartlett.
25. Hale TW, *Medications and Mothers' Milk*, Tenth Edition 2002, Pharmasoft Publishing, Amarillo Texas, ISBN 0-9636219-6-3
26. Morrison P, The ethics of infant feeding choice: do babies have the right to be breastfed, Australian Breastfeeding Association, Lactation Resource Centre, *Topics in Breastfeeding Set XVIII* March 2006
27. Hartmann P & Cregan M, Lactogenesis and the Effects of Insulin-Dependent Diabetes Mellitus and Prematurity. *J Nutrition* 2001;131(11);3016S-3020S http://jn.nutrition.org/content/131/11/3016S.full (accessed 3 November 2018) .
28. Van den Elsen LWJ, Garssen J, Burcelin R and Verhasselt V, Shaping the Gut Microbiota by Breastfeeding: The Gateway to Allergy Prevention? *Front. Pediatr*. 7:47.doi: 10.3389/fped.2019.00047 https://www.frontiersin.org/articles/10.3389/fped.2019.00047/full
29. Narvaez DW, Breastfeeding's Importance – What Science Tells Us: Misunderstanding of breastfeeding continues while scientific support increases. *Psychology Today*, 5 August 2019 https://www.psychologytoday.

com/gb/blog/moral-landscapes/201908/breastfeeding-s-importance-what-science-tells-us

30. Geddes D and Perella S, Editorial, Breastfeeding and Human Lactation, *Nutrients* 2019; 11, 802; doi:10.3390/nu11040802. https://www.mdpi.com/2072-6643/11/4/802/htm
31. Skebiel AL et al, The evolution of the nutrient composition of mammalian milks, *J Animal Ecol.* 2013;82(6):1254-1264, https://doi.org/10.1111/1365-2656.12095 (accessed 25 October 2018).
32. Dasgupta S, Seven of the Most Extreme Milks in the Animal Kingdom, Smithsonian.com, 14 Sept 2015. https://www.smithsonianmag.com/science-nature/seven-most-extreme-milks-animal-kingdom-180956588/ (accessed 25 October 2018).
33. *Breastfeeding and Human Lactation*, 4th Edition, p 79, Jan Riordan & Karen Wambach, Jones & Bartlett 2010, ISBN 978-0-7637-5432-7
34. Jenness R. The composition of human milk. *Semin Perinatol* 1979;3(3):225-39 https://www.ncbi.nlm.nih.gov/pubmed/392766 (accessed 17 November 2018)
35. Van der Ziel A, On the Work of the Swiss Zoologist, Adolf Portmann, Paper presented at the Eighth Annual Convention of the American Scientific Affiliation at Winona Lake, Indiana, September 1-3, 1953, *JASA* 1954; 6:5-9. https://www.asa3.org/ASA/PSCF/1954/JASA3-54VanderZiel.htmlnesota (accessed 4 November 2018).
36. Divecha D, What is a Secure Attachment? And Why Doesn't "Attachment Parenting" Get You There? *Developmental Science*, April 3, 2017 https://www.developmentalscience.com/blog/2017/3/31/what-is-a-secure-attachmentand-why-doesnt-attachment-parenting-get-you-there (accessed 21 August 2020)
37. Lucas A et al, Breast milk and subsequent intelligence quotient in children born preterm. *Lancet* 1992;339(8788):261-4. www.ncbi.nlm.nih.gov/pubmed/1346280 accessed 26 October 2018.
38. Rollins NC, Bhandari N, Hajeebhoy N, et al. Why invest, and what it will take to improve breastfeeding practices? *Lancet.* 2016;387(10017):491–504
39. Vandenplas Y et al. Human Milk Oligosaccharides: 2⊠-Fucosyllactose (2⊠-FL) and Lacto-N-Neotetraose (LNnT) in Infant Formula. *Nutrients* 2018;10(9);1161 at https://doi.org/10.3390/nu10091161 (accessed 29 October 2018).
40. A breakthrough in infant formula: 2'-FL HMO, Pioneering Abbott research helps bring its baby formula closer than ever to breast milk https://www.abbott.com/corpnewsroom/product-and-innovation/HMO-fundamentals.html (accessed 12 December 2018)
41. Looks can be deceiving, *Splash!* Dec 2018, http://milkgenomics.org/article/looks-can-be-deceiving-similar-gut-bacteria-have-different-functions-in-breast-fed-and-formula-fed-infants/ (accessed 5 Dec 2018)
42. Zivkovic AM, German JB, Lebrilla CB, Mills DA. Human milk glycobiome and its impact on the infant gastrointestinal microbiota. *Proc Natl Acad Sci USA.* 2011;108 Suppl 1:4653-8. https://www.ncbi.nlm.nih.gov/pubmed/20679197 (accessed 5 Nov 2018)
43. Jantscher-Krenn E[1], Bode L. Human milk oligosaccharides and their potential benefits for the breast-fed neonate. *Minerva Pediatr.* 2012 Feb;64(1):83-99. https://www.ncbi.nlm.nih.gov/pubmed/22350049 (accessed 29 October 2018)
44. Moukarzel S and Bode L, Human milk oligosaccharides and the preterm infant; a journey in sickness and in health. *Clin Perinatol* 2017;44(1):193-207, https://www.ncbi.nlm.nih.gov/pubmed/28159206 (accessed 4 November 2018).
45. Koletzko B, Human milk lipids, *Ann Nutr Metab* 2016;69(suppl 2):28–40 https://www.karger.com/Article/FullText/452819 (accessed 6 November 2018)
46. Hosseini et al, The role of infant sex on human milk composition. *Breastfeeding Medicine*, Feb 2020 Breastfeeding Medicine https://doi.org/10.1089/bfm.2019.0205 https://www.liebertpub.com/doi/abs/10.1089/bfm.2019.0205 (accessed 16 July 2020)
47. Daly SE et al, Degree of breast emptying explains changes in the fat content, but not fatty acid composition, of human milk. *Exp Physiol* 1993;78(6):741-55. https://www.ncbi.nlm.nih.gov/pubmed/8311942?dopt=Abstract (accessed 3 November 2018)
48. Owen CG et al, Infant Feeding and Blood Cholesterol: A Study in Adolescents and a Systematic Review. *Pediatrics* September 2002, 110 (3) 597-608; DOI: https://doi.org/10.1542/peds.110.3.597 https://pediatrics.aappublications.org/content/110/3/597
49. Almroth S and Bidinger PD, No need for water supplementation for exclusively breast-fed infants under hot and arid conditions, *Transactions of The Royal Society of Tropical Medicine and Hygiene* 1990;84(4):602-604. https://academic.oup.com/trstmh/article-abstract/84/4/602/1916687 (accessed 14 August 2018)
50. WHO website, Exclusive breastfeeding for six months best for babies everywhere http://www.who.int/mediacentre/news/statements/2011/breastfeeding_20110115/en/ (accessed 17 November 2018)
51. Beck KL, et al. Comparative proteomics of human and macaque milk reveals species-specific nutrition during postnatal development. *J Proteome Res.* 2015;14(5):2143-2157. https://www.ncbi.nlm.nih.gov/pubmed/25757574 (accessed 4 Nov 2018).
52. Pabst HF, Spady DW. Effect of breast-feeding on antibody response to conjugate vaccine. *Lancet.* 1990;336:269–70.
53. Hanson LA, Abstract: The newborn meets microbes and builds up its defense, while being protected by the mother:the role of breastfeeding GOLD Conference 2008.
54. W H Oddy et al. Breastfeeding, Childhood Asthma, and Allergic Disease. *Ann Nutr Metab* 2017;70 (suppl 2):26–36 https://www.karger.com/Article/Pdf/457920 (accessed 15 November 2018).

55. Oddy WH et al, Association between breastfeeding and asthma in 6 year old children: findings of a prospective birth cohort study, *BMJ* 1999;319;815-819, http://bmj.com/cgi/content/full/319/7213/815
56. Gdalevich M et al. M. Breast-feeding and the onset of atopic dermatitis in childhood: a systematic review and meta-analysis of prospective studies. *J Am Acad Dermatol.* 2001; 45: 520–527. https://www.jaad.org/article/S0190-9622(01)37990-2/abstract (accessed 16 November 2018)
57. Gdalevich M, et al. Breast-feeding and the risk of bronchial asthma in childhood: a systematic review with meta-analysis of prospective studies. *J Pediatr.* 2001; 139: 261–266 https://www.jpeds.com/article/S0022-3476(01)24448-5/abstract (accessed 17 November 2018)
58. Prameela KK & Mohamed Breast Milk Immunoprotection and the Common Mucosal Immune System: a Review, *AEK Mal J Nutr* 2010;16(1): 1 – 11. https://pubmed.ncbi.nlm.nih.gov/22691850/ (accessed 4 February 2021)
59. Goldman A. Evolution of Immune Functions of the Mammary Gland and Protection of the Infant. *Breastfeeding Medicine.* 2012;7(3):132-142. https://www.liebertpub.com/doi/abs/10.1089/bfm.2012.0025 (accessed 8 November 2018)
60. Goldman, A.S, Goldblum, R.M., Schmalstieg, F.C. Protective properties of human milk. Part III: Perinatal Nutrition. *Nutrition in Pediatrics: Basic Science and Clinical Applications*, 3rd Edition. W.A. Walker, ed. 32:551-561; 2003
61. Hanson LA, Breastfeeding provides passive and likely long-lasting active immunity. *Ann Allergy Asthma Immunol* 1998;81(6):523-33 https://www.ncbi.nlm.nih.gov/pubmed/9892025 (accessed 6 November 2018
62. L A Hanson et al. Breastfeeding protects against infections and allergy. *Breastfeeding Review*; Nov l988 , pp l9 – 22.
63. Garbes A. The More I Learn About Breast Milk, the More Amazed I Am, *The stranger*, 2015 https://www.thestranger.com/features/feature/2015/08/26/22755273/the-more-i-learn-about-breast-milk-the-more-amazed-i-am (accessed 13 November 2018).
64. Al-Shehri, Saad S., et al. Breastmilk-Saliva Interactions Boost Innate Immunity by Regulating the Oral Microbiome in Early Infancy. *PloS One* 10.9 (2015): e0135047
65. Lactation Matters blog, 14 February 2020. Ten things IBCLCs need to know about the gut microbiome, 14 February 2020 https://lactationmatters.org/2020/02/14/ten-things-ibclcs-need-to-know-about-the-gut-microbiome/ (accessed 27 February 2020
66. Queensland University of Technology, Breast milk and babies' saliva shape oral microbiome, 8 November 2018, https://medicalxpress.com/news/2018-11-breast-babies-saliva-oral-microbiome.html (accessed November 2019).
67. *Nutrition during Lactation*, Subcommittee on Nutrition during lactation, Committee on Nutritional Status dring pregnancy and lactation, Food and Nutrition Board, Institute of Medicine, National Academy of Sciencies, National Academy Press, Washington DC 1991. https://www.nap.edu/read/1577/chapter/1 (accessed 7 Nov 2018).
68. Goldman AS, Immunologic components in human milk during the second year of lactation. *Acta Paediatr Scand* 1983;72(3):461-2. https://www.ncbi.nlm.nih.gov/pubmed/6880736
69. Kellymom website, Immune factors in human milk, citing Iowa Extension Service, https://kellymom.com/nutrition/milk/immunefactors/ (accessed 6 Nov 2018)
70. Keller T et al, Intranasal breast milk for premature infants with severe intraventricular hemorrhage-an observation. *Eur J Pediatr* Nov 2018; doi: 10.1007/s00431-018-3279-7. [Epub ahead of print] https://www.ncbi.nlm.nih.gov/pubmed/30386923 (accessed 20 November 2018)
71. Akre J, *Infant feeding, the Physiological Basis, Bulletin of the World Health Organization, Supplement to Volume 67, 1989*, http://www.who.int/nutrition/publications/infantfeeding/9240686703/en/index.html (Accessed 6 January 2011).
72. Roy SK et al. Oral rehydration solution safely used in breast-fed children without additional water. *Journal of Tropical Medicine and Hygiene,* 1984;87:11-13. https://jhu.pure.elsevier.com/en/publications/oral-rehydration-solution-safely-used-in-breast-fed-children-with-3 (accessed 20 November 2018)
73. Human milk for tiny humans, http://www.human-milk.com/science.html accessed 25 October 2018
74. Hamlet Pharma, http://hamletpharma.com/en/hamlet/research/ (accessed 7 November 2018)
75. Mennella, J. A. (2007). The chemical senses and the development of flavor preferences in humans. In P.E.Hartmann & T. Hale (Eds.), *Textbook on Human Lactation* (pp. 403-414). Texas: Hale Publishing.
76. Beauchamp GK and Menella JA. Flavor Perception in Human Infants: Development and Functional Significance. *Digestion*. (2011): 1-5.
77. Dewar G, Flavors in breast milk: Can babies taste what their lactating mothers ate for lunch? Parenting Science, https://www.parentingscience.com/flavors-in-breast-milk.html (accessed 13 November 2018)
78. Palmer B, The influence of breastfeeding on the development of the oral cavity: a commentary. *Journal of Human Lactation* 1998;14(2):93-98 http://www.brianpalmerdds.com/bfeed_oralcavity.htm?fbclid=IwAR0EeammNtxwYxwr1YLfHNU9iWScjl7ebm07wNERr0zS1dxq6N9Gc_l9h8I (accessed 15 November 2018).
79. Kellymom website, Breastfeeding and Speech Development. https://kellymom.com/health/growth/speech-development/ (accessed 15 November 2018)

80. Broad FE, The effects of infant feeding on speech quality. *NZ Med* 1972;76(482):28-31. https://www.ncbi.nlm.nih.gov/pubmed/4508379
81. Ghozy S et al, Association of breastfeeding status with risk of autism spectrum disorder: A systematic review, dose-response analysis and meta-analysis *Asian Journal of Psychiatry* 2019 December 27, 48: 101916. https://read.qxmd.com/read/31923810/association-of-breastfeeding-status-with-risk-of-autism-spectrum-disorder-a-systematic-review-dose-response-analysis-and-meta-analysis
82. Kakulas F. (formerly Hassiotou). Even to the Brain: Yes, breastmilk stem cells do transfer to the organs of offspring. *SPLASH! Milk science update*: February 2019. http://milkgenomics.org/article/even-to-the-brain-yes-breastmilk-stem-cells-do-transfer-to-organs-of-offspring/
83. Pang WW et al, Nutrients or nursing? Understanding how breast milk feeding affects child cognition. *European Journal of Nutrition* https://doi.org/10.1007/s00394-019-01929-2, https://link.springer.com/content/pdf/10.1007%2Fs00394-019-01929-2.pdf
84. Victora CG, Horta BL, de Mola CL et al, Association between breastfeeding and intelligence, educational attainment, and income at 30 years of age: a prospective birth cohort study from Brazil, *Lancet* 2015;3(4);e199-e205, DOI: https://doi.org/10.1016/S2214-109X(15)70002-1 https://www.thelancet.com/journals/langlo/article/PIIS2214-109X(15)70002-1/abstract
85. World Alliance for Breastfeeding Action, 21 Dangers of Infant Formula. 2012. https://www.waba.org.my/whatwedo/advocacy/pdf/21dangers.pdf (accessed 1 Mar 2020)
86. Kent G. Comparing breastfeeding and feeding with infant formula, *World Nutrition*, Apr 2019, https://www.worldnutritionjournal.org/index.php/wn/article/view/612/550
87. Bartick MC and Reinhold 87A, The Burden of Suboptimal Breastfeeding in the United States: A Pediatric Cost Analysis. *Pediatrics*. 2010;125(5): e1048-56. http://www.breastfeedingor.org/wp-content/uploads/2012/10/burden-of-suboptimal-breastfeeding-in-the-us.-a-cost-analysis.pdf
88. Bartick MC et al, Suboptimal Breastfeeding in the United States, maternal and pediatric health ouctomes and costs. *Matern Child Nutr* 2017; 13: e12366 http://onlinelibrary.wiley.com/doi/10.1111/mcn.12366/epdf
89. Chen A et al, Breastfeeding and the Risk of Postneonatal Death in the United States. *Pediatrics* 2004;113:5 (May) 435-439. http://pediatrics.aappublications.org/content/113/5/e435
90. Ip S et al, Breastfeeding and Maternal and Infant Health Outcomes in Developed Countries. Rockville, Maryland: Agency for Healthcare Research and Quality, U.S. Department of Health and Human Services. 2007 https://archive.ahrq.gov/downloads/pub/evidence/pdf/brfout/brfout.pdf
91. Piwoz EG, Huffman SL. The Impact of Marketing of Breast-Milk Substitutes on WHO-Recommended Breastfeeding Practices. *Food and Nutrition Bulletin*. August 27 2015. http://fnb.sagepub.com/content/early/2015/08/26/0379572115602174.full.pdf+html
92. Payne S and Quigley MA. Breastfeeding and Infant Hospitalization: Analysis of the UK 2010 Infant Feeding Survey. *Maternal & Child Nutrition*. March 24, 2016 http://onlinelibrary.wiley.com/doi/10.1111/mcn.12263/abstract
93. Rollins N et al on behalf of The Lancet Breastfeeding Series Group. 2016. Why Invest, and What it Will Take to Improve Breastfeeding Practices. *Lancet*, January. 387 (10017). http://www.thelancet.com/pdfs/journals/lancet/PIIS0140-6736(15)01044-2.pdf
94. Stevens EE et al. A History of Infant Feeding. *Journal of Perinatal Education*.2009;18 (2): 32-39. https://www.ncbi.nlm.nih.gov/pmc/articles/PMC2684040/pdf/jpe-18-032.pdf
95. *Lancet Breastfeeding Series*, 29 January 2016 http://www.thelancet.com/series/breastfeeding
96. Thurow R The First 1,000 Days: A Crucial Time for Mothers and Children. Chicago Public Affairs 2016. https://www.thechicagocouncil.org/publication/first-1000-days (accessed 4 Sept 2020)
97. World Health Organization 2013. Short-Term effects of Breastfeeding: A Systematic Review on the Benefits of Breastfeeding on Diarrhoea and Pneumonia Mortality. Geneva: WHO. http://www.who.int/maternal_child_adolescent/documents/breastfeeding_short_term_effects/en/
98. World Health Organizagtion 2013, Long-Term Effects of Breastfeeding: A Systematic Review. Geneva: WHO. http://www.who.int/maternal_child_adolescent/documents/breastfeeding_long_term_effects/en/
99. Zimmerman R. Study: Breastfeeding Even More of a Health issue for Moms Than for Babies. *Common Health* September 29, 2016. http://www.wbur.org/commonhealth/2016/09/29/study-breastfeeding-moms-health
100. Strathearn L, Mamun AA, Najman JM, O'Callaghan MJ. Does breastfeeding protect against substantiated child abuse and neglect? A 15-year cohort study. *Pediatrics*. 2009 Feb;123(2):483-93.
101. Smith JP and Forrester R, Maternal time use and nurturing; analysis of the associaton between breastfeeding practice and time spent interacting with baby. *Breastfeed Med*. 2017 Jun;12:269-278. doi: 10.1089/bfm.2016.0118 https://www.ncbi.nlm.nih.gov/m/pubmed/28509564/ (accessed 1 March 2020)
102. Dieterich C et al Breastfeeding and Health Outcomes for the Mother-Infant Dyad. *Pediatric Clinics of North America*. 2013;60(1):31-48 https://www.ncbi.nlm.nih.gov/pmc/articles/PMC3508512/ (accessed 13 November 2018)
103. UNICEF 1991, Ten Steps to Successful Breastfeeding 1991, https://www.unicef.org/newsline/tenstps.htm

104. Kendall-Tackett K. Exclusively Breastfeeding Mothers Get More Sleep: Another Look at Nighttime Breastfeeding and Postpartum Depression. Science and Sensibility blog. October 19, 2011 Updated: February 15, 2017. https://www.scienceandsensibility.org/blog/exclusively-breastfeeding-mothers-get-more-sleep-another-look-at-nighttime-breastfeeding-and-postpartum-depression (accessed 15 November 2018).
105. Bosch OJ et al, Brain oxytocin correlates with maternal aggression, link to anxiety. J Neurosci 2005;25(29):6807-15. http://www.ncbi.nlm.nih.gov/pubmed/16033890 (accessed 1 November 2018)
106. Kerstin Uvnas Moberg, *The Oxytocin Factor, tapping the hormone of calm move and healing*, 2003, Pinter & Martin, ISBN 978-1-905177-34-9
107. Lester BM et al. Epigenetic Programming by Maternal Behavior in the Human Infant. *Pediatrics* 2018;142(4):e20171890. https://www.ncbi.nlm.nih.gov/pmc/articles/PMC6192679/ (accessed 13 November 2018)
108. Brown A. *Why breastfeeding grief and trauma matter*, published by Pinter & Martin 2019, ISBN978-1-78066-615-0
109. Borra C, Iacovou M, Sevilla A. New Evidence on Breastfeeding and Postpartum Depression: The Importance of Understanding Women's Intentions. *Maternal and Child Health Journal.* 2014;19(4):897-907. https://www.ncbi.nlm.nih.gov/pubmed/25138629 (accessed 15 November 2018)
110. Kendall-Tackett K, Why breastfeeeding is good for mothers' mental health, *Breastfeeding Today* 16 Jan 2019 https://www.llli.org/why-breastfeeding-is-good-for-mothers-mental-health/ (accessed 20 Jan 2019)
111. UNICEF BFI statement dated 6 December 2018. https://www.unicef.org.uk/babyfriendly/who-highlights-importance-of-safeguarding-breastfeeding-for-children-up-to-three-years-of-age/ (accessed 7 Jan 2018)
112. WHO-UNICEF Information Note, Clarification on the classification of follow-up formulas for children 6-36 months as breastmilk substitutes (undated) https://apps.who.int/iris/bitstream/handle/10665/275875/WHO-NMH-NHD-18.11-eng.pdf (accessed 1 March 2020).
113. Czosnykowska-Lukacka M, Breast milk macronutrient components in prolonged lactation. *Nutrients* 2018, 10, 1893; doi:10.3390/nu10121893. https://www.mdpi.com/2072-6643/10/12/1893/htm (Accessed 1 March 2020).
114. Ian Sample, Baby boys and girls receive different nutrients in breast milk, *The Guardian* 14 February, 2014, https://www.theguardian.com/science/2014/feb/14/baby-boys-girls-sex-formula-milk
115. Konner M, *Hunter-Gatherer Infancy and Childhood, The !Kung and Others*, Aldine, Hewlett & Lamb, https://www.wymagajace.pl/wp-content/uploads/2017/06/melkonner.pdf (accessed 26 March 2021)
116. Thai J and Gregory KE, Bioactive factors in human breast milk attenuate intestinal inflammation during early life. *Nutrients* 2020;*12*(2):581 https://doi.org/10.3390/nu12020581 https://www.mdpi.com/2072-6643/12/2/581/htm (accessed 2 March 2020).
117. Children's Hospital, Los Angeles, Necrotising Enterocolitis, https://www.chla.org/necrotizing-enterocolitis (accessed 4 February 2021)
118. Coutsoudis A, Coovadia HM, King J, The breastmilk brand: promotion of child survival in the face of formula-milk marketing. *Lancet* 2009;374(9687):423-5 https://pubmed.ncbi.nlm.nih.gov/19647609/ (accessed 3 June 2020)
119. Smith JP et al, 'Voldemort' and health professional knowledge of breastfeeding – do journal titles and abstracts accurately convey findings on differential health outcomes for formula fed infants? *ACERH Working Paper Number 4.* December 2008 Published by Australian Centre for Economic Research on Health (ACERH) http://www.acerh.edu.au
120. Valerie McClain, Human Milk Patent Pending", http://vwmcclain.blogspot.com
121. McClain V, Patents, Breastfeeding and HIV, AnotherLook 2001, http://www.anotherlook.org/papers/c/ (accessed 6 Nov 2018).
122. McClain, Human Milk Patent Pending, 2 May 2020, https://vwmcclain.blogspot.com/2020/05/the-cost-of-life-part-3.html
123. Ardythe L Morrow, David S Newburg, Guillermo M Ruiz-Palacios, Inventors http://patft.uspto.gov/netacgi/nph-Parser?Sect1=PTO1&Sect2=HITOFF&d=PALL&p=1&u=%2Fnetahtml%2FPTO%2Fsrchnum.htm&r=1&f=G&l=50&s1=7893041.PN.&OS=PN/7893041&RS=PN/7893041
124. McClain, Patents on life: a brief view of human milk component patenting, *World Nutrition* 2018;9(1) 57-69 https://worldnutritionjournal.org/index.php/wn/article/download/173/130/ (accessed 6 November 2018)
125. Bartick M, Reclaiming "breastfeeding" from "Human Milk": Politics, Public Health and the Power of Money, Breastfeeding Medicine Blog, 4 Nov 2018, https://bfmed.wordpress.com/2018/11/04/reclaiming-breastfeeding-from-human-milk-politics-public-health-and-the-power-of-money/ (accessed 5 November 2018)
126. Wikipedia, Milk Fat Globule Membrane, https://en.wikipedia.org/wiki/Milk_fat_globule_membrane (accessed 5 November 2018)
127. Smith JP, Lost Milk: Counting the Economic Value of Breast Milk in Gross Domestic Product, *J Hum Lact* published online 12 July 2013 DOI: 10.1177/0890334413494827. https://journals.sagepub.com/doi/10.1177/0890334413494827 (accessed 26 March 2021)
128. Miriam Labbok, personal communication
129. Ryland H, Breastfeeding rates in UK are the lowest in the world, British Science Association news. https://www.britishscienceassociation.org/news/breastfeeding-rates-in-uk-are-the-lowest-in-the-world (accessed 26

March 2021)

130. Infant Feeding Survey 2010: Chapter 2 – Incidence, Prevalence and Duration of Breastfeeding , Nov 2012. http://webarchive.nationalarchives.gov.uk/20180321190208/http://digital.nhs.uk/catalogue/PUB08694 (accessed 11 November 2018)
131. The Healthy Start Voucher scheme http://www.healthystart.nhs.uk/healthy-start-vouchers/what-to-buy-with-the-vouchers/ (accessed 11 November 2015)
132. Kent G, Letter to the Editor on Increasing Breastfeeding in WIC Participants: Cost of Formula as a Motivator, *Journal of Nutrition Education and Behavior* 2014; 46(5):e9
133. Department of Health, The Nursery Milk scheme, Frequently Asked Questions https://www.nurserymilk.co.uk/frequently-asked-questions (accessed 11 November 2018)
134. Costello A et al, Health professional associations and industry funding, *Lancet* 2017;389:597-8, https://www.thelancet.com/journals/lancet/article/PIIS0140-6736(17)30277-5/fulltext accessed 11 November 2018)
135. Royal College of Midwives, Infant Formula Advertising Statement, 28 May 2008. https://www.rcm.org.uk/news-views-and-analysis/news/infant-formula-advertising-statement (accessed 11 November 2018
136. The Global North generally includes the United States, Canada, Western Europe, developed countries in Asia, and Australia & New Zealand (the two countries are not located in the North, however share similar economic and cultural characteristics). On the other hand, Global South generally includes all the countries in Africa, Latin America, and developing parts of Asia (e.g. Middle East) https://medium.com/@vesabarileva/the-north-south-divide-of-countries-and-the-entire-world-e656ba588c8b (accessed 5 September 2020)
137. Hastings, G, Angus, K, Eadie, D et al. Selling second best: how infant formula marketing works. *Global Health* 16, 77 (2020). https://doi.org/10.1186/s12992-020-00597-w https://globalizationandhealth.biomedcentral.com/articles/10.1186/s12992-020-00597-w (accessed 3 September 2020)
138. Akre J. Chapter 1, From Grand Design to Change on the Ground: Going to Scale with a Global Feeding Strategy, *Infant and Young Child Feeding*, Dykes F & Moran VH, editors, John Wiley & Sons 2009.
139. WHO 2000, HIV and Infant Feeding Counselling: A training course, A Trainer's Guide, WHO/FCH/CAH/00.4 http://www.who.int/nutrition/publications/en/hiv_infant_feeding_course_trainer_eng.pdf (accessed 11 November 2018)
140. First Steps Nutrition Trust: Cost of infant milks marketed in the UK, February 2017. https://nhsforthvalley.com/wp-content/uploads/2014/03/Costs_of_Infant_Milks_Marketed_in_the_UK_February2017.pdf (accessed 11 November 2018)
141. UNICEF UK, Preventing disease and saving resources- the potential contribution of increaseing breastfeeding rates in the UK, October 2012. https://www.unicef.org.uk/babyfriendly/about/preventing-disease-and-saving-resources/preventing_disease_saving_resources/ (accessed 11 November 2018).
142. Labbok MH, Effects of breastfeeding on the mother. *Pediatr Clin North Am* 2001;48(1):143-58 https://www.ncbi.nlm.nih.gov/pubmed/11236722 (accessed 4 November 2018)
143. WHO Collaborative Study Team on the Role of Breastfeeding on the Prevention of Infant Mortality. Effect of breastfeeding on infant and child mortality due to infectious diseases in less developed countries: a pooled analysis. *Lancet*. 2000;355:451–455. http://www.ncbi.nlm.nih.gov/pubmed/10841125.
144. Bartick et al, Cost Analysis of Maternal Disease Associated With Suboptimal Breastfeeding *Obstet Gynecol* 2013;122(1):111-9. https://www.ncbi.nlm.nih.gov/pubmed/23743465 (accessed 8 Nov 2018).
145. Fox et al, Maternal breastfeeding history and Alzheimer's disease risk. *J Alzheimers Dis* 2013;37(4):809-21. https://www.ncbi.nlm.nih.gov/pubmed/23948914 (accessed 15 November 2018).
146. Victora C et al. Breastfeeding in the 21st century: epidemiology, mechanisms, and lifelong effect. *Lancet*. 2016;387(10017):475-490. https://www.ncbi.nlm.nih.gov/pubmed/26869575 (accessed 11 November 2018)
147. Walters DD, Phan LTH, Mathison R. The cost of not breastfeeding: global results from a new tool. *Health Policy and Planning* 2019;34(6):407-417. https://academic.oup.com/heapol/article/34/6/407/5522499 (accessed 28 June 2020)
148. Marsha Walker, page 51, Summary to Chapter 1: The design in Nature, *Breastfeeding Management for the Clinician, Using the Evidence,* Third Edition, Jones & Bartlett, 2014

Chapter 7: HIV in breastmilk

1. Thiry L, Sprecher-Goldberger S, Jonckheer T et al 1985, Isolation of AIDS virus from cell-free breast milk of three healthy virus carriers, *Lancet* 2(8583):981.
2. Ziegler JB, Cooper DA, Johnson RO, Gold J 1985, Postnatal transmission of AIDS-associated retrovirus from mother to infant. *Lancet,* I:896-898
3. Bucens M, Armstrong J, Stuckey M 1988, Virologic and electron microscopic evidence for postnatal HIV transmission via breastmilk. In: *Fourth International Conference on AIDS*, Stockholm. Frederick Md: University Publishing Group. Abstr #5099.
4. Datta P, Embree JE, Kreiss JK, Ndinya-Achola JO, Braddick M, Temmerman M, Nagelkerke NJ, Maitha G, Holmes KK, Piot P, et al. Mother-to-child transmission of human immunodeficiency virus type 1: report from the Nairobi Study. *J Infect Dis*. 1994 Nov 170(5):1134-40. http://www.jstor.org/

stable/30133531
5. Richardson BA, John-Stewart GC, Hughes JP, Nduati R, Mbori-Ngacha D, Overbaugh J and Kreiss JK, Breast-Milk Infectivity in Human Immunodeficiency Virus Type 1–Infected Mothers, *J Infect Dis.* 2003 Mar 1;187(5):736-40. https://www.ncbi.nlm.nih.gov/pmc/articles/PMC3382109/ (accessed 11 Feb 2020).
6. WHO/UNICEF 1992. Consensus statement from the WHO/UNICEF consultation on HIV transmission and breastfeeding. Geneva 30 April–1 May, 1992 https://apps.who.int/iris/handle/10665/61014 (accessed 5 March 2020)
7. Van de Perre P, Simonon A, Hitimana DG, Dabis F, Msellati P, Mukamabano B, Butera JB, Van Goethem C, Karita E, Lepage P. Infective and anti-infective properties of breastmilk from HIV-1-infected women. *Lancet* 1993 Apr 10;341(8850):914-8.
8. Baba TW, Kock J, Mittler M, et al. Mucosal infection of neonatal rhesus monkeys with cell-free SIV. *AIDS Research and Human Retroviruses* 1994;10(4):351-357.
9. Nduati RW et al, Human immunodeficiency virus type 1-infected cells in breast milk: association with immunosuppression and vitamin A deficiency. *J Infect Dis.* 1995 Dec;172(6):1461-8. https://www.ncbi.nlm.nih.gov/pmc/articles/PMC3358135/ (accessed 31 Aug 2020
10. Piatak M Jr, Saag MS, Yang LC, et al. High levels of HIV-1 in plasma during all stages of infection determined by competitive PCR. *Science.* 1993; 259:1749–54.
11. Lewis P, Nduati R, Kreiss JK, John GC, Richardson BA, Mbori-Ngacha D, Ndinya-Achola J, Overbaugh J. Cell-free human immunodeficiency virus type 1 in breast milk. *J Infect Dis.* 1998 Jan;177(1):34-9.
12. Ruff AJ, Halsey NA, Coberly J, Boulos R 1992, Breastfeeding and maternal-infant transmission of human immunodeficiency virus type 1. *J Pediatr* 121:325-29.
13. Embree JE, Njenga S, Datta P, Nagelkerke NJD, Ndinya-Achola JO, Mohammed Z, Ramdahin S, Bwayo JJ, Plummer F, Risk factors for postnatal mother-child transmission of HIV, *AIDS* 2000, 14:2535-2541.
14. Ekpini ER, Wiktor SZ, Satten GA, Adjorlolo-Johnson GT, Sibailly TS, Ou CY, Karon JM, Brattegaard K, Whitaker JP, Gnaore E, De Cock KM, Greenberg AE 1997, Late postnatal mother-to-child transmission of HIV-
15. John GC, Nduati RW, Mbori-Ngacha D, Overbaugh J, Welch M, Richardson BA, Ndinya-Achola J, Bwayo J, Krieger J, Onyango F, and Kreiss J. Genital Sheddiing of Human Immunodeficiency Virus Type 1 DNA during Pregnancy: Association with Immunosuppression, Abnormal Cervical or Vaginal Discharge, and Severe Vitamin A Deficiency. *J Infect Dis* 1997; 175:57-62. https://pubmed.ncbi.nlm.nih.gov/8985196/ (accessed 27 March 2021)
16. Garcia PM, Kalish LA, Pitt J, Minkoff H, Quinn TC, Burchett SK, Kornegay J, Jackson B, Moye J, Hanson C, Zorrilla C, Lew JF. Maternal levels of plasma human immunodeficiency virus type 1 RNA and the risk of peri-natal transmission. Women and Infants Transmission Study Group. *N Engl J Med.* 1999 Aug 5;341(6):394-402. https://pubmed.ncbi.nlm.nih.gov/10432324/ (accessed 27 March 2021)
17. John GC, Nduati RW, Mbori-Ngacha DA, Richardson BA, Panteleeff D, Mwatha A, Overbaugh J, Bwayo J, Ndinya-Achola JO, Kreiss JK. Correlates of mother-to-child human immunodeficiency virus type 1 (HIV-1) transmission: association with maternal plasma HIV-1 RNA load, genital HIV-1 DNA shedding, and breast infections. *J Infect Dis.* 2001 Jan 15;183(2):206-212.
18. Guay LA, Hom DL, Mmiro F, Piwowar EM, Kabengera S, Parsons J, Ndugwa C, Marum L, Olness K, Kataaha P, Jackson JB. Detection of human immunodeficiency virus type 1 (HIV-1) DNA and p24 antigen in breast milk of HIV-1-infected Ugandan women and vertical transmission. *Pediatrics.* 1996 Sep;98(3 Pt 1):438-44.
19. Koulinska IN, Villamor E, Chaplin B, Msamanga G, Fawzi W, et al. (2006) Transmission of cell-free and cell-associated HIV-1 through breast-feeding. *J Acquir Immune Defic Syndr* 41: 93–99.
20. Rousseau CM, Nduati RW, Richardson BA, John-Stewart GC, Mbori-Ngacha DA, et al. Association of levels of HIV-1-infected breast milk cells and risk of mother-to-child transmission. *J Infect Dis* 2004;190: 1880–1888.
21. Neveu D, Viljoen J, Bland RM, Nagot N, Danaviah S, Coutsoudis A, Rollins NC, Coovadia HM, van de Perre P and Newell M-L. et al. Cumulative exposure to cell-free HIV in breast milk, rather than feeding pattern per se, identifies postnatally infected infants. *Clin Infect Dis* 2011;52: 819–825. https://www.ncbi.nlm.nih.gov/pmc/articles/PMC3049337/ (accessed 10 Mar 2021)
22. Slyker JA, Chung MH, Lehman DA, Kiarie J, Kinuthia J, et al. (2012) Incidence and correlates of HIV-1 RNA detection in the breast milk of women receiving HAART for the prevention of HIV-1 transmission. *PLoS One* 7: e29777.
23. Valea D, Tuaillon E, Al Tabaa Y, Rouet F, Rubbo PA, et al. (2011) CD4+ T cells spontaneously producing human immunodeficiency virus type I in breast milk from women with or without antiretroviral drugs. *Retrovirology* 8: 34
24. Ndirangu J, Viljoen J, Bland RM, Danaviah S, Thorne C, Van de Perre P, Newell ML.Cell-Free (RNA) and Cell-Associated (DNA) HIV-1 and Postnatal Transmission through Breastfeeding. *PLoS One.* 2012;7(12):e51493. doi: 10.1371/journal.pone.0051493. Epub 2012 Dec 28. http://www.ncbi.nlm.nih.gov/pubmed/23284701
25. Lyimo MA, Howell AL, Balandya E, Eszterhas SK, Connor RI. Innate Factors in Human Breast Milk Inhibit Cell-Free HIV-1 but Not Cell-Associated HIV-1 Infection of CD4+ Cells. *J Acquir Immune Defic Syndr.* 2009 Apr 2.

26. Lee EJ, Kantor R, Zijenah L, Sheldon W, Emel L, Mateta P, Johnston E, Wells J, Shetty AK, Coovadia H, Maldonado Y, Jones SA, Mofenson LM, Contag CH, Bassett M, Katzenstein DA; HIVNET 023 Study Team. Breast-milk shedding of drug-resistant HIV-1 subtype C in women exposed to single-dose nevirapine. *J Infect Dis. 2005* Oct 1;192(7):1260-4. Epub 2005 Aug 23.
27. Lehman DA, Chung MH, John-Stewart GC, Richardson BA, Kiarie J, Kinuthia J, Overbaugh J. HIV-1 persists in breast milk cells despite antiretroviral treatment to prevent mother-to-child transmission.*AIDS.* 2008 Jul 31;22(12):1475-85.
28. Chung MH, Kiarie JN, Richardson BA, Lehman DA, Overbaugh J, Kinuthia J, Njiri F, John-Stewart GC. Highly active antiretroviral therapy versus zidovudine/nevirapine effects on early breast milk HIV type-1 RNA: a phase II randomized clinical trial. *Antivir Ther.* 2008;13(6):799-807.
29. McGuire MK et al. Best Practices for Human Milk Collection for COVID-19 Research. *Breastfeeding Medicine.* https://www.liebertpub.com/doi/full/10.1089/bfm.2020.0296 (accessed 11 Jan 2021)
30. Dunn DT, Newell ML, Ades AE, et al. Risk of human immunodeficiency virus type 1 transmission through breastfeeding. *Lancet* 1992; 340:585-8.
31. Kreiss J. Breastfeeding and vertical transmission of HIV-1. *Acta Paediatr Suppl* 1997;421:113-117.
32. Latham MC, Kisanga P, Current status of proection support and promotion of breastfeeding in four African countries: actions to protect, support and promote breastfeeding in Botswana, Kenya, Namibia and Uganda, based on a rapid review 2 Oct – 3 Nov 2000, Prepared for UNICEF ESARO March 2001.

Chapter 8: Breast and nipple problems: do they increase the risk?

1. WHO Exclusive breastfeeding for six months best for babies everywhere, 15 January 2011 https://www.who.int/mediacentre/news/statements/2011/breastfeeding_20110115/en/ (accessed 23 Jan 2020).
2. Piwoz E & Ross J, HIV and Infant Feeding, Knowledge Gaps and challenges for the future, Joint WABA/UNICEF HIV colloquium, Arusha, Tanzania 2002.
3. Margaret Neville, Milk secretion: an overview, 1998, available at http://mammary.nih.gov/reviews/lactation/Neville001/
4. D A Nguyen, M C Neville, Tight junction regulation in the mammary gland. *Journal of Mammary Gland Biology and Neoplasia* (impact factor: 6.74). 08/1998; 3(3):233-46. DOI:10.1023/A:1018707309361 available at http://www.researchgate.net/publication/12497525_Tight_junction_regulation_in_the_mammary_gland
5. Smith MM and Kuhn L, Exclusive breast-feeding: does it have the potential to reduce breast-feeding transmission of HIV-1?. *Nutrition Reviews* 2000;58(11):333-340.
6. Cox DB, Kent JC, Casey TM , Owens RA , Hartmann PE. Breast growth and the urinary excretionof lactose during human pregnancy and early lactation: endocrine relationships. *Exp Physiol* 1999;84:421-34.
7. Stelwagen K, Farr VC, McFadden HA, Prosser CG , Davis SR. Time course of milk accumulation – induced opening of the mammary tight junctions and blood clearance of milk components. *Am J Physiol Regul Integr Comp Physiol* 1997;273:R379-86.
8. Hartmann PE, Kulski JK. Changes in the composition of the mammary secretion of women after abrupt termination of breast feeding. *J Physiol.* 1978 Feb;275:1-11.
9. Fetherston CM, Lai CT, Mitoulas LR and Hartmann PE, Excretion of lactose in urine as a measure of increased permeability of the lactating breast during inflammation. *Acta Obstetricia et Gynecologica* 2006;85:20-25.
10. Desmarais L & Browne S. Inadequate weight gain in breastfeeding infants; assessments and resolutions, Lactation consultant Series Unit 8, 1990 La Leche League International
11. Tess BN, Rodrigues LC, Newell ML et al. Infant feeding and risk of mother-to-child transmission of HIV-1 in Sao Paulo State, Brazil. *J Acquir Immun Defic Syndr Hum Retrovirol* 1998;19:189-94.
12. Riordan J & Auerbach K, 1999. *Breastfeeding and Human Lactation, Second Edition*, 1999, Jones & Bartlett Publishers.
13. Ekpini ER, Wiktor SZ, Satten GA, Adjorlolo-Johnson GT, Sibailly TS, Ou CY, Karon JM, Brattegaard K, Whitaker JP, Gnaore E, De Cock KM, Greenberg AE 1997, Late postnatal mother-to-child transmission of HIV-1 in Abidjan, Cote d'Ivoire. *Lancet* 349(9058):1054-1059.
14. Miotti PG, Taha TE, Kumwenda NI, Broadhead R, Mtimavalye LA, Van der Hoeven L, Chiphangwi JD, Liomba G, Biggar RJ. HIV transmission through breastfeeding: a study in Malawi. *JAMA.* 1999 Aug 25;282(8):744-9.
15. Brodribb, W. (Ed.). *(2004). Breastfeeding management in Australia* (3rd ed.). Malvern 2004
16. Livingstone VH, Willis CE, Berkowitz J, Staphylococcus aureus and sore nipples. *Can Fam Physician.* 1996 Apr;42:654-9, available at http://www.breastfeedingclinic.com/ckfinder/userfiles/files/Staphylococcus.pdf
17. Kambarami RA, Kowo H, The prevalence of nipple disease among breastfeeding mothers of HIV seropositive infants. *Cent Afr J Med* 1997;43(1):20-2 https://www.ncbi.nlm.nih.gov/pubmed/9185375 (accessed 2 February 2020)
18. Hancock KF, Spangler AK. There's a fungus among us! *J Hum Lact* 9:179-80, 1993.
19. Odds FC: Ecology of candida and epidemiology of candidosis, chapter 7 in *Candida and candidosis: a review and bibliography,* 2nd ed London: Bailliere Tindall, 1988.

20. Amir LH, Forster DA, Lumley J, McLachlan H. A descriptive study of mastitis in Australian breastfeeding women: incidence and determinants. *BMC Public Health*. 2007;7:62. doi: 10.1186/1471-2458-7-62. https://www.ncbi.nlm.nih.gov/pmc/articles/PMC1868722/
21. WHO 2000, Mastitis, https://www.who.int/maternal_child_adolescent/documents/fch_cah_00_13/en/
22. Kinlay JR, O'Connell DL, Kinlay S. Incidence of mastitis in breastfeeding women during the firsrt six months after delivery: a prospectrive cohort stuyd. *Med J Aust* 1998:310-12
23. Connor, A. E. 1979. Elevated levels of sodium and chloride in milk from mastitic breast. *Pediatrics* 63:910–911
24. Neville MC, Keller RP, Seacat J, Casey CE, Allen JC, Archer P. Studies on human lactation. 1. Within feed and between-breast variation in selected components of human milk. *Am J Clin Nutr* 1984;40:635-46.
25. Abakada AO, Hartmann PE, Grubb WB. Sodium and serum albumin in milk: biochemical markers for human lactational mastopathy. *Proc Aust Biochem Soc* 1990; 22:SP52
26. Prentice A, Prentice AM, Lamb WH. Mastitis in rural Gambian mothers and the protection of the breast by milk antimicrobial factors. Transactions of the Royal Society of Tropical Medicine and Hygiene 1985;79:90-95
27. Filteau SM, Rice AL, Ball JJ et al. Breast milk immune factors in Bangladeshi women supplemented postpartum with retinol or beta-carotene. *Am J Clin Nutr* 1999;69:953-8.
28. Semba RD, Kumwenda N, Hoover DR, Taha TE, Quinn TC, Mtimavalye L, Biggar RJ, Broadhead R, Miotti PG, Sokoll LJ, van der Hoeven L, Chiphangwe JD. Human immunodeficiency virus load in breast milk, mastitis, and mother-to-child transmission of human immunodeficiency virus type 1. *J Infect Dis 1999*;180:93-98.
29. Semba RD, Kumwenda N, Taha TE, Hoover DR, Quinn TC, Yin Lan, Mtimavalye L, Broadhead R, Miotti PG, van der Hoeven L and Chiphangwi JD, Mastitis and immunological factors in breast milk of human immunodeficiencyh virus-infected women. *J Hum Lact* 1999;15(4):301-306.
30. Semba RD, Kumwenda N, Taha TE, Hoover DR, Yin Lan, Eisinger W, Mtimavalye L, Broadhead R, Miotti PG, van der Hoeven L, and Chiphangwi JD, Mastitis and immunological factors in breast milk of lactating women in Malawi, *Clin Diag Lab Immunology* 1999;6(5):671-674
31. Semba RD, Neville MC. Breast-feeding, mastitis, and HIV transmission: nutritional implications. *Nutr Rev*. 1999 May;57(5 Pt 1):146-53.
32. Lewis P, Nduati R, Kreiss JK, John GC, Richardson BA, Mbori-Ngacha D, Ndinya-Achola J, Overbaugh J. Cell-free human immunodeficiency virus type 1 in breastmilk. *J Infect Dis* 1998;177(1):34-39 available at http://www.ncbi.nlm.nih.gov/pmc/articles/PMC3358132/pdf/nihms-359821.pdf
33. Nussenblatt V, Kumwenda N, Lema V, Quinn T, Neville MC, Broadhead R, Taha TE, Semba RD. Effect of Antibiotic Treatment of Subclinical Mastitis on Human Immunodeficiency Virus Type 1 RNA in Human Milk. *J Trop Pediatr*. 2006 Apr 4;
34. ORC Macro, 2006. MEASURE DHS STATcompiler. http://www.measuredhs.com, accessed January 14 2006.
35. Coutsoudis A and Rollins N, Breast-feeding and HIV transmission: the jury is still out, *J Ped Gastroenterol and Nutr* 2003;36:434-442.
36. Gantt S et al, Laboratory Indicators of Mastitis Are Not Associated with Elevated HIV-1 DNA Loads or Predictive of HIV-1 RNA Loads in Breast Milk. *J Inf Dis* 2007; 196:570–6.
37. Willumsen JF, Filteau SM, Coutsoudis A, Uebel KE, Newell ML, Tomkins AM. Subclinical mastitis as a risk factor for mother-infant HIV transmission. *Adv Exp Med Biol.* 2000;478:211-23.
38. Willumsen JF, Newell ML, Filteau SM, Coutsoudis A, Dwarika S, York D, Tomkins AM, Coovadia HM. Variation in breastmilk HIV-1 viral load in left and right breasts during the first 3 months of lactation. *AIDS.* 2001 Sep 28;15(14):1896-8.
39. Flores M and Filteau S, Effect of lactation counselling on subclinical mastitis among Bangladeshi women. *Ann Trop Paediatr* 2002 Mar;22(1):85-8. doi: 10.1179/027249302125000210. https://pubmed.ncbi.nlm.nih.gov/11926056/ (accessed 5 July 2020)
40. Willumsen JF, Filteau SM, Coutsoudis A, Newell ML, Rollins NC, Coovadia HM, Tomkins AM, Breastmilk RNA viral load in HIV-infected South African women: effects of subclinical mastitis and infant feeding. *AIDS.* 2003 Feb 14;17(3):407-14.
41. Nussenblatt V, Lema V, Kumwenda N, Broadhead R, Neville MC, Taha TE, Semba RD. Epidemiology and microbiology of subclinical mastitis among HIV-infected women in Malawi. *Int J STD AIDS.* 2005 Mar;16(3):227-32.
42. Semrau K, Kuhn L, Brooks DR, Cabral H, Sinkala M, Kankasa C, Thea DM, Aldrovandi GM. Exclusive breastfeeding, maternal HIV disease, and the risk of clinical breast pathology in HIV-infected, breastfeeding women. *Am J Obstet Gynecol.* 2011 Oct;205(4):344.e1-8. Epub 2011 Jun 15.
43. WHO/UNAIDS/UNICEF, HIV and infant feeding counselling course, Geneva: World Health Organization, 2000. WHO document WHO/FCH/CAH/00.2-6.
44. BHIVA, HIV and breastfeeding your baby (Leaflet 1) (undated) https://www.bhiva.org/file/5bfd3080d2027/BF-Leaflet-1.pdf (accessed 6 December 2019)
45. Coutsoudis A, Pillay K, Spooner E, Kuhn L, Coovadia HM. Influence of infant-feeding patterns on early mother-to-child transmission of HIV-1 in Durban, South Africa: a prospective cohort study. South African Vitamin A Study Group. *Lancet* 1999 Aug 7;354(9177):471-6. https://www.ncbi.nlm.nih.gov/

pubmed/10465172 (accessed 10 December 2018)
46. Morbacher N, Stock J, *Breastfeeding Answer Book* Revised Edition, 1997, p 420. La Leche League International, Schaumburg, Illinois, USA
47. Kuhn L, Sinkala M, Kankasa C, Semrau K, Kasonde P, Scott N, Mwiya M, Cheswa V, Walter J, Wei-Yann T, Aldrovandi GM, and Thea DM. High Uptake of Exclusive Breastfeeding and Reduced Early Post-Natal HIV Transmission. *PLoS ONE* Dec 2007; 2(12): e1363. doi:10.1371/journal.pone.0001363
48. Fetherston C. Mastitis in lactating women: physiology or pathology? *Breastfeed Rev* 2001 Mar;9(1):5-12. https://pubmed.ncbi.nlm.nih.gov/11424519/ (accessed 27 March 2021)
49. Brodribb W (Ed) *Breastfeeding Management in Australia* (2nd ed) 1997, Nursing Mothers Association, Victoria, Australia.
50. Lunney KM, Iliff P, Kuda M et al, Associations between Breast Milk Viral Load, Mastitis, Exclusive Breast-Feeding, and Postnatal Transmission of HIV. *Clinical Infectious Diseases* 2010;50:762–769.
51. Kuhn L, Kim H-Y, Walter J, Thea DM, Sinkala M, Mwiya M, Kankasa C, Decker D, Aldrovandi GM, HIV-1 Concentrations in Human Breast Milk Before and After Weaning, *Sci Transl Med* Vol. 5, Issue 181, p. 181ra51, Sci. Transl. Med. DOI: 10.1126/scitranslmed.3005113, Apr 2013

Chapter 9: The importance of exclusive breastfeeding: why definitions matter

1. Lancet Child Survival Series, *Lancet*, Vol 361, January 4, 2003, http://www.who.int/child_adolescent_health/documents/lancet_child_survival/en/index.html (accessed 27 March 2021)
2. WHO Expert Consultation that completed the systematic review of the optimal duration of exclusive breastfeeding, A54/INF.DOC./4). See also resolution WHA54.2. (Geneva, 28–30 March 2001)
3. World Health Organization, Statement. Exclusive breastfeeding best for babies everywhere, 15 January 2011, https://www.who.int/mediacentre/news/statements/2011/breastfeeding_20110115/en/ accessed 8 July 2020).
4. de Paoli M, Manongi R, Helsing E, Klepp KI. Exclusive breastfeeding in the era of AIDS. *J Hum Lact* 2001;17(4); 313-320.
5. Kuhn L, Reitz C and Abrams EJ, Breastfeeding and AIDS in the developing world. *Current Opinion in Pediatrics* 2009;21:83–93.
6. Lawrence R, Lawrence R. *Breastfeeding: a guide for the medical profession*. St Louis, Missouri: Mosby, Inc. 1999.
7. Kent JC, Gardner H, Geddes DT, Breastmilk production in the first 4 weeks after birth of term infants. *Nutrients* 2016, *8*(12), 756 https://doi.org/10.3390/nu8120756 https://www.mdpi.com/2072-6643/8/12/756/htm (accessed 27 March 2021)
8. WHO 2001, Breastfeeding and replacement feeding practices in the context of mother-to-child transmission of HIV, an assessment tool for research, WHO/RHR/01.12, WHO/CAH/01.21 https://www.who.int/reproductivehealth/publications/maternal_perinatal_health/RHR_01_12/en/ (accessed 8 July 2020).
9. Catassi C, Bonucci A, Coppa GV et al. Intestinal permeability changes during the first month: effect of natural versus artificial feeding. *J Pedatr Gastroenterol Nutr* 1995;21:383-6.
10. Minchin M, *Milk Matters: infant feeding & immune disorder*, publisher Milk Matters Pty Ltd. Melbourne, 2015. ISBN 978095318319
11. Narayanan I, Prakash K, Murthy NS, Gujral W 1984, Randomized controlled trial of effect of raw and Holder pasteurised human milk and of formula supplements on incidence of neonatal infection. *Lancet* 2:1111-1113.
12. Black RF 1996, Transmission of HIV-1 in the breast-feeding process. *J Am Diet Assoc* 96:267-274.
13. Preble EA, Piwoz EG. *HIV and infant feeding: a chronology of research and policy advances and their implications for programs*. The LINKAGES Project. Washington, DC: Support for Analysis and Research in Africa (SARA) Project, September, 1998 . https://files.eric.ed.gov/fulltext/ED479277.pdf (accessed 2 Dec 2018)
14. Coutsoudis A, Pillay K, Spooner E, Kuhn L, Coovadia HM. Influence of infant-feeding patterns on early mother-to-child transmission of HIV-1 in Durban, South Africa: a prospective cohort study. South African Vitamin A Study Group. *Lancet.* 1999 Aug 7;354(9177):471-6 https://www.ncbi.nlm.nih.gov/pubmed/10465172 (accessed 10 December 2018)
15. Smith MM and Kuhn L, Exclusive breast-feeding: does it have the potential to reduce breast-feeding transmission of HIV-1?. Nutrition Reviews 2000;58(11):333-340.
16. Filteau SM, Rollins NC, Coutsoudis A, Sullivan KR, Willumsen JF, Tomkins AM. The effect of antenatal vitamin A and beta-carotene supplementation on gut integrity of infants of HIV-infected South African women. *J Pediatr Gastroenterol Nutr*. 2001 Apr;32(4):464-70.
17. Smith A and Heads J, Breast Pathology, in Walker M (Ed) *Core curriculum for lactation consultant practice, 2002.* Jones & Bartlett Inc and International Lactation Consultant Association.
18. Lawrence RA and Lawrence RM, 1999, *Breastfeeding: a guide for the medical profession,* 5th ed, Mosby Inc, St Louis, Missouri.
19. Amir L, Hoover K, Mulford C. Candidiasis & Breastfeeding, *Lactation Consultant Series* Unit 18, La Leche League International 1995.

20. Lake AM. Dietary protein enterocolitis. *Curr Allergy Rep*. 2001 Jan;1(1):76-9.
21. Fetherston C. Mastitis in lactating women: physiology or pathology? *Breastfeed Rev* 2001 Mar;9(1):5-12.
22. Iliff PJ, Piwoz EG, Tavengwa NV, Zunguza CD, Marinda ET, Nathoo KJ, Moulton LH, Ward BJ, the ZVITAMBO study group and Humphrey JH. Early exclusive breastfeeding reduces the risk of postnatal HIV-1 transmission and increases HIV-free survival. *AIDS* 2005, 19:699–708 https://www.ncbi.nlm.nih.gov/pubmed/15821396 (accessed 10 December 2018)
23. Coovadia HM, Rollins NC, Bland RM, Little K, Coutsoudis A, Bennish ML, Newell M-L. Mother-to-child transmission of HIV-1 infection during exclusive breastfeeding in the first 6 months of life: an intervention cohort study. *Lancet* 2007 March 31;369:1107-16. https://www.ncbi.nlm.nih.gov/pubmed/17398310 (accessed 19 Jan 2020)
24. Morbacher N, Stock J, *Breastfeeding Answer Book Revised Edition, 1997*, La Leche League International, Schaumburg, Illinois, USA.
25. Haider R, Kabir I, Huttly SR, Ashworth A. Training peer counselors to promote and support exclusive breastfeeding in Bangladesh. *J Hum Lact*. 2002 Feb;18(1):7-12.
26. Morrow AL, Guerrero ML, Shults J, Calva JJ, Lutter C, Bravo J, Ruiz-Palacios G, Morrow RC, Butterfoss FD. Efficacy of home-based peer counselling to promote exclusive breastfeeding: a randomised controlled trial. *Lancet*. 1999 Apr 10;353(9160):1226-31.
27. Almroth S and Bidinger PD, No need for water supplementation for exclusively breast-fed infants under hot and arid conditions. *Transactions of The Royal Society of Tropical Medicine and Hygiene*, 1990;84(4):602-604, https://doi.org/10.1016/0035-9203(90)90056-K
28. Ashraf RN, Jalil F, Aperia A et al Additional water is not needed forhealthy breastfed babies in a hot climate. *Acta Paediatr Scand* 1993;82:1007-1011.
29. Healthline, Parenthood, https://www.healthline.com/health/parenting/extrusion-reflex#development Accessed 9 July 2020
30. Is baby ready for solid foods? (Developmental signs of readiness) Kellymom, https://kellymom.com/nutrition/starting-solids/solids-when/ (accessed 9 July 2020)
31. Labbok M. What is the Definition of Breastfeeding? *Breastfeeding Abstracts*, February 2000, Volume 19, Number 3, pp. 19-21. La Leche League International. http://www.lalecheleague.org/ba/feb00.html (no longer found)
32. Labbok M and Krasovec K. Towards Consistency in Breastfeeding Definitions. *Studies in Family Planning* July/August 1990; 21(4):226-230.
33. *The Womanly Art of Breastfeeding*, Second Edition 166 pages, published 1976 by La Leche League International.
34. WHO 2001. The optimal duration of exclusive breastfeeding. Report of an expert consultation. Geneva, WHO (WHO/NH D/01.09, WHO/FCH/CAH/01.24) March 2001.
35. Italian Register for HIV infection in children 1994, Human immunodeficiency virus type 1 infection and breast milk. *Acta Paediatrica supplement* 400:51-58.
36. Gabiano C, Tovo PA, de Martino M Galli L, Giaquinto C, Loy A Schoeller MC, Giovannini M, Ferranti G, Rancilio L et al 1992, Mother-to-child transmission of human immunodeficiency virus type 1: Risk of infection and correlates of transmission. *Pediatrics* 90(3):369-74.
37. Dunn DT, Newell ML, Ades AE, Peckham CS 1992, Risk of human immunodeficiency virus type 1 transmission through breastfeeding, *Lancet* 340(8819)585-588.
38. Nduati R, John G, Mbori-Ngacha D, Richardson B, Overbaugh J, Mwatha A, Ndinya-Achola J, Bwayo J, Onyango FE, Hughes J, Kreiss J. Effect of breastfeeding and formula feeding on transmission of HIV-1: a randomized clinical trial. *JAMA*. 2000 Mar 1;283(9):1167-74, https://www.ncbi.nlm.nih.gov/pubmed/10703779 (accessed 28 October 2018)
39. Coutsoudis A, Breast-feeding and HIV transmission *Nutrition Research Reviews* (2001), 14, 191–206 DOI: 10.1079/NRR200123
40. Coutsoudis A, Pillay K, Spooner E, Kuhn L, Coovadia HM. Influence of infant-feeding patterns on early mother-to-child transmission of HIV-1 in Durban, South Africa: a prospective cohort study. South African Vitamin A Study Group. *Lancet*. 1999 Aug 7;354(9177):471-6.
41. Bobat R, Moodley D, Coutsoudis A, Coovadia HM. Breastfeeding by HIV-1-infected women and outcome in their infants: a cohort study from Durban, South Africa. *AIDS* 1997; 11: 1627 – 33.
42. Tess BH, Rodrigues LC, Newell ML, Dunn DT, Lago TD. Infant feeding and risk of mother-to-child transmission of HIV-1 in Sao Paulo State, Brazil. Sao Paulo Collaborative Study for vertical transmission of HIV-1. *J Acquir Immune Defic Syndr Hum Retrovirol* 1998; 19: 189–94 .
43. Coutsoudis A, Pillay K, Kuhn L, Spooner E, Tsai W-Y, Coovadia HM for the South African Vitamin A Study Group. Method of feeding and transmission of HIV-1 from mothers to children by 15 months of age: prospective cohort study from Durban, South Africa. *AIDS* 2001;15:379-387
44. World Health Organization 2003. Department of Child and Adolescent Health and Development, HIV and infant feeding data analysis, Workshop report, Recommendation for research studies, WHO/FCH/CAH/04.9. Geneva, 12-14 November 2003. http://apps.who.int/iris/bitstream/handle/10665/68749/WHO_FCH_CAH_04.9.pdf (accessed 18 November 2018.
45. Vnuk, A. Just one bottle. *Breastfeeding Review* 1993;11(8):358.
46. Smith J, Dunstone M, Elliott-Rudder. Health Professional Knowledge of Breastfeeding: Are the Health

Risks of Infant Formula Feeding Accurately Conveyed by the Titles and Abstracts of Journal Articles? *J Hum Lact* 2009; 25; 350 originally published online Apr 15, 2009; DOI: 10.1177/0890334409331506 http://jhl.sagepub.com/cgi/content/abstract/25/3/350

Chapter 10: Components in breastmilk that protect against HIV

1. Hanson LA, Adlerberth I, Carlsson, Castrignano SB, Hahn-Zoric M, Dahlgren U, Jalil F, Nilsson K, Roberton D. Breastfeeding protects against infections and allergy. *Breastfeeding Review* 1988;13:19-22.
2. Udall JN, Colony P, Fritze L, Pang K, Trier JS, Walker JA. Development of the gastrointestinal mucosal barrier: the effect of natural versus artificial feeding on intestinal permeability to macromolecules. *Pediatr Res* 1981;15: 245–49.
3. Planchon SM, Martins CAP, Guerrant RL, Roche JK. Regulation of intestinal epithelial barrier function. *J Immunol* 1994;153: 5730 – 39.
4. Newburg DS, Viscidi RP, Ruff A, Yolken RH 1992, A human milk factor inhibits binding of human immunodeficiency virus to the CD4 receptor. *Pediatr Res* 31(1):22-28.
5. Newburg, D et al. Human milk glycosaminoglycans inhibit HIV glycoprotein gp 120 binding to its host cell CD4 receptor. *J Nutr* 1995;125:419-24.
6. Duprat C, Mohammed Z, Datta P et al 1994, Human immunodeficiency virus type 1 IgA antibody in breast milk and serum. *Pediatr Infect Dis* J 13(7):603-608.
7. Van de Perre P, Simonon A, Hitimana D et al 1993, Infective and anti-infective properties of breastmilk from HIV-1 infected women. *Lancet* 341:914-18.
8. Orloff SL, Wallingford JC, McDougal JS 1993, Inactivation of human immunodeficiency virus type 1 in human milk: effects of intrinsic factors in human milk and of pasteurization. *J Hum Lact* 9(1):13-17.
9. Morrison P, HIV and infant feeding: to breastfeed or not to breastfeed: the dilemma of competing risks. Part 1. *Breastfeed Rev.* 1999 Jul;7(2):5-13, https://www.ncbi.nlm.nih.gov/m/pubmed/10453705/?i=6&from=/12179305/related
10. Morrison P, HIV and infant feeding: to breastfeed or not to breastfeed: the dilemma of competing risks. Part 2. *Breastfeed Rev.* 1999 Nov;7(3):11-20. https://www.ncbi.nlm.nih.gov/m/pubmed/10943427/?i=2&from=/10453705/related
11. Arnold LDW 1993, Currents in Human Milk Banking,: HIV and Breastmilk: What it means for milk banks. *J Hum Lact* 9(1): 47-48
12. Kabara JJ 1980, Lipids as host-resistance factors of human milk. *Nutr Rev* 38:65-73.
13. Sarkar NH, Charney J, Dion AS, Moor DH 1973, Effect of human milk on the mouse mammary tumor virus. *Cancer Res* 33:626-29.
14. Welsh JK, Arsenakis M, Coelen RJ et al 1979, Effect of antiviral lipids, heat and freezing on the activity of viruses in human milk. *J Infec Dis* 140:322-28.
15. Isaacs C, Thormar H, Pessolano T. Membrane-disruptive effect of human milk; inactivation of enveloped viruses. *J Infect Dis* 1986;154:966-71.
16. Thormar H, Isaacs CE, Brown HR, Bashatzky MR, et al, Inactivation of enveloped viruses and killing of cells by fatty acids and monoglycerides. *Antimicrob Agents Chemother* 1987;31:27-31.
17. McDougal, JS 1990, Pasteurization of human breast milk and its effect on HIV infectivity. Presentation at the annual meeting of the Human Milk Banking Assocation of North America, Lexington, Kentucky, October 15.
18. Isaacs, CE and Thormar, H; Human milk lipids inactivate enveloped viruses. In Atkinson, SA, Hanson, LA and Chandra, RK, eds: *Breastfeeding, nutrition, infection and infant growth in developed and emerging countries,* St John's Newfoundland, Canada, 1990, ARTS Biomedical Publisher, Canada:161-174.
19. Nduati RW, John GC, Richardson BA, Overbaugh J, Welch M, Ndinya-Achola J, Moses S, Holmes K, Onyango F and Kreiss JK 1995, Human immunodeficiency virus type 1-infected cells in breast milk: association with immunosuppression and vitamin A deficiency. *J Infect Dis* 1995;172:1461-8.
20. Lewis P, Nduati R, Kreiss JK, John GC, Richardson BA, Mbori-Ngacha D, Ndinya-Achola J, Overbaugh J, Cell-free human immunodeficiency virus type 1 in breastmilk. *Infect Dis* 1998;177(1):34-39.
21. Hoffman IF, Martinson FE, Stewart PW, Chilongozi DA, Leu SY, Kazembe PN, Banda T, Dzinyemba W, Joshi P, Cohen MS, Fiscus SA Human immunodeficiency virus type 1 RNA in breast-milk components. *J Infect Dis.* 2003 Oct 15;188(8):1209-12. Epub 2003 Oct 1.
22. Valerie McClain, Blog, https://vwmcclain.blogspot.com/2012/12/the-bitter-pill-of-human-milk-banking.html accessed 20 Jan 2020
23. Isaacs CE, Litov RE, Thormar H, Antimicrobial activity of lipids added to human milk, infant formula and bovine milk, *Journal of Nutritional Biochemistry* 1995;6(7):362-366. https://www.sciencedirect.com/science/article/abs/pii/095528639580003U (accessed 17 February 2020).
24. Newburg DS and Grave G, Recent advances in human milk glycobiology, *Pediatr Res* 2014;75(5):675-679. https://www.ncbi.nlm.nih.gov/pmc/articles/PMC4125201/ (accessed 17 February 2020)
25. Valerie McClain, personal communication, Aug 2010.
26. Newburg D and Walker WA, Protection of the neonate by the innate immune system of developing gut and of human milk. *Pediatr Res* 2007;61: 2–8, https://www.nature.com/articles/pr20073 (accessed 3 September 2020)

27. Lars Bode et al. Human milk oligosaccharide concentration and risk of postnatal transmission of HIV through breastfeeding. *Am J Clin Nutr* 2012. doi: 10.3945/ajcn.112.039503. https://www.ncbi.nlm.nih.gov/pmc/articles/PMC3441110/ (accessed 4 July 2020)
28. Kuhn L et al, Alpha-defensins in the prevention of HIV-transmission among breastfed infants. *J Acquir Immune Defic Syndr* 2005;39:138–142
29. Moussa S et al. Adaptive HIV-specific B cell-derived humoral immune defenses of the intestinal mucosa in children exposed to HIV via breast-feeding. *PLoS One*. 2013 May 21;8(5):e63408. doi: 10.1371/journal.pone.0063408. Print 2013. http://www.ncbi.nlm.nih.gov/pubmed/23704905
30. Palaia JM et al. Neutralization of HIV subtypes A and D by breast milk IgG from women with HIV infection in Uganda. *Journal of Infection* 2014;68(3):264-272. http://www.journalofinfection.com/article/S0163-4453(13)00332-0/abstract (accessed 3 September 2020)
31. Miller M, Iliff P et al, Breastmilk Erythropoietin and Mother-To-Child HIV Transmission Through Breastmilk, *Lancet* 2002 Oct 19;360(9341):1246-8. doi: 10.1016/S0140-6736(02)11277-3 . https://pubmed.ncbi.nlm.nih.gov/12401271/
32. Arsenault JE et al, Association between breast milk erythropoietin and reduced risk of mother-to-child transmission of HIV. *J Infect Dis*. 2010 Aug 15;202(3):370-3. doi: 10.1086/653706. https://pubmed.ncbi.nlm.nih.gov/20557236/
33. Henrick BM et al, Breastfeeding Behaviors and the Innate Immune System of Human Milk: Working Together to Protect Infants against Inflammation, HIV-1, and Other Infections. *Front Immunol.* 2017;8:1631. https://pubmed.ncbi.nlm.nih.gov/29238342/ (accessed 3 September 2020)
34. Prameela KK, HIV transmission through breastmilk: the science behind the understanding of current trends and future research. *Med J Malaysia*, Dec 2012;67(6):644-650. https://pubmed.ncbi.nlm.nih.gov/23770969/ (accessed 4 July 2020)
35. Shapiro RL, Lockman S, Kim S et al (2007) Infant morbidity, mortality, and breast milk immunologic profiles among breast-feeding HIV-infected and HIV-uninfected women in Botswana. *J Infect Dis* 196:562–565 https://pubmed.ncbi.nlm.nih.gov/17624842/ (accessed 4 July 2020)
36. Kuhn L, Aldrovandi G. Pendulum Swings in HIV-1 and Infant Feeding Policies: Now Halfway Back. *Adv Exp Med Biol.* 2012;743:273-87. http://www.ncbi.nlm.nih.gov/pubmed/22454357

Chapter 11: Pasteurised breastmilk as a replacement feed for the babies of HIV-positive mothers

1. Latham MC, Kisanga P, Current status of proection support and promotion of breastfeeding in four African countries: actions to protect, support and promote breastfeeding in Botswana, Kenya, Namibia and Uganda, based on a rapid review 2 Oct – 3 Nov 2000, Prepared for UNICEF ESARO March 2001.
2. Arnold LDW 1993, Issues in Human milk banking, *Breastfeeding and Human Lactation*, Riordan J and Auerbach KG, Editors, Jones & Bartlett, London & Boston, p 600 - 603.
3. Orloff SL, Wallingford JC, McDougal JS, Inactivation of human immunodeficiency virus type 1 in human milk: effects of intrinsic factors in human milk and of pasteurization. *J Hum Lact* 1993; 9(1):13-17. https://www.ncbi.nlm.nih.gov/pubmed/8489717 (accessed 18 Nov 2018)
4. McDougal, JS 1990, Pasteurization of human breast milk and its effect on HIV infectivity. Presentation at the annual meeting of the Human Milk Banking Assocation of North America, Lexington, Kentucky, October 15.
5. Isaacs, CE and Thormar, H; Human milk lipids inactivate enveloped viruses. In Atkinson, SA, Hanson, LA and Chandra, RK, eds: *Breastfeeding, nutrition, infection and infant growth in developed and emerging countries,* St John's Newfoundland, Canada, 1990, ARTS Biomedical Publisher, Canada:161-174.
6. Chantry CJ, Morrison P, Panchula J, Rivera C, Hillyer G, Zorilla C, Diaz C. Effects of lipolysis or heat treatment on HIV-1 provirus in breast milk. *J Acquir Immune Defic Syndr* 2000;24(4):325-9, http://www.ncbi.nlm.nih.gov/pubmed/11015148
7. Israel-Ballard KA, Maternowska MC, Abrams BF, Morrison P, Chitibura L, Chipato T, Chirenje ZM, Padian NS, Chantry CJ, Acceptability of Heat-treating Breast milk to Prevent Mother-to-Child Transmission of HIV in Zimbabwe: A Qualitative Study, *J Hum Lact* 2006; 22(1):48-60 https://pubmed.ncbi.nlm.nih.gov/16467287/ (accessed 1 July 2020)
8. Kiersten Israel-Ballard, https://globalhealth.washington.edu/faculty/kiersten-israel-ballard (accessed 2 July 2020
9. Walls T, Breastfeeding in mothers with HIV. *Journal of Paediatrics and Child Health* 2010; 46:349–352
10. LACTNET Archives, an email listserv for Lactation Professionals, LACTNET@PEACH.EASE.LSOFT.COM
11. WHO (World Health Organization). 2003. The global strategy for infant and young child feeding. Available at http://www.who.int/child_adolescent_health/documents/9241562218/en/index.html
12. Zimbabwe Ministry of Health and Child Welfare, Infant Feeding and HIV/AIDS; guidelines for health workers in Zimbabwe; June 12, 2000.
13. Israel-Ballard K, Coutsoudis A, Chantry CJ, Sturm AW, Karim F, Sibeko L, Abrams B. Bacterial safety of flash-heated and unheated expressed breastmilk during storage. *J Trop Pediatr*. 2006;52:399–405.
14. Israel-Ballard K, Donovan R, Chantry C, Coutsoudis A, Sheppard H, Sibeko L and Abrams B. Flash heat inactivation of HIV-1 in human milk. A potential method to reduce postnatal transmission in developing

countries. *J Acquir Immun Defic Syndr* 2007;45 (3): 318-323, 2007
15. Rollins N, Meda N, Becquet R, Coutsoudis A, Humphrey J, Jeffrey B, Kanshana S, Kuhn L, Leroy V, Mbori-Ngacha D, McIntyre J, Newell ML; Ghent IAS Working Group on HIV in Women and Children.
16. Israel-Ballard KA et al. Vitamin content of breast milk from HIV-1–infected mothers before and after flash-heat treatment. *J Acquir Immune Defic Syndr* 2008;48: 444–449.
17. Chantry CJ, Israel-Ballard K, Moldoveanu Z, Peerson J, Coutsoudis, Sibeko L and Abrams B. Effect of Flash-heat Treatment on Immunoglobulins in Breastmilk. *J Acquir Immune Defic Syndr*. 2009 July 1; 51(3): 264–267. doi:10.1097/QAI.0b013e3181aa12f2. http://www.ncbi.nlm.nih.gov/pmc/articles/PMC2779733/pdf/nihms126967.pdf (accessed 5 December 2010)
18. Volk ML, Hanson CV, Israel-Ballard K, Chantry CJ, Inactivation of Cell-Associated and Cell-Free HIV-1 by Flash-Heat Treatment of Breast Milk. *J Acquir Immune Defic Syndr* 2010;53(5):665-666.
19. Chantry, CJ, Wiedeman J, Buehring G, Peerson JM, Hayfron K, K'Aluoch O, Lonnerdal B, Israel-Ballard K, Coutsoudis A,7 and Abrams B. Effect of Flash-Heat Treatment on Antimicrobial Activity of Breastmilk. *Breastfeeding Medicine* 2011; 6(3), DOI DOI: 10.1089/bfm.2010.0078
20. Mbuya MNN, Humphrey JH, Majo F, Chasekwa B, Jenkins A, Israel-Ballard K, Muti M, Paul KH, Madzima RC, Moulton LH and Stoltzfus RJ. Heat treatment of expressed breast milk is a feasible option for feeding HIV-exposed, uninfected children after 6 months of age in rural Zimbabwe. *J Nutr* 2010, Epub ahead of print June 23, 2010 as doi: 10.3945/jn.110.122457
21. Jeffery BS, Mercer KG, Pretoria pasteurisation: a potential method for the reduction of postnatal mother to child transmission of the human immunodeficiency virus, *J Trop Pediatr* 2000;46(4):219-23.
22. Jeffery BS, Webber L, Mokhondo KR and Erasmus D, Determination of the Effectiveness of Inactivation of Human Immunodeficiency Virus by Pretoria Pasteurization, *J Trop Pediatr* 2001; 47(6):345-349.
23. Jeffery BS, Soma-Pillay P, Makin J and Mooman G, The effect of Pretoria pasteurization on bacterial contamination of hand-expressed human breastmilk. *J Trop Pediatr* 2004;49(4):240-244.
24. Reimers P, personal communication in GOLD10 Forum, www.goldconf.com May 2010
25. Rollins N, Meda N, Becquet R, Coutsoudis A, Humphrey J, Jeffrey B, Kanshana S, Kuhn L, Leroy V, Mbori-Ngacha D, McIntyre J, Newell ML; Ghent IAS Working Group on HIV in Women and Children. Preventing postnatal transmission of HIV-1 through breast-feeding: modifying infant feeding practices. *J Acquir Immune Defic Syndr*. 2004 Feb 1;35(2):188-95. https://pubmed.ncbi.nlm.nih.gov/14722453/ (accessed 2 July 2020).
26. Chantry CJ, Young SL, Rennie W, Ngonyani M, Mashi C, Israel-Ballard K, Peerson J, Nyambo MD, Matee M, Ash D, Dewey K and Koniz-Booher P. Feasibility of Using Flash-heated Breastmilk as an Infant Feeding Option for HIV-exposed, Uninfected Infants after 6 Months of Age in Urban Tanzania *J Acquir Immune Defic Syndr* 2012 , DOI: 10.1097/QAI.0b013e31824fc06e https://www.ncbi.nlm.nih.gov/pmc/articles/PMC3380080/ (accessed 3 September 2020)
27. Wills ME, Han VEM, Harris DA, et al. Short-time, low-temperature pasteurization of human milk. *Early Hum Dev*. 1982;7:71–80.
28. Israel-Ballard K, Chantry C, Dewey K et al. Viral, nutritional and bacterial safety of flash-heated and Pretoria pasteurized beast milk to prevent mother-to-child transmission of HIV in resource-poor countries: a pilot study. *J Acquir Immune Defic Syndr*. 2005;40:175-181.
29. Israel-Ballard K, Flash-heated and Pretoria Pasteurized destroys HIV in breast milk & Preserves Nutrients! *Advanced Biotech* Sept 2008, available at http://www.advancedbiotech.in/51%20Flash%20heated.pdf
30. TenHam WH, Heat treatment of expressed breast milk as in-home procedure to limit mother-to-child transmission of HIV: A systematic review. Submitted to School of Nursing Science, North-West University, Potchefstroom, South Africa November 2009 available at http://dspace.nwu.ac.za/bitstream/10394/3745/1/TenHam_HW.pdf
31. Brusseau R 1998, Analysis of refrigerated human milk following infant feeding (unpublished study).
32. See demo video at http://www.berkeley.edu/news/media/releases/2007/05/21_breastmilk-video.shtml
33. WHO 2006, Weight for age percentiles for girls, birth to 2 years http://www.who.int/childgrowth/standards/cht_wfa_girls_p_0_2.pdf
34. WHO 2006, Weight for age percentiles for boys, birth to 2 years http://www.who.int/childgrowth/standards/cht_wfa_boys_p_0_2.pdf

Chapter 12: Global policy on HIV and breastfeeding 1996–2009: formula for disaster

1. Ziegler JB et al. Postnatal transmission of AIDS-associated retrovirus from mother to infant. *Lancet*. 1985 Apr 20;i(8434):896-8. https://www.ncbi.nlm.nih.gov/pubmed/2858746 (accessed 21 Oct 2018).
2. Centers for Disease Control and Prevention. Recommendations for assisting in the prevention of perinatal transmission of human T lymphotropic virus type III/lymphadenopathy-associated virus and acquired immunodeficiency syndrome. *Morb Mortal Wkly Rep*.1985;34:721726, 731732. https://www.ncbi.nlm.nih.gov/pubmed/2999576 (accessed 24 November 2018)
3. Jelliffe, DB and Jelliffe EF, *Human Milk in the Modern World*, Chapter 6 International Concern. Oxford University Press 1978
4. World Health Assembly Resolution, Geneva, 27.43, page 20, 7-23 May 1974 http://apps.who.int/iris/bitstream/handle/10665/85874/Official_record217_eng.pdf?sequence=1&isAllowed=y (accessed 24

November 2018)
5. World Health Organization, *International Code of marketing of breast-milk substitutes*, Geneva 1981 http://www.who.int/nutrition/publications/code_english.pdf (accessed 24 November 2018)
6. Baby Feeding Law Group. *Organisations funded by the breastmilk substitute industry* June 2019 https://static1.squarespace.com/static/5c6bb04a65a70771b7cbc916/t/5d07df0ddac3c80001227 6e2/1560796942265/Websites_and_organisations_June19final.pdf (accessed 15 March 2020)
7. World Health Organization, Special Programme on AIDS statement, Breast-feeding/Breast milk and Human Immunodeficiency Virus (HIV) WHO/SPA/INF/87.8. http://apps.who.int/iris/bitstream/handle/10665/60788/WHO_SPA_INF_87.8.pdf (accessed 24 November 2018)
8. United Nations *Convention on the Rights of the Child*, 1989-1990, https://www.unicef.org.uk/wp-content/uploads/2010/05/UNCRC_united_nations_convention_on_the_rights_of_the_child.pdf (accessed 24 November 2018)
9. UNICEF. *Innocenti Declaration on the protection, promotion and support of breastfeeding*, Florence, Italy, 1 August 1990 http://worldbreastfeedingweek.org/2018/wp-content/uploads/2018/07/1990-Innocenti-Declaration.pdf (accessed 24 November 2018)
10. United Nations, World Summit for Children, New York, https://www.un.org/en/development/devagenda/children.shtml
11. WHO/UNICEF Consultation on HIV Transmission and Breast-Feeding 30 April – 1 May ⊠1992: Geneva, Switzerland. http://www.who.int/iris/handle/10665/61014 (accessed 25 November 2018)
12. Baby-Friendly USA: The Baby-Friendly Hospital Initiative, (https://www.babyfriendlyusa.org/about (accessed 11 January 2022)
13. UNICEF *Ten Steps to Successful Breastfeeding*, https://www.unicef.org/newsline/tenstps.htm (accessed 25 November 2018)
14. WHO/UNICEF. *Breastfeeding counseling: a training course*. Geneva: WHO, 1993. Accessed at https://www.who.int/maternal_child_adolescent/documents/who_cdr_93_3/en/ (accessed 10 February 2021)
15. UNAIDS, UNICEF and WHO HIV and Infant Feeding - A Policy Statement developed collaboratively by UNAIDS, UNICEF and WHO (UNAIDS, 1997, 12 p.) https://www.ncbi.nlm.nih.gov/pubmed/10453706 (accessed 28 March 2020)
16. UNICEF. *The Baby Friendly Hospital Initivative Newsletter*. Sept/Oct 1998 p. 6. Reprinted in SCN News, No. 17 Nutrition and HIV/AIDS, December 1998 https://www.unscn.org/resource-center-archives (accessed 10 May 2020)
17. Latham M, Greiner T, *Lancet* 1998; 352:9129 29 August (letter)
18. Latham M and Greiner T, Is the United Nations making wise recommendations on how to deal with HIV and breastfeeding? *Birth Issues* 1998;7(3)93-4. http://figshare.com/articles/Is_the_United_Nations_making_wise_recommendations_on_how_to_deal_with_HIV_and_breastfeeding_/1335668 (accessed 14 March 2015)
19. Nduati R et al, Effect of breastfeeding and formula feeding on transmission of HIV-1, a randomized clinical trial. *JAMA* 2000;283(9):1167-1174. doi:10.1001/jama.283.9.1167. https://jamanetwork.com/journals/jama/fullarticle/192449 (accessed 3 December 2018)
20. Francois Dabis, (updated April 2015) http://www.who.int/hiv/mediacentre/news/Francois_Dabis.pdf
21. Dabis F, Estimating the rate of mother-to-child transmission of HIV. Report of a workshop on methodological issues Ghent (Belgium), 17-20 February 1992. The Working Group on Mother-to-Child Transmission of HIV, AIDS 1993;7(8):1139-1148 http://discovery.ucl.ac.uk/1366336/
22. Dunn DT et al, Risk of human immunodeficiency virus type 1 transmission through breastfeeding. *Lancet* 1992;340(8819):585-8] https://www.ncbi.nlm.nih.gov/pubmed/1355163 (accessed 3 December 2018)
23. Global Programme on AIDS, Consensus Statement from the WHO/UNICEF Consultation on HIV transmission and breastfeeding Geneva 30 April – 1 May 1992. WHO/GPA/UBF/92.1. https://apps.who.int/iris/handle/10665/61014 (accessed 26 March 2020)
24. Chapter 5, Routes of Infection, Mother to Child transmission
25. Dabis F et al, Methodology of intervention trials to reduce mother to child transmission of HIV with special reference to developing countries, *AIDS* 1995; 9 (Suppl A)567-574. https://jhu.pure.elsevier.com/en/publications/methodology-of-intervention-trials-to-reduce-mother-to-child-tran-3 (accessed 28 November 2018)
26. Dabis F and The Working Group on Mother-to-child transmission of HIV, Rates of Mother-to-Child Transmission of HIV-1 in Africa, America, and Europe: Results from 13 Perinatal Studies. *Journal of Acquired Immune Deficiency Syndromes and Human Retrovirology* 1995;8:8506-510 https://pdfs.semanticscholar.org/6461/7d7f3284d2b5ab0fb3a56edf87c3f75e6034.pdf (accessed 23 March 2020).
27. Zunguza C, personal communication.
28. Connor EM et al, Reduction of Maternal-Infant Transmission of Human Immunodeficiency Virus Type 1 with Zidovudine Treatment, *New England Journal of Medicine*, 1994;331(18):1173-1180 https://www.nejm.org/doi/full/10.1056/NEJM199411033311801 (accessed 28 November 2018)
29. Mofensen L, Short-course zidovudine for prevention of perinatal infection, *Lancet* 1999;353:766-767.
30. CDC Recommendations of the U.S. Public Health Service Task Force on the Use of Zidovudine to Reduce Perinatal Transmission of Human Immunodeficiency Virus. *MMWR* 1994;43 (no. RR-11). https://www.cdc.gov/mmwr/preview/mmwrhtml/00032271.htm (accessed 3 December 2018)

31. Shaffer N, Bhiraleus P, Chinayon P, et al. High viral load predicts perinatal HIV-1 subtype E transmission, Bangkok, Thailand {Abstract}. Vancouver, Canada: XIth International Conference on AIDS, July1996.
32. CDC Studies of AZT to Prevent Mother-to-Child HIV Transmission in Developing Countries, AIDSInfo, 1 June 1997. https://aidsinfo.nih.gov/news/363/cdc-studies-of-azt-to-prevent-mother-to-child-hiv-transmission-in-developing-countries (accessed 29 November 2018).
33. Shaffer N, Chuachoowong R, Mock PA, Bhadrakom C, Siriwasin W, Young NL, Chotpitayasunondh T, Chearskul S, Roongpisuthipong A, Chinayon P, Karon J, Mastro TD, Simonds RJ. Short-course zidovudine for perinatal HIV-1 transmission in Bangkok, Thailand: a randomised controlled trial. Bangkok Collaborative Perinatal HIV Transmission Study Group. *Lancet.* 1999 Mar 6;353(9155):773-80.) https://www.thelancet.com/pdfs/journals/lancet/PIIS0140673698104117.pdf (accessed 29 November 2018)
34. Dabis F et al, 6-month efficacy, tolerance, and acceptability of a short regimen of oral zidovudine to reduce vertical transmission of HIV in breastfed children in Côte d'Ivoire and Burkina Faso: a double-blind placebo-controlled multicentre trial. DITRAME Study Group. Diminution de la Transmission Mère-Enfant. *Lancet* 1999;353(9155:786-92) https://www.ncbi.nlm.nih.gov/pubmed/10459959 (accessed 1 December 2018)
35. Wiktor SZ et al, Ekpini Randomized clinical trial of a short course of oral zidovudine to prevent mother-to-child transmission of HIV–1 in Abidjan, Côte d'Ivoire. *Lancet* 1999; 353: 781–5. https://www.thelancet.com/journals/lanonc/article/PIIS0140-6736(98)10412-9/fulltext (accessed 3 December 2018.
36. Kreiss J 1997, Breastfeeding and vertical transmission of HIV-1. *Acta Paediatr Suppl* 421:113-117.
37. De Wagt A & Clark D, Nutrition Section, United Nations Children's Fund, New York, USA. UNICEF's Support to Free Infant Formula for Infants of HIVInfected Mothers in Africa: A Review of UNICEF Experience. Presented at the LINKAGES Art and Science of Breastfeeding Presentation Series, April 14, 2004, Washington, DC. http://www.waba.org.my/whatwedo/hcp/pdf/r-unicef-free.pdf Accessed 10 December 2018.
38. Medscape, Ten years of HAART 2006, https://www.medscape.org/viewarticle/523119 (accessed 3 March 2020)
39. Julio Montaner, interview 2009, talking retrospectively about the pivotal change brought about by the International AIDS Conference held in Vancouver in 1996, https://www.youtube.com/watch?v=bM6514q3j-Y
40. Meier B, Mother's dilemma, special report. In War against AIDS, battle over baby formula reignites, *New York Times*, 8 June 1997 http://www.nytimes.com/1997/06/08/business/in-war-against-aids-battle-over-baby-formula-reignites.html (accessed 7 December 2018)
41. Gray G. McIntyre JA, Lytons SF. The effect of breastfeeding on vertical transmission of HIV-1 in Soweto, South Africa. *Int Conf AIDS* 1996; July 7-12;11(2):237 (abstract Oral Th.C415.)
42. Dr Glenda Gray, personal verbal communication, AIDS conference, Toronto, 2006.
43. UNAIDS, the first ten years, UNAIDS/07.20E / JC1262E, 2008
44. Baumslag N, Tricks of the Infant Food Industry, Health Topics – Children's Health, *Wise Traditions in Food, Farming and the Healing Arts*, the quarterly magazine of the Weston A Price Foundation, Volume 2, Number 3, Fall 2001. Available at http://www.westonaprice.org/childrens-health/325-tricks-of-the-infant-food-industry.html (accessed 26 December 2010 but unavailable on 7 March 2020).
45. UNAIDS 1996, Second International Consultation on HIV/AIDS and Human Rights (Geneva, 23-25 September 1996) http://data.unaids.org/publications/irc-pub03/3797_en.html (accessed 25 March 2020)
46. UNAIDS (Joint United Nations Programme on HIV/AIDS) HIV and infant feeding: an interim statement, Weekly Epidemiological Record 27 Sept 1996;71:289-291. https://apps.who.int/iris/bitstream/handle/10665/229839/WER7129.PDF (accessed 25 November 2020)
47. Bobat R, Moodley D, Coutsoudis A, Coovadia H. Breastfeeding by HIV-1-infected women and outcome in their infants: a cohort study from Durban, South Africa. *AIDS.* 1997 Nov;11(13):1627-33. https://www.ncbi.nlm.nih.gov/pubmed/9365768 (accessed 10 May 2020)
48. Gray GE (2010) Adolescent HIV—Cause for Concern in Southern Africa. Feb 2, 2010. *PLoS Med* 7(2): e1000227. https://doi.org/10.1371/journal.pmed.1000227 https://journals.plos.org/plosmedicine/article?id=10.1371/journal.pmed.1000227 (accessed 28 March 2021)
49. Craig Timberg, In Botswana, step to cut AIDS proves a formula for disaster, *Washington Post* 23 July 2007, http://www.washingtonpost.com/wp-dyn/content/article/2007/07/22/*AR2007072201204*_pf.html accessed 5 May 2019)
50. White E, *Breastfeeding and HIV/AIDS; the research, the politics and women's responses.* 1999. McFarland & Company, inc, publishers, North Carolina, USA,
51. Kuhn L, Aldrovandi G. Pendulum Swings in HIV-1 and Infant Feeding Policies: Now Halfway Back. *Adv Exp Med Biol.* 2012;743:273-87. http://www.ncbi.nlm.nih.gov/pubmed/22454357
52. Dabis F et al, Prevention of mother-to-child transmission of HIV in developing countries; recommendations for practice. Health Policy and Planning 2000; 15(1): 34–42 https://watermark.silverchair.com/150034.pdf (accessed 30 November 2018)
53. IATT WHO UNICEF, Introduction to Toolkit, Expanding and Simplifying Treatment for Pregnant Women Living with HIV: Managing the Transition to Option B/B+, https://www.childrenandaids.org/sites/default/files/2017-05/IATT-Toolkit-Dec-2014_JR-1-28-15-Web1.pdf (accessed 21 November 2021)
54. UNICEF 2005, PMTCT Report Card, Monitoring Progress on the Implementation of Programs

to Prevent Mother to Child Transmission of HIV, http://www.unicef.org/ufc_PMTCTreportcard.pdf (accessed 19 November 2008) (page not found on 25 June 2020)
55. UNAIDS, Prevention of HIV Transmission from Mother to Child Planning for Programme Implementation Report from a Meeting, Geneva, 23-24 March 1998. http://data.unaids.org/publications/irc-pub05/mtctreport_en.pdf
56. De Cock KM, Fowler MG, Mercier E, De Vincenzi I, Saba J, Hoff E, Alnwick DJ, Rogers M, Shaffer N, Prevention of mother-to-child HIV transmission in resource-poor countries; translation research into policy and practice. *JAMA* 2000;283:1175-1182 available at https://www.ncbi.nlm.nih.gov/pubmed/10703780 (accessed 14 January 2020)
57. WHO/UNICEF/UNAIDS Technical Consultation on HIV and Infant Feeding. Implementation of Guidelines Report of a Meeting - Geneva, 20-22 April 1998 http://www.unaids.org/sites/default/files/media_asset/jc180-hiv-infantfeeding-4_en_0.pdf (accessed 8 December 2018)
58. UNAIDS/UNICEF/WHO. 1998. HIV and Infant Feeding: A review of HIV transmission through breastfeeding, WHO/FRH/NUT/CHD/98.3. http://data.unaids.org/publications/irc-pub03/hivmod3_en.pdf (accessed 7 December 2018)
59. UNAIDS/UNICEF/WHO 1998. HIV and Infant Feeding: Guidelines for decision-makers. WHO/FRH/NUT/CHD/98.1. http://data.unaids.org/publications/irc-pub01/jc180-hiv-infantfeeding_en.pdf (accessed 7 December 2018)
60. UNAIDS/UNICEF/WHO 1998. HIV and Infant Feeding: Guidelines for health care managers and supervisors. WHO/FRH/NUT/CHD/98.2. http://data.unaids.org/publications/irc-pub01/jc180-hiv-infantfeeding_en.pdf (accessed 7 December 2018).
61. Altman LK UN Plans to treat 30,000 HIV infected pregnant women, *New York Times*, June 30, 1998. http://www.nytimes.com/1998/06/30/us/un-plans-to-treat-30000-hiv-infected-pregnant-women.html
62. Preble EA and Piwoz EG, 1998, *HIV and infant feeding: A chronology of research and policy advances and their implications for programs*, The Linkages Project and the Support for Analysis and Research in Africa (SARA) Project, the Academy for Educational Development, USAID Bureau for Africa available at https://files.eric.ed.gov/fulltext/ED479277.pdf (accessed 2 Dec 2018)
63. Altman L, AIDS brings a shift on breast-feeding, *New York Times*, July 26, 1998. http://www.nytimes.com/1998/07/26/world/aids-brings-a-shift-on-breast-feeding.html?ref=lawrencekaltman (accessed 9 December 2018)
64. UNAIDS 1998 Technical Update, page 10, http://data.unaids.org/publications/irc-pub01/jc531-mtct-tu_en.pdf (accessed 12 February 2021)
65. Temmerman M, Piot P. The epidemiology of HIV infection and AIDS in developing countries: the impact on women's health. *Annales Nestlé* 1993,51:98-105.
66. Wyeth, Nestlé Offer Free Tins to Stem Spread of AIDS Children's Agency Balks, *Wall Street Journal* Tuesday December 5, 2000 https://www.wsj.com/articles/SB975978176677135549 (accessed 7 December 2018)
67. United States Permanent Representative to the European Office of the United Nations, Geneva (1993-1996) see https://www.cov.com/en/professionals/s/daniel-spiegel (accessed 5 August 2018)
68. See Baby Milk Action press release, http://archive.babymilkaction.org/press/presssept97.html.
69. *SCN News*, No. 17 December 1998 https://www.unscn.org/resource-center-archives (accessed 10 May 2020)
70. WHO accused of stifling debate about infant feeding. *BMJ* 2000;320:1362 https://www.bmj.com/content/320/7246/1362.1.full (accessed 9 May 2020)
71. Yamey G, The Milk of Human Kindness. *British Medical Journal* Jan 2001 http://www.bmj.com/cgi/content/full/322/7277/57 (accessed 9 May 2020)
72. See http://pfeda.univ-lille1.fr/Ethiop/Pub/0628sod.htm (accessed 12 May 2019)
73. Helen Armstrong, personal conversation
74. WHO Collaborative Study Team on the Role of Breastfeeding on the Prevention of Infant Mortality. Effect of breastfeeding on infant and child mortality due to infectious diseases in less developed countries: a pooled analysis. *Lancet*. 2000;355:451–455. http://www.ncbi.nlm.nih.gov/pubmed/10841125 (accessed 23 March 2020.
75. WHO Technical consultation on behalf of the UNFPA/UNICEF/WHO/UNAIDS Inter-Agency Task Team on Mother-to-Child Transmission of HIV, New Data on the prevention of mother-to-child transmission of HIV and their policy implications conclusions and recommendations, Geneva 11-13 October 2000 https://apps.who.int/iris/handle/10665/66851 (accessed 18 March 2020)
76. UNAIDS and World Health Organization. *AIDS epidemic update* – December 2001, Geneva https://www.who.int/hiv/facts/en/isbn9291731323.pdf (accessed 11 April 2020).
77. United Nations General Assembly Special Session on HIV/AIDS, 25-27 June 2001, New York, United Nations Declaration of Commitment on HIV/AIDS https://www.who.int/hiv/pub/advocacy/aidsdeclaration_en.pdf (accessed 11 Apr 2020)
78. WHO 2003. Global strategy for infant and young child feeding, Geneva: World Health Organization, 2003
79. Morrison P. Personal notes, reports and emails to ILCA, June and July 2001.
80. Coutsoudis A, Pillay K, Spooner E, Kuhn L, Coovadia HM. Influence of infant-feeding patterns on early mother-to-child transmission of HIV-1 in Durban, South Africa: a prospective cohort study. South

African Vitamin A Study Group. *Lancet.* 1999 Aug 7;354(9177):471-6. https://www.ncbi.nlm.nih.gov/pubmed/10465172 (accessed 10 December 2018)

81. Coutsoudis A, Pillay K, Kuhn L, Spooner E, Tsai W-Y, Coovadia HM for the South African Vitamin A Study Group. Method of feeding and transmission of HIV-1 from mothers to children by 15 months of age: prospective cohort study from Durban, South Africa. *AIDS* 2001;15:379-387
82. WHO 2003, Global strategy for infant and young child feeding, Geneva: World Health Organization, available from: http://whqlibdoc.who.int/publications/2003/9241562218.pdf
83. WHO 2002, Strategic approaches to the prevention of HIV infection in infants : report of a WHO meeting, Morges, Switzerland, 20-22 March 2002, https://apps.who.int/iris/handle/10665/42723 (accessed 9 April 2020)
84. WHO 2003, WHO/UNICEF/UNFPA/UNAIDS/World Bank/UNHCR/WFP/FAO/IAEA. HIV and infant feeding: framework for priority action, Geneva: World Health Organization, 2003, http://whqlibdoc.who.int/publications/2003/9241590777.pdf (accessed 31 August 2012)
85. WHO 2004, HIV and infant feeding: framework for priority action, ISBN 92 4 159077 7, Slideset https://www.who.int/maternal_child_adolescent/documents/pdfs/hiv_if_slide_set.pdf (accessed 19 March 2020)
86. WHO 2004. HIV & Infant Feeding: Guidelines for Decision makers http://www.who.int/child_adolescent_health/documents/9241591226/en/index.html (accessed 23 December 2008).
87. WHO 2004. HIV and infant feeding: A guide for health-care managers and supervisors , World Health Organization 2003 http://www.who.int/child_adolescent_health/documents/9241591234/en/index.html (accessed 23 December 2008)
88. WHO 2004. HIV Transmission through breastfeeding: a review of available evidence. http://www.who.int/child-adolescent-health/New_Publications/NUTRITION/ISBN_92_4_156271_4.pdf
89. Koniz-Booher P, Burkhalter B, de Wagt A, Iliff P, Willumsen J (eds) 2004. *HIV and infant feeding: a compilation of programmatic evidence.* Bethesda, MD, published for UNICEF and the US Agency for Inernational Development by the Quality Assurance Project (QAP) University Research Co., LLC (URC).
90. WHO 2005 HIV and Infant Feeding Counselling Tools, ISBN 92 4 159301 6, available from http://whqlibdoc.who.int/publications/2005/9241593016.pdf
91. *Zimbabwe Parliamentary Gazette.* Statutory Instrument 46 of 1998 (CAP.15:09) Public Health (Breast-milk Substitutes and Infant Nutrition) Regulations, 1998
92. Meier BM and Labbok M, From the bottle to the Grave, *Case W. Res. L. Rev.* 1073 2009-2010, http://bmeier.web.unc.edu/files/2010/11/Meier-Labbok-2010.pdf accessed 10 May 2020

Chapter 13: Implementing the policy through the HIV and Infant Feeding Counselling Course

1. Currently called Harare Hospital. Before independence in 1980 and for many years afterwards the spelling of this name was Harari, whereas the city was always spelled Harare.
2. Morrison P, Review: WHO HIV and Infant Feeding Counselling Course, *J Hum Lact* 2002;18(4):403 http://jhl.sagepub.com/cgi/reprint/18/4/403
3. BEST Services, http://www.bestservices.ie/index.php (accessed 5 April 2020)
4. P 148 Page WHO/UNAIDS/UNICEF HIV and Infant Feeding Counselling: A training course; Trainer's Guide. WHO 2000, WHO/FCH/CAH/00.3, UNICEF/PD/NUT/(J)00-2, UNAIDS/99.56E https://www.who.int/nutrition/publications/en/hiv_infant_feeding_course_trainer_eng.pdf (accessed 29 March 2020)
5. Page 148-150, WHO/UNAIDS/UNICEF HIV and Infant Feeding Counselling: A training course; Trainer's Guide. WHO 2000, WHO/FCH/CAH/00.3, UNICEF/PD/NUT/(J)00-2, UNAIDS/99.56E https://www.who.int/nutrition/publications/en/hiv_infant_feeding_course_trainer_eng.pdf (accessed 29 March 2021)
6. Page 151, WHO/UNAIDS/UNICEF HIV and Infant Feeding Counselling: A training course; Trainer's Guide. WHO 2000, WHO/FCH/CAH/00.3, UNICEF/PD/NUT/(J)00-2, UNAIDS/99.56E https://www.who.int/nutrition/publications/en/hiv_infant_feeding_course_trainer_eng.pdf (accessed 29 March 2021)
7. Page 156, WHO/UNAIDS/UNICEF HIV and Infant Feeding Counselling: A training course; Trainer's Guide. WHO 2000, WHO/FCH/CAH/00.3, UNICEF/PD/NUT/(J)00-2, UNAIDS/99.56E https://www.who.int/nutrition/publications/en/hiv_infant_feeding_course_trainer_eng.pdf (accessed 29 March 2020)
8. Page 146, WHO/UNAIDS/UNICEF HIV and Infant Feeding Counselling: A training course; Trainer's Guide. WHO 2000, WHO/FCH/CAH/00.3, UNICEF/PD/NUT/(J)00-2, UNAIDS/99.56E https://www.who.int/nutrition/publications/en/hiv_infant_feeding_course_trainer_eng.pdf (accessed 29 March 2020)
9. *Zimbabwe Statutory Instrument 46 of 1998 [CAP 15:09] Public Health (Breastmilk Substitutes and Infant Nutrition) Regulations, 1998*, pages 349-378, Supplement to the Zimbabwean Government Gazette dated 6 March, 1998.
10. Latham MC, February 1999, Alternative infant feeding methods for mothers with HIV, Presented at Meeting on Nutrition and HIV/AIDS – Challenges in the New Millennium. Perspectives From the ECSA Region Maputo, Mozambique

11. American Academy of Pediatrics 1992, Policy statement on the use of whole cow's milk in infancy*: AAP News* May 1992, p 18.
12. WHO 1981, International Code and subsequent WHA Resolutions (IBFAN), see http://www.ibfan.org/issue-international_code-full.html
13. Del Fante P, Jenniskens F, Lush L, Morona D, Moeller B, Lanata CF and Hayes R 1993, *Journal of Tropial Medicine and Hygiene* 96,203-211
14. Zimbabwe National Aids Co-ordination Project, Sentinel Surveillance Statistics, 1998
15. About Wellstart, https://wellstart.org/lam.html (accessed 29 March 2020)
16. Koniz-Booher P, Burkhalter B, de Wagt A, Iliff P, Willumsen J (eds) 2004. *HIV and infant feeding: a compilation of programmatic evidence.* Bethesda, MD, published for UNICEF and the US Agency for Inernational Development by the Quality Assurance Project (QAP) University Research Co., LLC (URC).
17. Coutsoudis A, Pillay K, Spooner E, Kuhn L, Coovadia HM. Influence of infant-feeding patterns on early mother-to-child transmission of HIV-1 in Durban, South Africa: a prospective cohort study. South African Vitamin A Study Group. *Lancet.* 1999 Aug 7;354(9177):471-6. https://www.ncbi.nlm.nih.gov/pubmed/10465172 (accessed 10 December 2018)
18. Coutsoudis A, Pillay K, Kuhn L, Spooner E, Tsai W-Y, Coovadia HM for the South African Vitamin A Study Group. Method of feeding and transmission of HIV-1 from mothers to children by 15 months of age: prospective cohort study from Durban, South Africa. AIDS 2001;15:379-387
19. Doherty T et al. Effect of the HIV epidemic on infant feeding in South Africa. When they see me coming with the tins they laugh at me. Bulletin of the World Health Organization. 2016:84:90-96 https://apps.who.int/iris/bitstream/handle/10665/73449/bulletin_2006_84%282%29_90-96.pdf (accessed 6 March 2020)
20. Dr Chantell Witten, personal communication.

Chapter 14: Outcomes from the first PMTCT pilot sites

1. UNICEF 2005, PMTCT Report Card, Monitoring Progress on the Implementation of Programs to Prevent Mother to Child Transmission of HIV, http://www.unicef.org/ufc_PMTCTreportcard.pdf (accessed 19 November 2008, no longer available on 25 June 2020)
2. Moland et al.: Breastfeeding and HIV: experiences from a decade of prevention of postnatal HIV transmission in sub-Saharan Africa. *International Breastfeeding Journal* 2010 5:10. doi:10.1186/1746-4358-5-10
3. Young SL, Mbuya MNN, Chantry CJ, Geubbels EP, Israel-Ballard K, Cohan D, Vosti SA and Latham MC, Current Knowledge and Future Research on Infant Feeding in the Context of HIV: Basic, Clinical, Behavioral, and Programmatic, *Adv. Nutr* 2011;2: 225–243, doi:10.3945/an.110.000224 available at http://www.ncbi.nlm.nih.gov/pmc/articles/PMC3090166/ (accessed 26 Oct 2019)
4. WHO 2001 Technical Consultation. New data on the prevention of mother-to-child transmission of HIV and their policy implications http://whqlibdoc.who.int/hq/2001/WHO_RHR_01.28.pdf
5. De Wagt A, Is there an alternative? Analysis of studies on knowledge and perceptions of health workers and communities on HIV transmission and infant feeding options for HIV-positive mothers. UNICEF Eastern and Southern Africa regional Office, 2000.
6. Julie Patricia Smith, personal communication 8 May 2020
7. WHO 1981, International Code and subsequent WHA Resolutions (IBFAN), see http://www.ibfan.org/issue-international_code-full.html
8. WHO, UNICEF. Acceptable medical reasons for use of breast-milk substitutes. Geneva, WHO, 2000. MHO/NMH/NHD/09.1, WHO/FCH/CAH/09.1. http://whqlibdoc.who.int/hq/2009/WHO_FCH_CAH_09.01_eng.pdf
9. Latham MC, Kisanga P, Current status of proection support and promotion of breastfeeding in four African countries: actions to protect, support and promote breastfeeding in Botswana, Kenya, Namibia and Uganda, based on a rapid review 2 Oct – 3 Nov 2000, Prepared for UNICEF ESARO March 2001.
10. *Cornell Chronicle*, April 2011, https://news.cornell.edu/stories/2011/04/international-nutritionist-michael-latham-dies (accessed 10 June 2020)
11. Derrick Jelliffe, described in *World Nutrition* February 2013, Volume 4, Number 2 https://worldnutritionjournal.org/index.php/wn/article/view/347/293
12. Michael Latham, WABA Tribute after his death in April 2011.
13. Koniz-Booher P, Burkhalter B, de Wagt A, Iliff P, Willumsen J (eds). HIV and infant feeding: a compilation of programmatic evidence. UNICEF, US Agency for International Development by the Quality Assurance Project (QAP) University Research Co., LLC (URC); 2004. https://www.usaidassist.org/resources/hiv-and-infant-feeding-compilation-programmatic-evidence. The individual studies included are cited within the larger document.
14. UNICEF 2004, Storms D, ...Labbok M, UNICEF and the Global Strategy on Infant and Young Child Feeding (GSIYCF) Understanding the Past – Planning the Future, UNICEF 2004 https://www.unicef.org/nutrition/files/FinalReportonDistribution.pdf (accessed 9 June 2020)
15. De Wagt A, Clark D, UNICEF's Support to Free Infant Formula for Infants of HIV Infected Mothers in Africa: A Review of UNICEF Experience, LINKAGES Art and Science of Breastfeeding Presentation Series, Washington DC, April 14 2004. http://global-breastfeeding.org/pdf/UNICEF.pdf
16. SCN News,No. 17 December 1998, NUTRITION AND HIV/AIDS https://www.unscn.org/resource-

center-archives (accessed 10 May 2020).
17. Connor EM, Sperling, RS, Gelber R et al. Reduction of maternal-infant transmission of human immunodeficiency virus type 1 with zidovudine treatment. *N Engl J Med* 1994;331:1173-1180.
18. UNAIDS, Technical Update 1998 http://files.unaids.org/en/media/unaids/contentassets/dataimport/publications/irc-pub01/jc531-mtct-tu_en.pdf (accessed 22 May 2020)
19. UNICEF 2003 Evaluation of United Nations-supported pilot projects for the prevention of mother-to-child transmission of HIV: overview of findings, United Nations Children's Fund, New York 2003 http://www.unicef.org/evaldatabase/files/Global_2003_UN_Supported_PMTCT_Projects.pdf
20. Rutenberg M, Baek C, Kalibala S, Rosen S, HIV/AIDS working paper, Evaluation of United Nations-supported pilot projects for the prevention of mother-to-child HIV Overview of findings. Populations Counsel, Horizons, UNICEF 2003 https://www.unicef.org/evaldatabase/files/Global_2003_UN_Supported_PMTCT_Projects.pdf (accessed 10 May 2020
21. Sullivan E et al, Botswana's Program for preventing Mother-to-Child transmission of HIV, *Global Health Delivery* https://www.globalhealthdelivery.org/files/ghd/files/ghd-07_botswanas_program_for_preventing.pdf (accessed 27 June 2020)
22. Willumsen JF, Rollins NC. Evaluation of infant feeding practices by mothers at pMTCT and non pMTCT sites in Botswana. pMTCT Advisory Group, Botswana Food and Nutrition Unit, Family Health Division, Ministry of Health, Botswana, 2001.
23. UNAIDS 1997, HIV and Infant Feeding - A Policy Statement developed collaboratively by UNAIDS, UNICEF and WHO http://www.nzdl.org/gsdlmod (accessed 26 April 2020)
24. Leshabari SC, Koniz-Booher P, Åstrøm AN, de Paoli MM4 and Moland KM. Translating global recommendations on HIV and infant feeding to the local context: the development of culturally sensitive counselling tools in the Kilimanjaro Region, Tanzania. *Implementation Science* 2006, 1:22 doi:10.1186/1748-5908-1-22.
25. Coutsoudis A, Goga AE, Rollins N, Coovadia HM. Free formula milk for infants of HIV-infected women: blessing or curse? *Health Pol and Planning* 2002;17(2):154-160. https://pubmed.ncbi.nlm.nih.gov/12000775/ (accessed 6 June 2020)
26. Schwartlander B, Stover J, Walker N et al Resource needs for HIV.AIDS *Science* 2001; 292:2434-6.
27. Wilkinson D, Floyd K, Gilks CF. National and provincial estimated costs and cost effectiveness of a programme to reduce mother-to-child HIV transmission in South Africa. Centre for Epidemiological Research in Southern Africa, Medical Research Council, Hlabisa, Kwazulu-Natal. PMID: 11022629 [pubmed - indexed for MEDLINE]
28. Manzi M, Zachariah R, Tech R, Hunendwa L, Kazima J, Bakali E, Firmenich P and Humblet P, Scaling-up of PMTCT requires a new way of thinking and acting! *Tropical Medicine and International Health* 2005;10(12):1242-1250.
29. Soderlund N et al, Prevention of vertical transmission of HIV: analysis of cost effectiveness of options available in South Africa. *BMJ* 1999;318:1650-1656. http://www.bmj.com/cgi/content/full/318/7199/1650
30. Piwoz EG, Iliff PJ, Tavengwa N, Gavin L, Marinda E, Lunney K, Zunguza C, Nathoo KJ, the ZVITAMBO Study Group and Humphrey JH. An Education and Counseling Program for Preventing Breast-Feeding–Associated HIV Transmission in Zimbabwe: Design and Impact on Maternal Knowledge and Behavior. *J. Nutr.* 135: 950–955, 2005
31. Iliff PJ, Piwoz EG, Tavengwa NV, Zunguza CD, Marinda ET, Nathoo KJ, Moulton LH, Ward BJ, the ZVITAMBO study group and Humphrey JH. Early exclusive breastfeeding reduces the risk of postnatal HIV-1 transmission and increases HIV-free survival. *AIDS* 2005, 19:699–708 https://www.ncbi.nlm.nih.gov/pubmed/15821396 (accessed 10 December 2018)
32. Tavengwa N, Piwoz E, Gavin L, Zunguza C, Marinda E, Iliff P, Humphrey J, ZVITAMBO Study Group. Conference presentation: "Education and counselling make a difference to infant feeding practices and those feeding practices make a difference to infant mortality." ZVITAMBO Project, University of Zimbabwe; Harare City Health Department, Zimbabwe. WABA Global Forum 2, Arusha, Tanzania. September 23-27 2002.
33. UNICEF 2000 State of the World's Children, New York https://www.unicef.org/reports/state-worlds-children-2000 (accessed 29 March 2021)
34. Smart T, Infant feeding policy debated at the Conference on Retroviruses and Opportunistic Infections *AIDSMAP HATIP* #82, 13th March 2007 http://www.aidsmap.com/en/news/1F9F2D35-099B-42A5-94EA-0FEC977756E6.asp
35. WHO – UNAIDS – UNICEF, Technical Consultation on HIV and Infant Feeding, Implementation of Guidelines, Report of a Meeting - Geneva, 20-22 April 1998 http://www.unaids.org/sites/default/files/media_asset/jc180-hiv-infantfeeding-4_en_0.pdf (accessed 2 June 2020)
36. Stephen Lewis, former UN Envoy on HIV-AIDS, "AIDS-FreeWorld", International AIDS Society Meeting, July 19-22, 2009 Cape Town, South Africa

Chapter 15: Problems with counselling, but scaling up anyway

1. Moland KMI, de Paoli M, Sellen DW, Van Esterik P, Leshabari SC and Blystad. Breastfeeding and

HIV: experiences from a decade of prevention of postnatal HI HIV transmission in sub-Saharan Africa. *Int Breastfeed J.* 2010; 5: 10, doi: 10.1186/1746-4358-5-10. October 26, 2010 http://www.internationalbreastfeedingjournal.com/content/5/1/10

2. WHO 2000, HIV and Infant Feeding Counselling: A training course, Director's Guide WHO/FCH/CAH/00.2 https://apps.who.int/iris/bitstream/handle/10665/66194/WHO_FCH_CAH_00.2.pdf (accessed 29 March 2021)
3. WHO 2000, HIV and Infant Feeding Counselling: A training course, Trainer's Guide WHO/FCH/CAH/00.4 https://www.who.int/nutrition/publications/en/hiv_infant_feeding_course_trainer_eng.pdf (accessed 29 March 2021)
4. Bassett MT, Psychosocial and community perspectives on alternatives to breastfeeding. *Ann N Y Acad Sci* 2000;918:128-35 https://www.ncbi.nlm.nih.gov/pubmed/11131696 (accessed 13 April 2020)
5. Rutenberg M, Baek C, Kalibala S, Rosen S, HIV/AIDS working paper, Evaluation of United Nations-supported pilot projects for the prevention of mother-to-child HIV Overview of findings. Populations Counsel, Horizons, UNICEF 2003, https://www.unicef.org/evaldatabase/files/Global_2003_UN_Supported_PMTCT_Projects.pdf accessed 18 September 2020.
6. De Wagt A & Clark D, Nutrition Section, United Nations Children's Fund, New York, USA. UNICEF's Support to Free Infant Formula for Infants of HIVInfected Mothers in Africa: A Review of UNICEF Experience Presented at the LINKAGES Art and Science of Breastfeeding Presentation Series, April 14, 2004, Washington, DC. http://www.waba.org.my/whatwedo/hcp/pdf/r-unicef-free.pdf Accessed 10 December 2018.
7. Koniz-Booher P, Burkhalter B, de Wagt A, Iliff P, Willumsen J (eds) 2004. *HIV and infant feeding: a compilation of programmatic evidence.* Bethesda, MD, published for UNICEF and the US Agency for Inernational Development by the Quality Assurance Project (QAP) University Research Co., LLC (URC). http://www.qaproject.org/strat/HIVinfantfeed1004screen.pdf accessed 13 May 2020
8. WABA/LLLI Symposium on Breastfeeding and HIV & AIDS, "Breastfeeding – Guarding Maternal & Child Health in an HIV & AIDS World", Washington, D.C. USA, July 2, 2005.
9. Manzi M, Zachariah R, Tech R, Hunendwa L, Kazima J, Bakali E, Firmenich P and Humblet P, Scaling-up of PMTCT requires a new way of thinking and acting! *Tropical Medicine and International Health* 2005;10(12):1242-1250. https://pubmed.ncbi.nlm.nih.gov/16359404/ (accessed 1 June 2020)
10. Baek C, Rodriguez MX, Escoto LR. Program evaluation. "Report on the Qualitative Rapid Assessment of the UN-Supported PMTCT Pilot Program in Honduras." December 2002.
11. Vilakati D and Shongwe N. Report: "Rapid situational analysis of the BFHI in Swaziland." May 2001.
12. Kankasa C, Mshanga A, Baek C, Kalibala S, Rutenberg N. Program Report: "Report on the Rapid Assessment of the UN-Supported PMTCT Pilot Program in Zambia." December 2002.
13. pMTCT Advisory Group, 2001. Draft report: "Evaluation of Infant Feeding Practices by Mothers at 1 and non-pMTCTSites in Botswana." pMTCT Reference Group, Botswana Food and Nutrition Unit, Family Health Division, Ministry of Health Botswana. 2001.
14. UNICEF Zambia. Report on the rapid assessment of the UN-supported PMTCT pilot program in Zambia. Pilot interventions at university teaching hospital, Chipata health center, Mbala district hospital, Tulemane health center, Monze mission hospital, and Keemba rural health center. December 2002.
15. Willumsen JF, Rollins NC. Evaluation of infant feeding practices by mothers at pMTCT and non pMTCT sites in Botswana. pMTCT Advisory Group, Botswana Food and Nutrition Unit, Family Health Division, Ministry of Health, Botswana, 2001
16. UNICEF Rwanda,. Report on the rapid assessment of the un-supported PMTCT initiative in Rwanda pilot interventions at Kicukiro, Muhura, and Gisenyi health centers. Draft document. December 2002
17. Coutsoudis A, Pillay K, Spooner E, Kuhn L, Coovadia HM. Influence of infant-feeding patterns on early mother-to-child transmission of HIV-1 in Durban, South Africa: a prospective cohort study. South African Vitamin A Study Group. *Lancet.* 1999 Aug 7;354(9177):471-6. https://www.ncbi.nlm.nih.gov/pubmed/10465172 (accessed 10 December 2018)
18. Chopra M, Schaay N, Sanders D, Puoane T, Piwoz E, Dunnett L. HIV and Infant feeding: Summary of findings and recommendations from a formative research study with the Khayelitsha MTCT programme, South Africa. Draft Report, May 2000.
19. Leshabari, Sebalda C, Blystad A, de Paoli M, and Moland KM. HIV and infant feeding counselling: challenges faced by nurse-counsellors in northern Tanzania. *Hum Resour Health,* July 24, 2007; 5(1): 18. http://highwire.stanford.edu/cgi/medline/pmid;17650310
20. Nkonki LL, Daniels KL, PROMISE-EB Study Group: Selling a service: experiences of peer supporters while promoting exclusive infant feeding in three sites in South Africa. *Int Breastfeed J* 2010; 5:17
21. Morrison P, Review: WHO HIV and Infant Feeding Counselling Course, *J Hum Lact* 2002;18(4):403 http://jhl.sagepub.com/cgi/reprint/18/4/403
22. Spotlight: Botswana: A timeline of HIV action, *PlusNews Johannesburg,* 18 January 2012, : http://www.plusnews.org/report.aspx?ReportID=94671
23. De Wagt A, Is there an alternative? Analysis of studies on knowledge and perceptions of health workers and communities on HIV transmission and infant feeding options for HIV-positive mothers. UNICEF Eastern and Southern Africa regional Office, 2000
24. Chopra M, Doherty T, Jackson D, Ashworth A.Preventing HIV transmission to children: Quality of

counselling of mothers in South Africa. *Acta Pædiatr*, 2005; 94: 357–363. https://pubmed.ncbi.nlm.nih.gov/16028656/ (accessed 10 June 2020)

25. Pham P, Musemakweri A, Stewart H. Program evaluation: "Report on the Rapid Assessment of the UN-Supported PMCT Initiative in Rwanda: Pilot interventions at Kicukiro, Muhura, and Gisenyi Health Centers." December 2002.
26. Seidel G, Sewpaul V, Dano B. Experiences of breastfeeding and vulnerability among a group of HIV positive women – discussions with a peer support group of HIV positive mothers at King Edward Hospital, Durban, KwaZulu-Natal, South Africa. *Health Policy and Planning* 2000 15(1):24-33. 2000.
27. de Paoli M, Manongi R, Klepp K-I. Counsellors' perspectives on antenatal HIV testing and infant feeding dilemmas facing women with HIV in northern Tanzania. *Reproductive Health Matters* Reproductive Health Matters, 10:20, 144-156, https://www.tandfonline.com/doi/full/10.1016/S0968-8080%2802%2900088-5
28. Rollins N, Meda N, Becquet R, Coutsoudis A, Humphrey J, Jeffrey B, Kanshana S, Kuhn L, Leroy V, Mbori-Ngacha D, McIntyre J, Newell ML; Ghent IAS Working Group on HIV in Women and Children. Preventing postnatal transmission of HIV-1 through breast-feeding: modifying infant feeding practices. *J Acquir Immune Defic Syndr*. 2004 Feb 1;35(2):188-95. https://pubmed.ncbi.nlm.nih.gov/14722453/ (accessed 3 July 2020)
29. Almroth S, When breastfeeding becomes a choice. Implementing informed choice regarding infant feeding in a national programme to prevent mother-to-child transmisson of HIV in India. Report on a qualitative study of the counselling, decision making and implementation of informed choice regarding infant feeding for HIV-positive women in urban India. UNICEF, New Delhi, India, April 2002.
30. Piwoz, EG, Owens-Ferguson Y, Bentley ME, Corneli AL, Moses A, Nkhoma J, Tohill BC, Mtimuni BM, Ahmed Y, Jamieson DJ, van der Horst C, Kazembe P. Differences between international recommendations on breastfeeding in the presence of HIV and the attitudes and counselling messages of health workers in Lilongwe, Malawi. *Int Breastfeed J* 2006, 1:2 doi:10.1186/1746-4358-1-2.
31. Sarna A. Program Report (under review, not for circulation): "Report on Discussions with National AIDS Control Organization and Visits to Two Pilot Program Sites." December 2002.
32. McCoy D, Besser M, Visser F, Doherty T. Interim findings on the National PMTCT pilot sites: lessons and recommendations. Durban: Health Systems Trust for National Department of Health; 2002. http://www.hst.org.za/publications/HST%20Publications/pmtctsummary.pdf
33. Isiramen V. MSc dissertation: "Early and Abrupt Cessation of Breastfeeding In The Nigerian Context: Is This An Option For HIV Positive Women?" Institute of Child Health, University College, London; Ahmadu Bello University Teaching Hospital, Kaduna, Nigeria. August 2002.
34. Koricho AT, Moland KM, Blystad A: Poisonous milk and sinful mothers: the changing meaning of breastfeeding in the wake of the HIV epidemic in Addis Ababa, Ethiopia. *Int Breastfeed J* 2010, 5:12
35. Haider R, Kabir I, Huttly SR, Ashworth A. Training peer counselors to promote and support exclusive breastfeeding in Bangladesh. *J Hum Lact*. 2002 Feb;18(1):7-12.
36. Morrison P, Latham M, Greiner T, UNAIDS policy ought to promote exclusive breastfeeding but instead may lead to its decline in Africa, *BMJ* 2001;322;7285:512e.
37. Horizons Program. Integrating HIV Prevention and Care into Maternal and Child Health Care Settings: Lessons Learned from Horizons Studies July 23-27, 2001 Maasai Mara and Nairobi, Kenya Consultation Report. The Population Council Inc.
38. Doherty T et al. Effect of the HIV epidemic on infant feeding in South Africa. When they see me coming with the tins they laugh at me. *Bulletin of the World Health Organization*. 2006:84:90-96 https://apps.who.int/iris/bitstream/handle/10665/73449/bulletin_2006_84%282%29_90-96.pdf (accessed 6 March 2020)
39. Moland KMI, de Paoli M, Sellen DW, Van Esterik P, Leshabari SC and Blystad. Breastfeeding and HIV: experiences from a decade of prevention of postnatal HI HIV transmission in sub-Saharan Africa. *Int Breastfeed J*. 2010; 5: 10, doi: 10.1186/1746-4358-5-10. October 26, 2010, http://www.internationalbreastfeedingjournal.com/content/5/1/10 (accessed 30 March 2021)
40. Ngoma-Hazemba A and Ncama BP, Analysis of experiences with exclusive breastfeeding among HIV-positive mothers in Lusaka, Zambia, *Global Health Action* 2016;9:: 10.3402/gha.v9.32362. https://www.ncbi.nlm.nih.gov/pmc/articles/PMC5136125/
41. Tavengwa N, Piwoz E, Gavin L, Zunguza C, Marinda E, Iliff P, Humphrey J, ZVITAMBO Study Group. Conference presentation: "Education and counselling make a difference to infant feeding practices and those feeding practices make a difference to infant mortality." ZVITAMBO Project, University of Zimbabwe; Harare City Health Department, Zimbabwe. WABA Global Forum 2, Arusha, Tanzania. September 23-27 2002.
42. Piwoz EG, Iliff PJ, Tavengwa N, Gavin L, Marinda E, Lunney K, Zunguza C, Nathoo KJ, the ZVITAMBO Study Group and Humphrey JH. An Education and Counseling Program for Preventing Breast-Feeding–Associated HIV Transmission in Zimbabwe: Design and Impact on Maternal Knowledge and Behavior. *J. Nutr.* 135: 950–955, 2005. https://www.ncbi.nlm.nih.gov/pubmed/11131696 (accessed 13 Apr 2020)
43. Morrow AL, Guerrero ML, Shults J, Calva JJ, Lutter C, Bravo J, Ruiz-Palacios G, Morrow RC, Butterfoss FD. Efficacy of home-based peer counselling to promote exclusive breastfeeding: a randomised controlled

trial. *Lancet* 1999 Apr 10;353(9160):1226-31. https://www.ncbi.nlm.nih.gov/pubmed/10217083 (accessed 13 April 2020)

44. Jackson DJ, Tylleskar T, chopra M, Doherty T et al, Preliminary results from the multi-center cluster-randomized behaviour intervention trial PROMISE EBF: Exclusive breastfeeding promotion in Sub-Saharan Africa, American Public Health Association Conference, Wednesday, November 11, 2009: 1:00 PM http://apha.confex.com/apha/137am/webprogram/Paper201963.html
45. Bland RM et al. (2007). Infant feeding counselling for HIV-infected and uninfected women: appropriateness of choice and practice. *Bulletin of the World Health Organization*, 85(4):289–296.
46. Becquet R et al, and ANRS DITRAME Plus Study Group, Infant feeding practices before implementing alternatives to prolonged breastfeeding to reduce HIV transmission through breastmilk in Abidjan, Cote d'Ivoire, *J Trop Pediatr*. 2005 December ; 51(6): 351–355. https://www.ncbi.nlm.nih.gov/pmc/articles/PMC2100154/ (accessed 25 April 2020)
47. Leroy V et al and the ANRS 1201/1202 Ditrame Plus Study Group. Acceptability of Formula-Feeding to Prevent HIV Postnatal, Transmission, Abidjan, Co^te d'Ivoire ANRS 1201/1202 Ditrame Plus Study *J Acquir Immune Defic Syndr* 2007;44:77–86 https://journals.lww.com/jaids/Fulltext/2007/01010/Acceptability_of_Exclusive_Breast_Feeding_With.12.aspx (accessed 26 April 2020)
48. WHO 2007, HIV and infant feeding : new evidence and programmatic experience : report of a technical consultation held on behalf of the Inter-agency Task Team (IATT) on prevention of HIV Infections in pregnant women, mothers and their infants, Geneva, Switzerland, 25-27 October 2006, ISBN 978 92 4 159597 1 https://www.who.int/hiv/pub/toolkits/PMTCT9789241596015_eng.pdf (accessed 18 Apr 2020)
49. Abiodun et al, Acceptability of measures aimed at preventing mother-to-child transmission of HIV among pregnant women. *J Natl Med Assoc*, April 1, 2008; 100(4): 406-10. https://www.ncbi.nlm.nih.gov/pubmed/18481479
50. Sibeko L, Coutsoudis A, Nzuza S and Gray-Donald K. Mothers' infant feeding experiences: constraints and supports for optimal feeding in an HIV-impacted urban community in South Africa. *Public Health Nutr* 2009;12(11):1983-90. doi: 10.1017/S1368980009005199 https://pubmed.ncbi.nlm.nih.gov/19323863/
51. Creek T, Arvelo W, Kim A, Lu L, Bowen A, Finkbeiner T, Zaks L, Masunge J, Shaffer N and Davis M. Role of infant feeding and HIV in a severe outbreak of diarrhea and malnutrition among young children, Botswana, 2006. Session 137 Poster Abstracts, Conference on Retroviruses and Opportunistic Infections, Los Angeles, 25-28 February, 2007. http://www.retroconference.org/2007/Abstracts/29305.htm
52. Sullivan E et al, Botswana's Program for preventing Mother-to-Child transmission of HIV, Global Health Delivery https://www.globalhealthdelivery.org/files/ghd/files/ghd-07_botswanas_program_for_preventing.pdf (accessed 27 June 2020)
53. Becquet R, Bequet L, Ekouevi DK, Viho I, Sakarovitch C, Fassinou P, et al. Two-year morbidity-mortality and alternatives to prolonged breast-feeding among children born to HIV-infected mothers in Cote d'Ivoire. *PLoS Med* 2007;4:e17. PMID:17227132 doi:10.1371/ journal.pmed.0040017
54. WHO 2005 HIV and Infant Feeding Counselling Tools, Reference Guide, ISBN 92 4 159301 6 http://whqlibdoc.who.int/publications/2005/9241593016.pdf (accessed 30 December 2018)
55. Joint FAO/WHO Expert Workshop on enterobacter sakazaakii and other microorganisms in Powdered Infant Formula 2004) https://www.who.int/foodsafety/publications/micro/summary2.pdf (accessed 16 September 2020)
56. Bergstrom, E. Bacterial Contamination and Nutrient Concentration of Infant Milk in South Africa: A Sub-study of the National PMTCT Cohort Study. Masters Thesis, Uppsala University, 2003. http://www.healthlink.org.za/publications/564
57. Andresen E, Rollins NC, Sturm AW, Conana N and Greiner T, Bacterial contamination and over-dilution of commercial infant formula prepared by HIV-infected mothers in a prevention of mother-to-child transmission (PMTCT) programme in South Africa. *J Trop Pediatr* 2007;53:410–4. https://pubmed.ncbi.nlm.nih.gov/18063653/ (accessed 3 June 2020)
58. UNICEF State of the World's children 2000.
59. Dunne EF et al. Is Drinking Water in Abidjan, Côte d'Ivoire, Safe for Infant Formula? *J Acquir Immune Defic Syndr* 2001;28:393-398 (https://www.cdc.gov/safewater/publications_pages/2001/dunne_2001.pdf (accessed 3 May 2020)
60. Omari AAA, Luo C, Kankasa et al. Infant feeding practices of mothers of known HIV status in Lusaka, Zambia. *Health Policy and Planning* 2003;18(2): 156–162. https://www.ncbi.nlm.nih.gov/pubmed/12740320 (accessed 1 May 2020)
61. The state of the world's children 2007. Women and children: The double dividend of gender equality. New York: UNICEF; 2006. https://www.unicef.org/media/84811/file/SOWC-2007.pdf (accessed 30 March 2021)
62. Human Development Report 2006. Beyond scarcity: power, poverty and the 4. global water crisis. New York: United Nations Development Programme; 2006.
63. Coutsoudis A, Coovadia HM & Wilfert CM, HIV, infant feeding and more perils for poor people: new WHO guidelines encourage review of formula milk policies, *Bulletin of the World Health Organization* 2008;86:210–214. https://pubmed.ncbi.nlm.nih.gov/18368208/ (accessed 4 June 2020)
64. UNICEF Supports Breast-Feeding, Alan Court, UNICEF program director, letter, *The Washington Post*, 8

June 2007 http://www.washingtonpost.com/wp-dyn/content/article/2007/08/05/AR2007080501319.html (accessed 7 September 2012)

65. Coutsoudis, A, Goga, AE, Rollins, N and Coovadia HM on behalf of the Child Health Group (2002) Free formula milk for infant of HIV-infected women: blessing or curse? *Health Policy and Planning*: 17(2): 154-160. Oxford University Press
66. Dabis F, Leroy V, Bequet L, et al. Assessment of peri-partum and post-partum interventions to prevent mother-to-child transmission (PMTCT) of HIV-1 and improve survival in Africa. Presented at the 3rd conference on Global Strategies for the prevention of HIV transmission from mothers to infants, Uganda, September 2001
67. WHO (2003) HIV and infant feeding: guidelines for decision-makers. UNICEF, UNAIDS, WHO, UNFPA Final draft, June 2003
68. Latham MC, Kisanga P, Current status of protection support and promotion of breastfeeding in four African countries: actions to protect, support and promote breastfeeding in Botswana, Kenya, Namibia and Uganda, based on a rapid review 2 Oct – 3 Nov 2000, Prepared for UNICEF ESARO March 2001
69. UNICEF, New York, Nutrition Section, Infant and Young Child Feeding Programme Review. Case Study: Uganda 2009 by Luann Martin for UNICEF/AED. http://www.aednutritioncenter.org/update_docs/IYCF_Feeding_Prog_Rev_Case_Study_Uganda.pdf (website shut down April 2020 summarized at https://www.comminit.com/la/content/infant-and-young-child-feeding-programme-review-case-study-uganda accessed 30 March 2021)
70. Mouzin E, Mercier E, Henderson P. United Nations-sponsored pilot projects on PMTCT: monitoring of intervention uptake in Africa. Abstract 332, Third conference on global strategies for the prevention of HIV transmission from mothers to infants, September, Kampala, Uganda, 2001.
71. Doherty TM, McCoy D, Donohue S. Health system constraints to optimal coverage of the prevention of mother-to-child HIV transmission programme in South Africa: lessons from the implementation of the national pilot programme. *Afr Health Sci.* 2005 Sep;5(3):213-8
72. UNICEF 2005, PMTCT Report Card, Monitoring Progress on the Implementation of Programs to Prevent Mother to Child Transmission of HIV, http://www.uniteforchildren.org/knowmore/files/ufc_PMTCTreportcard.pdf
73. UNICEF PMTCT Plus Brochure, September 2005
74. Besson MH, Dintruff R, Rabbw M, Ladner L, Muyingo S, Coovadia H, Saba J. Capacity building increases the impact of the PMTCT donations program to reach more mothers and their children in developing countries. ICASA poster presentation, Dec 2005, http://www.axios-group.com/en/library/posters/AbujaPMTCTPoster261105.pdf
75. WHO HIV and Infant Feeding Technical Consultation Held on behalf of the Inter-agency Task Team (IATT) on Prevention of HIV Infections in Pregnant Women, Mothers and their Infants Geneva, October 25-27, 2006 CONSENSUS STATEMENT, https://www.who.int/maternal_child_adolescent/documents/pdfs/who_hiv_infant_feeding_technical_consultation.pdf (accessed 18 Nov 2021)
76. *The Washington Post*, Letters to the Editor Monday August 6, 2007. http://www.washingtonpost.com/wp-dyn/content/article/2007/08/05/AR2007080501319.html (accessed 7 September 2012) (reported in Network News).
77. *All Africa News Service*. Prevention of Mother-to-Child Transmission to Reach All Clinics by December – Radebe. 12 March 2007 http://allafrica.com/stories/200703120679.html
78. Source: WHO 2010, PMTCT strategic vision 2010-2015, Preventing mother-to-child transmission of HIV to reach the UNGASS and Millennium Development Goals. https://www.who.int/hiv/pub/mtct/strategic_vision/en/ (accessed 2 May 2020)

Chapter 16: What we don't know about the outcomes from the PMTCT sites

1. UNAIDS, UNICEF and WHO HIV and Infant Feeding - A Policy Statement developed collaboratively by UNAIDS, UNICEF and WHO (UNAIDS, 1997. https://www.ncbi.nlm.nih.gov/pubmed/10453706 (accessed 28 March 2020
2. De Paoli M, Manongi R, Helsing E and Klepp K-I. Exclusive breastfeeding in the era of AIDS. *J Hum Lact* 2001;17:313-320.
3. Young SL, Mbuya MNN, Chantry CJ, Geubbels EP, Israel-Ballard K, Cohan D, Vosty SA and Latham MC, Current Knowledge and Future Research on Infant Feeding in the Context of HIV: Basic, Clinical, Behavioral, and Programmatic Perspectives, *Adv Nutr* 2011;2(3):225-243. https://www.ncbi.nlm.nih.gov/pmc/articles/PMC3090166/
4. Njunga J, Blystad A: 'The divorce program': gendered experiences of HIV positive mothers enrolled in PMTCT programs - the case of rural Malawi.Int *Breastfeed J* 2010, 5:14.
5. Engebretsen IMS, Moland KM, Nankunda J, Karamagi CA, Tylleskar T, Tumwine JK: Gendered perceptions on infant feeding in Eastern Uganda: continued need for exclusive breastfeeding support. *Int Breastfeed J* 2010, 5:13.
6. Israel-Ballard KA, Maternowska MC, Abrams BF, Morrison P, Chitibura L, Chipato T, Chirenje ZM, Padian NS, Chantry CJ, Acceptability of Heat-treating Breast milk to Prevent Mother-to-Child Transmission of HIV in Zimbabwe: A Qualitative Study, *J Hum Lact* 2006;22(1):48-60 https://pubmed.ncbi.nlm.nih.gov/16467287/ (accessed 19 June 2020)

7. Chopra M, Shaay N, Sanders D, Sengwana J, Puoane T, Piwoz E, Dunnett L. Research report: Summary of the findings and recommendations from a formative research study from the Khayelitsha MTCT programme, South Africa." University of the Western Cape Public Health Programme; USAID/SARA Project, DoH Provincial Authority of Western Cape. May 2000.
8. De Paoli MM, Manongi R and Klepp K-I. Counsellors' perspectives on antenatal HIV testing and infant feed-ing dilemmas facing women with HIV in Northern Tanzania. *Reproductive Health Matters* 2002;10:144-156.
9. Doherty T, Chopra M, Nkonki L, Jackson D, Greiner T. Effect of the HIV epidemic on infant feeding in South Africa: "When they see me coming with the tins they laugh at me". *Bull World Health Organ.* 2006 Feb;84(2):90-6. Epub 2006 Feb 23.
10. Ndola Demonstration Project to Integrate infant feeding counselling and HIV voluntary counselling and testing into health care and community services, HIV and Infant Feeding: A summary of the findings and recommendations from the formative research carried out in Lubuto, Main Masala, Twapia and Kabushi Health Centre areas of Ndola, Zambia. https://knowledgecommons.popcouncil.org/cgi/viewcontent.cgi (accessed 30 March 2021)
11. Timberg C and Halperin D, *Tinderbox: how the West sparked the AIDS epidemic and how the world can finally overcome it.* The Penguin Press, 2012. ISB 978-1-59420-327-5 (pages 143 and 343 (note 17)
12. John Cleland et al, *Sexual Behaviour and AIDS in the Developing World*, Geneva, WHO 1995 https://apps.who.int/iris/handle/10665/37152 (accessed 24 August 2020)
13. Omari AAA, Luo C, Kankasa et al. Infant feeding practices of mothers of known HIV status in Lusaka, Zambia. *Health Policy and Planning 2003*;18(2): 156–162. https://www.ncbi.nlm.nih.gov/pubmed/12740320 (accessed 1 May 2020)
14. De Wagt A, Clark D, UNICEF's Support to Free Infant Formula for Infants of HIV Infected Mothers in Africa: A Review of UNICEF Experience, LINKAGES Art and Science of Breastfeeding Presentation Series, Washington DC, April 14 2004
15. Coetzee D, Hilderbrand K, Boulle A, Draper B, Abdullah F, Goemaere E. Effectiveness of the first district-wide programme for the prevention of mother-to-child transmission of HIV in South Africa. *Bull World Health Organ.* 2005 Jul;83(7):489-94.
16. Das P. Feeding risk cut for HIV-infected women. *Lancet.* 2003 Jul 26;362(9380):300.
17. UNICEF Zambia. Report on the rapid assessment of the UN-supported PMTCT pilot program in Zambia. Pilot interventions at university teaching hospital, Chipata health center, Mbala district hospital, Tulemane health center, Monze mission hospital, and Keemba rural health center. December 2002
18. Tlou S, Nyblade L, Kiss R, Field ML, Rantona K, Sentumo S. Working report on community responses to initiatives to Prevent mother-to-child transmission of HIV in Botswana. Findings from a qualitative study conducted in Bontleng community, Gaborone, Botswana from November 1999 to May 2000 .June 2000
19. Horizons Program. Integrating HIV Prevention and Care into Maternal and Child Health Care Settings: Lessons Learned from Horizons Studies July 23-27, 2001 Maasai Mara and Nairobi, Kenya Consultation Report. The Population Council Inc
20. Mugivhi MR, Problems experienced by mothers who opted for replacement infant feeding in a prevntion of mother-to-child transmission programme in Makhado Municipality, Limpopo Prov ince, South Africa, Master of Art Thesis, University of South Africa, November 2020 http://uir.unisa.ac.za/bitstream/handle/10500/4872/dissertation_mugivhi_mr.pdf (accessed 3 May 2020)
21. Nyblade L, Field ML. Synthesis paper: Women, Communities, and the Prevention of Mother-to-Child Transmission of HIV: Issues and Findings from Community Research in Botswana and Zambia The International Center for Research on Women. July 2000
22. Oladokun RE et al. Infant-feeding pattern of HIV-positive women in a prevention of mother-to-child transmission (PMTCT) programme. *AIDS Care.* 2010 Mar 12:1-7, https://pubmed.ncbi.nlm.nih.gov/20229369/ (accessed 29 May 2020)
23. WHO 2004. HIV and infant feeding: A guide for health-care managers and supervisors , World Health Organization 2003 https://www.who.int/nutrition/publications/HIV_IF_guide_for_healthcare.pdf (accessed 18 June 2020)
24. Rutenberg M, Baek C, Kalibala S, Rosen S, HIV/AIDS working paper, Evaluation of United Nations-supported pilot projects for the prevention of mother-to-child HIV Overview of findings. Populations Counsel, Horizons, UNICEF 2003, available at https://www.unicef.org/evaldatabase/files/Global_2003_UN_Supported_PMTCT_Projects.pdf accessed 18 September 2020.
25. Koniz-Booher P, Burkhalter B, de Wagt A, Iliff P, Willumsen J (eds) 2004. HIV and infant feeding: a compilation of programmatic evidence. Bethesda, MD, published for UNICEF and the US Agency for Inernational Development by the Quality Assurance Project (QAP) University Research Co., LLC (URC). http://www.qaproject.org/strat/HIVinfantfeed1004screen.pdf accessed 13 May 2020
26. UNICEF Rwanda,. Report on the rapid assessment of the un-supported PMTCT initiative in Rwanda pilot interventions at Kicukiro, Muhura, and Gisenyi health centers. Draft document. December 2002.
27. Pham P, Musemakweri A, Stewart H. Program evaluation (under review, not for circulation): "Report on the Rapid Assessment of the UN-Supported PMCT Initiative in Rwanda: Pilot interventions at Kicukiro, Muhura, and Gisenyi Health Centers." December 2002.
28. TRAC Tulane, results of reliability study, May 2006, http://payson.tulane.edu/cdc_utap/Results%20

only%20of%20reliability%20study%20TRAC-Tulane%20for%2002may2006%20presentation%20final.ppt
29. Axios Customer Satisfaction Survey Dec 2004, http://www.pmtctdonations.org/ftp/SatisfactionSurveyJan-05.pdf
30. UNICEF 2003 Evaluation of United Nations-supported pilot projects for the prevention of mother-to-child transmission of HIV: overview of findings, United Nations Children's Fund, New York 2003 http://www.unicef.org/evaldatabase/files/Global_2003_UN_Supported_PMTCT_Projects.pdf (accessed 14 June 2020)
31. WHO 2004, (prepared by Ellen Piwoz) What are the options? Using formative research to adapt global recommendations on HIV and infant feeding to the local context. ISBN 92 4 159136 6 https://apps.who.int/iris/bitstream/handle/10665/42882/9241591366.pdf (accessed 17 April 2004)
32. WHO 2004 National guide to monitoring and evaluating programmes for the prevention of HIV in infants and young children ISBN 92 4 159184 6 https://www.who.int/hiv/pub/prev_care/en/nationalguideyoungchildren.pdf (accessed 4 June 2020)
33. Theo Smart, *AIDSMAP News*, HIV surveillance at immunisation clinics reveals weakness in KwaZulu Natal's PMTCT programme, Wednesday, September 06, 2006, http://www.aidsmap.com/en/news/74A5B372-0FAF-4EB1-8825-F84DDAB7D367.asp
34. UNICEF 2007, Children and the Millennium Development Goals: Progress towards A World Fit for Children https://www.unicef.org/publications/index_42124.html (accessed 14 May 2020).
35. Holmes WR and Savage F, Exclusive breastfeeding and HIV, *Lancet* 2007;Vol 369:1065-1066 https://pubmed.ncbi.nlm.nih.gov/17398292/ (accessed 4 June 2020)
36. WHO 2009 Towards Universal Access, Scaling up priority HIV/AIDS interventions in the health sector, Progress Report 2009 https://www.who.int/hiv/pub/2009progressreport/en/ (accessed 13 May 2020)
37. Kalembo FW, Zgambo M, Loss to follow-up: a maor challenge to successful implementation of prevention of mother-to-child transmission of HIV-1 programs in sub-Saharan Africa, *International Scholarly Research Network AIDS* 2012, Article ID 589817 doi:10.5402/2012/589817 http://downloads.hindawi.com/archive/2012/589817.pdf (accessed 1 June 2020)
38. Rollins N, Little K, Mzolo S, Horwood C, Newell ML. Surveillance of mother-to-child transmission prevention programmes at immunization clinics: the case for universal screening. *Rev Med Virol.* 2007.
39. Theo Smart. HIV surveillance at immunisation clinics reveals weakness in KwaZulu Natal's PMTCT programme. *AIDSMAP Summary*, Wednesday, September 06, 2006 http://www.aidsmap.com/en/news/74A5B372-0FAF-4EB1-8825-F84DDAB7D367.asp
40. Manzi M, Zachariah R, Tech R, Hunendwa L, Kazima J, Bakali E, Firmenich P and Humblet P, Scaling-up of PMTCT requires a new way of thinking and acting! *Tropical Medicine and International Health* 2005;10(12):1242-1250. https://pubmed.ncbi.nlm.nih.gov/16359404/ (accessed 1 June 2020)
41. Miya RM, A broad literature overview of hiv prevention of mother to child transmission: male inclusion *Indian Journal of Medical Research and Pharmaceutical Sciences*, 2016;3(2) :11-45 http://www.ijmrps.com/February-2016.html accessed 4 May 2020
42. Rosen S et al. Patient retention in antiretroviral therapy programs in sub-Saharan Africa: A systematic review. *PLoS Med* 2007;4(10):e298. https://journals.plos.org/plosmedicine/article?id=10.1371/journal.pmed.0040298 (accessed 14 May 2020)
43. Susan Burger, IBCLC in New York, personal communication March 2009.
44. Preble EA and Piwoz EG, 1998, HIV and infant feeding: *A chronology of research and policy advances and their implications for programs,* The Linkages Project and the Support for Analysis and Research in Africa (SARA) Project, the Academy for Educational Development, USAID Bureau for Africa.
45. Pitt J et al. HIV vertical transmission rate determinations are subject to differing definitions and therefore different rates. The Pediatric Pulmonary and Cardiovascular Complications of Vertically Transmitted HIV Infection Study Group. *J Clin Epidemiol* 1998;51(2):159–64.
46. Ioannidis JP et al Predictors and impact of losses to follow-up in an HIV-1 perinatal transmission cohort in Malawi *Int J Epidemiol.* 1999 Aug;28(4):769-75. https://pubmed.ncbi.nlm.nih.gov/10480709/ (accessed 2 June 2020)
47. Sullivan E et al, Botswana's Program for preventing Mother-to-Child transmission of HIV, Global Health Delivery https://www.globalhealthdelivery.org/files/ghd/files/ghd-07_botswanas_program_for_preventing.pdf (accessed 27 June 2020)
48. De Haas AD et al. HIV transmission and retention in care among HIV-exposed children enrolled in Malawi's prevention of mother-to-child transmission programme. *J Int AIDS Soc* 2017, 20:21947 http://www.jiasociety.org/index.php/jias/article/view/21947
49. Cesar JA, Victora CG, Barros FC, Santos IS, Flores JA. Impact of breast feeding on admission for pneumonia during postneonatal period in Brazil: nested case-control study. *BMJ* 1999 May 15;318(7194):1316-20. https://www.ncbi.nlm.nih.gov/pmc/articles/PMC27869/ (accessed 17 July 2020)
50. Rollins N, Meda N, Becquet R, Coutsoudis A, Humphrey J, Jeffrey B, Kanshana S, Kuhn L, Leroy V, Mbori-Ngacha D, McIntyre J, Newell ML; Ghent IAS Working Group on HIV in Women and Children. Preventing postnatal transmission of HIV-1 through breast-feeding: modifying infant feeding practices. *J Acquir Immune Defic Syndr.* 2004 Feb 1;35(2):188-95. https://pubmed.ncbi.nlm.nih.gov/14722453/ (accessed 3 July 2020)

51. WABA HIV and Infant Feeding Global Planning Meeting, Lusaka, Zambia, 2004. https://www.waba.org.my/whatwedo/hiv/zambia2004.htm (accessed 28 April 2020)
52. Latham MC, Kisanga P, Current status of proection support and promotion of breastfeeding in four African countries: actions to protect, support and promote breastfeeding in Botswana, Kenya, Namibia and Uganda, based on a rapid review 2 Oct – 3 Nov 2000, Prepared for UNICEF ESARO March 2001

Chapter 17: Botswana, poster child of the PMTCT programme

1. Monteiro AC, Weaning Africans off Coca Cola, *Pediatrics* 2010, https://pediatrics.aappublications.org/content/weaning-africans-coca-cola
2. Sullivan E et al, Botswana's Program for preventing Mother-to-Child transmission of HIV, Global Health Delivery https://www.globalhealthdelivery.org/files/ghd/files/ghd-07_botswanas_program_for_preventing.pdf (accessed 27 June 2020)
3. Stuart-Macadam P and Dettwyler KA, *Breastfeeding: Biocultural Perspectives*, ISBN 0-202-01192-5, Aldine de Gruyter, New York, 1995.
4. Spotlight: Botswana: A timeline of HIV action, *PlusNews Johannesburg*, 18 January 2012, http://www.plusnews.org/report.aspx?ReportID=94671
5. *AIDSMAP*, Safer infant feeding, Part 1, 12 Sept 2006. http://www.aidsmap.com/news/sep-2006/safer-infant-feeding-update (accessed 29 June 2020)
6. Thior I, Lockman S, Smeaton LM, et al. Breastfeeding plus infant zidovudine prophylaxis for 6 months vs formula feeding plus infant zidovudine for 1 month to reduce mother-to-child HIV transmission in Botswana: a randomized trial: the Mashi Study. *JAMA.* Aug 16 2006;296(7):794-805
7. UNICEF Press Release. Major Increase in Services Needed for Pregnant HIV-Positive Women to Stop Virus Being Passed to Children, Abuja, Nigeria, 30 November 2005.
8. Creek T, Arvelo W, Kim A, Lu L, Bowen A, Finkbeiner T, Zaks L, Masunge J, Shaffer N and Davis M. Role of infant feeding and HIV in a severe outbreak of diarrhea and malnutrition among young children, Botswana, 2006. Session 137 Poster Abstracts, Conference on Retroviruses and Opportunistic Infections, Los Angeles, 25-28 February, 2007. http://www.retroconference.org/2007/Abstracts/29305.htm
9. Creek T, Morbidity and mortality of Botswana Infants. Powerpoint presentation, CDC 2006
10. Creek T. 11. Role of infant feeding and HIV in a severe outbreak of diarrhoea and malnutrition among young children – Botswana, 2006. Presented at the President's Emergency Plan for AIDS Relief Emergency Meeting/2006 HIV/AIDS Implementers' Meeting, Durban, South Africa; 2006.
11. Creek TL, Kim A, Lu L, Bowen A, Masunge J, Arvelo W, Smit M, Mach O, Legwaila K, Motswere C, Zaks L, Finkbeiner T, Povinelli L, Maruping M, Ngwaru G, Tebele G, Bopp C, Puhr N, Johnston SP, Dasilva AJ, Bem C, Beard RS and Davis MK. Hospitalization and Mortality Among Primarily Non-breastfed Children During a Large Outbreak of Diarrhea and Malnutrition in Botswana, 2006, *J Acquir Immune Defic Syndr.* 2010 Jan 1;53(1):14-9. https://www.ncbi.nlm.nih.gov/pubmed/19801943
12. Coutsoudis A, Coovadia HM & Wilfert CM, HIV, infant feeding and more perils for poor people: new WHO guidelines encourage review of formula milk policies, *Bulletin of the World Health Organization* 2008;86:210–214. https://pubmed.ncbi.nlm.nih.gov/18368208/ (accessed 4 June 2020)
13. Timberg C, In Botswana, Step to cut AIDS proves a formula for disaster, *Washington Post*, 23 July 2007 http://www.washingtonpost.com/wp-dyn/content/article/2007/07/22/AR2007072201204_pf.html (accessed 5 May 2019)

Chapter 18: Early cessation of breastfeeding

1. Ekpini ER, Wiktor SZ, Satten GA, Adjorlolo-Johnson GT, Sibailly TS, Ou CY, Karon JM, Brattegaard K, Whitaker JP, Gnaore E, De Cock KM, Greenberg AE. Late postnatal mother-to-child transmission of HIV-1 in Abidjan, Cote d'Ivoire. *Lancet.* 1997 Apr 12;349(9058):1054-9.
2. Van de Perre P, Meda N, Cartoux, Leroy V, Dabis F. Late postnatal transmission of HIV-1 and early weaning. Lancet 1997;350:221 (letter)
3. WHO Collaborative Study Team on the Role of Breastfeeding on the Prevention of Infant Mortality. Effect of breastfeeding on infant and child mortality due to infectious diseases in less developed countries: a pooled analysis. *Lancet.* 2000 Feb 5;355(9202):451-5, http://www.ncbi.nlm.nih.gov/pubmed/10841125
4. Black RE et al, Global, regional, and national causes of child mortality in 2008: a systematic analysis, *Lancet* 2010;375(9730:1969 – 1987. https://www.who.int/immunization/monitoring_surveillance/resources/Lancet_2010_withAppendix.pdf (accessed 2 May 2020)
5. De Wagt A, Clark D, UNICEF's Support to Free Infant Formula for Infants of HIV Infected Mothers in Africa: A Review of UNICEF Experience, LINKAGES Art and Science of Breastfeeding Presentation Series, Washington DC, April 14 2004.
6. Becquet R, Ekouevi DK, Viho I, Sakarovitch C, Toure H, Castetbon K, Coulibaly N, Timite-Konan M, Bequet L, Dabis F, Leroy V. Acceptability of Exclusive Breast-Feeding With Early Cessation to Prevent HIV Transmission Through Breast Milk, ANRS 1201/1202 Ditrame Plus, Abidjan, Cote d'Ivoire. *J Acquir Immune Defic Syndr.* 2005 Dec 15;40(5):600-608.
7. Coetzee D, Hilderbrand K, Boulle A, Draper B, Abdullah F, Goemaere E. Effectiveness of the first district-wide programme for the prevention of mother-to-child transmission of HIV in South Africa. *Bull World*

Health Organ. 2005 Jul;83(7):489-94.
8. WHO 2005 HIV and Infant Feeding Counselling Tools, ISBN 92 4 159301 6 http://whqlibdoc.who.int/publications/2005/9241593016.pdf
9. WHO 2003. HIV and infant feeding: A guide for health-care managers and supervisors, World Health Organization 2003. https://www.who.int/nutrition/publications/HIV_IF_guide_for_healthcare.pdf (accessed 28 April 2020)
10. WHO 2006, Infant and Young Child Feeding Counselling: An Integrated Course ISBN 92 4 159475 6, http://www.who.int/nutrition/iycf_intergrated_course/en/index.html
11. Latham MC, Kisanga P, Current status of proection support and promotion of breastfeeding in four African countries: actions to protect, support and promote breastfeeding in Botswana, Kenya, Namibia and Uganda, based on a rapid review 2 Oct – 3 Nov 2000, Prepared for UNICEF ESARO March 2001.
12. Goldman, A.; Goldblum, R.; Garza, C., Immunologic components in human milk during the second year of lactation. *Acta Paediatrica* 1983, 72, (3), 461-462.
13. Bradley J; Baldwin S; Armstrong H. Breastfeeding: a neglected household-level weaning-food resource. In: UNICEF 1987 with SIDA and International Development Research Centre, Canada. *Improving young child feeding in eastern and southern Africa. Household-level food technology. Proceedings of a workshop held in Nairobi, Kenya, 12-16 October 1987*, edited by D. Alnwick, S. Moses and O.G. Schmidt. Ottawa, Canada, International Development Research Centre, 1988. 7-33. (IDRC-265e). Full-text of workshop available at http://idl-bnc.idrc.ca/dspace/bitstream/10625/17651/1/28523_p7-33.pdf
14. WHO 1998. Complementary feeding of young children in developing countries: a review of current scientific knowledge. WHO/NUT/98.1.
15. Dewey KG, Cohen RJ, Brown KH, Rivera LL. Age of introduction of complementary foods to low birth weight breastfed infants: a randomized intervention study in Honduras. *Am J Clin Nutr* 1999;69:679-686.
16. Fongillo EA, Habicht J-P, Investigating the weanling's dilemma: lessons lfrom Honduras. *Nutr Rev* 1997;55:390-395.
17. Brahmbhatt H, Gray RH, Child mortality associated with reasons for non-breastfeeding and weaning: is breastfeeding best for HIV-positive mothers? *AIDS*. 2003 Apr 11;17(6):879-85.
18. Haggerty P, Rutstein SO. Breastfeeding and complementary infant feeding, and the postpartum effects of breastfeeding. *Demographic and Health Surveys*, Comparative Studies No.30. Calverton, MD: Macro International Inc.; 1999.
19. Chinkonde JR et al, The difficulty with responding to policy changes for HIV and infant feeding in Malawi *Int Breastfeed J* 2010, 5:11 doi:10.1186/1746-4358-5-11. http://www.internationalbreastfeedingjournal.com/content/5/1/11
20. Gribble KD, Mental health, attachment and breastfeeding: implications for adopted children and their mothers *Int Breastfeed J 2006*, 1:5 doi:10.1186/1746-4358-1-5
21. Small MF: *Our Babies Ourselves: How Biology and Culture Shape the Way We Parent*. New York: Anchor Books; 1998.
22. Piwoz EG, Huffman SL, Lusk D, Zehner ER, O'Gara C, Issues, Risks, and Challenges of Early Breastfeeding Cessation to Reduce Postnatal Transmission of HIV in Africa, For the Support for Analysis and Research in Africa (SARA) Project, Operated by the Academy for Educational Development, 2001. https://pdfs.semanticscholar.org/da62/aa8ffd13b771c34ca4c6b72400c9bf379a67.pdf (accessed 28 May 2020)
23. Howie, P.W., McNeilly, A.S., Houston, M.H. et al. Effect of supplementary food on suckling patterns and ovarian activity during lactation. *BMJ* 1981;283, 757-759.
24. Schleifer SJ, Scott B, Stein M, Keller SE: Behavioral and developmental aspects of immunity. *J Am Acad Child Psychiatry* 1986, 6:751-763.
25. Maunder RG, Hunter JJ: Attachment and psychosomatic medicine: development contributions to stress and disease. *Psychosom Med* 2001, 63:556-567.
26. Drummond PD, Hewson-Bower B: Increased psychosocial stress and decreased mucosal immunity in children with recurrent upper respiratory tract infections. *J Psychosom Res* 1997, 43:271-278
27. Wilson ME, Megel ME, Fredrichs AM, McLaughlin P: Physiologic and behavioral responses to stress, temperament, and incidence of infection and atopic disorders in the first year of life: A pilot study. *J Pediatr Nurs* 2003, 18:257-266.
28. Dettwyler KA: A time to wean: the hominid blueprint for the natural age of weaning in modern human populations. In *Breastfeeding: Biocultural Perspectives*. Edited by Stuart-Macadam P, Dettwyler KA. New York: Aldine de Gruyter; 1995:39-73.
29. Young SL, Mbuya MNN, Chantry CJ, Geubbels EP, Israel-Ballard K, Cohan D, Vosty SA and Latham MC, Current Knowledge and Future Research on Infant Feeding in the Context of HIV: Basic, Clinical, Behavioral, and Programmatic Perspectives, *Adv Nutr* 2011;2(3):225-243. https://www.ncbi.nlm.nih.gov/pmc/articles/PMC3090166/ (accessed 20 May 2020)
30. Willumsen JF, Rollins NC. Evaluation of infant feeding practices by mothers at pMTCT and non pMTCT sites in Botswana. pMTCT Advisory Group, Botswana Food and Nutrition Unit, Family Health Division, Ministry of Health, Botswana, 2001.
31. De Paoli MM, Manongi R and Klepp K-I. Counsellors' perspectives on antenatal HIV testing and

infant feeding dilemmas facing women with HIV in Northern Tanzania. *Reproductive Health Matters* 2002;10:144-156.
32. Bakaki PM, Lessons and experiences with early abrupt cessation of breastfeeding among HIV infected women in Kampala, Uganda. Makerere University-Johns Hopkins University Research Collaboration, January 2002.
33. Rutenberg N, Kalibala S, Mwai C, Rosen J, Integrating HIV Prevention and Care into Maternal and Child Health Care Settings: Lessons learned from HORIZONS studies. (July 23-27 2001, Maasai Mara, Kenya, February 2002.
34. Ndola (Zambia) District Health Management Team. Ndola Demonstration Project to integrate infant feeding counselling and HIV voluntary counseling and testing into health care and community services: A summary of the findings and recommendations from the formative research carried out in Lubuto, Main Masala Twapia and Kabushi Health Center areas, Ndola, Zambia. National Food and Nutrition Commission, LINKAGES, SARA. 1999.
35. Kuhn L and Aldrovandi G, Survival and Health Benefits of Breastfeeding Versus Artificial Feeding in Infants of HIV-Infected Women: Developing Versus Developed World. *Clin Perinatol* 37 (2010) 843–862 https://www.perinatology.theclinics.com/article/S0095-5108(10)00104-1/abstract (accessed 17 March 2020)
36. Brahmbhatt H, Gray RH. Child mortality associated with reasons for non-breastfeeding and weaning: is breastfeeding best for HIV-positive mothers? *AIDS* 2003;17:879–85
37. Kagaayi J, Gray RH, Brahmbhatt H, et al. Survival of infants born to HIV-positive mothers by feeding modality in Rakai, Uganda. *PLoS One* 2008;3:e3877
38. Homsy J, Moore D, Barasa A, et al. Breastfeeding, mother-to-child HIV transmission, and mortality among infants born to HIV-Infected women on highly active antiretroviral therapy in rural Uganda. *J Acquir Immune Defic Syndr* 2010;53:28–35
39. Peltier CA, Ndayisaba GF, Lepage P, et al. Breastfeeding with maternal antiretroviral therapy or formula feeding to prevent HIV postnatal mother-to-child transmission in Rwanda. *AIDS* 2009;23:2415–23
40. Nyandiko WM, Otieno-Nyunya B, Musick B, et al. Outcomes of HIV-exposed children in western Kenya: efficacy of prevention of mother to child transmission in a resource-constrained setting. *J Acquir Immune Defic Syndr* 2010;54:42–50.
41. Phadke MA, Gadgil B, Bharucha KE, et al. Replacement-fed infants born to HIVinfected mothers in India have a high early postpartum rate of hospitalization. *J Nutr* 2003;133:3153–7
42. Thomas T, Masaba R, van Eijk A, et al. Rates of diarrhea associated with early weaning among infants in Kisumu, Kenya [abstract # 774]. In: 14th Conference on Retroviruses and Opportunistic Infections. Los Angeles (CA): 25–28 February; 2007.
43. Kafulafula G, Thigpen M, Hoover DR, et al. Post-weaning gastroenteritis and mortality in HIV-uninfected African infants receiving antiretroviral prophylaxis to prevent MTCT of HIV-1 [abstract # 773]. In: 14th Conference on Retroviruses and Opportunistic Infections. Los Angeles (CA), February 25–28, 2007.
44. Kourtis AP, Fitzgerald D, Hyde L. et al. Diarrhea in uninfected infants of HIV-infected mothers who stop breastfeeding at 6 months: the BAN study experience [abstract # 772]. In: 14th Conference on Retroviruses and Opportunistic Infections. Los Angeles (CA), February 25–28, 2007.
45. Onyango C, Mmiro F, Bagenda D et al. Early breastfeeding cessation among HIV-exposed negative infants and risk of serious gastroenteritis: findings from a perinatal prevention trial in Kampala, Uganda [abstract # 775]. In: 14th Conference on Retorviruses and Opportunistic Infections. Los Angeles (CA), February 25–28, 2007.)
46. Creek T. Role of infant feeding and HIV in a severe outbreak of diarrhea and malnutrition among young children - Botswana, 2006. PEPFAR Implementers Meeting, Durban, South Africa, Abstract #LB1, 2006.
47. Creek T, Arvelo W, Kim A, Lu L, Bowen A, Finkbeiner T, Zaks L, Masunge J, Shaffer N and Davis M. Role of infant feeding and HIV in a severe outbreak of diarrhea and malnutrition among young children, Botswana, 2006. Session 137 Poster Abstracts, Conference on Retroviruses and Opportunistic Infections, Los Angeles, 25-28 February, 2007. http://www.retroconference.org/2007/Abstracts/29305.htm
48. Marquis G, Diaz J, Bartolini R, Creed de Kanashiro H, Rasmussen K. Recognizing the reversible nature of child-feeding decisions: breastfeeding, weaning, and relactation patterns in a shanty town community of Lima, Peru. *Soc Sci Med 1998*; 47(5):645-56. https://pubmed.ncbi.nlm.nih.gov/9690847/ (accessed 28 May 2020)
49. Smart T, *AIDSMAP*, Safer infant feeding update, part 2, 21 September 2006 https://www.aidsmap.com/news/sep-2006/safer-infant-feeding-update-part-2 (accessed 20 September 2020)
50. Tavengwa N, Is early breastfeeding cessation AFASS in rural Zimbabwe? PATH Satellite Powerpoint presented at IAC 2006, Toronto http://www.path.org/files/Naume_Tavengwa.pdf
51. de Paoli MM, Mkwanazi DB, Rollins NC. Rapid cessation of breastfeeding - a safe and feasible PMTCT strategy? Sixteenth International AIDS Conference, Toronto, Abstract CDC0535, 2006.
52. Alfieri C et al. Early weaning: a challenge for mothers in Burkina Faso. Sixteenth International AIDS Conference, Toronto, Abstract CDC0540, 2006.
53. Leshabari, Sebalda C et al. HIV and infant feeding counselling: challenges faced by nurse-counsellors in northern Tanzania. *Hum Resour Health*, July 24, 2007; 5(1): 18 available at http://www.human-resources-health.com/content/pdf/1478-4491-5-18.pdf

54. Buskens J. Woman´s inhumanity to woman in infant feeding counseling in southern Africa. Sixteenth International AIDS Conference, Toronto, Abstract THPE0605, 2006.
55. Kagoda B, Bakaki P. Health and socio-economic experiences of HIV-infected women and their infants in the era PMTCT: case reports from the breast milk study. Sixteenth International AIDS Conference, Toronto, Abstract CDC0577, 2006.
56. Thomas RM et al. Evaluation of mothers' experiences using a ready-to-use therapeutic food to aid in early breastfeeding cessation of infants of HIV-infected mothers: the BAN study in Lilongwe, Malawi. Sixteenth International AIDS Conference, Toronto, Abstract CDC0526, 2006.
57. Cames C et al. A sustainable baby food support for HIV-1-infected mothers. The Kesho Bora study (KB) initiative in Burkina Faso. Sixteenth International AIDS Conference, Toronto, Abstract TUPE0356, 2006. http://www.mpl.ird.fr/epiprev/actu.html
58. Ternier R et al. Nutritional support for infants of non-breastfeeding, HIV-positive mothers. Sixteenth International AIDS Conference, Toronto, Abstract THPE0185, 2006.
59. Kuhn L, Aldrovandi G. Pendulum Swings in HIV-1 and Infant Feeding Policies: Now Halfway Back. *Adv Exp Med Biol.* 2012;743:273-87. http://www.ncbi.nlm.nih.gov/pubmed/22454357
60. Kuhn L, Aldrovandi GM, Sinkala M et al. Effects of early, abrupt cessation of breastfeeding on HIV-free survival of children in Zambia. *N Engl J Med* 2008;359:130–141
61. Kuhn L, Aldrovandi GM, Sinkala M et al Differential effects of early weaning for HIV-free survival of children born to HIV-infected mothers by severity of maternal disease. *PLoS One* 2009;4:e6059. doi: 10.1371/journal.pone.0006059
62. Kuhn L, Sinkala M, Semrau K et al Elevations in mortality due to weaning persist into the second year of life among uninfected children born to HIV-infected mothers. *Clin Infect Dis* 2010;54:437–444
63. Arpadi SM, Fawzy A, Aldrovandi GM et al (2009) Growth faltering due to breastfeeding cessation among uninfected children born to HIV-infected mothers in Zambia. *Am J Clin Nutr* 90:344–350
64. Fawzy A, Arpadi S, Kankasa C et al (2011) Early weaning increases diarrhea morbidity and mortality among uninfected children born to HIV-infected mothers in Zambia. *J Infect Dis* 203:1222–1230
65. Gray S. Ecology of weaning among nomadic Turkana Pastoralists of Kenya: maternal thinking, maternal behavior and human adaptive strategies. Hum Biol 1996;68(3):437-65. https://pubmed.ncbi.nlm.nih.gov/8935324/ (accessed 28 May 2020)
66. Williams CD, Kwashiorkor: a nutritional disease of children associated with a maize diet, 1935 *Bull of the World Health Organ* 2003:81(12):912-913. https://www.ncbi.nlm.nih.gov/pmc/articles/PMC2572388/ (accessed 28 May 2020)
67. Brown A, *Why breastfeeding grief and trauma matter*, Pinter & Martin, London, 2019. ISBN 978-1-78066-615-0.
68. Kuhn L, Kim H-Y, Walter J, Thea DM, Sinkala M, Mwiya M, Kankasa C, Decker D, Aldrovandi GM, HIV-1 Concentrations in Human Breast Milk Before and After Weaning, *Sci Transl Med* Vol. 5, Issue 181, p. 181ra51, Sci. Transl. Med. DOI: 10.1126/scitranslmed.3005113, Apr 2013 available at http://stm.sciencemag.org/content/5/181/181ra51.full.html
69. Kuhn L and Aldrovandi G, Survival and Health Benefits of Breastfeeding Versus Artificial Feeding in Infants of HIV-Infected Women: Developing Versus Developed World. *Clin Perinatol* 2010;37:843–862 https://www.perinatology.theclinics.com/article/S0095-5108(10)00104-1/abstract (accessed 17 March 2020)
70. Van de Perre et al, How evidence based are public health policies for prevention of mother to child transmission of HIV? *BMJ* 2013;346:f3763 doi: 10.1136/bmj.f3763 (Published 20 June 2013)

Chapter 19: Animal milks: errors, omissions and experiments

1. WHO 1998. WHO – UNAIDS - UNICEF, Technical Consultation on HIV and Infant Feeding Implementation of Guidelines Report of a Meeting - Geneva, 20-22 April 1998 http://www.unaids.org/sites/default/files/media_asset/jc180-hiv-infantfeeding-4_en_0.pdf (accessed 18 February 2021).
2. WHO 2000, HIV and Infant Feeding Counselling: A training course, Director's Guide WHO/FCH/CAH/00.2 https://www.who.int/nutrition/publications/en/hiv_infant_feeding_course_director_eng.pdf (accessed 12 May 2020)
3. WHO 2006, Infant and Young Child Feeding Counselling: An Integrated Course, Participants Manual, ISBN 92 4 159475 6, available at http://www.who.int/nutrition/iycf_intergrated_course/en/index.html (accessed 23 December, 2008)
4. Papathakis PC et al. Are WHO/UNAIDS/UNICEF-recommended replacement milks for infants of HIV-infected mothers appropriate in the South African context? *Bulletin World Health Organization*, 2004, 82:164–171. https://apps.who.int/iris/handle/10665/72311 (accessed 11 May 2020)
5. Sarna A. "Report on Discussions with National AIDS Control Organization and Visits to Two Pilot Program Sites." December 2002
6. de Paoli M, Manongi R, Helsing E, Klepp KI. Exclusive breastfeeding in the era of AIDS. *J Hum Lact* 17(4); 313-320. July 2001
7. Oguta TJ. "Infant feeding practices and breastmilk alternatives for infants born to HIV-infected mothers in Homa-Bay District." MSc Thesis, June 2001.

8. Williams C, Zin MM, Mon AA. UNICEF Consultant Report "Country Adaptation of Global HIV and Infant Feeding Guidelines and Development of Replacement Feeding Guidelines for Myanmar, 2001-2003. Stage II: Formative research and development of replacement feeding guidelines for site 1: Monywa." January 2003
9. Briend A, Home-modified animal milk for replacement feeding: Is it feasible and safe? A technical paper prepared for HIV and Infant Feeding Techical Consultation 25-27 October 2006, https://www.ennonline.net/attachments/516/animal-milk-modification-who-discussion-paper-oct-2006.pdf (accessed 9 May 2020)
10. Parents Choice, What should we feed baby? http://www.parentschoiceformula.com/articles/Infant-Formula-Timeline-What-Should-we-Feed-Baby.aspx (accessed 17 April 2020)
11. Brouard C, Espie E, Weill FX, Kerouanton A, Brisabois A, Forgue AM, et al. 12. Two consecutive large outbreaks of Salmonella enterica serotype Agona infections in infants linked to the consumption of powdered infant formula. *Pediatr Infect Dis J* 2007; 26: 148-52. PMID:17259878 doi:10.1097/01.inf.0000253219.06258.23
12. Weir E. Powdered infant formula and fatal infection with 13. Enterobacter sakazakii. *Can Med Assoc J* 2002; 166: 1570.
13. Threlfall EJ, Ward LR, Hampton MD, Ridley AM, Rowe B, Roberts D, et al. 14. Molecular fingerprinting defines a strain of Salmonella enterica serotype anatum responsible for an international outbreak associated with formula-dried milk. *Epidemiol Infect* 1998; 121: 289-93. PMID:9825779 doi:10.1017/S0950268898001149
14. Sue Jarman, personal communication 17 April 2020.
15. Code Watch 25 Years of protecting Breastfeeding, WABA 2006:
16. First Steps Nutrition Trust, *Infant Milks in the UK* , page 36, June 2013 page 2 http://www.firststepsnutrition.org/pdfs/Infant_milks_a_simple_guide_England_Feb16.pdf
17. Coutsoudis A, Coovadia HM & Wilfert CM, HIV, infant feeding and more perils for poor people: new WHO guidelines encourage review of formula milk policies, *Bulletin of the World Health Organization* 2008;86:210–214. https://pubmed.ncbi.nlm.nih.gov/18368208/ (accessed 4 June 2020)
18. Marler B, About Enterobacter Sakazakii (E. Sakazakii) *Food Poison Journal*, October 30, 2010 https://www.foodpoisonjournal.com/food-poisoning-information/about-enterobacter-sakazakii-e-sakazakii/ (accessed 17April 2020)
19. Agostoni C, Axelsson I, Goulet O, Koletzko B, Michaelsen KF, Puntis JW, Rigo J, Shamir R, Szajewska H, Turck D, Vandenplas Y, Weaver LT.Preparation and Handling of Powdered Infant Formula: A Commentary by the ESPGHAN Committee on Nutrition. *J Pediatr Gastroenterol Nutr*. 2004 Oct;39(4):320-322. https://pubmed.ncbi.nlm.nih.gov/15448416/ (accessed 10 July 2020).
20. WHO 2006. Safe preparation, storage and handling of powdered infant formula Guidelines https://www.who.int/foodsafety/publications/micro/pif_guidelines.pdf (accessed 17 Apr 2020)
21. Duvehage, Kathy, personal communication
22. Browne, Gill, personal communication
23. Piwoz EG, Huffman SL, Lusk D, Zehner ER, O'Gara C, *Issues, Risks, and Challenges of Early Breastfeeding Cessation to Reduce Postnatal Transmission of HIV in Africa*, For the Support for Analysis and Research in Africa (SARA) Project, Operated by the Academy for Educational Development, 2001.
24. Flax V et al, Lipid-Based Nutrient Supplements Are Feasible As a Breastmilk Replacement for HIV-Exposed Infants from 24 to 48 Weeks of Age. *J. Nutr*. 143: 701–707, 2013.
25. Morrison P, Breastmilk costs peanuts! AnotherLook, December 2009, available at http://www.anotherlook.org/papers/j/english.pdf
26. Arie S, Hungry for Profit, *BMJ* 2010;341:c5221
27. Making peanut butter gets stickier, UNICEF is Plmpynut's biggest client, *Irin*, Johannesburg, 11 November 2009. http://www.irinnews.org/report.aspx?ReportID=86979
28. Parker ME et al, BAN Study Team. The health of HIV-exposed children after early weaning. *Matern Child Nutr* 2013 Apr;9(2):217-32. doi: 10.1111/j.1740-8709.2011.00369.x. Epub 2011 Nov 20
29. Medlineplus, Cotrimoxazole, *US National Library of US Medicine* https://medlineplus.gov/druginfo/meds/a684026.html (accessed 9 July 2020)
30. Sulfonamide, Oral route, *Mayo Clinic* https://www.mayoclinic.org/drugs-supplements/sulfonamide-oral-route/before-using/drg-20069536 (accessed 9 July 2020
31. UNICEF 2007, Children and the Milennium Development Goals, progress towards a world fit for children, http://www.reliefweb.int/rw/lib.nsf/db900SID/EMAE-79LN8U/$FILE/UNICEF_Children%20and%20the%20MDGs_Dec%202007.pdf
32. Coutsoudis A, Pillay K, Spooner E, Coovadia HM, Pembrey L, Newell ML. Routinely available cotrimoxazole prophylaxis and occurrence of respiratory and diarrhoeal morbidity in infants born to HIV-infected mothers in South Africa. *S Afr Med J*. 2005 May;95(5):339-45
33. Akre J, editor: Infant Feeding, the Physiological Basis, *Bulletin of the World Health Organization,* Supplement to Vol 67, 1989, http://apps.who.int/iris/bitstream/handle/10665/39084/bulletin_1989_67(supp).pdf (accessed 28 Oct 2018)
34. Coutsoudis A et al. Impact of cotrimoxazole prophylaxis on the health of breastfed HIV exposed negative infants in a resource-limited setting. *AIDS* 25, doi: 10.1097/QAD.0b013e32834ad699, 2011.
35. Carole Leach-Lemens, Cotrimoxazole in HIV-exposed but uninfected infants may undermine benefits

of breastfeeding; trial needed, say paediatricians. *Aidsmap.* 09 August 2011 http://www.aidsmap.com/page/2037662/

36. Kourtis AP, Role of intestinal mucosal integrity in HIV transmission to infants through breast-feeding: the BAN study. *J Infect Dis.* 2013 Aug 15;208(4):653-61. doi: 10.1093/infdis/jit221. Epub 2013 May 17.
37. WHO 2014, Guidelines on post-exposure prophylaxis for HIV and the use of co-trimoxazole prophylaxis for HIV-related infections among adults, adolescents and children: Recommendations for a public health approach, December 2014 supplement to the 2013 consolidated guidelines on the use of antiretroviral drugs for treating and preventing HIV infection https://apps.who.int/iris/bitstream/handle/10665/145719/9789241508193_eng.pdf (accessed 9 July 2020)
38. Lockman S, Effect of co-trimoxazole on mortality in HIV-exposed but uninfected children in Botswana (the Mpepu Study): a double-blind, randomised, placebo-controlled trial. *Lancet Glob Health.* 2017 May; 5(5): e491–e500. doi:10.1016/S2214-109X(17)30143-2 https://europepmc.org/backend/ptpmcrender.fcgi (accessed 1 Aug 2020)
39. Coutsoudis A, Coovadia H et al, New Co-trimoxazole recomments for HIV-exposed infants. *Bulletin of the World Health Organization* 2010. http://www.who.int/bulletin/volumes/88/12/10-076422/en/index.html
40. Daniels B, Coutsoudis, A, Moodley-Govender E, Mulol H, Spooner E, Kiepiela P et al. Effect of co-trimoxazole prophylaxis on morbidity and mortality of HIV-exposed, HIV-uninfected infants in South Africa: a randomised controlled, non-inferiority trial. *Lancet Glob Health.* 2019;7(12):PE1717-E1727, DOI: 10.1016/S2214109X(19)30422-X.)

Chapter 20: Already HIV-infected infants and babies who escape infection

1. UNICEF *State of World's Children 1998*:30. https://www.unicef.org/reports/state-worlds-children-1998 (accessed 31 March 2021)
2. Miller MF, Humphrey JH , Iliff PJ, Malaba LC, Mbuya NV, the ZVITAMBO Study Group and Stoltzfus RJ, Neonatal erythropoiesis and subsequent anemia in HIV-positive and HIV-negative Zimbabwean babies during the first year of life: a longitudinal study. *BMC Infectious Diseases* 2006, 6:1 doi:10.1186/1471-2334-6-1.
3. Obimbo EM, Mbori-Ngacha DA, Ochieng JO, Richardson BA, Otieno PA, Bosire R, Farquhar C, Overbaugh J, John-Stewart GC. Predictors of early mortality in a cohort of human immunodeficiency virus type 1-infected african children. *Pediatr Infect Dis J.* 2004 Jun;23(6):536-43.
4. Richardson BA, Mbori-Ngacha D, Lavreys L, John-Stewart GC, Nduati R, Panteleeff DD, Emery S, Kreiss JK, Overbaugh J. Comparison of human immunodeficiency virus type 1 viral loads in Kenyan women, men, and infants during primary and early infection. *J Virol.* 2003 Jun;77(12):7120-3.
5. Taha TE, Graham SM, Kumwende NI, et al. Morbidity among HIV-1 infected children and uninfected African children. *Pediatrics* 2000;106:e77.
6. Dickover RE, Dillon M Gillette SG, Deveikis A, Keller M, Plaeger-Marshall S, Chen I, Diagne A, Steihm ER, Bryson Y 1994, Rapid increases in load of human immunodeficiency virus correlate with early disease progression and loss of CD4 cells in vertically infected infants. *J Infect Dis* 170(5):1279-84.
7. Sharland M, Gibb DM and Tudor-Williams G. Advances in the prevention and treatment of paediatric HIV infection in the United Kingdom *Arch Dis Child* 2002;87:178-180 https://adc.bmj.com/content/archdischild/87/3/178.full.pdf (accessed 11 July 2020)
8. Kuhn L, Aldrovandi G. Pendulum Swings in HIV-1 and Infant Feeding Policies: Now Halfway Back. *Adv Exp Med Biol.* 2012;743:273-87. http://www.ncbi.nlm.nih.gov/pubmed/22454357
9. Kuhn L and Aldrovandi G, Survival and Health Benefits of Breastfeeding Versus Artificial Feeding in Infants of HIV-Infected Women: Developing Versus Developed World. *Clin Perinatol* 2010;37(4):843-x. https://www.ncbi.nlm.nih.gov/pmc/articles/PMC3008406/ (accessed 11 July 2020)
10. Kuhn, L. et al. (2007) High Uptake of Exclusive Breastfeeding and Reduced Early Post-Natal HIV Transmission. *PloS One.* 2 (12): e1363.
11. Kuhn L, Aldrovandi GM, Sinkala M, Kankasa C, Semrau K, Mwiya M, Kasonde P, Scott N, Vwalika C, Walter J, Bulterys M, Tsai W-Y and Thea DM for the Zambia Exclusive Breastfeeding Study. Effects of early, abrupt weaning for HIV-free survival of children in Zambia *N Engl J Med* 2008;359:130–141 http://content.nejm.org/cgi/reprint/NEJMoa073788v1.pdf
12. Lockman et al, "Morbidity and mortality among infants born to HIV-infected mothers and randomized to breastfeeding versus formula-feeding in Botswana (Mashi study)", XVI International AIDS Conference (Abstract no. TUPE0357), August 2006
13. WHO 2016, Consolidated guidelines on the use of antiretroviral drugs for treating and preventing HIV infection: recommendations for a public health approach – 2nd ed. ISBN 978 92 4 154968 4, http://www.who.int/hiv/pub/arv/arv-2016/en/
14. Violari A, Cotton MF, Gibb DM et al (2008) Early antiretroviral therapy and mortality among HIV-infected infants. *N Engl J Med* 359:2233–2244
15. Tozzi AE, Pazzotti P and Greco D 1990, Does breastfeeding delay progression to AIDS in HIV-infected children? Letter to the editor. *AIDS* 4:1493-94.
16. Kambarami RA & Kowo H 1997, The prevalence of nipple disease among breast feeding mothers of HIV

seropositive infants. *Central African J Med* 43(1):20-23.
17. Dr Greg Powell, Harare Paediatrician, PMTCT Partners' meeting.
18. Taha TE, Kumwenda NI, Hoover DR et al (2006) The impact of breastfeeding on the health of HIV-positive mothers and their children in sub-Saharan Africa. *Bulletin of the World Health Organization* WHO 84:546–554
19. WHO 2010, When to start Antiretroviral Therapy for HIV Infection in Infants and Children: Towards Universal Access: Recommendations for a Public Health Approach: 2010 Revision. Geneva: World Health Organization; 2010. https://www.ncbi.nlm.nih.gov/books/NBK138590/ (accessed 31 March 2021)
20. WHO HIV/AIDS, Key Facts, *The Conversation*, 6 July 2020 https://www.who.int/news-room/fact-sheets/detail/hiv-aids (accessed 12 July 2020)
21. New estimates show 14.8 million children globally are HIV-exposed but uninfected. *The Conversation* January 12, 2020. https://theconversation.com/new-estimates-show-14-8-million-children-globally-are-hiv-exposed-but-uninfected-128475 (accessed January 2020)
22. Slogrove AL et al, Estimates of the global population of children who are HIV-exposed and uninfected, 2000-18: a modelling study. *Lancet Global Health* 2019; pii: S2214-109X(19)30448-6. doi: 10.1016/S2214-109X(19)30448-6. https://www.ncbi.nlm.nih.gov/pubmed/31791800 Accessed 22 Sept 2020.
23. HIV.gov website, https://www.hiv.gov/hiv-basics/overview/data-and-trends/global-statistics accessed 12 July 2020
24. Sugandhi N et al, HIV-exposed infants: rethinking care for a lifelong condition. *AIDS* 2013, 27 (Suppl 2):S187–S195 https://www.ncbi.nlm.nih.gov/pmc/articles/PMC4089095 (accessed 12 July 2020).
25. Shapiro R, Lockman S. Mortality among HIV-exposed infants: the first and final frontier. *Clin Infect Dis* 2010; 50:445–447
26. Newell ML, Coovadia H, Cortina-Borja M, Rollins N, Gaillard P, Dabis F, et al. Mortality of infected and uninfected infants born to HIV-infected mothers in Africa: a pooled analysis. *Lancet* 2004; 364:1236–1243.
27. Ndirangu J, Newell M, Thorne C, Bland R. Treating HIV-infected mothers reduces under 5 years of age mortality rates to levels seen in children of HIV-uninfected mothers in rural South Africa. *Antiviral Therapy* 2012; 17:81–90.
28. Kuhn L, Kasonde P, Sinkala M, Kankasa C, Semrau K, Scott N, Tsai WY, Vermund SH, Aldrovandi GM, Thea DM. Does severity of HIV disease in HIV-infected mothers affect mortality and morbidity among their uninfected infants? *Clin Infect Dis.* 2005 Dec 1;41(11):1654-61. Epub 2005 Oct 27.
29. Futata E, Fusaro A, De Brito C, Sato M. The neonatal immune system: immunomodulation of infections in early life. *Rev Anti-Infect Therapy* Mar 2012; 10:289–298.
30. Horta BL, Bahl R, Martines JC, Victora CG. Evidence on the long-term effects of breastfeeding.World Health Organization; 2007. https://www.who.int/maternal_child_adolescent/documents/9241595230/en/ (accessed 31 March 2021)
31. Le Roux S, Abrams EJ et al, Infectious morbidity of breastfed, HIV-exposed uninfected infants under conditions of universal antiretroviral therapy in South Africa: a prospective cohort study. *Child & Adolescent Health* 2020 4(3). DOI:https://doi.org/10.1016/S2352-4642(19)30375-X, https://www.thelancet.com/journals/lanchi/article/PIIS2352-4642(19)30375-X/fulltext (accessed 12 July 2020)1
32. Babies of South African mothers taking HIV therapy have worse health in early months – unless they are vaccinated and consistently breastfed, *AIDSMAP*, 11 February 2020, https://www.aidsmap.com/news/feb-2020/babies-south-african-mothers-taking-hiv-therapy-have-worse-health-early-months-unless (accessed 12 July 2020)
33. Filteau S. The HIV-exposed, uninfected African child. *Trop Med Int Health* 2009; 14:276–287.
34. Rotherham-Borus M-J et al. Outcomes of HIV-exposed but uninfected children in South Africa over 5 years: Comparison to un-exposed peers. 23rd International AIDS Conference, abstract no 6968, 2020 as reported by *AIDSMAP*, 8 July 2020, https://www.aidsmap.com/news/jul-2020/aged-five-uninfected-children-hiv-positive-mothers-do-just-well-children-hiv-negative (accessed 12 July 2020).

Chapter 21: HIV-free survival

1. Morrison P, HIV and infant feeding: to breastfeed or not to breastfeed: the dilemma of competing risks. Part 1. *Breastfeed Rev.* 1999 Jul;7(2):5-13 https://pubmed.ncbi.nlm.nih.gov/10453705/ (accessed 31 March 2021)
2. Morrison P, HIV and infant feeding: to breastfeed or not to breastfeed: the dilemma of competing risks. Part 2. *Breastfeed Rev.* 1999 Nov;7(3):11-20. https://pubmed.ncbi.nlm.nih.gov/10943427/ (accessed 31 March 2021)
3. WHO Collaborative Study Team on the Role of Breastfeeding on the Prevention of Infant Mortality. Effect of breastfeeding on infant and child mortality due to infectious diseases in less developed countries: a pooled analysis. *Lancet.* 2000;355:451–455. http://www.ncbi.nlm.nih.gov/pubmed/10841125.
4. WHO 2003, Global Strategy on Infant and Young Child Feeding, https://apps.who.int/iris/bitstream/handle/10665/42590/9241562218.pdf (accessed 1 June 2020)
5. *The Lancet Child Survival Series* 2003 https://www.thelancet.com/series/child-survival (accessed 30 May 2020).

6. Black RE, Morris SS & Bryce J (2003) Where and why are 10 million children dying every year? *Lancet* 361, 2–10. https://pubmed.ncbi.nlm.nih.gov/12842379/ (accessed 30 May 2020)
7. Rollins N, Little K, Mzolo S, Horwood C, Newell ML. Surveillance of mother-to-child transmission prevention programmes at immunization clinics: the case for universal screening. *Rev Med Virol.* 2007 Jun 1. https://pubmed.ncbi.nlm.nih.gov/17545711/ (accessed 19 Feb 2021)
8. Bahl R, Frost C, Kirkwood BR, Edmond K, Martines J, Bhandari N, & Arthur P. Infant Feeding patterns and risks of death and hospitalization in the first half of infancy: multicentre cohort study. *Bull World Health Organization 2005*;83:418-426.
9. Noel F et al, Contribution of Bacterial Sepsis to Morbidity in Infants Born to HIV-Infected Haitian Mothers Acquir Immune Defic Syndr 2006;43:313–319, https://pubmed.ncbi.nlm.nih.gov/17079993/ (accessed 4 June 2020)
10. Latham MC, Kisanga P, Current status of proection support and promotion of breastfeeding in four African countries: actions to protect, support and promote breastfeeding in Botswana, Kenya, Namibia and Uganda, based on a rapid review 2 Oct – 3 Nov 2000, Prepared for UNICEF ESARO March 2001
11. Ross JS and Labbok MH. Modeling the effects of different infant feeding strategies on infant survival and mother-to-child transmission of HIV. *Am J Pub Health* 2004; 94(7)1174-1180. https://www.ncbi.nlm.nih.gov/pmc/articles/PMC1448417/ (accessed 30 May 2020)
12. Coutsoudis A, Goga AE, Rollins N, Coovadia HM. Free formula milk for infants of HIV-infected women: blessing or curse? *Health Pol and Planning* 2002;17(2):154-160. https://pubmed.ncbi.nlm.nih.gov/12000775/ (accessed 6 June 2020) https://watermark.silverchair.com/170154.pdf
13. Thior I, Lockman S, Smeaton LM, Shapiro RL, Wester C; Heymann SJ, et al. 15. Breastfeeding plus infant zidovudine prophylaxis for 6 months vs formula feeding plus infant zidovudine for 1 month to reduce mother-to-child HIV transmission in Botswana: a randomized trial: the Mashi Study. *JAMA* 2006; 296: 794-805. PMID:16905785 doi:10.1001/jama.296.7.794
14. Young SL, Mbuya MNN, Chantry CJ, Geubbels EP, Israel-Ballard K, Cohan D, Vosty SA and Latham MC, Current Knowledge and Future Research on Infant Feeding in the Context of HIV: Basic, Clinical, Behavioral, and Programmatic Perspectives, *Adv Nutr* 2011;2(3):225-243. https://www.ncbi.nlm.nih.gov/pmc/articles/PMC3090166/ (accessed 20 May 2020)
15. Kuhn L, Aldrovandi G. Pendulum Swings in HIV-1 and Infant Feeding Policies: Now Halfway Back. *Adv Exp Med Biol.* 2012;743:273-87. http://www.ncbi.nlm.nih.gov/pubmed/22454357
16. Coovadia H et al. Transmission rates, infant mortality outcomes, and effective counselling, in HIV infected mothers who breastfed exclusively: implications for review of UN guidelines on infant feeding. Sixteenth International AIDS Conference, Toronto, abstract CDC0544, 2006.
17. Homsy J et al. Mother-to-child HIV transmission and infant mortality among women receiving highly active antiretroviral therapy (HAART) in rural Uganda. Sixteenth International AIDS Conference, Toronto, Abstract no. TUPE0, 2006
18. Adejuyigbe E et al. The influence of infant feeding choice on morbidity and mortality in HIV-exposed infants in southwestern Nigeria. Sixteenth International AIDS Conference, Toronto, Abstract no. 2006.
19. Theo Smart, Infant Feeding policy debate at the conference on Retroviruses and Opportunistic Infections, HATIP #82, *AIDSMAP* 13th March 2007, https://www.aidsmap.com/news/mar-2007/croi-early-weaning-and-formula-feeding-puts-hiv-exposed-infants-resource-limited (accessed 19 February 2021)
20. Kuhn L and Aldrovandi G, Survival and Health Benefits of Breastfeeding Versus Artificial Feeding in Infants of HIV-Infected Women: Developing Versus Developed World. *Clin Perinatol* 2010;37:843–862 https://www.perinatology.theclinics.com/article/S0095-5108(10)00104-1/abstract (accessed 17 March 2020)
21. Nduati R, John G, Mbori-Ngacha D, et al. Effect of breastfeeding and formula feeding on transmission of HIV-1: A randomized clinical trial. *JAMA* 2000;283:1167–1174.
22. Phadke MA, Gadgil B, Bharucha KE, et al. Replacement-fed infants born to HIV-infected mothers in India have a high early postpartum rate of hospitalization. *J Nutr* 2003;133:3153–3157.
23. Creek T, Arvelo W, Kim A, et al. Role of infant feeding and HIV in a severe outbreak of diarrhea and malnutrition among young children, Botswana, 2006. 14th Conference on Retroviruses and Opportunistic Infections; 25–28 February; 2007; Los Angeles, CA. (Abstract # 770).
24. Creek TL, Kim A, Lu L, et al. Hospitalization and mortality among primarily nonbreastfed children during a large outbreak of diarrhea and malnutrition in Botswana, 2006. *J Acquir Immune Defic Syndr* 2010;53:14–19.
25. Taha TE, Kumwenda NI, Hoover DR, et al. The impact of breastfeeding on the health of HIVpositive mothers and their children in sub-Saharan Africa. *Bull World Health Organization* 2006;84:546–554.
26. Taha TE, Hoover, DR, Chen S, Kumwenda NI, Mipando L, Nkanaunena K, Thigpen MC, Taylor A, Fowler MG and Mofenson LM. Effects of Cessation of Breastfeeding in HIV-1–Exposed, Uninfected Children in Malawi. *Clinical Infectious Diseases* 2011;53(4):388–395
27. Thomas, T.; Masaba, R.; van Eijk, A., et al. Rates of diarrhea associated with early weaning among infants in Kisumu, Kenya. 14th Conference on Retroviruses and Opportunistic Infections; 25–28 February; 2007; Los Angeles, CA. (Abstract # 774) ed.
28. Doherty T, Chopra M, Jackson D, Goga A, Colvin M, Persson LA. Effectiveness of the WHO/UNICEF guidelines on infant feeding for HIV-positive women: results from a prospective cohort study in South Africa. *AIDS* 2007;21:1791–1797

29. Becquet R, Bequet L, Ekouevi DK, et al. Two-year morbidity-mortality and alternatives to prolonged breastfeeding among children born to HIV-infected mothers in Cote d'Ivoire. *PLOS Medicine* 2007;4:e17.
30. Onyango, C.; Mmiro, F.; Bagenda, D., et al. Early breastfeeding cessation among HIV-exposed negative infants and risk of serious gastroenteritis: findings from a perinatal prevention trial in Kampala, Uganda. 14th Conference on Retorviruses and Opportunistic Infections; 25–28 February; 2007; Los Angeles, CA. (Abstract #775) ed
31. Onyango-Makumbi C, Bagenda D, Mwatha A, et al. Early Weaning of HIV-Exposed Uninfected Infants and Risk of Serious Gastroenteritis: Findings from Two Perinatal HIV Prevention Trials in Kampala, Uganda. *J Acquir Immune Defic Syndr* 2010;53:20–27.
32. Medicins sans Frontieres, Africa's Miracle Food, Plumpynut (first appeared in *The Times*) 12 August 2005. https://www.msf.org/africas-miracle-food-plumpynut (accessed 15 July 2020).
33. Kourtis AP, Fitzgerald D, Hyde L et al. Diarrhea in uninfected infants of HIV-infected mothers who stop breastfeeding at 6 months: the BAN study experience. 14th Conference on Retroviruses and Opportunistic Infections; 25–28 February; 2007; Los Angeles, CA. (Abstract # 772) ed
34. Kafulafula, G; Thigpen, M; Hoover, DR, et al. Post-weaning gastroenteritis and mortality in HIV-uninfected African infants receiving antiretroviral prophylaxis to prevent MTCT of HIV-1. 14th Conference on Retroviruses and Opportunistic Infections; 25–28 February; 2007; Los Angeles, CA. (Abstract # 773) ed.
35. Kafulafula G, Hoover DR, Taha TE, et al. Frequency of Gastroenteritis and Gastroenteritis- Associated Mortality with Early Weaning in HIV-1-Uninfected Children Born to HIV-Infected Women in Malawi. *J Acquir Immune Defic Syndr* 2010;53:6–13
36. Kagaayi J, Gray RH, Brahmbhatt H, et al. Survival of infants born to HIV-positive mothers by feeding modality in Rakai, Uganda. *PLoS One* 2008;3:e3877. doi:10.1371/journal.pone.0003877.
37. Homsy J, Moore D, Barasa A, et al. Breastfeeding, mother-to-child HIV transmission, and mortality among infants born to HIV-Infected women on highly active antiretroviral therapy in rural Uganda. *J Acquir Immune Defic Syndr* 2010;53:28–35.
38. Peltier CA, Ndayisaba GF, Lepage P, et al. Breastfeeding with maternal antiretroviral therapy or formula feeding to prevent HIV postnatal mother-to-child transmission in Rwanda. *AIDS* 2009;23:2415–2423
39. Nyandiko WM, Otieno-Nyunya B, Musick B, et al. Outcomes of HIV-exposed children in western Kenya: efficacy of prevention of mother to child transmission in a resource-constrained setting. *J Acquir Immune Defic Syndr* 2010;54:42–50.
40. Cournil A et al for the Kesho Bora Study Group.Relationship between mortality and feeding modality among children born to HIV-infected mothers in a research setting: The Kesho Bora Study. *AIDS.* 2012 Dec 19. http://www.ncbi.nlm.nih.gov/pubmed/23262499
41. Kuhn L, Aldrovandi GM, Sinkala M, et al. Effects of early, abrupt cessation of breastfeeding on HIV-free survival of children in Zambia. *N Engl J Med* 2008; 359:130–41.
42. Kuhn L, Aldrovandi GM, Sinkala M, et al. Differential effects of early weaning for HIV-free survival of children born to HIV-infected mothers by severity of maternal disease. *PLoS One* 2009;4:e6059.
43. Kuhn L, Sinkala M, Semrau K, et al. Elevations in mortality due to weaning persist into the second year of life among uninfected children born to HIVinfected mothers. *Clin Infect Dis* 2010;54:437–44.
44. Arpadi SM, Fawzy A, Aldrovandi GM, et al. Growth faltering due to breastfeeding cessation among uninfected children born to HIV-infected mothers in Zambia. *Am J Clin Nutr* 2009;90:344–50.
45. Fawzy A, Arpadi S, Aldrovandi GM, et al. Diarrhea morbidity and mortality increases with weaning prior to 6 months among uninfected infants born to HIV-infected mothers in Zambia. In: International AIDS Society Conference in Cape Town, July 19–22, 2009; TUAC104.
46. Coovadia H & Coutsoudis A, HIV, infant feeding and survival: old wine in new bottles, but brimming with promise. *AIDS* 2007;21(14):1837-1840
47. Lawrence RA. *Breastfeeding: A guide for the medical profession.* 4th ed. St Louis, Missouri: Mosby; 1994.
48. Cunningham AS, Jelliffe DB, Jelliffe EFP. Breastfeeding and Health in the 1098s: A global epidemiological review. *J Pediatr* 1991; 118:659-666
49. Jelliffe DB, Jelliffe EFP. *Human milk in the modern world.* Oxford: Oxford University Press; 1978.
50. Habicht JP, DaVanzo J, Butz WP. Does breastfeeding really save lives, or are potential benefits due to biases? *Am J Epidemiol* 1986; 123:279-290.
51. Bauchner H, Leventhal JM, Shapiro ED. Studies of breast-feeding and infection: How good is the evidence? *JAMA* 1986; 256:887-892.
52. Feachem RG, Koblinski MA. Interventions for the control of diarrhoea diseases among young children: Promotion of breastfeeding. *Bulletin World Health Organization* 1984; 62:271-291.
53. Victora CG. Infection and disease: The impact of early weaning. *Bulletin World Health Organisation* 1996;4:390-396.

Chapter 22: ART and breastfeeding

1. Delaney M, History of HAART – the true story of how effective multi-drug therapy was developed for treatment of HIV disease, *Retrovirology* 2006;3(supple 1):S6. https://www.ncbi.nlm.nih.gov/pmc/articles/PMC1716971/ (accessed 25 July 2020).

2. Newell M-L et al, Mortality of infected and uninfected infants born to HIV-infected mothers in Africa: a pooled analysis. *Lancet* 2004; 8;364(9441):1236-43. doi: 10.1016/S0140-6736(04)17140-7. https://pubmed.ncbi.nlm.nih.gov/15464184 (accessed 19 July 2020)
3. Msellati P., Newell M-L., Dabis F., Rates of mother-to-child transmission of HIV-1 in Africa, America and Europe: Results from 13 perinatal studies *J Acquired Immune Defic Syndr* 1995;8:506-510.
4. De Cock, K.M., Fowler, M.G., Mercier, E., et al., Prevention of mother-to-child HIV transmission in resource-poor countries: translating research into policy and practice. *JAMA* 2000;283, 1175–1182
5. Kind C, Rudin C, Siegrist CA, et al. Prevention of vertical HIV transmission: additive protective effect of elective caesarean section and zidovudine prophylaxis. *AIDS* 1998;12:205-210
6. Maguire A, Sanchez E, Fortuny C, et al. Potential risk factors for vertical HIV-1 transmission in Catalonia, Spain: the protective role of caesarean section. *AIDS* 1997;11:1852-7.
7. Ometto L, Zanotto C, Maccabruni A, et. al. Viral phenotype and host-cell susceptibility to HIV-1 infection as risk factors for mother-to-child transmission. *AIDS* 1995; :427-434.
8. Lallemant M, Le Coeur S, Samba L, et al. Mother-to-child transmission of HIV-1 in Congo central Africa. *AIDS* 1994;8:1451-1456.
9. Roques P, Marce D, Courpotin C, et al. Correlation between HIV provirus burden and in utero transmission. *AIDS* 1993;7 (Supplement):S39-S43.
10. European Collaborative Study. Risk factors for mother-to-child transmission of HIV-1. *Lancet* 1992;339:1007-1012.
11. Blanche S, Rouzioux C, Moscatao M-LG, et al. A prospective study of infants born to women seropositive for human immunodeficiency virus type 1. *N Engl J Med* 1989;320:1643-1648.
12. International AIDS Conference, https://en.wikipedia.org/wiki/XVI_International_AIDS_Conference,_2006
13. International AIDS Conference, https://www.iasociety.org/Web/WebContent/File/Policy%20Report.pdf
14. United States Department of Health and Human Services Guidelines for the Use of Antiretroviral Agents in Adults and Adolescents Living with HIV. https://aidsinfo.nih.gov/guidelines/html/1/adult-andadolescent-arv/0.
15. McLaughlin M et al. The Evolution of Antiretroviral Therapy: Past, Present, and Future. *American Academy of HIV Medicine*. April 18, 2018 https://www.thebodypro.com/article/the-evolution-of-antiretroviral-therapy-past-prese (accessed 25 July 2020).
16. FDA-Approved HIV Medicines. https://aidsinfo.nih.gov/understanding-hiv-aids/factsheets/21/58/fda-approved-hiv-medicines
17. Trickey A, May M, Vehreschild J et al. Survival of HIV-positive patients starting antiretroviral therapy between 1996 and 2013: a collaborative analysis of cohort studies. *Lancet HIV* 2017; 4: e349–e356.
18. Weber R and the Swiss Cohort Study, Decreasing mortality and changing patterns of causes of death in the Swiss HIV Cohort Study, *HIV Medicine* 2013;14:195-207 https://onlinelibrary.wiley.com/doi/epdf/10.1111/j.1468-1293.2012.01051.x (accessed 1 April 2021)
19. Ashley Scheibelhut. The oldest person with HIV turns 100. *HIVPlus Mag* 16 pril 2019. https://www.hivplusmag.com/uu/2019/4/16/oldest-person-living-hiv-turns-100 (accessed 21 April 2019).
20. Garcia PM, Kalish LA, Pitt J, Minkoff H, Quinn TC, Burchett SK, Kornegay J, Jackson B, Moye J, Hanson C, Zorrilla C, Lew JF. Maternal levels of plasma human immunodeficiency virus type 1 RNA and the risk of perinatal transmission. Women and Infants Transmission Study Group. *N Engl J Med. 1999* Aug 5;341(6):394-402.
21. Shaffer N, Roongpisuthipong A, Siriwasin W, Chotpitayasunondh T, Chearskul S, Young NL, Parekh B, Mock PA, Bhadrakom C, Chinayon P, Kalish ML, Phillips SK, Granade TC, Subbarao S, Weniger BG, Mastro TD. Maternal virus load and perinatal human immunodeficiency virus type 1 subtype E transmission, Thailand. Bangkok Collaborative Perinatal HIV Transmission Study Group. *J Infect Dis.* 1999 Mar;179(3):590-9.
22. Mofenson LM, Lambert JS, Stiehm ER, Bethel J, Meyer WA 3rd, Whitehouse J, Moye J Jr, Reichelderfer P, Harris DR, Fowler MG, Mathieson BJ, Nemo GJ. Risk factors for perinatal transmission of human immunodeficiency virus type 1 in women treated with zidovudine. Pediatric AIDS Clinical Trials Group Study 185 Team. *N Engl J Med.* 1999 Aug 5;341(6):385-93.
23. John GC, Nduati RW, Mbori-Ngacha DA, Richardson BA, Panteleeff D, Mwatha A, Overbaugh J, Bwayo J, Ndinya-Achola JO, Kreiss JK. Correlates of mother-to-child human immunodeficiency virus type 1 (HIV-1) transmission: association with maternal plasma HIV-1 RNA load, genital HIV-1 DNA shedding, and breast infections. *J Infect Dis.* 2001 Jan 15;183(2):206-212. Epub 2000 Dec 15.
24. Cooper ER, Charurat M, Mofenson L et al. Combination antiretroviral strategies for treatment of pregnant HIV-infected women and prevention of perinatal HIV-1 transmission. *J Acquir Immune Defic Syndr* 2002;29:484-494.
25. Alice Park, The Story behind the first AIDS drug. *Time* 17 March 2017
26. Ruprecht RM, O'Brien LG, Rossoni LD, Nusinoff-Lehrman S. Suppression of mouse viraemia and retroviral disease by 3'-azido-3'-deoxythymidine. *Nature* 1986;323:467-469.
27. Van Rompay KK, Marthas ML, Ramos RA, et al. Simian immunodeficiency virus (SIV) infection of infant rhesus macaques as a model to test antiretroviral drug prophylaxis and therapy: oral 3'-azido-3'-deoxythymidine prevents SIV infection. *Antimicrob Agents Chemother* 1992;36:2381-2386

28. ZA Brown & DH Watts, Antiviral therapy in pregnancy, *Clin Obstet Gynecol* 1990;33(2):276-89 https://pubmed.ncbi.nlm.nih.gov/2190731/ (accessed 21 July 2020)
29. Sperling RS, Stratton P, O'Sullivan MJ, et al. A survey of zidovudine use in pregnant women with human immunodeficiency virus infection. *N Engl J Med* 1992;326:857-861
30. O'Sullivan MJ, Boyer PJ, Scott GB, et al. The pharmacokinetics and safety of zidovudine in the third trimester of pregnancy for women infected with human immunodeficiency virus and their infants: phase I acquired immunodeficiency syndrome clinical trials group study (protocol 082). *Am J Obstet Gynecol* 1993;168:1510-1516)
31. Connor EM et al, Reduction of Maternal-Infant Transmission of Human Immunodeficiency Virus Type 1 with Zidovudine Treatment, *New Engl J Med*, 1994;331(18):1173-1180 https://www.nejm.org/doi/full/10.1056/NEJM199411033311801 (accessed 28 November 2018)
32. CDC Recommendations of the U.S. Public Health Service Task Force on the Use of Zidovudine to Reduce Perinatal Transmission of Human Immunodeficiency Virus. *MMWR* 1994;43 (no. RR-11). https://www.cdc.gov/mmwr/preview/mmwrhtml/00032271.htm (accessed 3 December 2018)
33. Sperling RS, Shapiro DE, Coombs RW et al. Maternal viral load, zidovudeine tratment and the risk of transmission of human immunodeficiency virus type 1 from mother to infant. *N Engl J Med* 335:1621-1629, 1996.
34. Pediatric AIDS Clinical Trials Group brochure available at http://www.aids-alliance.org/resources/publications/pediatricaids.pdf
35. CDC Studies of AZT to prevent mother to child HIBV transmission in Developing countries. AIDSInfo June 1997. https://aidsinfo.nih.gov/news/363/cdc-studies-of-azt-to-prevent-mother-to-child-hiv-transmission-in-developing-countries (accessed 29 November 2018).
36. Shaffer N, Chuachoowong R, Mock PA, Bhadrakom C, Siriwasin W, Young NL, Chotpitayasunondh T, Chearskul S, Roongpisuthipong A, Chinayon P, Karon J, Mastro TD, Simonds RJ. Short-course zidovudine for perinatal HIV-1 transmission in Bangkok, Thailand: a randomised controlled trial. Bangkok Collaborative Perinatal HIV Transmission Study Group. *Lancet.* 1999 Mar 6;353(9155):773-80. https://www.thelancet.com/journals/lanonc/article/PIIS0140-6736(98)10411-7/fulltext (accessed 19 July 2020)
37. Dabis F et al, 6-month efficacy, tolerance, and acceptability of a short regimen of oral zidovudine to reduce vertical transmission of HIV in breastfed children in Côte d'Ivoire and Burkina Faso: a double-blind placebo-controlled multicentre trial. DITRAME Study Group. Diminution de la Transmission Mère-Enfant. *Lancet* 1999;353(9155:786-92) https://www.ncbi.nlm.nih.gov/pubmed/10459959 (accessed 1 December 2018)
38. Wiktor SZ et al, Ekpini Randomized clinical trial of a short course of oral zidovudine to prevent mother-to-child transmission of HIV–1 in Abidjan, Côte d'Ivoire. *Lancet* 1999; 353: 781–5. https://www.thelancet.com/journals/lanonc/article/PIIS0140-6736(98)10412-9/fulltext (accessed 3 December 2018.
39. Wilfert CM and McKinney RE, When Children Harbor HIV, Defeating AIDS: what will it take? *Scientific American* Special Report, 1998.
40. Nicoll A & Newell ML 1996, Preventing Perinatal transmission of HIV: The effect of breast-feeding (letter and reply) *JAMA* 276;19:1552.
41. Preble EA and Piwoz EG, HIV and infant feeding: *A chronology of research and policy advances and their implications for programs*, 1998 The Linkages Project and the Support for Analysis and Research in Africa (SARA) Project, the Academy for Educational Development, USAID Bureau for Africa.
42. Dunn DT , Tess BH, Rodrigues LC, Ades AE 1998, Mother to child transmission of HIV: implications of variation in maternal infectivity. *AIDS* 12:2211-2216.
43. WHO 2007 HIV Transmission Through Breastfeeding A Review of Available Evidence An Update from 2001 to 2007 https://www.who.int/nutrition/topics/Paper_5_Infant_Feeding_bangkok.pdf (accessed 25 Apr 2020)
44. Dabis F et al. (2000). Preventing mother-to-child transmission of HIV in Africa in the year 2000. *AIDS*, 14:1017–1026.
45. Mofensen L. Short-course zidovudine for prevention of perinatal infection, *Lancet* 1998;353(9155):766-767 https://www.thelancet.com/journals/lancet/article/PIIS0140-6736(99)90028-4/fulltext (accessed 19 July 2020)
46. Italian Register for Human Immunodeficiency Virus Infection in Children. Determinants of mother-to-infant human immunodeficiancy virus 1 transmissio before and after the introduction of zidovudine prophylaxis. *Arch Pediatr Adolesc Med* 2002;156:915-21. https://jamanetwork.com/journals/jamapediatrics/fullarticle/203871 (accessed 23 July 2020)
47. Guay LA, Musoke P, Fleming T et al. Intrapartum and neonatal single-dose nevirapine ompared with zidovudine for prevention of mother-to-child transmission of HIV-1 in Kampala, Uganda: HIVNET012 randomised trial. *Lancet*1999;354:795–802.
48. HIV Prevention Trials Network https://www.hptn.org/research/studies/2 (accessed 23 July 2020)
49. WHO 2006. Antiretroviral drugs for treating pregnant women and preventing HIV infection in infants: towards universal access. Recommendations for a public health approach. Geneva: World Health Organization. http://www.who.int/hiv/pub/mtct/pmtct/en
50. Moodley D, Moodley J, Coovadia H, et al. A multicenter randomized controlled trial of nevirapine versus a combination of zidovudine and lamivudine to reduce intrapartum and early postpartum mother-to-child

transmission of HIV-1. *J Infect Dis* 2003; 187: 725–35

51. Lallemant M, Jourdain G, Le Coeur S et al. A trial of shortened zidovudine regimens to prevent mother-to-child transmission of human immunodeficiency virus type 1. Perinatal HIV Prevention Trial (Thailand) Investigators. *N Engl J Med* 2000;343:982–91.
52. Mofensen L. A tale of two epidemics, the continuing challenge of preventing mother-to-child transmission of human immunodeficiency virus. *J Inf Dis* 2003;187:721-4.
53. Boeke CE, Jackson JB. Estimate of infant HIV-free survival at 6 to 8 weeks of age due to maternal antiretroviral prophylaxis in sub-Saharan Africa, 2004–2005. *J Int Assoc Physicians AIDS Care* (Chic Ill) 2008;7:133–140.
54. Eshleman SH, Hoover DR, Chen S, et al. Nevirapine (NVP) resistance in women with HIV-1 subtype C, compared with subtypes A and D, after the administration of single-dose NVP. *J Infect Dis* 2005; 192: 30–6.
55. Johnson JA, Li JF, Morris L, et al. Emergence of drug-resistant HIV1 after intrapartum administration of single-dose nevirapine is substantially underestimated. *J Infect Dis* 2005; 192:16–23.
56. Quaghebeur A, Mutunga L, Mwanyumba F, Mandaliya K, Verhofstede C, Temmerman M. Low efficacy of nevirapine (HIVNET012) in preventing perinatal HIV-1 transmission in a real-life situation. *AIDS*. 2004 Sep 3;18(13):1854-6
57. Jourdain G, Ngo-Giang-Huong N, Le Coeur S, et al. Intrapartum exposure to nevirapine and subsequent maternal responses to nevirapinebased antiretroviral therapy. *N Engl J Med* 2004; 351:229–40.
58. Lockman S, Shapiro RL, Smeaton LM, et al. Response to antiretroviral therapy after a single, peripartum dose of nevirapine. *N Engl J Med* 2007; 356:135–47.
59. Eure C, Bakaki P, McConnell M, et al. Effectiveness of Repeat Singledose Nevirapine in Subsequent Pregnancies among Ugandan Women [abstract 125]. In: Program and abstracts of the 13th Conference on Retroviruses and Opportunistic Infections 2006 (Denver). Reported by I-Base, https://i-base.info/htb/5676
60. Zijenah L, Kadzirange G, Rusakaniko S, et al. Community-based generic ART following single-dose nevirapine or short-course zidovudine in Zimbabwe [abstract 544]. In: Program and abstracts of the 13th Conference on Retroviruses and Opportunistic Infections 2006 (Denver). Reported by I-Base, https://i-base.info/htb/3425
61. Westreich D et al, Survival in Women Exposed to Single-Dose Nevirapine for Prevention of Mother-to-Child Transmission of HIV: A Stochastic Model. *J Infect Dis* 2007;195(6):837-846 https://academic.oup.com/jid/article/195/6/837/877735 (accessed 24 July 2020)
62. The Petra study team. Efficacy of the three short-course regimens of zidovudine and lamivudine in preventing early and late transmission of HIV-1 from mother to child in Tanzania, South Africa and Uganda (Petra Study): a randomized, double-blind, placebocontrolled trial. *Lancet* 2002; 359:1178–86.
63. Jackson B, Musoke P, Fleming T, et al. Intrapartum and neonatal single-dose nevirapine compared with zidovudine for prevention of mother-to-child transmissionofHIV-1 in Kampala, Uganda: 18-month follow-up of the HIVNET 012 randomized trial. *Lancet* 2003; 362: 859–67.
64. Leroy V, Karon JM, Alioum A, et al. 24-month efficacy of a maternal short-course zidovudine regimen to prevent mother-to-child transmission of HIV-1 in West Africa. *AIDS* 2002; 16: 631–41.
65. Chaisilwattana P, Chokephaibulkit K, Chalermchockcharoenkit A, et al. Short-course therapy with zidovudine plus lamivudine for prevention of mother-to-child transmission of human immunodeficiency virus type 1 in Thailand. *Clin Infect Dis* 2002; 35:1405–13.
66. Lallemant M, Jourdain G, Le Coeur S, et al. A randomized, double-blind trial assessing the efficacy of single-dose perinatal nevirapine added to a standard zidovudine regimen for the prevention of mother-to-child transmission of HIV-1 in Thailand [abstract 40LB]. In:Program and abstracts of the 11th Conference on Retroviruses and Opportunistic Infections (San Francisco).Alexandria, VA: Foundation for Retrovirology and Human Health, 2004:91.
67. Dabis F, Ekouevi DK, Rouet F, et al. Effectiveness of a short course of zidovudine + lamivudine and peripartumnevirapine to prevent HIV-1 mother-to-child transmission: the ANRS DITRAME Plus trial, Abidjan, Cote d'Ivoire [abstract 219]. *Antivir Ther* 2003; 8 (Suppl 1):S236–7.
68. CDC HIV and AIDS Timeline, https://npin.cdc.gov/pages/hiv-and-aids-timeline (accessed 23 Sept 2020)
69. Kumwenda NI, Hoover DR, Mofenson LM, Thigpen MC, Kafulafula, Li Q, Mipando L, Nkanaunena K, Mebrahtu T, Bulterys M, Fowler MG and Taha TE, Extended Antiretroviral Prophylaxis to Reduce Breast-Milk HIV-1 Transmission, *N Engl J Med* 2008;10.1056/nejmoa0801941, http://content.nejm.org/cgi/reprint/NEJMoa0801941v1.pdf
70. Bedri A, Gudetta B, Isehak A, et al, and the Six Week Extended-Dose Nevirapine (SWEN) Study Team. Extended-dose nevirapine to 6 weeks of age for infants to prevent HIV transmission via breastfeeding in Ethiopia, India, and Uganda: an analysis of three randomised controlled trials. *Lancet* 2008; 372: 300–13.
71. Coovadia HM, Brown ER, Fowler MG, Chipato T, Moodley D, Manji K, Musoke P, Stranix-Chibanda L, Chetty V, Fawzi W, Nakabiito C, Msweli L, Kisenge R, Guay L, Mwatha A, Lynn DJ, Eshleman SH, Richardson P, George K, Andrew P, Mofenson LM, Zwerski S, Maldonado Y; HPTN 046 protocol team. Efficacy and safety of an extended nevirapine regimen in infant children of breastfeeding mothers with HIV-1 infection for prevention of postnatal HIV-1 transmission (HPTN 046): a randomised, double-blind, placebo-controlled trial. *Lancet.* 2012 Jan 21;379(9812):221-8. https://www.thelancet.com/pdfs/journals/lancet/PIIS014067361161653X.pdf (accessed 1 Apr 2021)

72. Becquet R and Ekouevi DK, Breastfeeding, triple ARV prophylaxis, and MTCT prevention *Lancet Infect Dis*. 2011 Mar;11(3):154-5. Epub 2011 Jan 14, DOI:10.1016/S1473-3099(10)70299-1
73. WHO 2010. Guidelines on HIV and Infant Feeding. 2010. Principles and recommendations for infant feeding in the context of HIV and a summary of evidence. ISBN 978 92 4 159953 5. http://whqlibdoc.who.int/publications/2010/9789241599535_eng.pdf
74. Cooper ER, Charurat M, Mofenson L et al. Combination antiretroviral strategies for treatment of pregnant HIV-infected women and prevention of perinatal HIV-1 transmission. *J Acquir Immune Defic Syndr* 2002;29:484-494
75. Bulterys M et al . Advances in the prevention of mother-to-child transmission: current issues, future challenges. *AIDScience* 2002;2(4), February 2002 http://www.aidscience.org/Articles/aidscience017.asp (accessed 23 July 2020)
76. Townsend C, Cortina-Borja M, Peckham C, Tookey P. Trends in management and outcome of pregnancies in HIV-infected women in the UK and Ireland, 1990–2006. *BJOG* 2008;11:1078–1086
77. The Breastfeeding and HIV International Transmission Study (BHITS) Group. Late postnatal transmission of HIV-1 in breast-fed children:an individual patient datameta-analysis. *J Infect Dis* 2004; 189:2154-66
78. WHO/UNICEF/UNAIDS, Global HIV/AIDS response. Epidemic update and health sector progress towards Universal Access – Progress Report 2011, p153 http://whqlibdoc.who.int/publications/2011/9789241502986_eng.pdf
79. Palombi L, Marazzi MC, Voetberg A, Magid NA and the DREAM Program Prevention of Mother-to-Child Transmission Team. Treatment acceleration program and the experience of the DREAM program in prevention of mother-to-child transmission of HIV. AIDS. 2007 Jul;21 Suppl 4:S65-71.
80. Hoffman RM, Black V, Technau K, van der Merwe KJ, Currier J, Coovadia A, Chersich M. Effects of Highly Active Antiretroviral Therapy Duration and Regimen on Risk for Mother-to-Child Transmission of HIV in Johannesburg, South Africa. *J Acquir Immune Defic Syndr*. 2010 May 1; 54(1): 35–41. doi: 10.1097/QAI.0b013e3181cf9979, http://www.ncbi.nlm.nih.gov/pmc/articles/PMC2880466/
81. Chibwesha CJ, Giganti MJ, Putta N, Chintu N, Mulindwa J, Dorton BJ, Chi BH, Stringer JS, Stringer EM. Optimal Time on HAART for Prevention of Mother-to-Child Transmission of HIV. *J Acquir Immune Defic Syndr*. 2011 Oct 1;58(2):224-8. doi: 10.1097/QAI.0b013e318229147e, http://www.ncbi.nlm.nih.gov/pubmed/21709566
82. Kuhn L and Aldrovandi G, Survival and Health Benefits of Breastfeeding Versus Artificial Feeding in Infants of HIV-Infected Women: Developing Versus Developed World. *Clin Perinatol* 2010;37:843–862 https://www.perinatology.theclinics.com/article/S0095-5108(10)00104-1/abstract (accessed 17 March 2020)
83. Tonwe-Gold B, Ekouevi DK, Viho I, et al. Antiretroviral treatment and prevention of peripartum and postnatal HIV transmission in West Africa: evaluation of a two-tiered approach. PLOS Medicine 2007;4:e257.
84. Kuhn L, Aldrovandi GM, Sinkala M, Kankasa C, Mwiya M, Thea DM. Potential impact of new World Health Organization criteria for antiretroviral treatment for prevention of mother-to-child HIV transmission. *AIDS* 2010;24:1374–1371.
85. Cavarelli M and Scarlatti G, Human immunodeficiency virus type 1 mother-to-child transmission and prevention: successes and controversies. *J Int Med*, 2011. doi: 10.1111/j.1365-2796.2011.02458.x
86. Ngoma M, Raha A, Elong A, Pilon R, Mwansa J, Mutale W, Yee K, Chisele S, Wu S, Chandawe M, Mumba S and Silverman MS Interim Results of HIV Transmission Rates Using a Lopinavir/ritonavir based regimen and the New WHO Breast Feeding Guidelines for PMTCT of HIV International Congress of Antimicrobial Agents and Chemotherapy (ICAAC) Chicago Il, Sep19,2011. H1-1153, available at http://www.icaac.org/index.php/component/content/article/9-newsroom/169-preliminary-results-of-hiv-transmission-rates-using-a-lopinavirritonavir-lpvr-aluvia-based-regimen-and-the-new-who-breast-feeding-guidelines-for-pmtct-of-hiv-
87. The Kesho Bora Study Group. Triple antiretroviral compared with zidovudine and single-dose nevirapine prophylaxis during pregnancy and breastfeeding for prevention of mother-to-child transmission of HIV-1 (Kesho Bora study): a randomised controlled trial. *Lancet Infect Dis* 2011;Jan 14. DOI:10.1016/S1473-3099(10)70288-7 .
88. Chasela CS, Hudgens MG, Jamieson DJ, et al. Maternal or infant antiretroviral drugs to reduce HIV-1 transmission. *N Engl J Med* 2010;362: 2271–81.
89. Shapiro RL, Hughes MD, Ogwu A, et al. Antiretroviral regimens in pregnancy and breast-feeding in Botswana. *N Engl J Med* 2010;362: 2282–94.
90. WHO 2010. Recommendations for use of antiretroviral drugs for treating pregnant women and preventing HIV infection in infants. Guidelines on care, treatment and support for women living with HIV/AIDS and their children in resource-constrained settings, available at http://www.who.int/hiv/pub/mtct/guidelines/en/
91. Thistle P, Bolotin S, Lam E, Schwarz D, Pilon R, Ndawana B, Simor AE, Silverman M. Highly active anti-retroviral therapy in the prevention of mother-to-child transmission of HIV in rural Zimbabwe during the socio-economic crisis. *Med Confl Surviv*. 2011 Jul-Sep;27(3):165-76, DOI: 10.1080/13623699.2011.631752
92. WHO 2011, Global Health Sector Strategy on HIV/AIDS 2011-2015 https://apps.who.int/iris/bitstream/handle/10665/44606/9789241501651_eng.pdf (accessed 27 July 2020)

93. Kilewo C, Karlsson K, Ngarina M, et al. Prevention of mother-to-child transmission of HIV-1 through breastfeeding by treating mothers with triple antiretroviral therapy in Dar es Salaam, Tanzania: the Mitra Plus study. *J Acquir Immune Defic Syndr.* 2009; 52:406–16.
94. Peltier CA, Ndayisaba GF, Lepage P, et al. Breastfeeding with maternal antiretroviral therapy or formula feeding to prevent HIV postnatal mother-to-child transmission in Rwanda. *AIDS.* 2009; 23:2415–23.
95. Thomas TK, Masaba R, Borkowf CB, et al. Triple-antiretroviral prophylaxis to prevent mother-to-child HIV transmission through breastfeeding—the Kisumu Breastfeeding Study, Kenya: a clinical trial. *PLoS Med.* 2011; 8:e1001015
96. Six Week Extended-Dose Nevirapine (SWEN) Study Team. Extended-dose nevirapine to 6 weeks of age for infants to prevent HIV transmission via breastfeeding in Ethiopia, India, and Uganda: an analysis of three randomised controlled trials. *Lancet.* 2008; 372:300–13.
97. Thior I, Lockman S, Smeaton LM, et al. Breastfeeding plus infant zidovudine prophylaxis for 6 months vs formula feeding plus infant zidovudine for 1 month to reduce mother-to-child HIVtransmission in Botswana: a randomized trial: the Mashi Study. *JAMA.* 2006; 296:794–805.
98. Omer SB, Six Week Extended-Dose Nevirapine Study Team. Twelve-month follow-up of Six Week Extended Dose Nevirapine randomized controlled trials: differential impact of extended dose nevirapine on mother-to-child transmission and infant death by maternal CD4 cell count. *AIDS.* 2011; 25:767–76.
99. WHO 2009, Rapid advice: use of antiretroviral drugs for treating pregnant women and preventing HIV infection in infants http://www.who.int/hiv/pub/mtct/advice/en/index.html, (accessed 20 April 2010 as reported on p 19 of the WHO 2010 Guidelines on HIV and Infant feeding, see next paragraphs of this chapter).
100. WHO-UNICEF 2016, Guideline: Updates on HIV and Infant Feeding, http://apps.who.int/iris/bitstream/10665/246260/1/9789241549707-eng.pdf
101. WHO 2012, Programmatic update; Use of antiretroviral drugs for treating pregnant women and preventing HIV infection in infants, Executive Summary April 2012, http://whqlibdoc.who.int/hq/2012/WHO_HIV_2012.8_eng.pdf
102. World Health Organization. Treat all people living with HIV, offer antiretrovirals as additional prevention choice for people at "substantial" risk. www.who.int/mediacentre/news/releases/2015/hiv-treat-allrecommendation/en/.
103. WHO 2016, Consolidated guidelines on the use of antiretroviral drugs for treating and preventing HIV infection: recommendations for a public health approach – 2nd ed. ISBN 978 92 4 154968 4 available at http://www.who.int/hiv/pub/arv/arv-2016/en/

Chapter 23: EBF + ART, a winning combination

1. Shapiro et al, Low adherence to recommended infant feeding strategies among HIV-infected women: results from the pilot phase of a randomized trial to prevent mother-to-child transmission in Botswana. *AIDS Education and Prevention*, 2003;15(3), 221–230.
2. Coutsoudis A, Pillay K, Spooner E, Kuhn L, Coovadia HM. Influence of infant-feeding patterns on early mother-to-child transmission of HIV-1 in Durban, South Africa: a prospective cohort study. South African Vitamin A Study Group. *Lancet.* 1999 Aug 7;354(9177):471-6. https://www.ncbi.nlm.nih.gov/pubmed/10465172 (accessed 10 December 2018)
3. Iliff PJ, Piwoz EG, Tavengwa NV, Zunguza CD, Marinda ET, Nathoo KJ, Moulton LH, Ward BJ, the ZVITAMBO study group and Humphrey JH. Early exclusive breastfeeding reduces the risk of postnatal HIV-1 transmission and increases HIV-free survival. *AIDS* 2005, 19:699–708 https://www.ncbi.nlm.nih.gov/pubmed/15821396 (accessed 10 December 2018)
4. Harvard University, TH Chan School of Public Health, https://www.hsph.harvard.edu/roger-shapiro/ (accessed 3 August 2020)
5. Shapiro RL, Hughes MD, Ogwu A et al (2010). Antiretroviral regimens in pregnancy and breast-feeding in Botswana. *New England J Med* 362(24):2282–94
6. Shapiro R, Hughes M, Ogwu A, Kitch D, Lockman S, Moffat C, Makhema J, Moyo S, Thior I, McIntosh K, van Widenfelt E, Leidner J, Powis K, Asmelash A, Tumbare E, Zwerski S, Sharma U, Handelsman E, Jayeoba O, Moko E, Souda S, Lubega E, Akhtar M, Wester C, Snowden W, Martinez-Tristani M, Mazhani L, Essex M, The Mma Bana Study Team. A randomized trial comparing highly active antiretroviral therapy regimens for virologic efficacy and the prevention of mother-to-child HIV transmission among breastfeeding women in Botswana (The Mma Bana Study). Oral presentation WELBB101 at 5th IAS Conference on HIV Pathogenesis, Treatment and Prevention, Cape Town, South Africa, 19-22 July 2009 (presented by R Shapiro) (websites accessed February 2013 but no longer available) http://www.ias2009.org/pag/Abstracts.aspx?SID=2435&AID=3821 Webcast of this session at http://www.ias2009.org/pag/webcasts/?sessionid=2435 Powerpoint at http://www.ias2009.org/PAGMaterial/WELBB101_Shapiro_1.ppt see Slides 12 and 16.
7. Kahlert C et al, Is breastfeeding an equipoise option in effectively treated HIV-infected mothers in a high-income setting? *Swiss Med Wkly.* 2018;148:w14648 https://smw.ch/article/doi/smw.2018.14648 accessed 4 November 2020.
8. Ngoma M, Raha A, Elong A, Pilon R, Mwansa J, Mutale W, Yee K, Chisele S, Wu S, Chandawe M,

Mumba S and Silverman MS Interim Results of HIV Transmission Rates Using a Lopinavir/ritonavir based regimen and the New WHO Breast Feeding Guidelines for PMTCT of HIV International Congress of Antimicrobial Agents and Chemotherapy (ICAAC).51st Interscience Conference on Antimicrobial Agents and Chemotherapy (ICAAC): Session 164, Abstract H1-1153. Presented September 19, 2011. Chicago Il, Sep19,2011. H1-1153

9. Daniel Keller, Medscape HAART Prevents HIV Transmission During Breastfeeding, Medscape September 29, 2011 https://www.medscape.com/viewarticle/750634 (accessed 6 August 2020)
10. The 47th Interscience Conference on Antimicrobial Agents and Chemotherapy ICAAC 2007 Study Summaries: Michael Silverman, M.D. *The Body* September 2007 http://www.thebody.com/content/art43608.html
11. Ngoma MS et al. Efficacy of WHO recommendation for continued breastfeeding and maternal cART for prevention of perinatal and postnatal HIV transmission in Zambia Journal of the International AIDS Society 2015, 18:19352, http://www.jiasociety.org/index.php/jias/article/view/19352 http://dx.doi.org/10.7448/IAS.18.1.19352
12. Gartland MG et al, Field effectiveness of combination antiretroviral prophylaxis for the prevention of mother-to-child HIV transmission in rural Zambia, *AIDS* 2013 May 15; 27(8): doi:10.1097/QAD.0b013e32835e3937, https://www.ncbi.nlm.nih.gov/pmc/articles/PMC3836017/pdf/nihms521144.pdf/ accessed 5 August 2020
13. Luoga E et al, No HIV Transmission From Virally Suppressed Mothers During Breastfeeding in Rural Tanzania *J Acquir Immune Defic Syndr* 2018 Sep 1;79(1):e17-e20. doi: 10.1097/QAI.0000000000001758. https://pubmed.ncbi.nlm.nih.gov/29781882/ (accessed 6 Aug 2020)
14. WHO. Guideline on When to Start Antiretroviral Therapy and on Preexposure Prophylaxis for HIV. Geneva, Switzerland: World Health Organization; 2015. http://apps.who.int/iris/bitstream/
15. Mmiro FA, Aizire J, Mwatha AK, et al. Predictors of early and late mother-to-child transmission of HIV in a breastfeeding population: HIV Network for Prevention Trials 012 experience, Kampala, Uganda. *J Acquir Immune Defic Syndr.* 2009;52:32–39.
16. Mandelbrot L et al for the ANRS Study Group, No perinatal HIV-1 transmission from women with effective antiretroviral therapy starting before conception *Clin Infect Dis* 2015 Dec 1;61(11):1715-25. doi: 10.1093/cid/civ578. Epub 2015 Jul 21 https://pubmed.ncbi.nlm.nih.gov/26197844/ (accessed 6 August 2020)
17. Townsend CL, Cortina-Borja M, Peckham CS, de Ruiter A, Lyall H, Tookey PA. Low rates of mother-to-child transmission of HIV following effective pregnancy interventions in the United Kingdom and Ireland, 2000-2006. *AIDS* 2008 May 11;22(8):973-81. https://www.ncbi.nlm.nih.gov/pubmed/18453857
18. American Academy of Pediatrics: Policy Statement: Infant Feeding and Transmission of Human Immunodeficiency Virus in the United States COMMITTEE ON PEDIATRIC AIDS, Pediatrics 2013; 131:2 391-396; published ahead of print January 28, 2013, doi:10.1542/peds.2012-3543 https://pediatrics.aappublications.org/content/131/2/391 (accessed 4 August 2020) Reaffirmed April 2016 (https://pediatrics.aappublications.org/content/138/2/e20161650
19. British HIV Association guidelines for the management of HIV in pregnancy and postpartum 2018 (2019 interim update) Section 9.4 Infant feeding, page 88 https://www.bhiva.org/file/5bfd30be95deb/BHIVA-guidelines-for-the-management-of-HIV-in-pregnancy.pdf (accessed 18 January 2020), BHIVA HIV and breastfeeding your baby https://www.bhiva.org/file/5bfd3080d2027/BF-Leaflet-1.pdf, BHIVA General Info on infant feeding, https://www.bhiva.org/file/5bfd308d5e189/BF-Leaflet-2.pdf
20. Greiner T, Morrison P. Breastfeeding by HIV-infected women in the USA e-response to AAP Policy Statement, Infant Feeding and Transmission of HIV in the USA, Pediatrics online, 5 Mar 2013 https://pediatrics.aappublications.org/content/131/2/391.short/reply#pediatrics_el_55196 or http://bit.ly/1wLtBj3 [Accessed 23 October 2014, no longer available]. This article is a published response to American Academy of Pediatrics: Policy Statement: Infant Feeding and Transmission of Human Immunodeficiency Virus in the United States COMMITTEE ON PEDIATRIC AIDS Pediatrics 2013; 131:2 391-396; published ahead of print January 28, 2013, doi:10.1542/peds.2012-3543
21. Chibwesha CJ, Giganti MJ, Putta N et al (2011). Optimal Time on HAART for prevention of mother-to-child transmission of HIV. *J Acquired Immunodefic Syndromes.* 58(2):224-8.
22. WHO 2011 Policy Brief on Kesho Bora Study,. https://www.who.int/reproductivehealth/publications/rtis/KeshoBora_study.pdf (accessed 8 August 2020)
23. Kesho Bora Study Group, Triple antiretroviral compared with zidovudine and single-dose nevirapine prophylaxis during pregnancy and breastfeeding for prevention of mother-to-child transmission of HIV-1 (Kesho Bora study): a randomised controlled trial, *Lancet* 2011; DOI:10.1016/S1473-3099(10)70288-7. https://www.thelancet.com/journals/laninf/article/PIIS1473-3099
24. Peltier CA, Ndayisaba GF, Lepage P et al. Breastfeeding with maternal antiretroviral therapy or formula feeding to prevent HIV postnatal mother-to child transmission in Rwanda. *AIDS* 2009;23(18):2415–23.
25. Kilewo C, Karlsson K, Massawe A et al. Prevention of mother-to-child transmission of HIV-1 through breast-feeding by treating infants prophylactically with lamivudine in Dar es Salaam, Tanzania: the Mitra Study. *J Acquired Immune Defic Syndr* 2008;48(3):315–23.
26. Marazzi MC, Nielsen-Saines K, Buonomo E, Scarcella P, Germano P, Majid NA, Zimba I, Ceffa S, Palombi L. Increased Infant Human Immunodeficiency Virus-Type One Free Survival at One Year of Age in Sub-Saharan Africa With Maternal Use of Highly Active Antiretroviral Therapy During Breast-Feeding.

Pediatr Infect Dis J 2009;28: 483–487 https://pubmed.ncbi.nlm.nih.gov/19483516/ (accessed 8 August 2020)

27. Thomas TK, Masaba R, Borkowf CB et al (2011). Triple-antiretroviral prophylaxis to prevent mother-to-child HIV transmission through breastfeeding -the Kisumu Breastfeeding Study, Kenya: a clinical trial. PLoS Medicine 8(3):e1001015. http://1.usa.gov/1wCtovS [Accessed 23 October 2014.
28. Johnson G et al, Should providers discuss breastfeeding with women living with HIV in high-income countries? An ethical analysis. *Clin Infect Dis* 2016 Nov 15;63(10):1368-1372. doi: 10.1093/cid/ciw587. Epub 2016 Aug 29. https://pubmed.ncbi.nlm.nih.gov/27572099/ (accessed 8 August 2020)
29. Carole Leach Lemens, Exclusive breastfeeding hampered by infant illnesses, follow up of mothers with HIV shows. NAM *AIDSMAP* 7 December 2012 https://www.aidsmap.com/news/dec-2012/exclusive-breastfeeding-hampered-infant-illnesses-follow-mothers-hiv-shows
30. Bork KA et al. Morbidity in relation to feeding mode in African HIV-exposed, uninfected infants during the first 6 mo of life: the Kesho Bora study. *Am J Clin Nutr* 2014;100:1559–68. doi:10.1097/QA1,0b013e318277005e, 2012
31. WHO 2004. HIV and infant feeding: A guide for health-care managers and supervisors , World Health Organization 2003 https://www.who.int/nutrition/publications/HIV_IF_guide_for_healthcare.pdf (accessed 18 June 2020)
32. Correspondence with Gareth Tudor-Williams, January and February 2011

Chapter 24: International HIV and infant feeding policy comes full circle

1. Morrison P, Taking another look at policy on HIV and infant feeding, 1985 - 2008, AnotherLook 26 March, 2009, http://www.anotherlook.org/papers/h/english.pdf
2. Creek et al, Hospitalization and Mortality Among Primarily Nonbreastfed Children During a Large Outbreak of Diarrhea and Malnutrition in Botswana, 2006. *J Acquir Immune Defic Syndr*.2010;53(1):14-19.
3. Kuhn L, Aldrovandi GM, Sinkala M, Kankasa C, Semrau K, Mwiya M, Kasonde P, Scott N, Vwalika C, Walter J, Bulterys M, Tsai W-Y and Thea DM for the Zambia Exclusive Breastfeeding Study. Effects of early, abrupt weaning for HIV-free survival of children in Zambia *N Engl J Med* 2008;359. Available at http://content.nejm.org/cgi/reprint/NEJMoa073788v1.pdf
4. UNICEF/WHO, Baby Friendly Hospital Initiative: Revised, Updated and Expanded for Integrated Care, Preliminary Version for Country Implementation, January 2006, http://www.unicef.org/nutrition/files/BFHI_Revised_Section1.pdf (accessed 23 December 2008)
5. WHO 2006, Infant and Young Child Feeding Counselling: An Integrated Course ISBN 92 4 159475 6, available at http://www.who.int/nutrition/iycf_intergrated_course/en/index.html (accessed 23 December, 2008).
6. WHO 2006. HIV and Infant Feeding Technical Consultation held on behalf of the inter-agency task team on prevention of HIV infections in pregnant women, mothers and their infants. http://www.who.int/child-adolescent-health/New_Publications/NUTRITION/consensus_statement.pdf
7. WHO, UNICEF, UNAIDS, UNFPA 2007, HIV and infant feeding, new evidence and programmatic experience, Report of a Technical Consultation held on behalf of the Inter-agency Task Team (IATT) on prevention of HIV infections in pregnant women, mothers and their infants, Geneva, Switzerland, 25-27 October 2006, ISBN 978 92 4 159597 1 http://whqlibdoc.who.int/publications/2007/978241595971_eng.pdf
8. WHO, UNICEF, UNAIDS, UNFPA 2007, HIV and infant feeding, Update, based on the technical consultation held on behalf of the Inter-agency Task Team (IATT) on Prevention of HIV infection in pregnant women, mothers and their infants, Geneva, 25-27 October 2006. ISBN 978 92 4 159596 4. http://whqlibdoc.who.int/publications/2007/9789241595964_eng.pdf
9. WHO, UNICEF, UNAIDS, UNFPA 2007, HIV Transmission Through Breastfeeding: a review of available evidence, HIV Transmission through breastfeeding, 2007 update, ISBN 978 92 4 159659 6. http://whqlibdoc.who.int/publications/2008/9789241596596_eng.pdf
10. WHO 2007 Guidance on global scale-up of the prevention of mother to child transmission of HIV: towards universal access for women, infants and young children and eliminating HIV and AIDS among children / Inter-Agency Task Team on Prevention of HIV Infection in Pregnant Women, Mothers and their Children, see page 8, available at http://www.unfpa.org/upload/lib_pub_file/736_filename_guidance.pdf
11. WHO 2007, How to prepare powdered infant formula in care settings http://www.who.int/foodsafety/publications/micro/PIF_Care_en.pdf
12. WHO 2007, How to prepare formula for cup-feeding at home. http://www.who.int/foodsafety/publications/micro/PIF_Cup_en.pdf
13. WHO 2007, How to prepare formula for bottle-feeding at home. http://www.who.int/foodsafety/publications/micro/PIF_Bottle_en.pdf
14. WHO 2008, HIV and Infant Feeding counselling tools: Orientation Guide for Trainers ISBN 978 92 4 159653 4, http://whqlibdoc.who.int/publications/2008/9789241596534_eng.pdf
15. WHO 2009, Infant and young child feeding: Model Chapter for textbooks for medical students and

allied health professionals, http://www.who.int/child_adolescent_health/documents/9789241597494/en/index.html

16. Theo Smart, Infant feeding policy debate at the Conference on Retroviruses and Opportunistic Infections. HATIP #82, *AIDSMAP* 13th March 2007 http://www.aidsmap.com/en/news/1F9F2D35-099B-42A5-94EA-0FEC977756E6.asp
17. Onyango C, Mmiro F, Bagenda D, Mubiro K, Musoke P, Fowler M, Jackson J, Early Breastfeeding Cessation among HIV-exposed Negative Infants and Risk of Serious Gastroenteritis: Findings from a Perinatal Prevention Trial in Kampala, Uganda Poster Session 138, 14th Conference on Retroviruses and Opportunistic Infections, Los Angeles, 25-28 February, 2007 http://www.retroconference.org/2007/Abstracts/29008.htm
18. Kafulafula G, Thigpen M, Hoover D, Li Q, Kumwenda, Mipando L, Taha T, Mofenson L and Fowler M, Post-weaning Gastroenteritis and Mortality in HIV-uninfected African Infants Receiving Antiretroviral Prophylaxis to Prevent MTCT of HIV-1, Poster Session 138, 14th Conference on Retroviral and Opportunistic Infections, Los Angeles, 25-28 February, 2007
19. Thomas T, Masaba R, van Eijk A, Ndivo R, Nasokho P, Thigpen M and Fowler M. Rates of Diarrhea Associated with Early Weaning among Infants in Kisumu, Kenya, Poster Session 138, 14th Conference on Retroviruses and Opportunistic Infections, Los Angeles, 25-28 February, 2007 http://www.retroconference.org/2007/Abstracts/29105.htm
20. Sinkala M, Kuhn L, Kankasa C, Kasonde P, Vwalika C, Mwiya M, Scott N, Semrau K, Aldrovandi G, Thea D and Zambia Exclusive Breastfeeding Study Group (ZEBS) No Benefit of Early Cessation of Breastfeeding at 4 Months on HIV-free Survival of Infants Born to HIV-infected Mothers in Zambia: The Zambia Exclusive Breastfeeding Study, Session 136, Poster Session, 14th Conference on Retroviruses and Opportunistic Infections, Los Angeles 25-28 February, 2007 http://www.retroconference.org/2007/Abstracts/28331.htm
21. Kagaayi J, Gray RH, Brahmbhatt H, Kigozi G, Nalugoda F, et al. (2008) Survival of Infants Born to HIV-Positive Mothers, by Feeding Modality, in Rakai, Uganda. *PLoS ONE* 2008;3(12): e3877. doi:10.1371/journal.pone.0003877 http://www.plosone.org/article/info:doi/10.1371/journal.pone.0003877
22. Kuhn L, Sinkala M, Kankasa C, Semrau K, Kasonde P, Scott N, Mwiya M, Cheswa V, Walter J, Wei-Yann T, Aldrovandi GM, and Thea DM. High Uptake of Exclusive Breastfeeding and Reduced Early Post-Natal HIV Transmission. *PLoS ONE* Dec 2007;2(12): e1363. doi:10.1371/journal.pone.0001363
23. Coovadia HM, Rollins NC, Bland RM, Little K, Coutsoudis A, Bennish ML, Newell M-L. Mother-to-child transmission of HIV-1 infection during exclusive breastfeeding in the first 6 months of life: an intervention cohort study. *Lancet* 2007 March 31;369:1107-16.
24. Palombi L, Marazzi MC, Voetberg A, Magid NA. Treatment acceleration program and the experience of the DREAM program in prevention of mother-to-child transmission of HIV. *AIDS.* 2007 Jul;21 Suppl 4:S65-71.
25. Thomas T, Masaba R, Ndivo R, Zehl C, Borkowf C, Thigpen M, De Cock K, Amornkul P, Greenberg A, Fowler M and Kisumu Breastfeeding Study Team, Prevention of Mother-to-Child Transmission of HIV among Breastfeeding mothers using HAART, Kisumu, Kenya 2003-2007, Oral abstract presented at the 15th Conference on Retroviruses and Opportunistic Infections, Boston, USA, 3-6 February 2008, see http://www.retroconference.org:8888/2008/Abstracts/33397.htm
26. Kilewo C et al. Prevention of mother-to-child transmission of HIV-1 through breast-feeding by treating infants prophylactically with lamivudine in Dar es Salaam, Tanzania: the Mitra Study. *J Acquir Immune Defic Syndr.* 2008 Jul 1;48(3):315-23.
27. Kilewo C et al. Prevention of mother-to-child transmission of HIV-1 through breastfeeding by treating mothers with triple antiretroviral therapy in Dar es Salaam, Tanzania: the Mitra Plus study. *J Acquir Immune Defic Syndr.* 2009 Nov 1;52(3):406-16.
28. Marazzi MC, Nielsen-Saines K, Buonomi E, Scarcella P, Germano P, Majid NA, Zimba I, Ceffa S and Palombi L, Increased infant human immunodeficiency virus-type one free survival at one year of age in sub-Saharan Africa with maternal use of Highly Active Antiretroviral Therapy during breast-feeding. *Pediatr Infect Dis J* 2009;28: 483–487
29. Chasela C et al. Both maternal HAART and daily infant nevirapine (NVP) are effective in reducing HIV-1 transmission during breastfeeding in a randomized trial in Malawi: 28 week results of the Breastfeeding, Antiretroviral and Nutrition (BAN) Study. Oral presentation WELBC103 at 5th IAS Conference on HIV Pathogenesis, Treatment and Prevention, Cape Town, South Africa, 19-22 July 2009
30. Peltier CA et al Breastfeeding with maternal antiretroviral therapy or formula feeding to prevent HIV postnatal mother-to-child transmission in Rwanda, *AIDS* 2009, 23:2415–2423.
31. Shapiro R et al. M, The Mma Bana Study Team. A randomized trial comparing highly active antiretroviral therapy regimens for virologic efficacy and the prevention of mother-to-child HIV transmission among breastfeeding women in Botswana (The Mma Bana Study). Oral presentation WELBB101 at 5th IAS Conference on HIV Pathogenesis, Treatment and Prevention, Cape Town, South Africa, 19-22 July 2009. Webcast of this session available at http://www.ias2009.org/pag/webcasts/?sessionid=2435
32. Chetty T, Naidu KK, Newell ML. Evidence summaries of individual reports identified through a systematic review of HIV-free survival by infant feeding practices from birth to 18-24 months, WHO 16 October 2009, Summary 5 to HIV and infant feeding. Principles and recommendations for infant feeding in the

context of HIV, WHO 2010. http://www.who.int/child_adolescent_health/documents/9789241599535_annex_5.pdf

33. WHO 2009, Rapid advice: use of antiretroviral drugs for treating pregnant women and preventing HIV Infection in infants, http://www.who.int/hiv/pub/mtct/rapid_advice_mtct.pdf
34. Palombi L, Marazzi MC, Voetberg A, Magid NA and the DREAM Program Prevention of Mother-to-Child Transmission Team. Treatment acceleration program and the experience of the DREAM program in prevention of mother-to-child transmission of HIV. *AIDS*. 2007 Jul;21 Suppl 4:S65-71.
35. Townsend CL, Cortina-Borja M, Peckham CS, de Ruiter A, Lyall H, Tookey PA. Low rates of mother-to-child transmission of HIV following effective pregnancy interventions in the United Kingdom and Ireland, 2000–2006. *AIDS* 2008; 22: 973–981
36. WHO 2009, Rapid advice: revised WHO principles and recommendations on infant feeding in the context of HIV http://whqlibdoc.who.int/publications/2009/9789241598873_eng.pdf
37. Morrison P, The ethics of infant feeding choice: do babies have the right to be breastfed, *Australian Breastfeeding Association, Lactation Resource Centre, Topics in Breastfeeding* Set XVIII March 2006. Reprinted by Breastfeeding Advocacy Australia, August 2020. https://storage.googleapis.com/wzukusers/user-34970444/documents/6198a5c0feb34b3ab6e9d0dd96b3a49e/Morrison-P-Ethics-of-infant-feeding-choice-Mar-2006-1.pdf (accessed 18 Oct 2020)
38. Nduati R, Research experiences with infant feeding interventions, WHO-UNAIDS-UNICEF 1998, Technical Consultation on HIV and Infant Feeding Implementation of Guidelines Report of a Meeting - Geneva, 20-22 April 1998, pages 16-17.
39. Vaga BB et al, Reflections on informed choice in resource-poor settings: the case of infant feeding counselling in PMTCT programmes in Tanzania, *Soc Sci Med*, 2014 Mar;105:22-9. https://pubmed.ncbi.nlm.nih.gov/24508717/ (accessed 18 Oct 2020)
40. Griswold M et al, Women Living With HIV in High Income Countries and the Deeper Meaning of Breastfeeding Avoidance: A Metasynthesis, *J Hum Lact* Jan 2020;1-9 https://journals.sagepub.com/doi/10.1177/0890334419886565 (accessed 18 Oct 2020)
41. Gross MS et al, Breastfeeding with HIV, Evidence for new policy, *J Law, Med & Ethics* 2019. https://journals.sagepub.com/doi/abs/10.1177/1073110519840495
42. Brewster D, Science and ethics of human immunodeficiency virus/acquired immunodeficiency syndrome controversies in Africa, *Journal of Paediatrics and Child Health* 47 (2011) 646–655
43. WHO 2009, Acceptable Medical Reasons for the use of Breastmilk Substitutes. http://apps.who.int/iris/bitstream/10665/69938/1/WHO_FCH_CAH_09.01_eng.pdf (accessed 18 Oct 2020)
44. The British Pregnancy Advisory Service https://www.bpas.org/get-involved/campaigns/briefings/breastfeeding-and-formula-feeding/ (accessed 19 October 2020)
45. Morrison P, How Often does breastfeeding really fail? *Breastfeeding Today*, 19 February 2016, https://www.llli.org/how-often-does-breastfeeding-really-fail/
46. Chisenga M et al Determinants of infant feeding choices by Zambian mothers: a mixed quantitative and qualitative study *Maternal & Child Nutrition*, 2011;7:148–159 http://onlinelibrary.wiley.com/doi/10.1111/j.1740-8709.2010.00264.x/pdf
47. Orloff SL, Wallingford JC, McDougal JS 1993, Inactivation of human immunodeficiency virus type 1 in human milk: effects of intrinsic factors in human milk and of pasteurization. *J Hum Lact* 9(1):13-17.
48. Chantry CJ, Morrison P, Panchula J, Rivera C, Hillyer G, Zorilla C, Diaz C. Effects of lipolysis or heat treatment on HIV-1 provirus in breast milk. *J Acquir Immune Defic Syndr* 2000;24(4):325-9.
49. Jeffery BS, Mercer KG, Pretoria pasteurisation: a potential method for the reduction of postnatal mother to child transmission of the human immunodeficiency virus, *J Trop Pediatr* 2000;46(4):219-23.
50. Jeffery BS, Webber L, Mokhondo KR and Erasmus D, Determination of the Effectiveness of Inactivation of Human Immunodeficiency Virus by Pretoria Pasteurization, *J Trop Pediatr* 2001; 47(6):345-349.
51. Jeffery BS, Soma-Pillay P, Makin J and Mooman G, The effect of Pretoria pasteurization on bacterial contamination of hand-expressed human breastmilk. *J Trop Pediatr* 2004;49(4):240-244.
52. Israel-Ballard K, Chantry C, Dewey K et al. Viral, nutritional and bacterial safety of flash-heated and Pretoria pasteurized beast milk to prevent mother-to-child transmission of HIV in resource-poor countries: a pilot study. *J Acquir Immune Defic Syndr*. 2005;40:175-181.
53. Israel-Ballard KA, Maternowska MC, Abrams BF, Morrison P, Chitibura L, Chipato T, Chirenje ZM, Padian NS, Chantry CJ, Acceptability of Heat-treating Breast milk to Prevent Mother-to-Child Transmission of HIV in Zimbabwe: A Qualitative Study, *J Hum Lact* 2006; 22(1):48-60.
54. Israel-Ballard K, Coutsoudis A, Chantry CJ, Sturm AW, Karim F, Sibeko L, Abrams B. Bacterial safety of flash-heated and unheated expressed breastmilk during storage. *J Trop Pediatr*. 2006;52:399–405.
55. Chantry CJ, Abrams BF, Donovan RM, Israel-Ballard KA, Sheppard HW, Breastmilk pasteurization: appropriate assays to detect HIV inactivation (letter). *Inf Dis Obstet and Gynecol* 2006;95938:1–2, DOI 10.1155/IDOG/2006/95938
56. Israel-Ballard K, Donovan R, Chantry C, Coutsoudis A, Sheppard H, Sibeko L and Abrams B. Flash heat inactivation of HIV-1 in human milk. A potential method to reduce postnatal transmission in developing countries. *J Acquir Immun Defic Syndr* 2007;45 (3): 318-323
57. Israel-Ballard, demo video at http://www.berkeley.edu/news/media/releases/2007/05/21_breastmilk-video.shtml

58. Israel-Ballard KA et al. Vitamin content of breast milk from HIV-1–infected mothers before and after flash-heat treatment. *J Acquir Immune Defic Syndr* 2008;48: 444–449.
59. Israel-Ballard K, Flash-heated and Pretoria Pasteurized destroys HIV in breast milk & Preserves Nutrients!, *Advanced Biotech* Sept 2008, http://www.advancedbiotech.in/51%20Flash%20heated.pdf
60. TenHam WH, Heat treatment of expressed breast milk as in-home procedure to limit mother-to-child transmission of HIV: A systematic review. Submitted to School of Nursing Science, North-West University, Potchefstroom, South Africa November 2009 http://dspace.nwu.ac.za/bitstream/10394/3745/1/TenHam_HW.pdf
61. Chantry CJ, Israel-Ballard K, Moldoveanu Z, Peerson J, Coutsoudis, Sibeko L and Abrams B. Effect of Flash-heat Treatment on Immunoglobulins in Breastmilk. *J Acquir Immune Defic Syndr*. 2009 July 1; 51(3): 264–267. doi:10.1097/QAI.0b013e3181aa12f2. http://www.ncbi.nlm.nih.gov/pmc/articles/PMC2779733/pdf/nihms126967.pdf (accessed 5 December 2010)
62. Volk ML, Hanson CV, Israel-Ballard K, Chantry CJ, Inactivation of Cell-Associated and Cell-Free HIV-1 by Flash-Heat Treatment of Breast Milk. *J Acquir Immune Defic Syndr* 2010;53(5):665-666.
63. Mbuya MNN, Humphrey JH, Majo F, Chasekwa B, Jenkins A, Israel-Ballard K, Muti M, Paul KH, Madzima RC, Moulton LH and Stoltzfus RJ. Heat treatment of expressed breast milk is a feasible option for feeding HIV-exposed, uninfected children after 6 months of age in rural Zimbabwe. *J Nutr* 2010, Epub ahead of print June 23, 2010 as doi: 10.3945/jn.110.122457
64. Young SL, Israel-Ballard KA, Dantzer EA, Ngonyani MM, Nyambo MT, Ash DM, Chantry CJ. Infant feeding practices among HIV-positive women in Dar es Salaam, Tanzania, indicate a need for more intensive infant feeding counselling. *Public Health Nutr*. 2010 Dec;13(12):2027-33. doi: 10.1017/S1368980010001539. Epub 2010 Jun 29. https://pubmed.ncbi.nlm.nih.gov/20587116/
65. Coutsoudis I, Nair N, Adhikari M, Coutsoudis A. Feasibility and safety of setting up a donor breastmilk bank in a neonatal prem unit in a resource limited setting: An observational, longitudinal cohort study. *BMC Public Health* 2011, 11:356 doi:10.1186/1471-2458-11-356. http://www.biomedcentral.com/1471-2458/11/356
66. WHO 2010. Guidelines on HIV and infant feeding. 2010. Principles and recommendations for infant feeding in the context of HIV and a summary of evidence. 1.Breast feeding 2.Infant nutrition 3.HIV infections – in infancy and childhood. 4.HIV infections – transmission. 5.Disease transmission, Vertical – prevention and control. 6.Infant formula. 7.Guidelines. I.World Health Organization. ISBN 978 92 4 159953 5 available at http://www.who.int/child_adolescent_health/documents/9789241599535/en/index.html (accessed 24 July 2010)
67. UNICEF 2010, Facilitator Guide, The Community Infant and Young Child Feeding Counselling Package, available at http://motherchildnutrition.org/healthy-nutrition/pdf/mcn-Facilitator-Guide.pdf session 17 HIV, pp 126-136.
68. WHO 2020, Infant feeding for the prevention of mother-to-child transmission of HIV, https://www.who.int/elena/titles/hiv_infant_feeding/en/ (accessed 20 November 2021).

Chapter 25: If undetectable equals untransmissable, what about breastfeeding?

1. The evidence for U=U: why negligible risk is zero risk, *I-Base* https://i-base.info/htb/32308 (accessed 22 February 2021)
2. Beckerman K et al. Control of maternal HIV-1 disease during pregnancy. *Int Conf AIDS* 1998 Jun 28-Jul 3; 12:41. Poster abstract 459. https://i-base.info/ttfa/wp-content/uploads/2012/05/Beckerman-Abs459-IAS-geneva-1998.pdf
3. U.S. Department of Health and Human Services (DHHS). Guidelines for the Use of Antiretroviral Agents in HIV-1-Infected Adults and Adolescents. December 1998. https://aidsinfo.nih.gov/ContentFiles/AdultandAdolescentGL12011998012.pdf
4. Quinn TC et al. Viral load and heterosexual transmission of HIV type 1. Rakai Project Study Group. *N Engl J Med* 2000; 342: 921-929. http://www.nejm.org/doi/full/10.1056/NEJM200003303421303
5. Castilla J et al. Effectiveness of highly active antiretroviral therapy in reducing heterosexual transmission of HIV. *J Acquir Immune Defic Syndr*. 2005;40:96-101. https://pubmed.ncbi.nlm.nih.gov/16123689 (accessed 28 October 2020)
6. Vernazza P et al. HIV-positive individuals not suffering from any other STD and adhering to an effective antiretroviral treatment do not transmit HIV sexually. (Les personnes séropositives ne souffrant d'aucune autre MST et suivant un traitment antirétroviral efficace ne transmettent pas le VIH par voie sexuelle). *Bulletin des médecins suisses* 2008;89 (5). Included with English translation. http://www.giv.org.br/divulgacao/intransmissivel/BullSuisse2008-05-089.pdf
7. Cohen MS et al for the HPTN 052 Study Team. Prevention of HIV-1 infection with early antiretroviral therapy. *New Engl J Med* 2011; 365:493-505. http://www.nejm.org/doi/full/10.1056/NEJMoa1105243
8. Cohen MS et al. Final results of the HPTN 052 randomized controlled trial: antiretroviral therapy prevents HIV transmisosion. IAS 2015, 19 – 22 July 2015, Vancouver. MOAC0101LB. http://dx.doi.org/10.7448/IAS.18.5.20482
9. Rodger AJ et al for the PARTNER study group. Sexual activity without condoms and risk of HIV transmission in serodifferent couples when the HIV-positive partner is using suppressive antiretroviral

therapy. *JAMA,* 2016;316(2):1-11. DOI: 10.1001/jama.2016.5148. http://jama.jamanetwork.cm/article.aspx?doi=10.1001.jama.2016.5148

10. Rodger A, Bruun T, Weait M, et al. Partners of people on ART-a new evaluation of the risks (the PARTNER study): design and methods. *BMC Public Health* 2012; 12: 296 https://bmcpublichealth.biomedcentral.com/articles/10.1186/1471-2458-12-296 (accessed 1 Apr 2021)
11. Rodger A et al. HIV transmission risk through condomless sex if HIV+ partner on suppressive ART: PARTNER Study. 21st CROI, 3-6 March 2014, Boston. Oral late breaker abstract 153LB. http://www.croiwebcasts.org/console/player/22072 (webcast)
12. Bavington BM et al for the Oposites Attract Study Group. The Opposites Attract Study of viral load, HIV treatment and HIV transmission in serodiscordant homosexual male couples: design and methods, *BMC Public Health* 2014;14:917. Published online 2014 Sep 4. doi:10.1186/1471-2458-14-917 https://www.ncbi.nlm.nih.gov/pmc/articles/PMC4168197/ (accessed 29 October 2020)
13. Grulich A et al. HIV treatment prevents HIV transmission in male serodiscordant couples in Australia, Thailand and Brazil. IAS 2017, Paris. Oral abstract TUAC0506LB. http://programme.ias2017.org/Abstract/Abstract/5469 (accessed 29 October 2020)
14. Rodger AJ et al, Risk of HIV transmission through condomless sex in serodifferent gay couples with the HIV positive partner taking suppressive antiretroviral therapy (PARTNER): final results of a multicentre, prospective, observational study, https://doi.org/10.1016/S0140-6736(19)30418-0 *Lancet* 2019;393:2428-2438 https://www.thelancet.com/journals/lancet/article/PIIS0140-6736(19)30418-0/fulltext (accessed 19 Sept 2019)
15. Rodger A et al. Risk of HIV transmission through condomless sex in MSM couples with suppressive ART: The PARTNER2 Study extended results in gay men. *AIDS* 2018, 23-27 July 2018, Amsterdam. Late breaker oral abstract WEAX0104LB. http://programme.aids2018.org/Abstract/Abstract/13470 https://tinyurl.com/y6tweapv
16. HIV transmission and the criminal law, *NAMLIFE,* http://namlife.org/cms1255092.aspx (accessed 10.8.2010).
17. Dear colleague: national gay men's HIV/AIDS awareness day. *US CDC News.* (27 September 2017) https://www.cdc.gov/nchhstp/dear_colleague/2017/dcl-092717-National-Gay-Mens-HIV-AIDS-Awareness-Day.html (accessed 29 October 2020)
18. The Swiss Statement, *I-Base* https://i-base.info/guides/pregnancy/swiss-statement (accessed 27 October 2020)
19. Schweizerische Ärztezeitung / *Bulletin des médecins suisses* / Bollettino dei medici svizzeri /2008; 89:5 http://www.aids.ch/e/fragen/pdf/swissguidelinesART.pdf
20. Edwin J. Bernard, Swiss experts say individuals with undetectable viral load and no STI cannot transmit HIV during sex, *AIDSMAP,* 30 January 2008 http://www.aidsmap.com/Swiss-experts-say-individuals-with-undetectable-viral-load-and-no-STI-cannot-transmit-HIV-during-sex/page/1429357/
21. Community partners, https://www.preventionaccess.org/community
22. Rebekah Webb, Feeding your baby when you have HIV, *AIDSMAP,* December 2019.
23. Shapiro RL et al. Antiretroviral regimens in pregnancy and breast-feeding in Botswana. *N Engl J Med.* 2010;362(24):2282–94.
24. Moseholm E & Weiss N, Women living with HIV in high-income settings and breastfeeding, *J Int Med* 2019, https://onlinelibrary.wiley.com/doi/full/10.1111/joim.12986 (accessed 31 December 2019)
25. Bispo S, Chikhungu L, Rollins N, Siegfried N, Newell M-L, Postnatal HIV transmission in breastfed infants of HIV-infected women on ART: a systematic review and meta-analysis. *J Int AIDS Soc* 2017, 20:21251. https://onlinelibrary.wiley.com/doi/epdf/10.7448/IAS.20.1.21251 http://dx.doi.org/10.7448/IAS.20.1.21251
26. Flynn PM et al for the PROMISE Study Team, Prevention of HIV-1 Transmission Through Breastfeeding: Efficacy and Safety of Maternal Antiretroviral Therapy Versus Infant Nevirapine Prophylaxis for Duration of Breastfeeding in HIV-1-Infected Women With High CD4 Cell Count (IMPAACT PROMISE): A Randomized, Open-Label, Clinical Trial. *J Acquir Immune Defic Syndr* 2018;77(4):383-392. doi: 10.1097/QAI.0000000000001612. https://www.ncbi.nlm.nih.gov/pubmed/29239901
27. Stranix-Chibanda L et al for the PROMISE study team. Slow Acceptance of Universal Antiretroviral Therapy (ART) Among Mothers Enrolled in IMPAACT PROMISE Studies Across the Globe. *AIDS Behav* 2019: 23(9): 2522–2531. From https://www.ncbi.nlm.nih.gov/pmc/articles/PMC6766470/
28. Kahlert CR et al, Review article: Biomedical intelligence Is breastfeeding an equipoise option in effectively treated HIV-infected mothers in a high-income setting? *Swiss Med Wkly.* 2018;148:w14648
29. Moseholm E & Weiss N, Women living with HIV in high-income settings and breastfeeding, *J Int Med* 2019, https://onlinelibrary.wiley.com/doi/full/10.1111/joim.12986 (accessed 31 December 2019)
30. Danaviah S, Evidence of Long-Lived Founder Virus in Mother-to-Child HIV Transmission. *PLoS ONE* 10(3): e0120389.doi:10.1371/journal.pone.0120389
31. Van de Perre P et al, HIV-1 reservoirs in breast milk and challenges to elimination of breast-feeding transmission of HIV-1. *Sci Transl Med* 2012 Jul 18;4(143):143sr3. doi: 10.1126/scitranslmed.3003327. https://pubmed.ncbi.nlm.nih.gov/22814853/ (accessed 1 Nov 2020)
32. Shapiro RL, Ndung'u T, Lockman S, Smeaton LM, Thior I, Wester C, Stevens L, Sebetso G, Gaseitsiwe S, Peter T, Essex M. Highly active antiretroviral therapy started during pregnancy or postpartum suppresses

HIV-1 RNA, but not DNA, in breast milk. *J Infect Dis.* 2005 Sep 1;192(5):713-9.

33. Lehman DA, Chung MH, John-Stewart GC, Richardson BA, Kiarie J, Kinuthia J, Overbaugh J. HIV-1 persists in breast milk cells despite antiretroviral treatment to prevent mother-to-child transmission. *AIDS* 2008 Jul 31;22(12):1475–85
34. Milligan C, Overbaugh J. The role of cell-associated virus in mother-to-child HIV transmission. *J Infect Dis.* 2014 Dec 15;210 Suppl 3:S631-640.
35. Dufour C, Gantner P, Fromentin R and Chomont N. The multifaceted nature of HIV latency, *J Clin Invest.* 2020;130(7):3381–3390. https://doi.org/10.1172/JCI136227.
36. Chun TW, Finzi D, Margolick J, Chadwick K, Schwartz D, Siliciano RF. In vivo fate of HIV-1-infected T cells: quantitative analysis of the transition to stable latency. *Nat Med.* 1995;1(12):1284–1290
37. Siliciano JD, et al. Long-term follow-up studies confirm the stability of the latent reservoir for HIV-1 in resting CD4+ T cells. *Nat Med.* 2003;9(6):727–728.
38. Crooks AM, et al. Precise quantitation of the latent HIV-1 reservoir: implications for eradication strategies. *J Infect Dis.* 2015;212(9):1361–1365
39. Blankson JN, Persaud D, Siliciano RF. The challenge of viral reservoirs in HIV-1 infection. *Ann Rev Med.* 2002;53:557–593
40. Eisele E, Siliciano RF. Redefining the viral reservoirs that prevent HIV-1 eradication. *Immunity.* 2012;37(3):377–388.
41. Ho DD, Neumann AU, Perelson AS, Chen W, Leonard JM, Markowitz M. Rapid turnover of plasma virions and CD4 lymphocytes in HIV-1 infection. *Nature.* 1995;373(6510):123–126.
42. Wei X, et al. Viral dynamics in human immunodeficiency virus type 1 infection. *Nature* 1995;373(6510):117–122.
43. Wong JK, et al. Recovery of replication-competent HIV despite prolonged suppression of plasma viremia. Science. 1997;278(5341):1291–1295.
44. Finzi D, et al. Identification of a reservoir for HIV-1 in patients on highly active antiretroviral therapy. *Science.* 1997;278(5341):1295–1300.
45. Chun TW, et al. Presence of an inducible HIV-1 latent reservoir during highly active antiretroviral therapy. *Proc Natl Acad Sci USA.* 1997;94(24):13193–13197.
46. Siliciano JM and Siliciano R, The Remarkable Stability of the Latent Reservoir for HIV-1 in Resting Memory CD4 T Cells, The Journal of Infectious Diseases 2015;212(9):1345–1347, https://doi.org/10.1093/infdis/jiv219
47. Thiry L, Sprecher-Goldberger S, Jonckheer T, et al. Isolation of AIDS virus from cell-free breast milk of three healthy virus carriers. *Lancet* 1985; 2:891–2.
48. Gray L, Fiscus S, Shugars D. HIV-1 variants from a perinatal transmission pair demonstrate similar genetic and replicative properties in tonsillar tissues and peripheral blood mononuclear cells. *AIDS Res Hum Retroviruses* 2007; 23:1095–104
49. Lewis P, Nduati R, Kreiss JK, et al. Cell-free human immunodeficiency virus type 1 in breast milk. *J Infect Dis* 1998; 177:34–9.
50. AVERT HIV science overview https://www.avert.org/professionals/hiv-science/overview (accessed 29 October 2020)
51. Crooks AM , Bateson R , Cope AB et al. . Precise quantitation of the latent HIV-1 reservoir: implications for eradication strategies. *J Infect Dis* 2015; 212:1361–5.
52. Graf EH, et al. Gag-positive reservoir cells are susceptible to HIV-specific cytotoxic T lymphocyte mediated clearance in vitro and can be detected in vivo [corrected]. *PLoS One.* 2013;8(8):e71879.
53. Pardons M, et al. Single-cell characterization and quantification of translation-competent viral reservoirs in treated and untreated HIV infection. *PLoS Pathog.* 2019;15(2):e1007619.
54. Chun TW & Fauci A, HIV reservoirs: pathogenesis and obstacles to viral eradication and cure . *AIDS* 2012 Jun 19;26(10):1261-8. doi: 10.1097/QAD.0b013e328353f3f1 https://pubmed.ncbi.nlm.nih.gov/22472858/ (accessed 30 Oct 2020)
55. Gandhi RT, et al. The effect of raltegravir intensification on low-level residual viremia in HIV-infected patients on antiretroviral therapy: a randomized controlled trial. PLoS Med. 2010;7(8):e1000321
56. Dinoso JB, et al. Treatment intensification does not reduce residual HIV-1 viremia in patients on highly active antiretroviral therapy. *Proc Natl Acad Sci U S A.* 2009;106(23):9403–9408.
57. Hatano H, et al. A randomized, controlled trial of raltegravir intensification in antiretroviral-treated, HIV-infected patients with a suboptimal CD4+ T cell response. *J Infect Dis.*2011;203(7):960–968.
58. McMahon D, et al. Short-course raltegravir intensification does not reduce persistent low-level viremia in patients with HIV-1 suppression during receipt of combination antiretroviral therapy. *Clin Infect Dis.* 2010;50(6):912–919.
59. WHO 2016, Consolidated guidelines on the use of antiretroviral drugs for treating and preventing HIV infection: recommendations for a public health approach – 2nd ed. ISBN 978 92 4 154968 4 available at http://www.who.int/hiv/pub/arv/arv-2016/en/
60. Benjamin Ryan, POZ, Treatment News, Viral Rebound Chance is Low for those on successful HIV treatment, June 12, 2017 https://www.poz.com/article/viral-rebound-chance-low-successful-hiv-treatment
61. O'Connor J et al on behalf of the UK Collaborative HIV Cohort (CHIC) Study, Durability of viral suppression with first-line antiretroviral therapy in patients with HIV in the UK: an observational cohort

study, *Lancet* HIV 2017;4:e295-302, May 4 2017, http://dx.doi.org/10.1016/

62. Fowler MG, Flynn P and Aizire J. Current opinion: what's new in perinatal HIV prevention? *Current Opin Pediatr* 2018:30(1):144-151, https://www.ncbi.nlm.nih.gov/pmc/articles/PMC6112766/ (accessed 4 November 2020)
63. Myer L, Phillips TK, Hsiao NY, et al. Plasma viremia in HIV-positive pregnant women entering antenatal care in South Africa. *J Int AIDS Soc.* 2015;18:20045
64. Waitt C, Low N, Van de Perre, Lyons F, Loutfy M et al, Does U=U for breastfeeding mothers and infants? Breastfeeding by mothers on effective treatment for HIV infection in high-income settings. *Lancet HIV* 2018; S2352-3018(18)30098-5, http://dx.doi.org/10.1016/
65. Haberl L et al, Not recommended, but done: Breastfeeding with HIV in Germany. *AIDS Patient Care STDS*, 2021;35(2):33-38, doi: 10.1089/apc.2020.0223
66. WHO 2016. Guideline. Updates on HIV and infant feeding: the duration of breastfeeding and support from health services to improve feeding practices among mothers living with HIV.
67. National Surveillance of HIV in Pregnancy and Childhood https://www.ucl.ac.uk/nshpc/hiv-exposed-and-hiv-positive-children (accessed 7 November 2020)
68. Francis K, Thorne C, Sconza R, Horn A, Peters H. Supported breastfeeding among women with diagnosed HIV in the UK- the current picture, Population, Policy and Practice Programme, UCL Great Ormond Street Institute of Child Health, poster presentation, International AIDS Conference, Mexico, July 2019. https://www.ucl.ac.uk/nshpc/sites/nshpc/files/peters_supported_breastfeeding_among_women_with_diagnosed_hiv_in_the_uk_190703.pdf (accessed 7 October 2020)
69. White AB, Mirjahangir JF, Horvath H, Anglemyer A, Read JS. Antiretroviral interventions for preventing breast milk transmission of HIV. *Cochrane Database Syst Rev.* 2014;10(10):CD011323
70. Prazuck T, Chaillon A, Avettand-Fènoël V, Caplan A-L, Sayang C, Guigon A, et al. HIV-DNA in the genital tract of women on long-term effective therapy is associated to residual viremia and previous AIDS defining illnesses. *PLoS One.* 2013;8(8):e69686. doi: http://dx.doi.org/10.1371/journal.pone.0069686
71. King CC, Ellington SR, Davis NL, Coombs RW, Pyra M, Hong T, et al.; Partners in Prevention HSV/HIV Transmission Study and Partners PrEP Study Teams. Prevalence, Magnitude, and Correlates of HIV-1 Genital Shedding in Women on Antiretroviral Therapy. *J Infect Dis.* 2017;216(12):1534–40. doi: http://dx.doi.org/10.1093/infdis/jix550

Chapter 26: Breastfeeding by HIV-positive women in the global north

1. Centers for Disease Control and Prevention (1985). Current trends recommendations for assisting in the prevention of perinatal transmission of human T lymphotropic virus type III/lymphadenopathy-associated virus and acquired immunodeficiency syndrome. *MMWR Weekly* 34(48) http://1.usa.gov/1wEQ11H
2. Socialstyrelsen (1987) The Social Welfare Board's Directive on the use of breast milk etc [in Swedish] Stockholm: Welfare NBoHa.
3. Burdge DR, Money DM, Forbes JC et al (2003). Canadian consensus guidelines for the management of pregnancy, labour and delivery and for postpartum care in HIV-positive pregnant women and their offspring (summary of 2002 guidelines). *Canadian Medical Association Journal* (CMAJ) 168(13):1671-4.
4. de Ruiter A, Mercey D, Anderson J et al. British HIV Association and Children's HIV Association guidelines for the management of HIV infection in pregnant women *HIV Medicine* 2008;9: 452-502 http://bit.ly/1FV61Tq [Accessed 21 October 2014].
5. Australian Government, NHMRC (2013). Eat for Health. Infant Feeding Guidelines. SUMMARY. http://bit.ly/1xDUP7W
6. Townsend CL, Cortina-Borja M, Peckham CS, Tookey PA. Trends in management and outcome of pregnancies in HIV-infected women in the UK and Ireland, 1990-2006. *BJOG* 2008 Aug;115(9):1078-86. Epub 2008 May 22.
7. Public Health England. Progress towards ending the HIV epidemic in the United Kingdom p 17. https://assets.publishing.service.gov.uk/government/uploads/system/uploads/attachment_data/file/821273/Progress_towards_ending_the_HIV_epidemic_in_the_UK.pdf accessed 25 Oct 220)
8. *NAM /AIDSMAP* https://www.aidsmap.com/about-hiv/feeding-your-baby-when-you-have-hiv, accessed 23 October 2020
9. Avert website, http://www.avert.org/hiv-aids-europe.htm
10. Thorne CN et al. Presentation with late stage HIV disease at diagnosis of HIV infection in pregnancy. 5th IAS Conference, Cape Town, South Africa.19-22 July 2009. Poster abstract TUAC103. http://www.ias2009.org/pag/Abstracts.aspx?AID=1155
11. UNAIDS/WHO 2009, *AIDS Epidemic Update* http://data.unaids.org/pub/Report/2009/2009_epidemic_update_en.pdf
12. Haberl L, Not Recommended, but done, Breastfeeding with HIV in Germany, #50 presented at the Tenth International workshop on HIV and women, 6 March 2020 http://regist2.virology-education.com/presentations/2020/HIVWomen/20_haberl.pdf (accessed 13 February 2021)
13. Haberl L et al, Not Recommended, But Done: Breastfeeding with HIV in Germany, *AIDS Patient Care and STDs* 2021;35(2)33-38 https://pubmed.ncbi.nlm.nih.gov/33571048/ (accessed 13 February 2021).
14. KFF, HIV/AIDS Fact sheet, epidemic in the US, . https://www.kff.org/hivaids/fact-sheet/the-hivaids-

epidemic-in-the-united-states-the-basics/
15. Fenton KA, The XI International AIDS Conference in Vancouver: perspectives from epidemiology and public health, Genitourin Med 1996;72:370-373 https://www.ncbi.nlm.nih.gov/pmc/articles/PMC1195708/pdf/genitmed00011-0064.pdf accessed 23 Oct 2020
16. Panel on Treatment of Pregnant Women with HIV Infection and Prevention of Perinatal Transmission, Recommendations for Use of Antiretroviral Drugs in Transmission in the United States, http://aidsinfo.nih.gov/contentfiles/lvguidelines/PerinatalGL.pdf
17. At Least 3 Percent of D.C. Residents Have HIV or AIDS, City Study Finds; Rate Up 22% From 2006, Jose Antonio Vargas and Darryl Fears, *Washington Post*, Sunday, March 15, 2009 http://www.washingtonpost.com/wp-dyn/content/article/2009/03/14/AR2009031402176_pf.html (accessed 23 June 2011)
18. Jeremy Olson, With help, Minnesota moms keep babies HIV-free A state medical collaboration has nearly eliminated infections for newborns, *St. Paul Pioneer Press*, April 4, 2010, http://www.twincities.com/ci_14812180?nclick_check=1
19. Number of mother-to-child HIV transmissions in Canada now almost zero, *The Star*. 22 July 2015. http://www.thestar.com/news/canada/2015/07/22/number-of-mother-to-child-hiv-transmissions-in-canada-now-almost-zero.html
20. Health Canada. (2006). HIV/AIDS in Canada -Surveillance Report to June 30, 2006. Ottawa.
21. McCall J, Vicol L, Pharm G, Healthy Mothers, Healthy Babies: Preventing Vertical Transmission of HIV/AIDS Nursing BC, Registered Nurses Association of British Columbia Apr 2009, http://findarticles.com/p/articles/mi_qa3916/is_200904/ai_n31964419/?tag=content;col1
22. Screening in pregnancy key to eliminating mother-to-child HIV transmission, *UBC News*, Jul 22, 2015 https://news.ubc.ca/2015/07/22/screening-in-pregnancy-key-to-eliminating-mother-to-child-hiv-transmission/
23. Money D, Tulloch K, Boucoiran I, et al. Guidelines for the care of pregnant women living with HIV and interventions to reduce perinatal transmission: executive summary. *J Obstet Gynaecol Can* 2014;36:721–34.
24. Views from the front lines, Interview with Dr Mona Loutfy, *CATIE Prevention in Focus* Spring 2018 https://www.catie.ca/en/pif/spring-2018/front-lines-pregnancy-and-infant-feeding (accessed 24 October 2020)
25. Australian Medical Association, Antenatal testing and intervention are saving babies from HIV infection, 19 April 2009 available at http://ama.com.au/node/4574 (accessed 19 June 2011)
26. HIV on the rise in straight Australian men, Kirby Institute report, *The Sydney Morning Herald*, 23 September 2018. https://www.smh.com.au/healthcare/hiv-on-the-rise-in-straight-australian-men-kirby-institute-report-20180920-p50501.html (accessed 3 April 2021)
27. The *Sydney Morning Herald*, October 2010.
28. McDonald, Karalyn. '"You don't grow another head": The experience of stigma among HIV-positive women in Australia". *HIV Australia*. 9 (4): 14–17.
29. Machon K, Women living with HIV in Australia: Overview of current issues and services 10/03/2020 https://www.napwha.org.au/wp-content/uploads/2020/03/NAPWHA_NDWLHIV2020_Kirsty-Machon.pdf
30. Australian Government, National Health and Medical Research Council, Department of Health and Aging Eat for Health, Infant Feeding Guidelines, Information for Healthworkers Summary, Page 6 (https://www.eatforhealth.gov.au/sites/default/files/files/the_guidelines/n56b_infant_feeding_summary_130808.pdf (accessed 25 October 2020)
31. New Zealand Ministry of Health Breastfeeding by women with HIV infection https://www.health.govt.nz/our-work/diseases-and-conditions/hiv-and-aids/breastfeeding-women-hiv-infection
32. Kent G, "HIV/AIDS, Infant Feeding, and Human Rights," in Wenche Barth Eide and Uwe Kracht, eds., *Food and Human Rights in Development. Volume I. Legal and Institutional Dimensions and Selected Topics* (Antwerp, Belgium: Intersentia, 2005), pp. 391-424, http://www2.hawaii.edu/~kent/HIVAIDS,%20Infant%20Feeding%20and%20Human%20Rights.doc (accessed 5 July 2009)
33. Kent G, Tested in court, the right to breastfeed, *SCN News*, No. 18, July 1999. http://www2.hawaii.edu/~kent/TESTED%20IN%20COURT%20THE%20RIGHT%20TO%20BREASTFEED.pdf (accessed 8 October 2020)
34. Wikipedia, https://en.wikipedia.org/wiki/Death_of_Eliza_Jane_Scovill
35. Greene, S., Ion, A., Elston, D., Kwaramba, G., Smith, S., Carvalhal, A., & Loutfy, M. (2014). "Why aren't you breastfeeding?": How mothers living with HIV talk about infant feeding in a "breast is best" world. *Health Care for Women International*, epub ahead of print. doi: 10.1080/07399332.2014.888720
36. Pamela Morrison & Ted Greiner (2014) Letter to the Editor, *Health Care for Women International*, 35:10, 1109-1112, DOI: 10.1080/07399332.2014.954705 http://dx.doi.org/10.1080/07399332.2014.954705
37. Leicestershire and Rutland, Local Safeguarding Children Board, Practice Guidance, Child Protection and HIV, http://www.lscb-llr.org.uk/index/guidance/guidance_child_protection_hiv.htm (accessed 6 October 2011 but may no longer be available).
38. Pokhrel S, Quigley MA, Fox-Rushby J, et al, Potential economic impacts from improving breastfeeding rates in the UK. *Archives of Disease in Childhood* 2015;100:334-340. https://adc.bmj.com/content/100/4/334.abstract (accessed 6 October 2020)
39. Gross MS et al, Breastfeeding with HIV: An Evidence-Based Case for New Policy. *The Journal of Law,*

Medicine & Ethics 2019; 47:152-160. https://journals.sagepub.com/doi/full/10.1177/1073110519840495 (accessed 23 October 2020)
40. Walls T, Breastfeeding in mothers with HIV. Journal of Paediatrics and Child Health 2010;46:349–352 https://pubmed.ncbi.nlm.nih.gov/20642646/ (accessed 9 October 2020)
41. Morrison P, Israel-Ballard K, Greiner T, Informed choice in infant feeding decisions can be supported for HIV-infected women even in industrialized countries, *AIDS* 2011, 25:18071811 http://www.ncbi.nlm.nih.gov/pubmed/21811145
42. Tariq S et al, "It pains me because as a woman you have to breastfeed your baby": decision-making about infant feeding among African women living with HIV in the UK *Sex Transm Infect* 2016;92:331–336, http://sti.bmj.com/content/92/5/331 accessed on April 8, 2017
43. Ayugi de Masi J, Becoming an African Mum, *HIV Weekly* 19 Sept 2012. http://www.aidsmap.com/Jackies-back-and-shes-a-mother/page/2512977/?utm_source=NAM-Email-Promotion&utm_medium=hiv-weekly&utm_campaign=hiv-weekly (this article may no longer be available on the internet).
44. Griswold M and Pagano-Therrien J, Women Living With HIV in High Income Countries and the Deeper Meaning of Breastfeeding Avoidance: A Metasynthesis *Journal of Human Lactation* 2000; 1–9.
45. UK Department of Health, HIV and infant feeding: Guidance from the UK Chief Medical Officers' Expert Advisory Group on AIDS, 24 September 2004, available at http://www.dh.gov.uk/en/Publicationsandstatistics/Publications/PublicationsPolicyAndGuidance/DH_4089892?IdcService=GET_FILE&dID=12178&Rendition=Web (accessed 16 April 2009)
46. BHIVA & CHIVA guidelines for management of HIV infection in pregnant women 2008, available at http://www.bhiva.org/files/file1031055.pdf
47. The Children's Commissioner for England's follow up report to: The arrest and detention of children subject to immigration control (Executive summary) February 2010, available at https://www.childrenscommissioner.gov.uk/wp-content/uploads/2017/07/Follow-up-report-to-the-arrest-and-detention-of-children-subject-to-imm-control.pdf (accessed 8 October 2020)
48. Tudor-Williams G, Second Joint Conference of the British HIV Association (BHIVA) and the British Association for Sexual Health and HIV (BASHH), 20-23 April 2010, Manchester
49. BHIVA & CHIVA Position statement on infant feeding in the UK, Nov 2010 http://www.bhiva.org/documents/Publications/InfantFeeding10.pdf (accessed 30 January 2011)
50. Taylor GP, Anderson J, Clayden P, Gazzard BF, Fortin J, Kennedy J, Lazarus L, Newell M-L, OsoroB, Sellers S, Tookey PA, Tudor-Williams G, Williams and De Ruiter A for the BHIVA/CHIVA Guidelines Writing Group. British HIV Association and Children's HIV Association position statement on infant feeding in the UK 2011. *HIV Medicine* DOI: 10.1111/j.1468-1293.2011.00918.x
51. American Academy of Pediatrics Policy Statement, Testing and Prophylaxis to Prevent Mother-to-Child Transmission in the United States Committee on Pediatric AIDS, *Pediatrics* 122(5):1127-1134, (doi:10.1542/peds.2008-2175) November 2008 http://aappolicy.aappublications.org/cgi/content/abstract/pediatrics;122/5/1127?rss=1
52. Panel on Treatment of HIV-Infected Pregnant Women and Prevention of Perinatal Transmission. Recommendations for Use of Antiretroviral Drugs in Pregnant HIV-1-Infected Women for Maternal Health and Interventions to Reduce Perinatal HIV Transmission in the United States. May 24, 2010; pp 1-117. http://aidsinfo.nih.gov/ContentFiles/PerinatalGL.pdf accessed 19 June 2011
53. American Academy of Pediatrics, Committee on Pediatric AIDS, Infant feeding and transmission of HIV in the United States, COMMITTEE ON PEDIATRIC AIDS, *Pediatrics* 2013; 131:2 391-396; published ahead of print January 28, 2013, doi:10.1542/peds.2012-3543, https://pediatrics.aappublications.org/content/131/2/391 (accessed 23 February 2021)
54. Greiner T, Morrison P, Breastfeeding by HIV-infected women in the USA, *Pediatrics* e-response, published at http://pediatrics.aappublications.org/content/131/2/391.full/reply#pediatrics_el_55196
55. AAP Publications Reaffirmed or Retired, *Pediatrics* August 2016, 138 (2) e20161650; DOI: https://doi.org/10.1542/peds.2016-1650
56. Centers for Disease Control Human Immunodeficiency Virus (HIV) – 21st March 2018 https://www.cdc.gov/breastfeeding/breastfeeding-special-circumstances/maternal-or-infant-illnesses/hiv.html
57. European AIDS Clinical Society Guidelines, Version 10.1. October 2020 https://www.eacsociety.org/files/guidelines-10.1_5.pdf (accessed 6 Nov 2020)
58. BHIVA, HIV and breastfeeding your baby, using the Safer Triangle, https://www.bhiva.org/file/5bfd3080d2027/BF-Leaflet-1.pdf (accessed 7 October 2020)
59. Gartland GM et al, Field effectiveness of combination antiretroviral prophylaxis for the prevention of mother-to-child HIV transmission in rural Zambia. AIDS. 2013 May 15; 27(8): https://www.ncbi.nlm.nih.gov/pmc/articles/PMC3836017/pdf/nihms521144.pdf (accessed 8 Oct 2020)
60. Ngoma MS et al with Silverman MS. Efficacy of WHO recommendation for continued breastfeeding and maternal cART for prevention of perinatal and postnatal HIV transmission in Zambia. *J Int AIDS Soc* 2015, 18:19352 http://www.jiasociety.org/index.php/jias/article/view/19352 (accessed 8 October 2020)
61. Shapiro RL, Hughes MD, Ogwu A et al. Antiretroviral regimens in pregnancy and breast-feeding in Botswana. *New Engl J Med* 2010;362(24):2282–94.
62. Seery P, Lyall H, Foster C, Khan W, Dermont S, Raghunanan S, Marks M. Breastfeeding experiences of mothers with HIV from two UK centres, Abstract P145, from the 4th Joint Conference of the British

HIV Association (BHIVA) with the British Association for Sexual Health and HIV (BASHH) Edinburgh, UK 17–20 April 2018 https://www.bhiva.org/file/jhWlaZopMPYnm/AbstractBook2018.pdf accessed 16 January 2020
63. National Surveillance of HIV in Pregnancy and Childhood https://www.ucl.ac.uk/nshpc/hiv-exposed-and-hiv-positive-children (accessed 5 October 2020) (Renamed ISOSS in 2021)
64. Francis K, Thorne C, Sconza R, Horn A, Peters H. Supported breastfeeding among women with diagnosed HIV in the UK- the current picture, Population, Policy and Practice Programme, UCL Great Ormond Street Institute of Child Health, poster presentation, International AIDS Conference, Mexico, July 2019. https://www.ucl.ac.uk/nshpc/sites/nshpc/files/peters_supported_breastfeeding_among_women_with_diagnosed_hiv_in_the_uk_190703.pdf (accessed 7 October 2020)
65. Peters H et al, Vertical HIV Transmissions in the UK- insights into the current picture and remaining challenges, UCL GOSH Institute of Child Health, London. CHIVA conference presentation, September 2021, https://www.ucl.ac.uk/integrated-screening-outcomes-surveillance/sites/integrated_screening_outcomes_surveillance/files/peters_chiva_vertical_transmissions_2021.pdf (accessed 21 November 2021)
66. Email from the ISOSS Co-ordinator, 28 January 2021.
67. BHIVA Statement 25 March 2020, https://www.bhiva.org/management-of-a-woman-living-with-HIV-while-pregnant-during-Coronavirus-COVID-19
68. Didikoglu A et al, Early life factors and COVID-19 infection in England: A prospective analysis of UK Biobank participants *Early Human Development*, Jan 2021;155:105326 https://reader.elsevier.com/reader/sd/pii/S0378378221000220

Chapter 27: Mothers' stories

1. Breastfeeding with an undetectable viral load: some insights into the current UK situation, *AIDSMAP*, 26 April, 2019 https://www.aidsmap.com/news/apr-2019/breastfeeding-undetectable-viral-load-some-insights-current-uk-situation (accessed 7 October 2020)
2. WHO 2010, Guidelines on HIV and infant feeding. Principles and recommendations for infant feeding in the context of HIV and a summary of evidence, ISBN 978 92 4 159953 5 available at http://whqlibdoc.who.int/publications/2010/9789241599535_eng.pdf
3. Smith J, Dunstone M, Elliott-Rudder. Health Professional Knowledge of Breastfeeding: Are the Health Risks of Infant Formula Feeding Accurately Conveyed by the Titles and Abstracts of Journal Articles? *J Hum Lact* 2009; 25; 350 originally published online Apr 15, 2009; DOI: 10.1177/0890334409331506 http://jhl.sagepub.com/cgi/content/abstract/25/3/350
4. Morrison P and Faulkner Z, HIV and breastfeeding: the unfolding evidence, *Essentially MIDIRS*, Dec/Jan 2015;5(11):7-13, https://www.midirs.org/wp-content/uploads/2014/12/272-MID-EM-December-2014-p7-12.pdf
5. de Ruiter A, Taylor GP, Clayden P (2014). British HIV Association guidelines for the management of HIV infection in pregnant women 2012 (2014 interim review). *HIV Medicine* 15(supp 4):1-77.
6. Chibwesha CJ, Giganti MJ, Putta N et al (2011). Optimal Time on HAART for prevention of mother-to-child transmission of HIV. *J Acquir Immunodefic Syndr*. 58(2):224-8.
7. Morrison P, Greiner T, Letter to the Editor, *Health Care for Women International* 2014;0:1-4 http://dx.doi.org/10.1080/07399332.2014.954705
8. Townsend CL, Cortina-Borja M, Peckham CS et al (2008). Low rates of mother-to-child transmission of HIV following effective pregnancy interventions in the United Kingdom and Ireland, 2000-2006. *AIDS* 22(8):973-81.
9. UCL Great Ormond Street Institute of Child Health. Obstetric and paediatric HIV surveillance data from the UK Population, Policy and Practice Research and Training Department UCL Great Ormond Street Institute of Child Health July 2020 update. https://www.ucl.ac.uk/nshpc/sites/nshpc/files/isoss_slides_july_2020.pdf
10. Francis K, Thorne C, Sconza R, Horn A, Peters H. Supported breastfeeding among women with diagnosed HIV in the UK- the current picture, Population, Policy and Practice Programme, UCL Great Ormond Street Institute of Child Health, poster presentation, International AIDS Conference, Mexico, July 2019. https://www.ucl.ac.uk/nshpc/sites/nshpc/files/peters_supported_breastfeeding_among_women_with_diagnosed_hiv_in_the_uk_190703.pdf (accessed 7 October 2020)
11. HIV and breastfeeding Case Study *The Doula magazine* https://doula.org.uk/hiv-breastfeeding-case-study/ (acessed 30 September 2020)
12. Minchin M. *Milk Matters: Infant Feeding and Immune Disorder*, available for free download, at https://infantfeedingmatters.com/ (accessed 31 March 2020.
13. WABA, Understanding International Policy on HIV and Breastfeeding: A Comprehensive Resource, Second edition, published 14 July 2018, http://waba.org.my/understanding-international-policy-on-hiv-and-breastfeeding-a-comprehensive-resource/ and at http://www.hivbreastfeeding.org (accessed 24 July 2021)
14. Kesho Bora Study Group, Triple antiretroviral compared with zidovudine and single-dose nevirapine prophylaxis during pregnancy and breastfeeding for prevention of mother-to-child transmission of HIV-1 (Kesho Bora study): a randomised controlled trial, *Lancet* 2011; DOI:10.1016/S1473-3099(10)70288-7

https://www.thelancet.com/journals/laninf/article/PIIS1473-3099(10)70288-7/fulltext (accessed 21 Jan 2020)
15. WHO 2010, Guidelines on HIV and infant feeding. Principles and recommendations for infant feeding in the context of HIV and a summary of evidence, ISBN 978 92 4 159955 5 http://whqlibdoc.who.int/publications/2010/9789241599535_eng.pdf
16. WHO-UNICEF 2016, Guideline: Updates on HIV and Infant Feeding, http://apps.who.int/iris/bitstream/10665/246260/1/9789241549707-eng.pdf
17. WHO 2016, Consolidated guidelines on the use of antiretroviral drugs for treating and preventing HIV infection: recommendations for a public health approach – 2nd ed. ISBN 978 92 4 154968 4 https://www.who.int/hiv/pub/arv/arv-2016/en/

Chapter 28: Helping an HIV-positive mother who wants to breastfeed

1. Kahlert CR et al, Review article: Biomedical intelligence Is breastfeeding an equipoise option in effectively treated HIV-infected mothers in a high-income setting? Published 24 July 2018 | doi:10.4414/smw.2018.14648 *Swiss Med Wkly*. 2018;148:w14648

Chapter 29: Advocacy, politics, spillover and lessons learned

1. WHO, HIV/AIDS in Europe, Moving from death sentence to chronic disease management https://www.who.int/hiv/pub/idu/hiv_europe.pdf
2. Lubbe W, Botha E, Niela-Vilen H. et al. Breastfeeding during the COVID-19 pandemic – a literature review for clinical practice. *Int Breastfeed J* 2020;15, 82. https://doi.org/10.1186/s13006-020-00319-3 https://internationalbreastfeedingjournal.biomedcentral.com/articles/10.1186/s13006-020-00319-3
3. Morrison P. HIV and infant feeding: to breastfeed or not to breastfeed: the dilemma of competing risks. Part 1. *Breastfeed Rev*. 1999 Jul;7(2):5-13. PMID: 10453705. https://pubmed.ncbi.nlm.nih.gov/10453705/ (accessed 11 November 2020)
4. Morrison P. HIV and infant feeding: to breastfeed or not to breastfeed: the dilemma of competing risks. Part 2. *Breastfeed Rev.* 1999 Nov;7(3):11-20. PMID: 10943427. https://pubmed.ncbi.nlm.nih.gov/10943427/ (accessed 11 November 2020)
5. Tompson M, AnotherLook, Breastfeeding by HIV-1 positive mothers, *Lancet* Sept 29, 2001;358:1095, https://www.thelancet.com/journals/lancet/article/PIIS0140-6736(01)06203-1/fulltext (accessed 11 November 2020)
6. Morrison P, Latham M, Greiner T, UNAIDS policy ought to promote exclusive breastfeeding but instead may lead to its decline in Africa. *BMJ* electronic version (eBMJ) (letter) 3 March 2001 http://www.bmj.com/cgi/eletters/322/7285/512/e
7. Tompson M, LeVan Fram J, Eastman A, McClain VW, Morrison P. Exclusive breastfeeding is best in all cases. *Bull World Health Organ*. 2002;80(7):605. Epub 2002 Jul 30. https://pubmed.ncbi.nlm.nih.gov/12163929/ (accessed 11 November 2020)
8. Morrison P, Greiner T, Infant feeding choices for HIV-positive mothers, *Breastfeeding Abstracts* 2000;19(4):27-28.
9. Morrison P. Book Review. HIV and Infant Feeding Counselling: A Training Course (WHO) *J Hum Lact* 2002;18(4):403
10. Morrison P. Book review. The Milk of Human Kindness: Defending Breastfeeding from the Global Market & the AIDS Industry. *J Hum Lact* 2003:19:322.
11. Morrison P. Book review, Issues, Risks and Challenges of Early Breastfeeding Cessation to Reduce Postnatal Transmission of HIV in Africa *J Hum Lact* 2003:19:322-323.
12. Israel-Ballard K, Maternowska MC, Abrams BF, Morrison P, Chitibura L, Chipato T, Zvavahera MC, Padian NS, Chantry CJ. Acceptability of Heat-treating Breast milk to Prevent Mother-to-Child Transmission of HIV in Zimbabwe: A Qualitative Study *J Hum Lact* 2006 22(1):48-60.
13. Morrison P & Greiner T. Letter to the Editor, *Health Care for Women International* 26 Sept 2014. http://dx.doi.org/10.1080/07399332.2014.954705
14. Morrison P. Practice Update: HIV and breastfeeding, *Essentially MIDIRS* August 2014;5(7):38-9, http://www.midirs.org/em-aug2014-worldbreastfeedingweek/
15. Morrison P and Faulkner Z. HIV and breastfeeding: the unfolding evidence, *Essentially MIDIRS*, Dec/Jan 2015;5(11):7-13, http://www.midirs.org/em-decjan-hiv/
16. Morrison P. Greiner T, Israel-Ballard K. Informed choice in infant feeding decisions can be supported for HIV-infected women even in industrialized countries *AIDS* 2011, 25:1807–1811, e-pub ahead of print AIDS, 1 August 2011, final version 24 September 2011, http://www.ncbi.nlm.nih.gov/pubmed/21811145
17. Eastman A, Tomson M, Brussel C, Buchanan P, Crowe D, Le Van Fram J, Hathaway J, McClain V, Morrison P and Sachs M, Breastfeeding vs formula feeding among HIV-infected women in resource-poor areas, (letter), *JAMA*, 2002 Mar 6;287(9):1111; author reply 1112-3. https://pubmed.ncbi.nlm.nih.gov/11879099/ (accessed 11 November 2020)
18. Greiner T, Sachs S, Morrison P. The Choice by HIV-Positive Women to Exclusively Breastfeed Should Be Supported. *Archives of Pediatrics & Adolescent Medicine* 156(1):87-88, 2002

19. Greiner T, Grundmann C, Krasovec K, Pitter C, Wilfert C. Structural Violence and Clinical Medicine: Free Infant Formula for HIV-Exposed Infants. *PLoS Med* 2007;4(2):e87. https://doi.org/10.1371/journal.pmed.0040087 (accessed 25 Feb 2021)
20. Chantry CJ, Morrison P, Panchula J, Rivera C, Hillyer G, Zorilla C, Diaz C. Effects of Lipolysis or Heat Treatment on HIV-1 Provirus in Breast Milk. *J Acquir Immune Defic Syndr* 2000 August; 24 (4):325-9
21. Morrison P. The Ethics of infant feeding choice: do babies have the right to be breastfed? *Topics in Breastfeeding*, SET XVIII, Lactation Resource Centre, Australian Breastfeeding Association, March 2006.
22. Morrison P, Thinking positively about breastfeeding in the UK. *Treasure Chest* LCGB Newsletter 2008;49:8-9.
23. Morrison P. The risk of HIV transmission during breastfeeding: a table of Research findings, *AIDS-Star One*, USAID/PEPFAR, September 2010, available at http://www.aidstar-one.com/focus_areas/pmtct/HIV_transmission_through_breastfeeding
24. Morrison P, What HIV-positive women want to know about breastfeeding, *Fresh Start by Best Start*, pages 8-12, special World AIDS Day issue, 1 December 2013, http://issuu.com/freshstartbybeststart/docs/fresh_start_supplement_final
25. Morrison P. Breastfeeding for HIV-Positive Mothers, *Breastfeeding Today*, 1 November 2014;26:20-25, http://viewer.zmags.com/publication/17f8c1a9#/17f8c1a9/22
26. Morrison P. IBFAN-BPNI HIV and Infant Feeding Global Status of Policy and Programmes based on World Breastfeeding Trends Initiative assessment findings from 57 countries, *World Breastfeeding Trends Initiative, WBTi, Foreword page* 7-9, 2015. http://worldbreastfeedingtrends.org/docs/HIV-and-Infant-Feeding.pdf
27. Tompson ML, *Passionate Journey, My unexpected life*, 2011, Hale Publishing, Amarillo Texas.
28. Liles C, Perspectives on HIV/AIDS and Breastfeeding, La Leche League International Chicago, Illinois, 2001
29. Crowe D, Infectious HIV in Breastmilk: Fact or Fantasy? LLLI Conference in Chicago, 2001
30. Prof Miles W Cloyd, Detecting Infectious HIV Detecting Infectious HIV in Human Milk in Human Milk, La Leche League International Conference, San Francisco, 5 July, 2005.
31. Morrison P. First do no harm, counselling the HIV+ mother about infant feeding, La Leche League South Africa Area Conference, Port Elizabeth, South Africa. 8 July, 2000.
32. Morrison P. "Guilty until Proven Innocent, What is the risk of MTCT of HIV through breastfeeding?", and "First Do No Harm: Counselling the HIV+ mother about Infant Feeding", presented at the South Australia College of Lactation Consultants, Adelaide, Australia and at the College of Lactation Consultants of Western Australia, Perth, 6th and 12-13th May 2000.
33. Morrison P. Mother's milk and HIV, updated, Queensland College of Lactation Consultants Seminar, Mater Hospital, Brisbane, Australia, 18 October 2003
34. Morrison P, Mother's milk and HIV, further updated, Australian Breastfeeding Association Seminars for Health Professionals Sydney 10 May 2004, Sydney, 11 May 2004 Brisbane, 12 May 2004 Melbourne, 13 May 2004 Adelaide, and 15 May 2004, Perth
35. Morrison P, The ethics of infant feeding choice: do babies have the right to be breastfed?, Australian Lactation Consultants Association Conference, Sydney, 19 September 2004
36. Morrison P. The politics of infant feeding choice, transcultural issues, ALMA Conference, Melbourne, 18 November 2004
37. Morrison P, Mother's Milk and HIV, risks, rights and responsibilities, The Informative Breastfeeding Service 25th Anniversary Conference, Port-of-Spain, Trinidad. 16 November 2002
38. Liles C, Tompson M, Breastfeeding in the context of HIV/AIDS: where is the evidence base supporting policy recommendations? Toronto, ON: XVI Int AIDS Conference; 2006.
39. Morrison P, Counselling on HIV & Infant Feeding: Accountability towards Child Survival. WABA/York University Conference, Gender, Child Survival & HIV/AIDS, from evidence to policy, Founders College, York University, Toronto, Canada, 9 May 2006
40. Morrison P. A matter of life or death: the untold story of HIV, breastfeeding and child survival, Global Media Strategies on HIV & AIDS Conference, hosted by Asia-Pacific Institute for Broadcasting Development, Hotel Nikko, Kuala Lumpur, Malaysia 28 May 2007
41. Morrison P, How to support first world HIV+ mothers who want to breastfeed, La Leche League of Basque Country, Fourth International Breastfeeding Symposium on Breastfeeding in Special Circumstances, 15-16 November 2010, Bilbao, Spain
42. Morrison P, Ethics, breastfeeding and society, do babies have the right to be breastfed? Eighth Spanish Breastfeeding Congress on Building Health, Palacio Euskalduna, Bilbao, Spain, 26-28 February, 2015
43. Morrison P. "What do we need to consider about HIV and infant feeding?" Lactation Consultants of Great Britain, Breastfeeding Workshop on HIV and Managing Change, Brighton, East Sussex, England, 22 March 2011
44. Morrison P, Heat-treating human milk, La Leche League Great Britain National Conference on Global Issues in Breastfeeding: Infection,Treatment & Myth, Britannia Hotel, Coventry, England, 14 October 2011
45. Morrison P, Developments in HIV and breastfeeding, Association of Breastfeeding Mothers Conference on connecting, informing, empowering mothers. Thistle Birmingham City Hotel, 16 June, 2012

46. Morrison P, HIV and breastfeeding, Breastfeeding Festival, Manchester, England, 25-26 June 2016
47. Morrison P, "Breastfeeding and HIV, ONE policy for all babies, breastmilk ONLY could save ONE Million lives, GOLD07 Breastfeeding Conference Online (hosted by Health-e-Learning, Australia), 25 June 2007
48. Morrison P, "Breastfeeding: Choice of duty or duty of care?" GOLD08 Breastfeeding Conference Online (hosted by Health-e-Learning, Australia) 18 May 2008
49. Morrison P, New opportunities and obligations to support breastfeeding by HIV-positive mothers in the First World, GOLD10 Breastfeeding Conference Online (hosted by Health-e-Learning, Australia), 7 May 2010
50. Morrison P. Back to the future on HIV and breastfeeding, the findings that transformed policy, GOLD13 Breastfeeding Conference Online (hosted by International Conference Services Ltd. Vancouver, Canada) 26/27 April, 2013, repeated for Alumni Conference 27 Jan – 13 Feb 2014, www.hivbreastfeeding.org
51. Morrison P, The politics of HIV and breastfeeding, i-Lactation Online Conference, March 2017
52. WABA-UNICEF HIV Colloquium, https://www.waba.org.my/whatwedo/hiv/colloquium/ (accessed 12 November 2020).
53. Greiner T, The role of breastfeeding-supportive NGOs in HIV and infant feeding, UNICEF/WABA HIV Symposium, Arusha, Tanzania, 20 Sept 2002, http://global-breastfeeding.org/2002/09/20/the-role-of-breastfeeding-supportive-ngos-in-hiv-and-infant-feeding/#more-334
54 Stephen Lewis, Keynote speech at WABA-UNICEF HIV Colloquium 2002, https://www.waba.org.my/whatwedo/hiv/colloquium/programme.html (accessed 12 November 2020).
55. WABA Newsletter, April 2004 https://www.waba.org.my/resources/wabalink/pdf/Issue33/33.pdf
56. Gender, Child Survival and HIV/AIDS, From evidence to policy conference, http://www.yorku.ca/esterik/advocacy.html
57. New York Times, https://www.nytimes.com/2006/08/08/health/08docs.html
58. PATH, https://www.path.org/media-center/updates-from-the-xvi-international-aids-conference/
59. Dunn DT, Newell ML, Ades AE, Peckham CS. Risk of human immunodeficiency virus type 1 transmission through breastfeeding, Lancet 1992 Sep 5;340(8819)585-588. https://www.ncbi.nlm.nih.gov/pubmed/1355163 (accessed 14 Janury 2020)
60. Crowe D, Kent G, Morrison P, Greiner T, Commentary: Revisiting the Risk of HIV Infection from Breastfeeding, *AnotherLook website*, December 2006 http://www.anotherlook.org/papers/g/english.pdf (accessed 11 November 2020)
61. Griswold MK and Pagano-Therrien J, Women Living With HIV in High Income Countries and the Deeper Meaning of Breastfeeding Avoidance: A Metasynthesis, *J Hum Lact* 2020:1-9, DOI: 10.1177/0890334419886565
62. Taylor GP, Anderson J, Clayden P, Gazzard BF, Fortin J, Kennedy J, Lazarus L, Newell M-L, OsoroB, Sellers S, Tookey PA, Tudor-Williams G, Williams and De Ruiter A for the BHIVA/CHIVA Guidelines Writing Group. British HIV Association and Children's HIV Association position statement on infant feeding in the UK 2011. *HIV Medicine* DOI: 10.1111/j.1468-1293.2011.00918.x
63. American Academy of Pediatrics, Committee on Pediatric AIDS, Infant feeding and transmission of HIV in the United States, COMMITTEE ON PEDIATRIC AIDS, *Pediatrics* 2013; 131:2 391-396; published ahead of print January 28, 2013, doi:10.1542/peds.2012-3543, http://pediatrics.aappublications.org/content/early/2013/01/23/peds.2012-3543.full.pdf+html (accessed 28 January 2013)
64. Haberl L, Not Recommended, but done, Breastfeeding with HIV in Germany, #50 presented at the Tenth International workshop on HIV and women, 6 March 2020 http://regist2.virology-education.com/presentations/2020/HIVWomen/20_haberl.pdf (accessed 13 February 2021)
65. WABA, Understanding International Policy on HIV and Breastfeeding: A Comprehensive Resource, Second edition, 14 July 2018 http://waba.org.my/understanding-international-policy-on-hiv-and-breastfeeding-a-comprehensive-resource/ and at www.hivbreastfeeding.org
66. Lakshmi Menon, personal communication, 1 December 2018.
67. WHO 2009, HIV and infant feeding, Revised Principles and Recommendations. Rapid Advice, November 2009. Available at http://whqlibdoc.who.int/publications/2009/9789241598873_eng.pdf
68. Ted Greiner, personal communication.
69. Chasela C et al. 2009. Both maternal HAART and daily infant nevirapine (NVP) are effective in reducing HIV-1 transmission during breastfeeding in a randomized trial in Malawi: 28 week results of the Breastfeeding, Antiretroviral and Nutrition (BAN) Study. Paper presented at 5th IAS Conference on HIV Pathogenesis, Treatment and Prevention, Cape Town, South Africa, July 2009. Abstract no. WELBC103
70. Chasela CS et al, Maternal or Infant Antiretroviral Drugs to Reduce HIV-1 Transmission N Engl J Med 2010;362:2271-81, http://content.nejm.org/cgi/reprint/362/24/2271.pdf
71. Kilewo CK et al. 2008. Prevention of mother-to-child transmission of HIV-1 through breast-feeding by treating infants prophylactically with lamivudine in Dar es Salaam, Tanzania: the Mitra Study. *J Acquir Immune Defic Syndr* 48(3): 315–23.
72. Vyankandondera JS et al, 2003. Reducing risk of HIV-1 transmission from mother to infant through breastfeeding using antiretroviral prophylaxis in infants (SIMBA study). Paper presented at the 2nd International AIDS Society Conference on HIV Pathogenesis and Treatment, Paris, France, July 2003.

Abstract no. LB7 2003.
73. Thomas, T. et al. 2008. PMTCT of HIV-1 among breastfeeding mothers using HAART: the Kisumu breastfeeding study, Kisumu, Kenya, 2003-2007. Paper presented at the Fifteenth Conference on Retroviruses and Opportunistic Infections, February 2008, Boston, MA. Abstract no. 45aLB.
74. Kilewo CK 2009. Prevention of mother to child transmission of HIV-1 through breastfeeding by treating mothers with triple antiretroviral therapy in Dar es Salaam, Tanzania: the Mitra Plus study. *J Acquir Immune Defic Syndr* 52(3): 406-16.
75. Palombi, L., M.C. Marazzi, A. Voetberg, and N.A. Magid. 2007. Treatment acceleration program and the experience of the DREAM program in prevention of mother-to-child transmission of HIV. *AIDS* 21 (Suppl 4): S65–71.
76. Marazzi MC 2009. Increased infant human immunodeficiency virus-type one free survival at one year of age in sub-Saharan Africa with maternal use of Highly Active Antiretroviral Therapy during breast-feeding. *Ped Inf Dis J* 28: 483–487.
77. Peltier, C.A., G.F. Ndayisaba, P. Lepage, J. van Griensven, V. Leroy, C.O. Pharm, P.C. Ndimubanzi, O. Courteille, and V. Arendt. 2009. Breastfeeding with maternal antiretroviral therapy or formula feeding to prevent HIV postnatal mother-to child transmission in Rwanda. *AIDS* 23: 2415-23.
78. Shapiro RM. 2009. A randomized trial comparing highly active antiretroviral therapy regimens for virologic efficacy and the prevention of mother-to-child HIV transmission among breastfeeding women in Botswana (The Mma Bana Study). Paper presented at 5th IAS Conference on HIV Pathogenesis, Treatment and Prevention, Cape Town, South Africa, July 2009. Abstract no. WELBB101. Webcast of this session available at www.ias2009.org/pag/webcasts/?sessionid=2435. Powerpoint available at www.ias2009.org/PAGMaterial/WELBB101_Shapiro_1.ppt.
79. Homsy J 2010. Breastfeeding, Mother-to-Child HIV Transmission, and Mortality Among Infants Born to HIV-Infected Women on Highly Active Antiretroviral Therapy in Rural Uganda. *J Acquir Immune Defic Syndr* 53:28–35.
80. Morrison P, The risk of HIV transmission during breastfeeding: a table of research findings. USAID, PEPFAR, *AIDSTAR-One*, September 2010. http://www.aidstar-one.com/focus_areas/pmtct/HIV_transmission_through_breastfeeding (accessed 20 November 2010, may no longer be available).
81. Coutsoudis, A., K. Pillay, E. Spooner, L. Kuhn, and H.M. Coovadia (for the South African Vitamin A Study Group). 1999. Influence of infant-feeding patterns on early mother-to-child transmission of HIV-1 in Durban, South Africa: a prospective cohort study. *Lancet* 354(9177): 471–6.
82. Coutsoudis, A., K. Pillay, L. Kuhn, E. Spooner, W.-Y. Tsai, and H.M. Coovadia (for the South African Vitamin A Study Group). 2001. Method of feeding and transmission of HIV-1 from mothers to children by 15 months of age: prospective cohort study from Durban, South Africa. *AIDS* 15: 379–387.
83. NHS, who can give blood? https://www.blood.co.uk/who-can-give-blood/men-who-have-sex-with-men/ (accessed 26 February 2021)
84. Murray E, Essay on 'The social and cultural activities of young people vary in different contexts and societies. Explore the diverse and adverse lives of young people within a globalised world' citing Palmer G, *The politics of breastfeeding*, London: Harper Collins, 1993.
85. De Wagt A, Clark D, UNICEF's Support to Free Infant Formula for Infants of HIV Infected Mothers in Africa: A Review of UNICEF Experience, LINKAGES Art and Science of Breastfeeding Presentation Series, Washington DC, April 14 2004, available at http://global-breastfeeding.org/pdf/UNICEF.pdf (accessed 6 Mar 2011)
86. Moland KMI, de Paoli M, Sellen DW, Van Esterik P, Leshabari SC and Blystad. Breastfeeding and HIV: experiences from a decade of prevention of postnatal HIV transmission in sub-Saharan Africa. *Int Breastfeed J*. 2010; 5: 10, doi: 10.1186/1746-4358-5-10. October 26, 2010
87. Lake L et al Child health, infant formula funding and South African health professionals: Eliminating conflict of interest, *S Afr Med J* 2019;109(12):902-906. https://doi.org/10.7196/SAMJ.2019.v109i12.14336, http://www.samj.org.za/index.php/samj/article/view/12787/9055
88. Witten C, Why many South African mothers give up breastfeeding their babies so soon *The Conversation*, 5 October 2020, https://theconversation.com/why-many-south-african-mothers-give-up-breastfeeding-their-babies-so-soon-145557 (accessed 9 October 2020)
89. Maureen Minchin, personal communication 21 November 2020.
90. Nestlé Nutrition Institute, 14th Continuing Nutrition Education Symposium at the University of Pretoria, September 2019 https://www.Nestlé nutrition-institute.org/country/za/
91. Nestlé Nutrition Institute, Nurses Academy, Addis Ababa, Ethiopia, April 2019 https://www.Nestlé nutrition-institute.org/country/za/news/article/2019/04/25/expansion-of-the-the-first-1-000-days-nurses-academy-by-nestl%C3%A9-nutrition-institute-africa-east-africa (accessed 8 November 2020)
92. Tshwane declaration of support for breastfeeding in South Africa, South African *J Clin Nutr*, 2011;24(4):214, available at http://www.sajcn.co.za/index.php/SAJCN/article/viewFile/586/820
93. Gribble K, Mathison R, Ververs M-t and Coutsoudis A, Mistakes from the HIV pandemic should inform the COVID-19 response for maternal and newborn care, *Int Breastfeeding J* 2020;15:67 https://internationalbreastfeedingjournal.biomedcentral.com/track/pdf/10.1186/s13006-020-00306-8 (accessed 8 November 2020)
94. Humphrey JH, The risks of not breastfeeding. *J Acquir Immune Defic Syndr*. 2010 Jan 1;53(1):1-4.

Index

Abakada, A.O. 109
Abbott 89
Academy of Breastfeeding Medicine 401
acid labile viruses 127
acidity of stomach 127
ACTG 076 Protocol 150, 151, 295–7
acute HIV infection phase 15–16
adipose tissue 76
adopted babies 49, 51
AFASS conditions 184–5, 204, 226, 230, 263
African Summit on HIV/AIDS, Tuberculosis and Other Infectious Diseases 249
AIDS
  cases in babies 42
  diagnosis of 60
  history of the US epidemic 29
  incubation times 278
  progression of HIV to 19
  slow to manifest symptoms 15
AIDS Clinical Trials Group 150
AIDS denialism 357, 396
AIDS industry 10
AIDSMAP 340
Akre, James 92, 177
Aldrovandi, Grace 48, 133, 260, 266, 287–8, 291–2
Alfieri, Dr 262
Alipui, Nicholas 231
allergies 77–8
Alnwick, David 167
alpha-defensins 131
Altman, Lawrence 32
Amata study 290
American Academy of Pediatrics 314, 365–6, 401
American Foundation for AIDS Research 34
amniotic fluid 43–4
Angola 177
animal immunodeficiency virus 20–1 *see also* simian (monkey) immunodeficiency virus (SIV)
animal milks 267–76 *see also* formula-feeding
ankyloglossia 108
Annales Nestlé 168
Annan, Kofi 168
Anna's story 373–7
AnotherLook 318, 326, 395–6, 399
antenatal education 211 *see also* infant feeding counselling
antibiotic medications 107, 274–6
antibiotic properties of breastmilk 75–6
antibiotic resistance 276
antibodies
  antibody tests 16
  in breastmilk 51, 79, 80, 128, 133
  in colostrum 75, 103
  developing antibodies to HIV 17
  human immune system 13–14
  for mastitis 110
  maternal antibodies in babies' blood 56
  testing babies for 62–3
  testing for HIV 56, 57–8, 59
antifungals 108
antigen-antibody combination tests 57–61
antigens 119
antimicrobials 75–6, 79, 128–9, 138
antioxidants 114
anti-poverty interventions 199
antiretroviral prophylaxis (ARVs)
  given to children 210, 300
  HIV-free survival 290
  maternal health 301
  PMTCT project 208–9, 210, 232–3
  short-courses 298–9
  success in preventing MTCT 303
  WHO policy changes in 2009 322–3
antiretroviral therapy (ART)
  adherence to 349
  ART+EBF 49, 306–16, 322–3, 328, 332, 401
  assessment of disease progression for 60
  in Botswana 249
  and breastfeeding 293–305
  costs of 151, 295, 296, 300, 302
  early US and French research 150–1
  effect on transmission 48
  given to children 210, 281
  Global Strategy on Infant and Young Child Feeding 181–2
  HIV in breastmilk 98, 99
  and latency 344–5
  long-term adverse effects 280
  'lost to follow-up' statistics 244
  maternal health 301
  and MTCT 49, 152, 293–305, 321
  PMTCT project 208, 209–10
  in pregnancy 44, 279
  reduction in infectivity 295, 296–7
  short-courses 298–9
  success in African adults 38
  timing of 68, 101
  and transmissibility 333–51
  undetectable equals untransmittable (U=U) 337–41
  and viral reservoirs 347–9
  WHO policy changes in 2009 322–3
antiviral properties of human milk 119, 128, 129–30, 131, 135, 138
armed conflict 35
Armstrong, Helen 136, 173, 189, 199, 403
ART+EBF 49, 306–16, 322–3, 328, 332, 401
Asian Journal of Psychiatry 82
assay tests 57, 64, 65, 344
asthma 77–8
asylum seekers 362, 365
attachment (mother-child bond) 259, 264–5, 271
attachment (to the breast) 104, 107, 115, 211, 391
Australia 355, 359
Australian Time Use Survey of New Mothers 90, 136
autism 82

autoimmune disease 77–8
Avebury, Lord Eric 362, 401
AVERT website 346
AXIOS group 232
Ayugi de Masi, Jacquie 360

baby foods 263 *see also* solid foods, introduction of
Baby Friendly 7, 86, 124, 176, 178, 181, 238, 318, 394
baby spit backwash 79–80
bacterial breast/nipple infections 107
bacterial contamination of formula 226, 269–70
Bakaki, P. 263
BAN trial 263, 274, 289
Bangladesh 112
Barré-Sinoussi, Françoise 34
Bartick, Melissa 89–90
bathhouses 31–2, 34
Baumslag, Naomi 154
Becker, Genevieve 189, 192, 201
Beckerman, Karen 333
Bellamy, Carol 39, 168, 169–70, 173
Bergman, Nils 271
Berlin patient 17
BHIVA guidelines 369, 371
BHIVA/CHIVA Position Statement on Infant Feeding in the UK 362–5
bias, counsellors' 220–1, 222
birth (intra-partum) transmission 44–5, 60–1, 97, 278, 307–8, 314, 348, 373
birth spacing 87, 138
biting 54
Black, Rebecca 119
Bland, Ruth 224
bleeding nipples 48
blister fluid 52
blocked ducts 109–10, 114, 116
blood barrier, maternal-infant 43, 44
blood transfusions 24, 29, 33–4, 42, 46, 403
blood-brain barrier 82
BLT (bone marrow, liver, thymic) mice 54–5
Bode, Lars 131
body fluids, presence of HIV in 15
bonding 84, 259, 264, 271
Botswana
  ART+EBF research 7, 306–7
  BOTUSA study 244
  breastfeeding in 156
  choice of infant feeding method 239
  cotrimazole 275
  Creek study 210
  flooding 11–12, 213, 228, 244, 250–3, 286, 287–8, 317, 405
  formula preparation facilities 226
  four-country review of HIV and infant feeding 206–8
  government-provided formula 209, 225
  HIV and Infant Feeding Counselling Course 218
  HIV-free survival 288
  PMTCT project 232, 248–53
  study on immunologic quality of breastmilk 133
  study on reducing viral load 61
bottle feeding *see also* expressing milk; formula-feeding
  cleaning bottles 185, 194, 197, 226, 271
  as cultural norm in many places 91–2
  of expressed milk 83
  expressed milk for wet-nursing 52
  Global Strategy on Infant and Young Child Feeding 180
  HIV and Infant Feeding Counselling Course 194–5
  as a sign of HIV-positive status 167
BOTUSA 244
Brabeck, Peter 168
brain development in babies 75, 82
Brazil 123
breast abcesses 48, 104, 106, 109, 112, 114, 259
breast compression techniques 115
breast engorgement 104–5, 114–15, 266
breast inflammation 48
breast involution 306
'breast is best' 156, 165, 172, 357, 361
breast physiology and milk production 74, 103
Breastfeeding Answer Book, The 113
Breastfeeding Counselling Course 190
breastfeeding support *see also* infant feeding counselling
  and the achievement of exclusive breastfeeding 121
  asylum seekers 362
  deteriorating 230
  emergency situations 72–3
  helping an HIV-positive mother who wants to breastfeed 388–93
  maternal mental health 86
  'safer breastfeeding' education 211
  solving breastfeeding problems 102, 105–6, 112, 116–17
  withholding of 220, 371
breastmilk *see also* transmissibility of HIV during breastfeeding
  antiviral properties of human milk 119, 128, 129–30, 131, 135, 138
  components that protect against HIV 128–33
  enzymes 81
  first detection of HIV in 42–3
  HIV in breastmilk 42–3, 96–101, 111, 346–7
  importance of breastfeeding generally 69–95
  patents 89
  unique specificity of 73–4
  viral loads 46, 66, 67
breastmilk feeding 52, 114, 122, 137, 141, 330, 383, 403 *see also* expressing milk; heat-treating breastmilk
breast/nipple problems 102–17
Brewster, D. 326
Briend, André 269, 274
Briony's story 372–87
British HIV Association 314, 370
British Medical Journal 23, 32, 171–2, 245
Brodribb, Wendy 114
Bronner, Andrée 161
Brown, Timothy Ray 17
Browne, Gill 136, 177
Bryson, Yvonne 63

buffalo milk 90, 164, 193, 198, 269
Bulletin of Swiss Medicine (*Bulletin des Médecins Suisses*) 336
Burger, Susan 244
Burkina Faso 151, 178, 224, 262, 263, 290, 297–8

cabergoline 368
Cadman, Hilary 130
caesarean births 44, 45, 301, 314, 379, 383
Cameroon 22–3
Canada 31, 153, 354–5
candida infections 108
carbohydrates in breastmilk 75, 86
cART (combination antiretroviral therapy) 300, 307, 350
CATIE (Canadian AIDS Treatment Information Exchange) 337, 354
CCR5-Delta32 deletion mutation 17
CCR5-expressing memory CD4 T-cells 132
CD4 T cells
  ART and breastfeeding 295, 304
  cell-associated vs cell-free virus 98
  and HIV 14, 18, 32
  HIV in breastmilk 100, 132
  and latency 344, 345
  reservoirs of 342
  testing for HIV 60, 66
CD8 cells 18, 344–5
CD8 cytotoxic lymphocytes 15
CDC (Centers for Disease Control and Prevention) 29, 31, 42, 53, 142, 250, 252, 317, 352, 368
cell-associated vs cell-free virus 98, 342, 346
cell-free HIV 43, 44, 98, 110, 342, 346
cervical fluids 43, 44, 60–1, 97
Chantry, Caroline 135, 138, 402
CHAT vaccine 25
Chibwesha, C.J. 302, 314
CHIC study 348
chickenpox 52
Chigwedere, Pride 38
child abuse and neglect 84, 264, 265
child protection and safeguarding 357–9
child to mother transmission 49–52
Chile 54
chimerism 82
chimpanzees 22, 25
China 88
Chisenga, Molly 328
chloride 103
Chopra, Mickey 240
Christiansen, Niels 157, 161, 171
Christina's story 381–7
circulating recombinant form (CRF) 23
Clarke, David 152, 162–3, 207, 226, 397
cognitive development 75, 83
co-infection/super-infection 16, 278
colonialism 24, 25
colostrum 46, 74–5, 97, 103, 128
commercial advocate, breastfeeding has no 118, 234
complementary foods *see* solid foods, introduction of
condoms 39, 335
Conference on Retroviruses and Opportunistic Infections (CROI) 26–7, 59, 251, 260, 287, 320, 334
confidentiality 146, 404
Congo 22–5, 28 *see also* Zaire
Connor, Edward 295–6
contaminated blood 33
contamination of formula 88, 119, 226, 250–3, 269–70
Convention on the Rights of the Child 143
Coovadia, H.M. 125–6, 213, 251, 291, 359, 398
cortisol 85
cost (financial) of not breastfeeding 92–4, 205 *see also* economic value of breastfeeding; risks of not breastfeeding
costs of formula-feeding 92–4, 163, 185, 208, 210–12, 235, 268–9, 405
costs of 'free' formula provision 302
costs of interventions to prevent breastfeeding 160, 167, 270
costs of treatment 151, 295, 296, 300, 302
Côte d'Ivoire 151, 218, 221, 225, 227, 289, 291
cotrimazole 274–6
counselling *see* infant feeding counselling
Counselling Tools 184–6, 255, 258, 320
Coutsoudis, Anna 88, 98, 119, 123–4, 127, 180, 196, 211, 219, 228, 252–3, 275, 286, 291, 380, 400
covert breastfeeding 229, 368
Covid-19/SARS-CoV-2 15, 20, 25, 99–100, 371, 394, 395, 403–4, 406
cow's milk 77, 269, 309
cradle of the AIDS pandemic 23
Creek, Tracy 64, 209, 244, 251, 252, 260, 320
CRF01 (subtype E) 28
CRF2-AG 50
criminalisation 334, 336, 361
cross-nursing 49, 51
crying 238, 258, 259, 262, 271
cultural norms about formula feeding (global north) 91–2, 327, 340, 357
cultural norms and breastfeeding
  in Africa generally 177–8, 198, 360–1
  exclusive breastfeeding 306
  and expressed milk 136
  global north 91–2
  infant feeding counselling 219
  maternal fidelity, breastfeeding as indicator of 201–2, 237–8
  no expectation of choice 201–2, 216
  older children 257–8
  PMTCT project 235–8
  taboos and stigma about not breastfeeding 94, 325–6
cultural norms and the provision of foods other than milk 120
cumulative risks 47–8, 98, 124, 298, 315
cup feeding 52, 140, 180, 185, 271–3
cures for HIV 17, 345
cytokines in breastmilk 77, 81
Czosnykowska-Lukacka, Matylda 86

da Silva, Regina 401

Dabis, François 148, 298
Danaviah, S. 342
Daniels, B. 275
Datta, Prathiba 96
De Cock, Kevin 47, 48, 49, 160, 166, 179
De Vincenzi, Isabelle 167
de Wagt, Arjan 152, 205, 207–8, 220, 226, 272
death certificates 37
deaths *see* infant deaths; maternal deaths
definitions of breastfeeding 47, 48, 99, 118–27, 312–13
dehydration 111, 264
delayed lactogenesis 104
deliberate infection with HIV 50 *see also* criminalisation
dendritic cells 343
depression 85, 86, 259, 265
detection of HIV 16
diarrhoea 80, 225, 245, 250–4, 260, 275, 277, 284, 320–1
disease progression 18, 60
DNA 14, 16, 22, 29, 98, 111, 346–7
Doherty, Tanya 202, 239
domino effect of lactation failure 105–6, 113
donor breastmilk 52, 136 *see also* milk banks
dose responses 47, 93, 127
Doula, The 376
draining breasts in early days, importance of 106, 115–16
DREAM study 301, 302, 308, 323
'drop-out bias' 244
drug resistance 278
drugs in breastmilk 72
dry sex 39
Dufour, Caroline 344, 347
Dugas, Gaëtan ('Patient Zero') 26, 29, 32
dummies 271
Dunn, David 46–7, 48, 49, 66, 123, 147, 179, 399
duration of breastfeeding *see also* early cessation of breastfeeding; exclusive breastfeeding; extended breastfeeding; weaning
  ART with breastfeeding to 12 months 308–14
  and autism 82
  cumulative risks 298
  measuring in studies 46, 47, 48
  recommendations on breastfeeding (2010s) 303–4
  shortening to lessen HIV transmission risk 254–66
  timing of mother's infection 46, 66, 100
  two years as 'gold standard' 73, 86–7, 102
  WHO Global Strategy 178

early cessation of breastfeeding 141, 179, 180, 212, 254–66, 271, 279, 290–1
Eastern Europe 35–6, 41
EBF+ART 49, 306–16, 328, 401
Ebola 15, 21
E.coli 226, 227
economic value of breastfeeding 84, 90, 92–4, 205, 358
eczema 78
Ekpini, Rene 100, 254
elafin 132
electricity supplies 249
ELISA test 57, 62–3, 65, 67
elite controllers 18, 353
Elizabeth Glaser Pediatric AIDS Foundation 34, 231
Embree, Joanne 96
emergency preparedness guidelines 51
Emerling, Carol 157
emotional benefits of breastfeeding 84–5, 257–8, 259
emotional effects of sudden weaning 264–6, 271–2
emtricitabine 341
engorgement 104–5, 114–15, 266
Enterobacter sakazakii 270
enzymes 14, 16, 81
epidermal growth factor 123, 128
epigenetics 85
episiotomy 44
epithelial barrier 43, 103, 107, 113, 119, 128, 132
erythropoietin (EPO) 132
ESPGHAN (European Society for Paediatric Gastroenterology, Hepatology and Nutrition) 270
essential fatty acids 129, 268, 269
Ethiopia 222
Europe
  European guidance on HIV-positive women and breastfeeding 368–9
  HIV-positive women and breastfeeding 353
  spread of AIDS to 30, 32, 41
  treatments for HIV 301
European AIDS Clinical Society 368–9
European Collaborative Study 353
European Communities AIDS Task Force 149
evaporated milk 193
exclusive breastfeeding
  in Africa generally 178
  'allowable lapses' 126–7
  benefits for mothers 112
  counsellors' knowledge of 220
  definitions of breastfeeding 47, 48, 99, 111, 118–27, 312–13
  EBF+ART 49, 306–16, 328, 401
  Framework for Priority Action on HIV and Infant Feeding 183
  frequency of counselling 223–4
  in the global north 327, 363–4
  global recommendation for all babies 102, 106
  Global Strategy on Infant and Young Child Feeding 178, 180, 181
  HIV Counselling Course 201
  importance of 118–27
  mothers' experiences with counselling 222
  and MTCT 49, 112–14, 212
  Nairobi study excludes 48
  PMTCT project 211
  policy changes in 2000s 319, 322
  as protective factor 123–4, 125, 132
  research showing no increased risk of transmission 196
Expert Advisory Group on AIDS 362
expressing milk *see also* pasteurisation
  cultural norms 136–7
  hand expression 106, 130, 137, 191

heat treating milk 116
to help with engorgement 115
policy changes in 2000s 329–30
professional scepticism about 136–7
recommendations for replacement feeding 184
seen as 'difficult' 137
as a sign of HIV-positive status 236
for testing for HIV 130
for wet-nursing 52
extended breastfeeding 47, 86, 254–66, 308–14

father-to-child transmission 52
fats in breastmilk 76, 86, 90, 129
fatty acids 129, 268, 269
FDA (Federal Drug Administration) 270, 295
Ferraro, Ms 169
Fetherston, Cathy 104–5, 114
Filteau, Suzanne 281
first cases of AIDS 23–4
first report of HIV through breastfeeding 42–3
First Steps Nutrition Trust 270
flash heating 135, 136, 137–8, 140–1
food, pre-chewed 53–5
food insecurity 180, 248, 280
food rations 263
food supplements 263, 267, 274
formula industry
exploiting window of opportunity 154, 168
and global policy-makers 168–73
jargon 404
marketing and branding 70, 71, 91–2, 142
and mothers' choice 326–7
patents 89
spillover effects into non-HIV populations 406
and the UN 168–9
'Voldemort effect' 88–9
formula-feeding *see also* mixed feeding
2006 policy change 319
as aberration 238–40
advice to formula feed to avoid HIV transmission 124, 208
AFASS conditions 184–5, 204, 226, 230, 263
autoimmune disease 78
coercion to formula-feed in global north 356–7, 359
contamination of formula 88, 119, 226, 250–3, 269–70
costs of 92–4, 163, 185, 208, 210–12, 235, 268–9, 405
as cultural norm in many places 91–2, 327, 340, 357
effect on intellectual development 75
feasibility versus safety of 204–5
formula mishaps 88
Framework for Priority Action on HIV and Infant Feeding 183
free supplies of 156–7, 168–9, 205–6, 208, 224–5, 229–30, 239, 245–6, 249–50, 394, 405
functional adequacy 83
Global Strategy on Infant and Young Child Feeding 181
government financial support for 75, 91
HIV and Infant Feeding Counselling Course 189–203, 215–16, 218–19
HIV-free survival rates 283–92
HIV-positive women in the global north 352–71
labelling 173, 240
lack of data on life-saving 241
mortality due to 11–12
politics of 403
potential for sensitivity to foreign proteins 77
as recommended preferred alternative 146–7, 168, 176–7, 183–4
and the risk of MTCT 125–6
risks of formula feeding 88–9, 92–4, 174, 200, 206, 226–8, 235, 248–53, 358, 406
safe preparation 166, 197, 206, 225–6, 249, 267–8, 320, 406
seen as 'almost as good' 70
as a sign of HIV-positive status 167, 236
spillover effects 404–6
sustainability of formula supplies 138, 225, 239, 251, 308–9, 362
UNAIDS 154–9
unbranded 173
'Voldemort effect' 88–9, 127
in WHO guidance 155
formula-feeding preparation training 191, 192–6, 197–8, 219
fortified flour 263
Fowler, Mary Glenn 349
Framework for Priority Action on HIV and Infant Feeding 182–4
France 150, 295–6
free fatty acids 129
frenulotomy 97, 108
frequency of feeding a baby 77, 87, 106, 115
fuel, access to 221, 235

Gabon 51
galactogogues 85, 381
galactose 75
Gallo, Robert 34–5
Gartland, M.G. 313
gastroenteritis 260, 320–1, 406
gay liberation movement 31–2
GDP, breastfeeding not counted in 90
Geddes, Donna 73
generalised risk estimates 49
Ghent working group 148–50, 158
ghrelin 81
Glaser, Elizabeth 33–4
Glaxo Wellcome 165, 171
global north, HIV-positive women and breastfeeding 352–71, 401
Global Plan Towards the Elimination of New HIV Infections Among Children by 2015 and Keeping Their Mothers Alive 158
global policy on HIV and breastfeeding 142–88, 317–32, 356, 402
Glover, Anne 376
glycan 17
glycosaminoglycans 128
Goldman, Armand 79

'good' mothers 200, 357, 360–1
gp120 17
grandmothers 39–40, 51, 178, 239, 264, 271
Grant, James 168
Gray, Glenda 153–4, 156
Greene, Saara 357
Greiner, Ted 122, 144, 197, 261, 314, 357, 359, 367, 396, 398
grief 85, 264, 265, 392
Griswold, Michele 361–2
Gross, Marielle 358
Group M HIV 22–3, 25, 27–8
Group O HIV 22–3, 26, 30
growth factors in breastmilk 81
growth stunting 280
Guay, Laura 298
Guinea-Bissau 23
gut microbiota 73, 75–6, 90, 119, 128, 132, 275 *see also* intestinal mucosal surfaces
gut permeability 119
gut-associated lymphoid tissue (GALT) 347

Haberl, L. 350
haemophiliacs 29, 32, 33–4
Haiti 25–6, 27, 30, 32, 263, 285
Halperin, Daniel 31, 237
HAMLET (human α-lactalbumin) 81
hand expression 106, 130, 137, 191
Hansen, Keith 70–1
Hanson, Lars 128
heat-treating breastmilk 134–41, 329–30, 402 *see also* pasteurisation
Henrick, B.M. 132
heterosexual transmission 28, 38–9, 41, 70, 237, 334
highly active antiretroviral therapy (HAART)
  Amata study 290
  ART+EBF research 307–8, 309–16
  guidelines on 348
  PMTCT projects 300
  during pregnancy 301–2
  PROMISE study (Promoting Maternal Infant Survival Everywhere) 341
  timing of treatment 302
  and transmissibility 44, 45, 49, 99, 334, 343
  WHO recommendations 305
HIV
  origins of HIV 20–30
  overview of virus 13–19
HIV and Infant Feeding Counselling Course 124–5, 189–203, 210, 215–34, 242, 256, 267
HIV and Infant Feeding Guidelines for Decision Makers/Health-care Managers and Supervisors (2004) 148, 182–3, 256
HIV Counselling Course 176–7
HIV Medicine 363
HIV-1 and HIV-2 22
HIV-exposed babies who escape infection 279–82
HIV-free survival 47–8, 212, 245, 252, 283–92, 319, 322, 328
HIV-infected clone cells 349
HIV-positive status
  criminalisation for non-disclosure 336
  disclosure to family 240
  formula feeding as 'forced disclosure' of 238, 360
  mothers not knowing 179, 211–12, 233
  not breastfeeding as indicator of HIV-positive status 160, 167
  psychosocial consequences of 236
Ho, David 67, 152
Hoffmann, I.F. 130
Holck, Dr 167
Holder pasteurisation 134–5
Holmes, Wendy 242
home-prepared formula 193–4, 212, 267
homosexual men 26, 28, 29, 30, 31–2, 36, 335
Honduras 159, 164, 220, 222, 231
Hooper, Edward 23, 25
Hormann, Elizabeth 199
HPTN 046 trial 300
HPTN 052 study 334
HTLV (human T-cell leukaemia viruses) 34–5
HTLV-III 35, 36, 42
Hudson, Rock 34
Human Development Report 228
Human Milk Banking Association of North America 130–1, 135
human milk fat globule membrane (HMFGM) 90
human milk fortifiers 88, 191
human milk industry 89–90, 130–1
human milk lipids 129–30
human milk oligosaccharides (HMOs) 75–6, 89, 130–1
human rights
  coercion to formula-feed in global north 357, 359
  human right to food 83
  mothers' right to choose 188, 201, 202, 235, 322, 362
  public health 163, 322
  right to life and right to privacy 162–3
  spillover effects 406
  UNAIDS 154–9
  WHO Rapid advice 324–8
Humphrey, Jean 406–7
Hunter, Susan 40

iatrogenic transfer 25
IBFAN 161, 163, 177
IgA 79, 81, 87, 112, 128, 131, 138
IgG 59, 79, 128, 131, 132
IgM 59, 79, 97, 128
Iliff, Peter 125, 132, 207, 397
immune system
  CD4 count 295
  components that protect against HIV in breastmilk 128–9
  and early exposure to HIV 280–1
  and early weaning 259
  effects of HIV on 133
  extended breastfeeding 256, 257
  and heat-treated milk 138
  and malnutrition 278
  preterm babies 87–8
  role of breastfeeding in 47–8, 69, 73, 75, 77–81, 86, 89, 119, 128–33, 277

and thrush 108
and viruses generally 13–14, 15
immunity to HIV 18–19
immunoglobulins 79, 81, 112
in utero transmission 43–4
India 64, 211, 221, 222, 231, 232, 268, 288
indirect fluorescent antibody (IFA) tests 57
induced lactation 51
infant deaths
in the 6-24 months period 255
from conditions that breastfeeding would protect from 284
due to formula-feeding 320–1
and early weaning 254–6, 260
and exclusive breastfeeding 118, 211
formula-fed babies 11–12, 251–3, 260
global infant mortality rates 285
HIV infection counted as equivalent to 292
lack of data in PMTCT project 240–1, 243–5, 252–3, 255
malnutrition 177, 284
from misguided efforts to prevent mother-to-child transmission 10
and mixed feeding 125
mortality risks of MTCT versus not breastfeeding 285
Nairobi study 48
risks of not breastfeeding 93, 150, 213
statistics on HIV-related mortality 210
and type of feeding 70
in untreated HIV-infected babies 277
'infant feeding' 404
infant feeding counselling
Counselling Tools 184–6, 255, 258, 320
early cessation of breastfeeding, as recommendation 261–3
exploring breastfeeding options 161, 179
frequency of 223–4
in the global north 216–18
guidance on provision of 175–6
HIV and Infant Feeding Counselling Course 124–5, 189–203, 210, 215–34, 242, 256, 267
integrated with post-test counselling 212
PMTCT project 209
and provision of formula supplies 156
scaling up of 215–34
Infant Food Manufacturers (IFM) 157, 161
infection control practices 50
infection rates across the world 35–8
infection routes of HIV in babies 42–55
informed choice
in African healthcare 216
counsellor confusion 220–1
and early weaning 255
ethics of 325–7
and the formula industry 326–7
global policy recommendations 169, 175–6, 183–4, 188
HIV and Infant Feeding Counselling Course 201, 211, 215–16
human rights 362
maternal rights *not* to breastfeed 235
mothers' experiences with counselling 222–3
mothers' right to choose 188, 201, 202, 235, 322, 362
mothers' understanding of relative risks 221
no expectation of choice in Africa 201–2
versus recommendations 325–8
Innocenti Declaration 144–5, 176, 181
integrase inhibitors 346, 348
Integrated Screening Outcomes Surveillance Service (ISOSS) 370
Interagency Group for Action on Breastfeeding (IGAB) 122
Interagency Task Team (IATT) for the Prevention and Treatment of HIV Infection in Pregnant Women, Mothers and Children 158–9, 174
interleukin-8 112
International AIDS Conferences 39, 50, 67, 151, 152–4, 261, 294, 333, 354, 370, 398
International Board Certified Lactation Consultant (IBCLC) 72–3, 137, 157, 189
International Breastfeeding Journal 405
International Code of Marketing of Breastmilk Substitutes (WHO code)
and the cost of alternatives to breastmilk 208
on donations of formula 206
early days of 71
formula purchasing abiding by the 173
global policy recommendations 142, 143, 161, 168, 169, 171, 176, 178, 181
HIV Counselling Course 198
and human rights 325
packaging 173, 240
and the PMTCT project 208
revised guidelines (2003) 230
International Committee on the Taxonomy of Viruses 35
International Lactation Consultant Association (ILCA) 177, 192, 318, 399–400
International Workshop on HIV and Women 353
Interscience Conference on Antimicrobial Agents and Chemotherapy (ICAAC) 308
intervention trials 149
interventions to prevent breastfeeding 160
intestinal damage 275, 285, 309, 342
intestinal mucosal surfaces 77, 97, 119, 128, 131
intra-partum (birth) transmission 44–5, 60–1, 97, 278, 307–8, 314, 348, 373
intravenous drug users 26, 28, 29, 30, 32, 34, 35
IQ 75, 83
Isaacs, C. 129
isolation of the HIV 29, 34–5
Israel-Ballard, Kiersten 136, 137, 177, 236, 287, 359, 402
Italian Register for HIV in Children 298
Ivory Coast 36, 297–8

Jackson, Thad 157
Jammet Dietetique Nouvelle SA 173
jargon 404
Jarman, Sue 269
Jeffery, Bridget 139
Jelliffe, Derrick 198, 207

Jelliffe, Dick and Patrice 71, 122
Jimbo, William 250
John, Grace 96, 97
Journal of Human Lactation 361, 399
Journal of Paediatrics and Child Health 359
Journal of Pediatrics 53
Journal of the American Medical Association 162
Journal of the International AIDS Society 312
journals 9–10, 127, 162, 396

Kagaayi, J. 321
Kagoda, B. 263
Kahlert, Christian 307, 348, 350, 351, 388
Kakulas, Foteini 82
Kaletra 308
Kambarami, Rose 108, 278
Kaposi's sarcoma 29, 31, 32
Kent, George 83, 356
Kenya 206–8, 211, 238, 260, 265, 269, 288–90, 321
Kesho Bora study group 263, 290, 302, 314–16, 385, 402
KIBS study 288–9
Kisanga, Pauline 67, 134, 177, 178–9, 180, 206, 207, 228, 230, 233–4, 245–6, 257, 285–6
Koniz Booher, Peggy 207, 226, 241
Kreiss, Joan 96, 100, 156
Kuhn, Louise 48, 113, 116, 119, 131, 133, 260, 263–4, 266, 278, 283, 287–8, 291–2
Kuiken, Carla 26
!Kung 87, 248
kwashiorkor 251, 265
Kyenkya-Isabirye, Margaret 122

La Leche League 7, 123, 144, 161, 199, 219, 318, 395
La Leche League International/WABA Symposium on HIV and Breastfeeding 219
Labbok, Miriam 118, 121–2, 188, 234
lactase deficiency 275
lactation consultants 72–3, 177, 235–6, 256, 275, 369, 388–93 *see also* International Board Certified Lactation Consultant (IBCLC)
lactation management 114–15
lactation suppression 266, 368
lactoferrin 81, 103, 110, 112, 128, 131, 132, 138
lactogenesis-II 103, 104, 109
lactoperoxidase 128
lactose content in human milk 75, 103
lactose in mother's urine 104–5
Lallemant, M. 299
lamivudine 174
Lancet 37, 42, 62, 70, 71, 88, 93, 96, 124, 147, 148, 174, 228, 242, 251, 284, 298, 348, 399
latent reservoirs 343–7
Latham, Michael 67, 134, 198, 206–7, 228, 230, 233–4, 245–6, 257, 285–6, 396
Lawrence, Ruth A. 71, 204
Le Roux, Dr 281
legal advisors for women wishing to breastfeed 390
lentiviruses 14, 15, 23
Leonard, Rod 157
leptin 81
Leshabari, Sebalda 219, 262
let-down reflex 84–5
leucocytes 80, 110, 111, 112, 119, 128
Lewis, Paul 96, 110
Lewis, Stephen 39, 203, 214, 397–8
Lhotska, Lida 163
Libya 50
LINKAGES 285, 397
lipids in breastmilk 76, 86, 90, 129
Little, Kirsten 50
Llotska, Lida 189
lobola (bride price) 201
Lockman, Shahin 275
long labours 44
long-term health effects of exposure to HIV 280
long-term non-progressors (LTNPs) 17–18
lopinavir 312
Los Angeles 31, 34
Los Angeles Times 31
Loutfy, Mona 354–5
Lunney, Kevin 114
Luoga, E. 311, 313
lymphadenopathy-associated virus (LAV) 29, 34
lymphocytes in breastmilk 132, 138, 342
lymphoid tissues 62, 79, 344, 345–6, 347
lysozyme 81, 110, 112, 128, 138

macrophages 14, 343, 346
Madzima, Rufaro 177, 206–7
Maggiore, Christine 357
Mahommed, A.E.K. 78–9
Makhema, Joe 249
malaria 276
Malawi
- BAN trial 289
- breastfeeding in 111
- early cessation of breastfeeding, as recommendation 260
- HIV testing 65
- HIV-free survival 288
- MTCT 66
- PMTCT project 236, 243, 244, 258, 274
- statistics on mortality from formula-feeding 320

male partners
- multiple sexual partners 237
- opinions on breastfeeding 236, 237, 239
- role in decisions about infant feeding 224–5

malnutrition
- Botswana flooding 250–1
- breastfeeding promotion to combat 70
- and breastmilk sodium 111
- consequences of not breastfeeding 247, 255, 264
- food supplements 274
- and formula-feeding 235
- and the immune system 278
- infant deaths 177, 284
- risk of 6-24 month old period in children 255

marasmus 251
marketing of breastmilk substitutes 70, 71, 88, 91–2, 142, 144, 147
MASHI study 249, 288, 343
mastitis 48, 99, 104, 106, 109–11, 112, 114–15,

116, 259, 266
maternal antibodies in babies' blood 62, 65
maternal deaths 94, 280, 281
maternal fidelity, breastfeeding as indicator of 201–2, 237–8
maternal health
 benefits of breastfeeding for 86
 risk of not breastfeeding to 92–4
maternal immunosuppression 100
Mbeki, Thabo 38
Mbori-Ngacha, Dorothy 96
McClain, Valerie 89, 130
McDougal, J.C. 129
Medscape 312
Meier, Barry 188
melamine contamination of formula 88
Mellors, John 67, 152
meta-analyses 46–7, 123, 147, 148, 160, 340, 399
micro-chimeriam 82
micronutrient sachets 267
milk banks 134–5, 184, 380, 394
milk ejection reflex (MER) 84–5
milk stasis 103, 104, 105, 113, 116
milk supply issues 72, 104
Miller, Maria 132
Milligan, C. 346
Minchin, Maureen 70, 77–8, 384
Miotti, P.G. 46
mixed feeding
 after 6 months 309
 definitions of breastfeeding 48, 99, 111
 Global Strategy on Infant and Young Child Feeding 180
 and increased maternal infectivity 113–14
 and the infant gut 119–20
 Kesho Bora study group 316
 as last resort for poorer mothers 223, 239
 mechanism for HIV transmission 120
 potential for breast problems/mastitis 104
 reasons for 120–1
 and the risk of MTCT 48, 104, 106, 123–4, 125
 risks of any infection 228–9
Mma Bana study 307, 309, 314, 340
Mofensen, Lynne 150, 298
Moland, Karen 405
molecular clocks 23, 29, 30
Montagnier, Luc 34, 35
Montaner, Julio 152–3
Morrison, Pamela 120
mortality *see* infant deaths; maternal deaths
mothering tool, breastfeeding as 72, 84, 259
mouth lesions 97, 108
Mozambique 178, 279, 308, 321, 323
MTCT (mother to child transmission)
 and antiretroviral therapy (ART) 49, 152, 293–305, 321
 ART+EBF research 306–16
 breastfeeding as risk for 97
 counsellors' knowledge of 220
 cumulative risks 46
 early US and French research on ART to reduce 150–1
 and exclusive breastfeeding 49, 112–14, 212
 and the formula-feeding 125–6
 human rights 163
 infection routes of HIV in babies 42–55
 mechanisms for blocking 298
 and mixed feeding 48, 104, 106, 123–4, 125
 mortality risks of MTCT versus not breastfeeding 285
 probability of infection via breastfeeding 96
 research on ART and untransmissibility 333
 risk of infection with HIV via breastfeeding 179
 statistics on MTCT 243, 276, 285–6, 293, 298, 301, 406
 Swiss statement on optimum scenario 350–1
 and viral load 307, 309, 312, 314, 333
mucosal surfaces 43, 97, 119, 285, 342
mucous membranes 44, 79
Mugivhi, Modipadi R. 239–40
multiple sexual partners 237
mutate, ability of HIV to 16
Myanmar 269

Nairobi study 48, 66, 100, 129–30, 147–8, 158, 288, 343, 346
Namibia 206–8, 262
Nastouli, E. 65
National Agency of Research on AIDS in France 150
National Cancer Institute 34–5
National Institutes of Health 64, 150, 365
National Surveillance of HIV in Pregnancy and Childhood (NSHPC) 370, 373, 404
Nature 18, 29
Nduati, Ruth 47, 48, 49, 96, 123, 147–8, 162, 179, 215, 325, 399
necrotising enterocolitis (NEC) 87–8, 132, 135, 270, 384
'negligible' versus 'zero' risk of transmission 339
Nestlé 72, 154, 156, 157, 161, 168, 169, 171–2, 406
neural development 75, 82, 264
neutrophils 80, 111
nevirapine 99, 111, 174, 210, 211, 233, 299, 300, 315, 341
New England Journal of Medicine 38, 299, 308, 314
New York 29–30, 31, 32, 34, 41
New York Times 31, 32, 153, 155–6, 157, 164, 165
New Zealand 355
Newburg, David 128, 130, 131
Ngoma, Mary 312, 313
Nicoll, Angus 156
Nigeria 208, 222, 225, 287
night feedings 197, 226, 229, 258
nipple problems 102–17
nipple shields 51
non-nucleoside reverse transcriptase inhibitors (NNRTIs) 99, 347
non-puerperal-induced lactation 51
nosocomial infection 24–6, 50
nucleic acid amplification test (NAAT) 58
nucleoside reverse transcriptase inhibitors (NRTIs) 347, 348
nucleotide analyses 29

nucleotide reverse transcriptase inhibitors (NnRTIs) 347
nucleotides in breastmilk 77
Nutrients 73
NUTRIFASO 263
Nutriset 274
nutritional supplementation 112
NVAZ study 289

obesity 81
Odhiambo, Dorothy 166
oligosaccharides 75–6, 89, 128, 130–1
One World One Hope *see* International AIDS Conferences
Opposites Attract study 335
oral thrush 48, 106, 108
origins of HIV 20–30
Orloff, S.L. 129
orphaned children 39–40, 50–1, 245, 271
Osborne, Connie 157, 397
Overbaugh, Julie 96, 346
oversupply of milk 104–6, 114–15
oxytocin 84–5, 103

p24 57, 132
pacifiers 271
PACTG 076 protocol 295–6, 297, 301
Pagano-Therrien, Jesica 361–2
Palaia, J.M. 131
Palmer, Gabrielle 69
Papathakis, C. 267
partial breastfeeding *see* mixed feeding
PARTNER study 334–5, 339
PARTNER2 study 335
Pasteur Institute 25, 29, 34
pasteurisation 129, 134–41, 160, 184, 212, 329–30, 380, 402
patents 89–90, 130–1
PATH Symposium 398
Patient Zero 26, 29, 32
PCR (polymerase chain reaction) testing 58, 62, 64, 65, 67, 135, 345
peanut paste 274
Pediatrics 54, 248, 314, 367
peer support programmes 219–20
Peeters, Martine 21, 22
PEPFAR 260
PEPI study 288, 289
Perella, Sharon 73
permeability of milk cells 103–4, 105, 110, 113
Peters, Helen 370
Phillips, Andrew N. 348
phylogenetic testing 29, 61
physiology of breastmilk synthesis 74, 103
Piot, Peter 21, 38, 96, 147, 154, 159–60, 161, 165, 166, 168, 172
Piwoz, Ellen 48–9, 110, 119, 123, 241–2, 259, 261, 264, 265, 271, 397
placenta 43, 69, 72, 74, 104, 133, 295
placental microtransfusion 44
Plumpy'Nut 263, 269, 274
PMTCT (Prevention of Mother to Child Transmission) Projects
  in Botswana 249–53
  HIV-free survival 283–92
  and the IATT 159
  lack of data in 278, 398
  lack of long-term follow-up 205–6, 213–14, 234, 235–47, 286, 317
  loss to follow-up 243–5
  mixed feeding 120–1
  monitoring and evaluation 240–3
  morbidity and mortality data 245–7
  outcomes from first pilots 204–14
  pilots 11, 149–50, 152, 164–5, 179, 180
  Quality Assurance Project 207
pneumocystis pneumonia 29, 31, 277, 357
polio vaccines 25
politics
  of breastfeeding 9–10
  facilitating spread of HIV from Congo 25
  global policy recommendations 402–3
  HIV and breastfeeding 394–5
  undetectable equals untransmittable (U=U) and breastfeeding 351
Portman, Adolf 75
Positive People's Forum 339
post-exposure prophylaxis (PEP) 61
postpartum depression 85, 86
potassium 111
poverty 94, 177, 180, 198, 206, 213, 222, 225
powdered animal milks 267–8
powdered formula, safety of 269–70
Powell, Greg 279
Prameela, K.K. 78–9, 132–3
Preble, E.A. 119, 123
pre-exposure prophylaxis (PrEP) 16, 61
pregnant women
  early research on ART 293–305
  infection of babies during pregnancy 43–4
  levels of infection in 39
  new infections during pregnancy 45
  research into ART 295–6
  universal treatment for 38
pre-masticated food 53–5
prescription formula 206
preterm babies 80, 87–8, 119, 132, 191, 307, 380, 383
Pretoria pasteurisation 136, 139–41
Prevention Access Campaign 337–9
primates 21–2
progenitor T-cells 343
progesterone 74
prolactin 74, 84–6, 259
PROMISE study (Promoting Maternal Infant Survival Everywhere) 341–2
PROMISE-EBF 224
prostitution 24, 35–6
protease/protease inhibitors 128
protein content of breastmilk 77–80, 86, 90
provirus 14
public health 32, 169, 284, 304, 322, 324
public relations 169
Puerto Rico 135

Quality Assurance Project 207
Raju, Tonse 69
Rakai project 333–4
randomised controlled trials 47, 123, 147, 150, 151
rapid testing 58
ready-to-feed formula 269–70
receptor-mimetic oligosaccharides 128
refrigeration 130, 135, 249, 320
Reimer, Penny 400
relactation 229, 239
'replacement feeding' *see* formula-feeding
replication-competent genomes 348
research
  'allowable lapses' 127
  on alternatives to breastfeeding 149
  on antiretroviral therapy 150–1
  on ART and untransmissability 333–51
  data collection problems 149, 188, 234, 240–3
  and the definition of breastfeeding 121–3, 125–6
  delays in publication 37
  difference in health outcomes between replacement feeding and breastfeeding 288–91
  'drop-out bias' 244
  early research into transmission via breastfeeding 147–88
  early research on ART 295–6
  ethical conduct 149–50, 160, 162, 165
  funding 149–50
  'grey literature' 207, 241
  HIV in breastmilk 99
  HIV-free survival 286–7
  informed consent 162–3
  journal submissions 9–10, 127, 162, 396
  lack of breastfeeding knowledge in researchers 306
  lack of collaboration with lactation professionals 117
  lack of data on breastfeeding 205
  lack of published data 207, 213
  learning-by-doing 161
  'lost to follow-up' statistics 244, 404
  measurement of policies versus measurement of treatment 150
  randomised controlled trials 47, 123, 147, 150, 151
  registry of mother-infant pairs to capture transmissions 350, 370
  used to recommend against breastfeeding 110–11
  using breastmilk samples 99–100
  'Voldemort effect' 88–9
reservoirs, viral 10, 16, 342–7
retained placenta 104
retroviruses 14, 21, 25, 34, 35, 346
reverse transcriptase 16, 22, 34, 347
Review of HIV through Breastfeeding 182–3
Review of Transmission through Breastfeeding 162
Richardson, Barbara 96
rights-based approaches 94 *see also* human rights
risk of infection with HIV via breastfeeding 96, 147, 148, 179, 188, 200
risks of formula feeding 88–9, 92–4, 174, 200, 206, 226–8, 235, 248–53, 358, 406
risks of mixed feeding 48, 104, 106, 113–14, 123–4, 125
risks of not breastfeeding 71–2, 83, 89–94, 167, 174, 199, 201, 245–7, 250, 284, 407
ritonavir 312
RNA
  and HIV generally 14, 29
  HIV in breastmilk 98, 111, 112, 346–7
  testing breastmilk for HIV 130
  testing for HIV 58, 62
Rollins, Nigel 98, 125–6, 127, 243, 262, 267
Romania 28
room temperature breastmilk 130, 135
Ross, Jay 49
Royal College of Midwives 91
Royal College of Paediatrics and Child Health 91
Royal Society 25
ruling out HIV 64–5
Russia 35, 36, 50
Rwanda 218, 220, 290

Saadeh, Randa 162, 177
Saba, Joseph 148, 159
'safer breastfeeding' education 211
Safer Triangle booklet 369–70
SAINT study 299
saliva 53–5, 79–80
Salmonella 80, 138, 250, 269, 270
San Francisco 29–30, 31, 32, 34
sanitation 219, 225, 284, 315
Savage, Felicity 163, 167, 176, 189, 192, 242, 318, 332, 401
Science 23, 35
SCN News 146, 171
Scovill, Eliza Jane 357
screening for HIV 33, 35
Seery, Paula 370
self-testing kits 59
Semba, R.D. 110–11
semen 39
Semrau, Katherine 112
sentinel surveillance testing 38, 179, 199
seroconversion 16, 46, 52, 56, 354
seroreversion 65
Serwadda, David 37
sex clubs 31–2, 34
sex tourism 26
sex workers 24, 35, 36, 37
sexual transmission 33
sexually transmitted diseases (other than HIV) 44, 335
Shaffer, Nathan 151
Shaffer, Neil 296
Shapiro, Roger 306–7, 343
Shaw, George 67
Sherry, Jim 169
Shilts, Randy 29, 34
shock-and-kill strategies 345
sIgA 78–9, 87, 103, 112, 128, 131
Silverman, Michael 308, 309, 312, 313
simian (monkey) immunodeficiency virus (SIV) 21–3, 43, 97

skimmed human milk 130
sleep 258
Smit, Molly 209
Smith, Julie 84, 88–9, 90, 127, 205
Smith, Melanie 113, 119
social media 91–2
social safety nets 94
socio-economic circumstances 48, 282, 315 *see also* poverty
sodium 103, 104, 105, 109, 110, 111, 114
solid foods, introduction of 119–20, 121, 123, 178, 263, 309
soluble toll-like receptor 2 (sTLR2) 132
sore nipples 107–9
South Africa
  ART research 299
  breastfeeding in 51
  cotrimazole 275
  Coutsoudis study 98, 123, 138
  early weaning studies 262
  government-provided formula 209
  Gray study 153–4
  health worker training 219
  HIV-free survival 287, 289
  home-prepared formula 269
  PMTCT project 221, 224, 226, 231–2
  pre-masticated food 54
  spillover effects 405
  spread of HIV in 37–8
  stigma over formula feeding 240
Spiegel, Daniel 169
spillover effects 167, 202, 224, 230–1, 240, 286, 404–6
Stamps, Timothy 144
Staphylococcus infections 107
statistics on children with HIV 176, 178, 243
statistics on HIV-exposed but uninfected babies 279–80
statistics on infections via breastfeeding 147, 148, 155, 168, 179, 208, 246, 277
statistics on MTCT 243, 276, 285–6, 293, 298, 301, 406
statistics on prevalence of HIV 39–41
stem cells 80, 82–3
Stewart, Grace John 325–6
stigma/ostracisation
  AIDS 32
  criminalisation 336
  formula-feeding 229, 235, 238–40
  HIV-positive status 37, 167, 209
  for not breastfeeding 94, 139, 236–7, 360
stress responses 85
subclinical mastitis 109–10, 111, 112, 132
subtype A 23, 36, 132
subtype B 26, 27–8, 29, 30, 64, 65
subtype C 28, 64
subtype D 28, 36, 132
subtype E (CRF01) 28
subtype F1 28
subtypes of HIV 22–3, 24, 27–8, 64, 65, 132
sucking, babies' need for 265, 271–3
sulfonamides 274
superinfection 16, 278
survival sex 39
sustainability of formula supplies 138, 225, 239, 251, 308–9, 362 *see also* AFASS conditions
Swanborg, Catharina 81
Swazi Observer 54
Swaziland 38, 40, 248, 262
Swiss Statement 336–7, 350–1
Swiss study on transmissibility 334, 342, 350
syringe/needle transmission 24, 34, 35, 50 *see also* intravenous drug users
systematic reviews 351 *see also* meta-analyses

T cells 14, 18, 32 *see also* CD4 T cells
taboos 39, 94, 136, 155, 238
Tanzania 37, 132, 218, 221, 239, 262, 269
T-cell maturation 77
teeth and dental development 82
Temmerman, Marleen 96
tenofovir 341
Ternier, Ralph 263
testing for HIV
  in adults 56–61
  availability of infant testing 279
  in babies 61–8
  in breastmilk 130
  HIV in breastmilk 99
  low uptake of 209
  PMTCT project 209, 232
  pregnant women 38
  sentinel surveillance testing 179
  stigma about 39
  subtypes of HIV 28, 64
  window periods for testing 16, 47, 57–9, 61, 65, 66
  ZVITAMBO project 212
Thailand 28, 151, 156, 208, 221, 296–7, 299
Thomas, T.K. 318
Thorley, Virginia 395
Thormar, H. 129
thrush 108
thymus 77
tight junctions 103, 104, 105, 109, 110
Timberg, Craig 31, 237, 251
timing of mother's infection 48, 65–8, 100, 133, 166
timing of treatment 302, 307, 340–1
Tlou, Sheila D. 156–7
Tompson, Marian 326, 395–6
tongue protrusion reflex 121
tongue tie 97, 108
transcriptase 14, 16
transcriptionally silent genomes 345
transforming growth factor X 128
transmissibility of HIV during breastfeeding 42, 45–6, 96, 340–2, 349–50, 388 *see also* undetectable equals untransmittable (U=U)
transmissibility studies 333–51
transmission network analysis 29
trauma 264, 361
Treatment Action Campaign 38
Treatment as Prevention 337
triglycerides 129

Tshabalala-Msimang, Manto 38
Tudor-Williams, Gareth 363
Tulloch, James 167
twins 45, 379–81
Tyson, Kathleen 356

Uganda
 cultural norms and breastfeeding 160
 early cessation of breastfeeding, as recommendation 260
 four-country review of HIV and infant feeding 206–8
 HIV in breastmilk study 98, 131
 HIV-free survival 287, 289
 multiple sexual partners 237
 PMTCT project 218, 224, 225
 Rakai project 333–4
 spread of HIV in 36–7
 statistics on mortality from formula-feeding 320, 321
UK HIV-positive women and breastfeeding 353, 357–9, 360, 361–3, 369, 370–1
UN (United Nations)
 in Africa generally 25
 Commission on Human Rights 154
 Convention on the Rights of the Child 143
 FAO (Food and Agriculture Organization) 270
 Interagency Task Team (IATT) for the Prevention and Treatment of HIV Infection in Pregnant Women, Mothers and Children 158–9, 174
 and Nestlé 168
 on reducing HIV in children 176
 World Summit for Children 144
UNAIDS (Joint United Nations Programme on HIV/AIDS)
 breastfeeding guidance 146, 154–67
 constitution of 146
 and the Ghent working group 148
 global spending on AIDS 10
 HIV Counselling Course 189–203
 maternal rights *not* to breastfeed 235
 meetings on human rights 154–9
 and the Nairobi study 96
 PMTCT project 204, 206, 242
 statistics on HIV-exposed but uninfected babies 279–80
 WHO/UNICEF/UNAIDS Technical Consultation on HIV and infant feeding 161–4
 on women with HIV 154
 workshop: how to promote and normalise formula-feeding 159–61
undetectable equals untransmittable (U=U) 337–41, 349–50, 368, 388, 403
UNESCO 26
UNGASS 319–20
UNICEF
 Baby Friendly 7, 86, 124, 144–5, 176, 178, 181, 238, 318, 394
 endorsement of contrimazole 274
 and the formula industry 168–70, 171, 172
 and free formula 229–30
 Global Strategy on Infant and Young Child Feeding 180–1
 HIV and Infant Feeding Counselling Course 189–203, 218
 and the IATT 159
 infant feeding guidance 70, 94, 136, 317–32
 maternal rights *not* to breastfeed 235
 micronutrient sachets 267
 and Nestlé 168–9
 PMTCT project 11, 205, 206, 207, 231–3, 241, 242, 243
 policy changes in 2010s 317–32
 Rapid advice (2010) 303
 and UNAIDS 146
 WABA-UNICEF HIV Colloquium 48, 110, 396–8
 WABA-UNICEF Symposium on HIV and Breastfeeding 207–8, 219
 on women with HIV 39
University of Nairobi 96, 100, 147–8
University of Western Australia 73–4, 82
US (United States)
 CDC (Centers for Disease Control and Prevention) 29, 31, 42, 53, 142, 250, 252, 317, 352, 368
 child protection and safeguarding 358
 FDA (Federal Drug Administration) 270, 295
 Guidelines for the Use of Antiretroviral Agents 294
 history of the US epidemic 29–30, 31, 34
 HIV and infant feeding recommendations 365–8
 HIV-positive women and breastfeeding 354, 401, 402
 introduction of HIV to 26
 National Institutes of Health 64, 150, 365
 research into ART 295–6
 research into MTCT 150

vaccination 79, 201, 280
vaginal fluid 39, 44, 97
Van de Perre, Philippe 128, 166, 254, 266, 342, 349–50
van Esterik, Penny 351, 398
Vernazza, Pietro 334, 336, 350
viraemia 18, 46, 54, 66, 100, 344, 347–8
viral complexity 28
viral diversity 13–14, 16, 49
viral eradication/cure 17, 345
viral load
 and ART 152, 294–5, 303, 314, 348
 in breastmilk 57, 67, 97, 98, 110, 111, 112, 119
 following abrupt cessation of breastfeeding 266
 and frequency of infant suckling 113
 infection routes of HIV in babies 48, 57, 67
 and MTCT 307, 309, 312, 333
 in plasma 46, 47, 48, 67, 114, 135, 313
 and testing for HIV 58
 timing of infection in baby 277
 timing of mother's infection 100
 undetectable 304, 305, 312–14, 333–51
 viral load testing 60–1, 66
 during weaning 116
viral rebound 295, 298, 348
viral reservoirs 10, 16, 342–7

Virodene 38
Vitamin A 66, 114, 124, 150, 177
vitamin supplementation 267, 269
'Voldemort effect' 88–9, 127
voluntary counselling and testing (VCT) 174

Wahl, Grace 54–5
Waitt, Catriona 349–50
Wall Street Journal 21, 168, 169
Washington Post 156, 233, 251
water, giving babies 120, 125
water content of breastmilk 76, 121
water supply 219, 221, 225–8, 235, 249, 250–3, 284
weaning
  consequences of abrupt 8, 104, 116, 245
  counselling 222
  early cessation of breastfeeding 141, 180, 212, 254–66, 271, 279, 290–1
  early weaning and mortality 254–6
  effects of early breastfeeding cessation on women 258–9
  emotional effects of sudden weaning 264–6, 271–2
  epithelial barrier 103
  Global Strategy on Infant and Young Child Feeding 178
  grief 85
  increased risk of HIV transmission 109, 116
  pre-masticated food 53
  providing support for 392
  solid foods, introduction of 119–20, 121, 123, 178, 263, 309
Wellstart Lactation Management Education Program 199
wet nursing 49, 50–2, 160, 184
White, Edith 157
WHO (World Health Organization)
  2010 Guidelines on HIV and Infant Feeding 330–2
  ART recommendations 314
  Breastfeeding Counselling Course 145
  Collaborative Study 174
  Consensus Statement 144
  Consultation on HIV transmission and breastfeeding 144, 148
  contaminated formula 270
  different advice for developed and developing countries 402
  in early days of HIV pandemic 26
  and the formula industry 171–2
  Global Programme on AIDS 149
  Global Strategy on Infant and Young Child Feeding 176–82, 284
  guidance on infant feeding 48, 63, 142, 144, 155, 226, 330–2
  guidance on reducing stigma 240
  Guide for Health Care Managers and Supervisors 148, 182–3, 256
  Guidelines for Decision-makers 148
  guidelines for the global north 352
  guidelines on ART for maternity 302, 303–4
  guidelines on safe preparation of formula 320
  guidelines on wet-nursing 51
  HIV and Infant Feeding Counselling Course 124, 189–203, 215–34, 320
  HIV and Infant Feeding Data Analysis Workshop 126
  HIV Counselling Course 173
  HIV-free survival 284
  importance of breastfeeding 70, 71, 86, 278
  Integrated Course on Infant and Young Child Feeding 267
  Integrated Infant and Young Child Feeding Counselling Course 318
  Kesho Bora study group 315
  maternal rights *not* to breastfeed 94, 235
  Model Chapter on Infant and Young Child Feeding 320
  PMTCT project 206, 232, 241–3
  policy changes in 2010s 317–32
  potential mechanisms for exclusive breastfeeding to reduce MTCT 118–19
  Rapid advice 303, 322–5, 328, 402
  recommendations on alternatives to breastfeeding 183–4
  recommendations on breastfeeding 70, 71, 86, 96–7, 118, 123, 126, 148, 303–4
  recommendations on HIV and infant feeding 142, 144
  recommending formula feeding 146–7
  report on sexual behaviour 237
  Review of the Evidence of Transmission of HIV through Breastfeeding 148
  revised (2006) training courses 317–18
  study on early weaning 254–6
  Technical Consultation 1998 157, 161–4, 267
  Technical Consultation 2000 174
  Technical Consultation 2006 269, 318–19
  Technical Consultation 2009 247, 303, 321–2
  and UNAIDS 146
  value of breastfeeding for HIV-infected infants 278
  Weekly Epidemiological Record 155
  WHO/Health Action International workshop 39
WHO code (International Code of Marketing of Breastmilk Substitutes)
  and the cost of alternatives to breastmilk 208
  on donations of formula 206
  early days of 71
  formula purchasing abiding by the 173
  global policy recommendations 142, 143, 161, 168, 169, 171, 176, 178, 181
  HIV Counselling Course 198
  and human rights 325
  packaging 173, 240
  and the PMTCT project 208
  revised guidelines (2003) 230
Williams, Cicely 71, 265
Willumsen, Juana 112, 207
Windeyer Institute 25
window periods for testing 16, 47, 57–9, 61, 65, 66
Witten, Chantell 405
women
  East Africa 37

impact of pandemic on 397–8
infection in women in the early stages of pandemic 32–3
infections in global north 352
patterns of infection in 1990s 38–9
statistics on infections 154
Women and AIDS Support Network (WASN) 8
World AIDS Conference 1998 164–7
World AIDS Conference 2006 287
World AIDS Day 322
World Alliance for Breastfeeding Action (WABA)
and the 2006 WHO Technical Consultation 318
on formula feeding 83, 163
La Leche League International/WABA Symposium on HIV and Breastfeeding 219
PMTCT project 207, 245
WABA HIV Kit 35–6, 400, 401
WABA-ILCA collaboration 399
WABA-UNICEF HIV Colloquium 48, 110, 396–8
WABA-UNICEF Symposium on HIV and Breastfeeding 207–8, 219
World Health Assembly 142, 168, 180, 208
Worobey, Michael 31
Wyeth 157, 169–70, 172

Yamey, Gavin 171–2
Yarl's Wood 362
Young, Sera 236, 260, 287

Zaire 26, 36 *see also* Congo
Zambia
ART research 302
ART+EBF research 308
cultural norms and breastfeeding 238
early cessation of breastfeeding 260
HIV and Infant Feeding Counselling Course 190
HIV-free survival 290
PMTCT project 218, 223
statistics on mortality from formula-feeding 321
studies into infant feeding and transmission 116, 157
water quality 227
ZEBS study 112, 278, 290, 317
'zero' versus 'negligible' risk of transmission 339
zidovudine
ART+EBF 312
Botswana 249
early research on ART 99, 150, 151, 156, 295–6, 297
Kesho Bora study group 315
PMTCT project 165, 210, 211
PROMISE study (Promoting Maternal Infant Survival Everywhere) 341
research on ART and untransmissibility 333
short-courses 174, 208, 299
Zimbabwe
Baby Friendly 145
blood transfusions 24
breastfeeding culture 7, 177–8, 191, 199–200, 235, 237
breastmilk at room temperature study 135, 136
costs of formula 211
early cessation of breastfeeding 260
early weaning studies 261
and formula donations 169–70
HIV in 9, 37
PMTCT project 218, 231
as test of policies 176, 189
viral load in breastmilk study 111
ZVITAMBO project 46, 67, 114, 124–5, 127, 132, 138–9, 211, 212, 223, 261, 397, 406–7
zoonotic diseases 20, 23, 25
Zunguza, Clare 124, 207

Also from Pinter & Martin

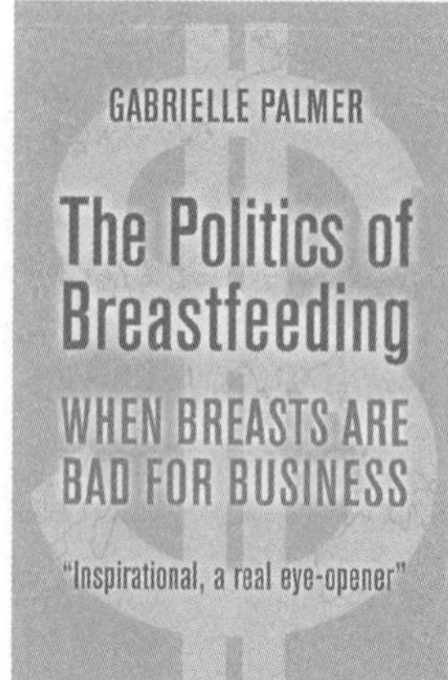

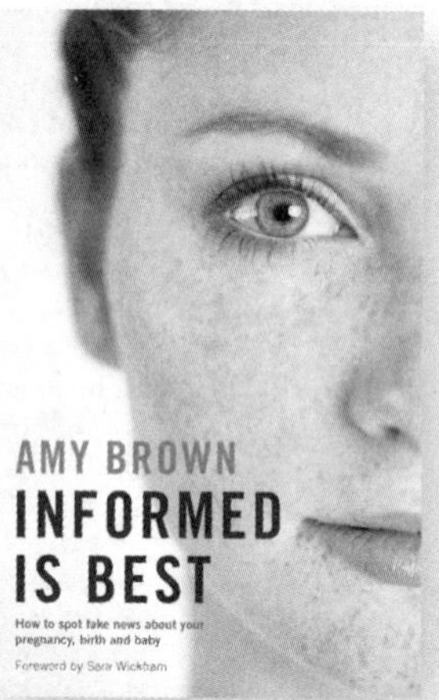

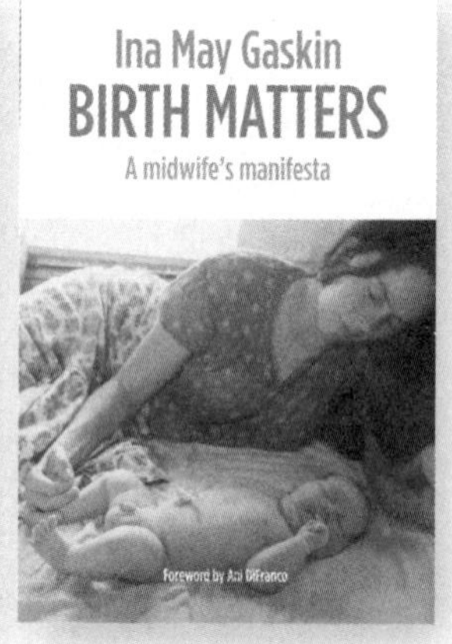

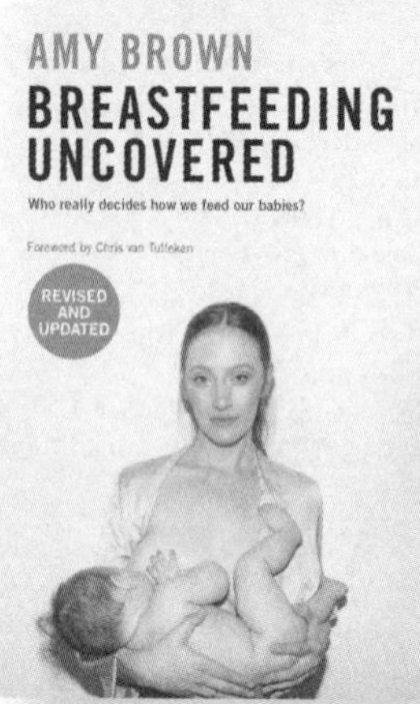

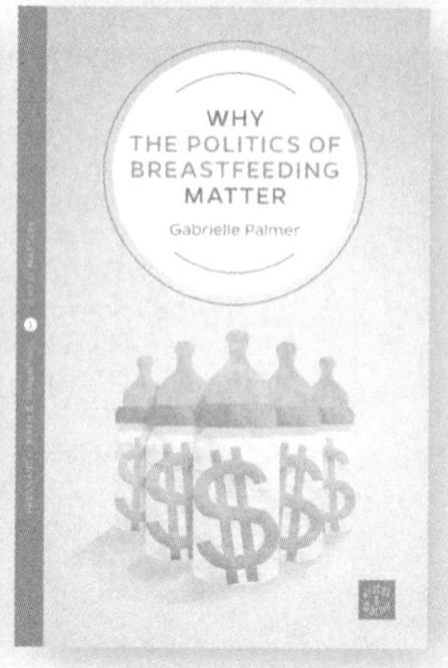

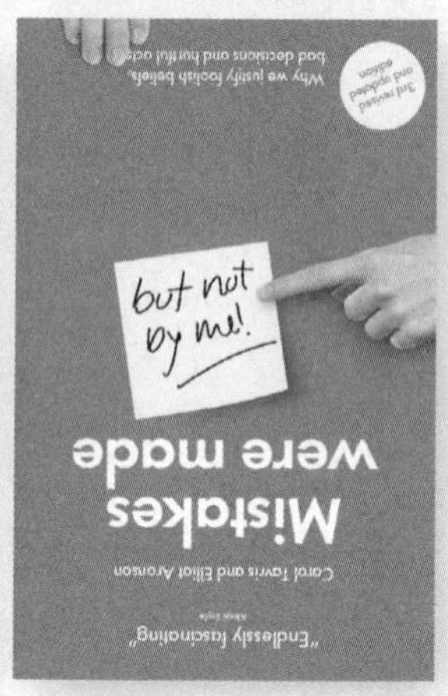

pinterandmartin.com

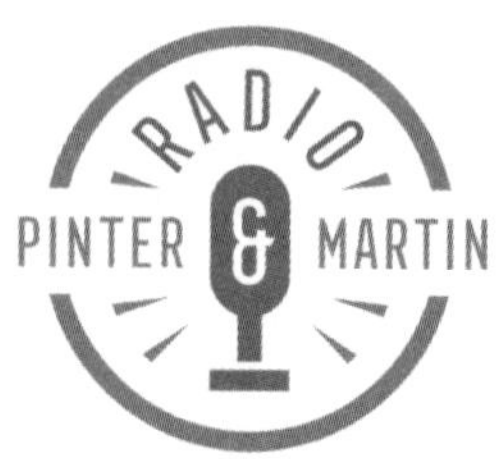

THE WORLD'S FIRST RADIO STATION DEDICATED
TO PREGNANCY, BIRTH & PARENTHOOD

pinterandmartin.radio